BACTERIAL PLASMIDS AND ANTIBIOTIC RESISTANCE

BACTERIAL PLASMIDS
AND
ANTIBIOTIC RESISTANCE

First International Symposium
INFECTIOUS ANTIBIOTIC RESISTANCE
Castle of Smolenice,
Czechoslovakia 1971

Editors

V. Krčméry, L. Rosival, T. Watanabe

1972

AVICENUM — Czechoslovak Medical Press · Prague
SPRINGER-VERLAG · Berlin · Heidelberg · New York

ISBN 978-3-642-49269-3   ISBN 978-3-642-49267-9 (eBook)
DOI 10.1007/978-3-642-49267-9
Library of Congress Catalog Card Number 72-77436

Publishers:

AVICENUM — CZECHOSLOVAK MEDICAL PRESS,
PRAGUE

SPRINGER VERLAG,
BERLIN — HEIDELBERG — NEW YORK

CONTENTS

II

1st INTERNATIONAL SYMPOSIUM
INFECTIOUS (transferable) ANTIBIOTIC RESISTANCE

Castle of Smolenice, Czechoslovakia
30th August 1971 — 2nd September 1971

Organizers:

THE SLOVAK MEDICAL SOCIETY
(President: Professor R. T. NIEDERLAND, M. D.)
(Secretary General: J. MARIANYI, M. D.)

CZECHOSLOVAK SOCIETY OF MICROBIOLOGY
(President: Professor J. ŠTEFANOVIČ, M. D.)

SLOVAK ACADEMY OF SCIENCES (President: Acad. Professor K. ŠIŠKA, M. D.)

RESEARCH INSTITUTE OF HYGIENE, Bratislava
(Director: Professor L. ROSIVAL, M. D.)

Secretary General of the Symposium:
Professor L. ROSIVAL, M. D.

Organizing Secretariat:
V. KRČMÉRY, Ph. D.
J. JANOUŠKOVÁ, Ph. D.
J. BARANYAI, M. D.

HONORARY CHAIRMEN of the SYMPOSIUM:
Professor Tsutomu WATANABE, M. D., Keio University, Tokyo
Professor G. LEBEK, M. D., University of Berne

INTERNATIONAL ORGANIZING COMITTEE:
Professor Tsutomu WATANABE (Tokyo)
Professor S. M. NAVAŠIN (Moskva)
Professor P. FREDERICQ (Liége)
Professor D. SMITH (Boston)
Professor U. TAUBENECK (Jena)
Professor S. W. GLOVER (Edinburgh)
Professor H. KNOTHE (Frankfurt)
Professor L. ROSIVAL (Bratislava)

CO-EDITORS OF THE PROCEEDINGS:
C. K. ELLIOTT, M. D.
E. ELLIOTT, M. D.

PREFACE

Antibiotics are one of the greatest benefits science ever gave to mankind and one of the few things that cannot be misused against the man. Thus, the starting point of all our efforts is highly humanistic, and is expressed by cordial athmosphere in which we all work and communicate on a wide international basis.

All our efforts are aimed to preserve the antibiotics as effective tools in medical treatment, and thus we must deal with *antibiotic resistance*. Owing to it many antibiotics are slowly retreating from the first line of the battle between the man and pathogens. But new drugs are coming and we must check them very carefully to assure their efficiency as long as possible. In this process of inactivation of antibiotics, *infectious resistance factors* are today on the scene not only of clinicians, epidemiologists or hygienists, but equally, if not more, of geneticists and molecular-biologists. This is why we all were together in Smolenice to exchange our ideas and experience.

Among other things, it is important to draw up specifications for, and to make a toxicological evaluation of *antibiotics used as food additives* and to assess the efficacy, direct and indirect potential health hazards of a number of antibiotics and chemotherapeutic agents that, under certain conditions, might leave residues in food of animal origin and/or cause the resistance to antibiotics. The Joint meeting of FAO/WHO Expert Committee on Food Additives, which convened in 1968, recommended the promotion of the research of antibiotic resistance transfer under the conditions of agricultural and veterinary use of antibiotics as well as long-term studies of the effects of antibiotic residues that are likely to occur in human food.

Our Research Institute of Hygiene in Bratislava pays much attention to the problems of R factors in Czechoslovakia. We have followed the recommendations of the so-called *SWANN's Report* to establish Reference laboratories to study and combat the spread of resistance factors among enterobacteriaceae and staphylococci. Thanks to the support of our Ministry of Health and to the initiative of the Commission for Effective Pharmacotherapy in our country, and Dr. Modr personally, a *Reference laboratory* for transferable resistance factors has been established in our Institute.

The Symposial discussions focussed attention onto various aspects of the above mentioned type of international research. I think that only by a clear definition of priorities and responsibilities our scientific problems of transferable resistance could be dealt with effectively. One of the first priorities should be a surveillance programme in regard to the infectious resistance from the scientific and practical point of view.

Together with the surveillance of R factors, however, well founded genetic and molecular-biological studies of these factors and other bacterial plasmids are urgently needed.

7

Our Symposium should be the first attempt for such a complex approach and could present the start for not only interdisciplinary but also *international* dealing with the problems of transferable resistance.

More than 80 participants were present in the Smolenice Symposium and nearly 50 papers were read and discussed. Participants were coming from all parts of the world indeed and everybody interested in R factors has had an equal opportunity to attend and to contribute to the programme. Thus, Symposium in Smolenice could be called the *First International Symposium* on R factors. An International Commission for study of bacterial plasmids has been established here by the Honourable President of the International Society of Chemotherapy, Professor WELSCH. Many participants offered their time and means to come from far distances and helped thus to give the Symposium its true significance and dignity. Others could not come but were equally interested, and some of them sent us their papers to be read in Smolenice. An admirably cordial atmosphere was thus created, both refreshing our minds ("helped to improve our mental health" as said by Stephen Seligman) and stimulating our discussions.

It is certainly a remarkable fact, that an International Commission studying bacterial plasmids, especially those associated with antibiotic resistance, was established here in the Castle of Smolenice during, and as a result of, our Symposium. We are especially thankful to Professor Maurice WELSCH, the President of International Society of Chemotherapy, for his coming here and inaugurating the new Commission. I don't think anybody would doubt that the establishment of the Commission was a highly needed and desirable event in the present difficult and complicated situation created by the all-over-the-world spread of strains with R factors. An international cooperation must be continuous and somehow directed if we should achieve an improvement of the present situation. I appreciate much also the interest of the research workers of many pharmaceutical companies producing antibiotics in the events in the fields of transferable resistance.

Finally, let me express out thanks and acknowledgment to the institutions who helped to organise the Symposium: to Slovak Medical Society and to the Academy of Science for giving the Castle at our disposal. But all of us, present and engaged in the Symposium, helped to make it fruitful and advanced. And, while many of us picked up so many new ideas and stimulation for future work, our next meeting on R factors will be again very valuable and instructive.

I should like to thank the AVICENUM, Czechoslovak Medical Press for their cooperation in producing this book.

The publication of the Proceedings was supported by Schering Corporation U.S.A. through ESSEX CHEMIE AG Lucerne, Switzerland.

Professor L. ROSIVAL, M. D., Sc. C.
Secretary General of the Symposium

OPENING LECTURES

FURTHER OUTLOOKS OF ANTIBIOTICS IN THE SHADOWS
OF RESISTANCE FACTORS

TSUTOMU WATANABE

Department of Microbiology, Keio University School of Medicine, Tokyo, Japan

Mr. President, honorable members of the Symposium, Ladies and Gentlemen!

It is a privilege and great honor for me to have an opportunity to give an Opening lecture at the occasion of the First International Symposium on Infectious Antibiotic Resistance in Smolenice.

As all of you know, R factors are extrachromosomal DNA elements of bacteria and confer drug resistances on their host bacteria. They can transfer themselves to other bacteria by causing conjugation, and can also be transferred by phage-mediated transduction in particular systems. There are some evidences that they can be attached to the host chromosomes, and thus we can call them either episomes or plasmids.

R factors can be transferred not only to *Enterobacteriaceae* but also to a variety of gram-negative bacilli, which include many pathogenic bacteria such as *Shigella*, *Salmonella*, enteropathogenic *Escherichia coli*, *Vibrio cholerae*, *Pasteurella*, *Pseudomonas* and several others. In fact, highly virulent strains of bacteria carrying R factors are causing infections in man and animals.

An important point with R factors is that many of them carry multiple drug resistance genes. Therefore, R factor-carrying multiple-drug-resistant bacteria can be selected for by any single drug concerned, thus causing an increase of R factor-carrying bacteria quite easily.

Some people have claimed that R factors are practically not important on the basis of the finding that *Salmonella* strains which have received R factors have lost their virulence. In other words, they claimed that R factors reduce the virulence of their host bacteria. But their interpretation was found incorrect. Our studies have shown that rough mutants act as much better recipients for R factors than the original smooth strain, and therefore spontaneous rough mutants contained in the wild type population selectively receive the R factors. In fact the *Salmonella* clones which showed reduced virulence as a result of acceptance of R factors were found to be rough mutants. Our recent studies with *Salmonella typhimurium* have shown that most R factors, if not all, do not significantly reduce the virulence of the host *S. typhimurium* as far as we use smooth type clones.

Clinical and epidemiological data also indicate that R factor-carrying strains and drug-sensitive strains are equally virulent. R factor-carrying rough mutant clones of bacteria may be occurring more frequently also in the natural conditions than R factor-carrying smooth bacteria but the formers may well be selected out in vivo by the defense mechanisms of the host organisms. A shocking news has recently been reported by Dr. Mata in Guatemala. That is about a terrible outbreak of epidemic of severe dysentery with

9

R factor-carrying, multiple-drug-resistant *Shigella dysenteriae*, and it is estimated that indeed more than fifteen thousand people have already died of dysentery for the past three years in Central America. This epidemic has apparently invaded Mexico and the southern part of the United States.

The first multiple-drug-resistant strain of *Shigella* was found in Japan in 1955. The presence of R factor was not studied with this particular strain, because R factors were not known at that time, but it is most likely that this strain carried R factor assuming from its drug resistance pattern. Similar multiple-drug-resistant strains of gram-negative bacilli have sharply increased in Japan since 1956. As you already know, the presence and sharp increase of R factor-carrying bacteria have been proved all over the world wherever they have been investigated.

The cause of the increase of R factor-carrying bacteria is, of course, due to the selective pressure by antibiotics and other chemotherapeutic agents. These drugs are nowadays being used not only for man but also for animals, cultured fish, fruits, vegetables and rice plants and even for honey bees. It has been shown that the use of antibiotics for animal and fish culturing greatly increase the pool of R factor-carrying bacteria in our environment. It seems likely that the use of antibiotics for other non-medical purposes also helps the increase of the reservoir of R factors.

There has been much debate for the past several years on the potential danger of the increase of R factor-carrying bacteria in animals as a result of antibiotic feeding. Particularly the so-called Swann Report of United Kingdom discussed on this point most systematicaly and recommended strict restriction of the use of antibiotics for animals. The Swann Report and other scientists have pointed out that bacteria of common pathogenicity to man and animals such as *Salmonella* carrying R factors may be transmitted to man from animals. Another danger pointed out is that R factors can be transferred to human pathogens by way of non-pathogenic bacteria such as *E. coli*. The Swann Report claimed that these events are really causing hazards to man.

Hypersensitive reactions of man to antibiotic residues is another problem. However, this problem can be solved rather easily by taking sufficient durations of withdrawal period, where antibiotics are not given to the animals, because antibiotics are excreted relatively rapidly.

A rather important problem or protest raised by the opponents against the Swann Report is "Are the R factors really transferred to man from animals? If so, how many percent of the human R factors have come from animals?" The latter question is technically extremely difficult to answer. But I think there is no doubt that at least some R factors are transferred from animals to man. As you know, infections of man with *Salmonella* species of animal origin occurs not infrequently. Therefore, the transmission of animal *E. coli* strains to man must be occurring even more frequently. If these *E. coli* strains carry R factors, there is a possibility that they are transferred to human pathogens in man.

It is true that the transfer of R factors in vivo does not occur as easily as in vitro, but we must recall the fact that various species of pathogenic bacteria carrying R factors are actually causing infections in man and animals indicating that R factors can be transferred to pathogenic bacteria in vivo even though the frequencies of their transfer may be low.

I have presented an hypothesis about a decade ago that the origin of R factors may be analogous to the formation of F' factors. In other words, the drug resistance genes of R factors may have originated from chromosomes of some bacteria and may have been picked up by some episomes. This hypothesis was not quite popular at that time, because the biochemical mechanisms of the drug resistances by R factors were thought entirely different from those of the chromosomal drug resistance genes, which were known at that time. The biochemical mechanisms of the drug resistances conferred by R factors are now known to be due to the production of specific drug-inactivating enzymes at least with some drugs. Recent studies with *Klebsiella*, *Proteus*, *Pseudomonas* etc. have indicated that similar drug-inactivating enzymes are produced by these bacteria without R factors. Thus my original hypothesis seems to be receiving a support.

If R factors have indeed developed as a result of gene pick-up, there is a possibility that more and more drug resistance genes might be added to the R factors. R factors with more drug resistance genes should have a greater selective advantage under the selective pressure of antibiotics which is currently observable. It is also quite probable that R factors with multiple drug resistance genes may arise through genetic recombination among R factors with less drug resistance genes. At any rate our experiences in the past seem to indicate that the possibility of the addition of new drug resistance genes to R factors is not only an imaginary fear.

I have been talking specifically about R factors but the situation with the drug resistances of *Staphylococcus aureus* is more or less similar. Penicillinase plasmids and other drug resistance plasmids can be transferred to other strains of *S. aureus* by phagemediated transduction. The differences of *Staphylococcus* plasmids from R factors are that they cannot be transferred by conjugation and that their host range is limited to *Staphylococcus*.

If pathogenic bacteria become resistant to some drugs, we are forced to use other drugs to which the bacteria are still sensitive in order to treat the infections. A difficulty with R factors is that the resistances conferred by R factors include the resistances to the most important drugs which are currently available. It is true that clinicians are now encountering serious difficulties because of R factors of gram-negative bacilli and drug resistance plasmids of *Staphylococcus*.

The discovery of new antibiotics and other synthetic chemotherapeutics is becoming more and more difficult.

Nobody could deny that these drug-resistant bacteria are casting dark shadows on chemotherapy. Chemotherapeutic agents are no longer magic bullets unlike in the days of Ehrlich, Fleming and Waksman. What should we do with these drug-resistant bacteria? Needless to say, more efforts should be made in searching for new chemotherapeutic agents. But our efforts should be directed also toward some other directions.

Antibiotics and other chemotherapeutic agents had originally been developed for treating human infections. To treat human infections and to save their lives are, so to say, supreme orders, and we must continue using chemotherapeutic agents for man, even if drug-resistant bacteria may be increasing. However, I do not mean by this statement that we may continue using chemotherapeutics as carelessly as we have done in the past. As you know, antibiotics have frequently been given to common cold patients for the purpose of preventing complications or for simple, non-specific diarrhea even without studying the specific, causative organisms. Similar uses of antibiotics have been carried out rather frequently.

Statistical data seem to indicate that the frequencies and drug resistance markers of R factor-carrying bacteria in various countries are dependent on the amounts and kinds of antibiotics used in these countries. For example, in Japan, chloramphenicol has been used for man in larger amounts perhaps than in most other countries, and most R factors found in Japan have chloramphenicol resistance marker and, if we take *Shigella* as an example, about 70 to 80 % of the total *Shigella* strains isolated in Japan have R factors.

The second question is what we should do about the non-medical use of antibiotics. The non-medical use of antibiotics aims at the economical profits, namely the increase of productivity. If the increase of the pool of R factor-carrying bacteria in our environment is really causing a serious hazard to our health, there is no question that we should immediately stop the non-medical use of antibiotics. At the present moment, however, we do not know yet, to what extent the R factors in our environment are causing hazards to our health.

One might argue that we should stop using antibiotics for non-medical purposes, if there is even a small possibility that they may be hazardous to man. But this argument seems impractical to me. Some sort of compromise should be necessary in this kind of argument. The situation may be somewhat similar to the air pollution by motor cars. It is well known that motor cars are the main cause of air pollution. But perhaps only few people may insist that the use of motor cars should be abandoned immediately. Most people may rather insist that the increase of motor car production should be reduced or that the motor cars should be improved so that air pollution is not caused by them.

The Swann Report has recommended to make efforts in developing effective drugs which can be specifically used for animals. They have also recommended that the use for animals of antibiotics which are being used as human medicines should be restricted and that the use of antibiotics which cause an increase of R factor-carrying bacteria or cross resistance to human antibiotics should not be used for animals.

Our recent discovery that flavomycin (also called moenomycin and phospholipol) specifically kills R factor-carrying bacteria seems quite hopeful in this regard. I will present a paper on the detail of our study with flavomycin later on in this Symposium.

There may be several other approaches to the control of R factors. Acridine dyes are known to cure R factors, although the efficiencies of curing are not yet satisfactory. It may be possible to discover better curing agents for R factors in the future. The search for agents which inhibit the transfer of R factors may also be found fruitful. Surface actants such as sodium dodecyl sulfate and agents which inhibit the synthesis of DNA such as acridine dyes, mitomycin C etc. are already known to inhibit the transfer of R factors.

Another important and promising approach has been reported by Dr. UMEZAWA at the Congress in Prague last week. He had disclosed the biochemical mechanism of inactivation of kanamycin by the enzyme produced by R factor-carrying bacteria. Then he chemically modified the site of action of the enzyme on the structure of kanamycin. In this way he has succeeded in obtaining deoxykanamycin B, which is effective against bacteria carrying kanamycin-resistance R factor.

In this lecture, I have mainly discussed on the practical aspects of R factors. But before closing my lecture, I should like to emphasize that purely basic studies must be also encouraged in parallel with the practical studies. We have already seen that Umezawa's deoxykanamycin B has become available only through the basic biochemical study of the mechanism of kanamycin resistance. Our studies with flavomycin have also been very much helped by the results of basic studies of bacterial conjugation and sex pili by Dr. Brinton, Drs. Meynells and their associates. We should not be too short-sighted in advancing our research. Even if the basic studies turn out not to be applicable to practical purposes, I think they are important and valuable as such, because they should contribute a great deal to the wisdom of mankind. I believe this should be the way of science.

I am very happy to learn from Professor Welsch about the establishment of the Commission of Bacterial Plasmids Governing Antibiotic Resistance and Other Properties under the International Society of Chemotherapy. The proposed activities of this Commission seem quite fruitful to me and I would like to work actively for this Commission to promote international cooperation in this field.

Finally, on behalf of the participants from abroad, I would like to express our deepest thanks to all of the people of Czechoslovakia who have worked in organizing this Symposium for their great efforts and also for their warm hospitality to us. We all wish the very great success of the Symposium. Thank you.

PROBLEMS OF TRANSFERABLE ANTIBIOTIC RESISTANCE
IN CZECHOSLOVAKIA

V. KRČMÉRY, L. ROSIVAL, F. VÝMOLA, M. HEJZLAR

Research Institute of Hygiene, Bratislava, Institute of Epidemiology and Microbiology,
Praha, Czechoslovakia

First investigations on transferable resistance factors were started in Czechoslovakia in 1964 and were discussed with Professor WATANABE when visiting Prague during the Mendelian Symposium in 1965. They were concerned with concomittant occurence of penicillinase, mercury resistance and tetracycline resistance plasmids in clinical strains of S. aureus. Our first publication on that topics appeared in 1966 (KRČMÉRY and VÝMOLA, 1966). In the same year, VONDRÁŠKOVÁ and STÁRKA (1966) successfully eliminated multiresistance determinants from E. coli strains obtained from patients with urogenital infections showing their extra-chromosomal nature.

First transfers of R factors in Czechoslovakia were performed in the Research Institute of Hygiene in 1966 and published in 1967 (MACÚCH et al., 1967). They showed the presence of transferable tetracycline resistance in strains of *Escherichia coli* isolated in agricultural farms where the animals were fed with this antibiotic. In the following five years of investigation of those problems, we isolated and tested many thousands E. coli strains from pig and poultry faeces, and we found (table 1), that

1. very high proportion of T-monoresistant strains (95 %) was found in farms with antibiotic feeding, in contrast to 15—20% resistance to T in control farms where anti-

Table 1

T-RESISTANCE OF ANIMAL ENTEROPATHOGENIC E. COLI

	Cow (Not fed with CTC)	Piggery	Poultry farm
		Fed with CTC	
Faeces	57/2	57/44/42	45/44/40
Soil	50/0	44/20	33/23

The total number of strains is followed by number of resistant strains and by number of R factor-bearing strains.

biotics were not regularly given. BARTOŠ (1971) also found that, in the chicken farms, the appearance of *susceptible* E. coli strains is extremely rare, and that they can be at present isolated merely from animals in wild nature,

2. In some of farms studied, the T-monoresistance was only partially transferable. However, non-transferable determinants of T resistance could be frequently mobilised

in triparental crosses described by ANDERSON (1966) if an external fertility factor has been introduced, thus showing

a) their extra-chromosomal nature,

b) their epidemiological and perhaps also ecological significance

It therefore may be concluded that a multistep selection by tetracyclines *in vivo*, exerted by continuous antibiotic feeding of animals, can, and does, provide strains with extra-chromosomal tetracycline resistance which *in vitro* could originate only by chance, e. g. by selecting in a number of susceptible strains carrying fertility factors,

3. Among strains of *E. coli* collected in that area, a surprisingly high percentage of colicinogenic strains was observed (up to 30 %, see KRČMÉRY and JANOUŠKOVÁ, 1969). The colicinogenic factors in these strains were, in many instances, able to act as mobilising agents for such and other resistance determinants.

Similar findings were also collected in our studies of hospital strains from two large hospitals (KRČMÉRY et al., 1971). It appeared, that

1. Multi-resistant strains are now more numerous than monoresistant or susceptible ones,

2. Many strains among the susceptible ones carry a transferable Col factor or other fertility factor,

3. Several strains out of those non transferring their resistance determinants possess mobilisable and thus extra-chromosomal genetic determinants of resistance.

Several authors dealt with the problems of transferable resistance in Czechoslovakia (BOHUŠ and BALÁŽ, 1968, HORÁK, 1969, BOHUŠ, 1971). To get better review of the present situation in this country, we started to perform a nationwide surveillance of transferable multiresistance in following groups of strains of Enterobacteria and staphylococci:

In strains from enteric epidemics.

In strains from selected groups of hospitalised patients with parenteral infections caused by Enterobacteriaceae.

In strains from *healthy persons*, mainly children.

In strains from food samples collected both in production and in their distribution.

Table 2

R FACTORS IN E. COLI STRAINS FROM HEALTHY CHILDREN

No. of resistant strains		No. of strains		
		R^+	R^+Tcol^+	R^+col^-
T	9	6	3	3
T + A	4	4	2	2
T + S	2	2	0	2
T + C	1	1	0	1
T + A + N/K	2	2	1	0
Total	18	15	6	8

Table 2 shows preliminary results obtained in healthy children examined in maternity schools. 18 out of 100 children examined had an appraciable number of antibiotic-resistant *E. coli* in their stools, and 15 of them transferred their resistance to recipient strains.

Table 3 shows that 72 out of 100 children with a diagnosis of pyelonephritis had antibiotic-resistant strains *E. coli* in their urine. 33 of them carried an R factor.

In both groups of strains mentioned, a significant proportion carried a transferable colicinogenic factor (Tcol) often associated with rather complex resistance determinants. In exchange of resistant strains and their circulation among various ecological systems,

Table 3

R FACTORS IN E. COLI STRAINS FROM THE URINE OF CHILDREN
WITH PYELONEPHRITIS

No. of resistant strains		No. of strains		
		R+	R+Tcol+	R+col−
A	2	1	0	0
T	36	12	4	6
T + C	3	2	0	1
T + C + S	5	4	3	0
T + C + N/K	9	4	3	0
T + C + A	7	3	2	1
T + C + A +S	6	3	0	3
T + S + N/K	4	4	1	3
Total	72	33	13	14

e. g. hospital wards, agricultural farms, food-producing plants and the population, food of animal origin could be an important carrier, as showed before by several authors. Our preliminary results from food samples show (Table 4) that antibiotic-resistant strains can be frequently isolated from food samples leaving food-producing plants. The dairy products, including milk, contained sometimes ampicillin-resistant strains of *E. coli,*

Table 4

RESISTANT STRAINS E. COLI IN FOOD SAMPLES
SEPT. 1970 – DECEMBER 1971

Total number of strains examined		784
Susceptible to all antibiotics		251
Resistant to one or more drugs		533
No. of strains from *milk* and dairy products	Total	232
Resistant to ampicillin		128 (5)
Resistant to A plus other drug		25 (5)
Susceptible		68
No. of strains from *meat* and meat products	Total	417
Resistant to tetracycline		128 (11)
Resistant to T and other drug		112 (10)
Susceptible		124
No of strains from other food	Total	135
Resistant		76 (1)
Susceptible		59

No. in parenthesis = Transferable resistance

the meat products, however, the tetracycline-resistant ones. In several strains from this material the transferability of antibiotic resistance was demonstrated.

According the recomendations of so-called SWANN'S Report, the Czechoslovak Comission for Pharmacotherapy recommended to establish a National Reference Laboratory for study of transferable antibiotic resistance. This was already established in February 1971 at the Research Institute of Hygiene in Bratislava.

We consider the present situation with R factors-bearing strains in many ecological systems, as hospitalised patients, children in city and country population, food and nutrition articles, and, of course, agricultural farms, to be serious and feel that several antibiotics, mostly tetracyclines and penicillins, are especially threatened by the spread of R-factor-bearing strains. An international cooperation is obviously needed to improve the present situation and the unfavourable outlooks, if the effectiveness of many antibiotics should be secured *pro futuro*.

REFERENCES

ANDERSON, E. S. (1968): The ecology of transferable drug resistance. — Annual Review of Microbiology *22*, 131—181.

BARTOŠ, J. (1968): Sensitivity of Escherichia coli isolated from various animals to tetracycline (in Czech). — Veterinární medicina *13*, 63—68.

BOHUŠ, J., BALÁŽ, M. (1968): Role of some members of Enterobacteriaceae family in maintaining and spreading of the transferable polyresistance. — Folia microbiologica *13*, 275—9.

BOHUŠ, J. (1971): Acceptance of R factor by a Shigella sonnei strain from commensal E. coli strains during dysentery. — Journal of Hygiene, Epidemiology and Microbiology *15*, 225—7.

KRČMÉRY, V., VÝMOLA, F. (1966): Concomittant occurence of penicillinase and tetracycline resistance plasmids in S. aureus. — Journal of Hygiene, Epidemiology and Microbiology *11*, 104—108.

KRČMÉRY, V. and JANOUŠKOVÁ, J. (1969): Mutual relations of colicinogenic factors and resistance determinants in E. coli. — Zeitschrift für allgemeine Mikrobiologie *9*, 191—7.

MACŮCH, P., SEČKÁROVÁ, A., PARRÁKOVÁ, E., KRČMÉRY, V., VÝMOLA, F. (1967): Transfer of tetracycline resistance from E. coli. — Zeitschrift für allgemeine Mikrobiologie *7*, 159—163.

VONDRÁŠKOVÁ, M., STÁRKA, J. (1966): Multiple resistant strains of E. coli isolated from urinary tract. — Journal of Hygiene, Epidemiology and Microbiology *10*, 174—8.

I.

PUBLIC-HEALTH AND CLINICAL ASPECTS
OF RESISTANCE
AND OF R FACTORS

Moderators:

G. LEBEK (Berne)
S. M. NAVAŠIN (Moskva)
P. GUINÉE (Bilthoven)
F. VÝMOLA (Prague)
H. KNOTHE (Frankfurt)

IN VIVO TRANSFER OF A PLASMID GOVERNING GENTAMYCIN RESISTANCE

Y. A. CHABBERT and J. L. WITCHITZ.

Institut Pasteur — Bacteriologie Médicale, Paris, France.

Bacterial resistance to Gentamycin has been described for the first time in France by CHRISTOL, BURE, BOUSSOUGANT and WITCHITZ (1971) and the extrachromosomal location of the relevant gene (s) was demonstrated by WITCHITZ and CHABBERT (1971 a). Biochemical mechanism of plasmid-mediated Gentamycin resistance has been shown to be an adenylating process by BENVENISTE and DAVIES (1971).

This kind of bacteria is more and more frequently isolated in French hospitals (WITCHITZ, CHABBERT, 1971 b.). We are intending to present here some evidence of in vivo transfer of plasmid governing Gentamycin resistance.

MATERIAL AND METHODS

Donor strains:

a) K. pneumoniae 69/433 isolated 1st. November 1969 from urine of a patient hospitalized for tetanus. This patient was treated by 240 mg per day of Gentamycin.

b) *E. coli 69/516*
P. mirabilis: 69/178
Providencia: 69/504
Ps. aeruginosa: 69/268.

These four strains have been isolated 26th. 12, 1969 from a peritoneal dialysis liquid of a patient suffering of acute hemolysis post abortum. The liquid was containing Gentamycin.

Recipient strains:

E. coli K12 LA115: resistant to sodium azide of E. coli K12 IP54.117 F⁻ lac⁺ (L. Le Minor).

E. coli K12 LA116 and LA255: resistant mutants to sodium azide of E. coli K12 C600 F⁻lac⁻thr⁻leuc⁻bio⁻(E. WOLLMAN).

E. coli K12 LA290: resistant mutant to sodium azide of E. coli K12 J5F⁻ (N. DATTA).

E. coli K12 LA106: resistant mutant to Rifampicin of E. coli K12 Hfr. IP6553 (F. JACOB).

Methods for transfer and transduction used have been described by CHABBERT and BAUDENS (1967) et by BOUANCHAUD and CHABBERT (1969).

RESULTS

Results of transfers from *K. pneumoniae* 69/433, P. mirabilis 69/178, *Ps. aeruginosa* 69/268, *Providencia* 69/504 and *E. coli* 69/516 to *E. coli* K12 can be seen in table 1. Different strains of *E. coli* K12 were used as three recipients and these recipients were selected on different drugs. The resistant patterns of donor strains are different, but all of them were able to transfer mostly or uniquely the following markers: Ampicillin (A), Chloramphenicol (C), Sulfonamides (Su), Gentamycin (Gk), Kanamycin (Kp). The Gk and Kp markers have been previously described by WITCHITZ and CHABBERT (1971a). When the following markers: A, C, Su, Gk were transfered to an Hfr strain of E. coli, the Hfr strain remained sensitive to f2 and MS2 phages, so the plasmid (s) carrying the A, C, Su, Gk characters can be described as R(fi⁻) factors.

The same four markers were also transduced "en bloc" by phage P, 1 Kc from *E. coli* K12 to *E. coli* LA 255, so they likely belong to a same genetic element, the R (fi⁻) (A, C, Su, Gk) factor.

Table 1

Original strain	Resistance pattern	Recipient	Selecting antibiotics	Transfered characters				
K. pneumoniae 69/433	ACSuKpGk	LA 115	G	A C	Su		Gk	R 55
		LA 116	G	A C	Su		Gk	
		LA 290	G	A C	Su		Gk	
		LA 115	K	A C	Su		Gk	
		LA 116	K	A C	Su		Gk	
		LA 290	K	A C	Su		Gk	
		LA 115	C	A C	Su		Gk	
		LA 115	A	A C	Su		Gk	
E. coli 69/516	ACTSuSKpGk	LA 115	G	A C	Su		Gk	R 56
			G	A C T	Su	Kp	Gk	
		LA 290	K	T		Kp		
		LA 290	C	A C	Su		Gk	
			C	A C T	Su	Kp	Gk	
		LA 290	T	T		Kp		
			T	A C T	Su	Kp	Gk	
		LA 290	A	A C	Su		Gk	
				A C T	Su	Kp	Gk	
P. mirabilis 69/178	ACTSuGk	LA 115	G	A C	Su		Gk	R 98
Providencia 69/504	ACTSuSKpGk	LA 290	G	A C	Su		Gk	R 92
			K	A C	Su		Gk	
			C	A C	Su		Gk	
			A	A C	Su		Gk	
Ps. aeruginosa 69/268	ACTSuKpGk	LA 115	G	A C	Su		Gk	R 64
		LA 290	G	A C	Su		Gk	
		LA 115	A	A C	Su		Gk	

DISCUSSION

Transferable Gentamycin Resistance Gk has been observed for the first time in November 1969 in an hospital in Paris. From December 1969 to June 1971 several hundred strains harbouring a plasmid governing Gentamycin resistance have been isolated from different hospitals by WITCHITZ and CHABBERT (1971b). We are reporting here the results of resistance transfers obtained from the wild strains isolated from the two first patients harbouring Gentamycin resistant strains.

The first strain isolated in November 1969 from urine of a tetanic patient was a Klebsiella strain. Two months later four other species were isolated from the same sample of peritoneal dialysis liquid. These species were: E. coli, P. mirabilis, Providencia, Pseudomonas aeruginosa. All these strains are transferring Gentamycin resistance to E. coli K12. As reported in table 1 four strains of Klebsiella, Providencia, P. mirabilis and Pseudomonas are transferring only the resistance pattern: A, C, Su, Gk. From the wild strain of E. coli this pattern was also transferred alone or associated with the both characters T and Kp. In addition the characters A, C, Su, Gk have been transduced "en bloc" by phage P1 from E. coli K12. So this transfer factor might be considered as fi⁻.

What we should like to discuss here is the probability the five first strains harboured the same plasmid. It seems highly unlikely that the second patient has been contaminated simultaneously by four bacterial species harbouring the same plasmid R fi⁻(A, C, Su, Gk). At that time this plasmid has never been observed among resistant Enterobacteria and Pseudomonas.

Furthermore the Gk character conferring a high level of resistance: 128 mcg/ml (WITCHITZ and CHABBERT, 1971a) and governing Gentamycin C adenylation (BENVENISTE and DAVIES, 1971) has never been described before. The level of transferable Gentamycin resistance observed by D. H. SMITH (1969) was below 2 mcg/ml. Other cases of intermediate (32/64 mcg/ml) Gentamycin resistants have been described among Providencia and Pseudomonas (CHABBERT and ACAR, 1969) but transfers have never been successful.

In addition resistance to Ampicillin, Chloramphenicol and Sulfonamides are frequently plasmid-mediated but the pattern A, C, Su is very unfrequent. In an independent study of resistance transfers from the same species studied here, Providencia, Proteus, Pseudomonas, (BAUDENS, unpublished data) the pattern A, C, Su has not been obtained among recipient bacteria.

A third characteristic of plasmids studied here is the combination of a Chloramphenicol resistance character with a fi⁻ transfer factor. This combination has never been described before.

For all these reasons the probability of contamination by independent strains is very low.

An alternative possibility could be the simultaneous and independant formation of four identical plasmids in these four strains. Origin of plasmids is still a speculative question, but genetical events involved in plasmid formation and/or evolution are obviously too rare to happen simultaneously in four bacterial species.

The most likely hypothesis is that the resistance characters have been transferred by conjugation in situ from one strain to the three other strains. The origin of the plasmid in this first strain is unknown. It could be the result of a recombination, picking up, mutation or any other event involved in plasmid formation. We can consider that the second patient was contaminated by only one strain harbouring the plasmid. The fact that a Klebsiella strain carrying the plasmid has been previously isolated support the later possibility.

Experimental studies have established the possibility of in vivo transfer. But clinical situations where these transfers have been unequivocally demonstrated are still rare. Epidemiological consequences of in vivo transfer have been predicted by ANDERSON (1968) in Salmonella epidemics.

It seems that the fact we reported is one good example of such in vivo transfer and is likely the first where transfer occured between several strains of different species. The

21

peritoneal dialysis liquid was probably able to mimic experimental in vivo environment for the conjugating bacterias allowing the formation of a "ménage á quatre".

The wide spread of Gentamycin resistance among hundreds of strains in a few months could have its origin in one unique initial event.

REFERENCES

ANDERSON, E. S. (1968): The ecology of transferable drug resistance in the enterobacteria. Ann. Rev. of Microbiology, *22*, 132.

BENVENISTE, R. and DAVIES, J. (1971): R factor mediated gentamicin resistance: a new enzyme which modifies aminoglycoside antibiotics FEBS Letters, *14*, 293.

BOUANCHAUD, D. H. and CHABBERT, Y. A. (1969): Stable coexistence of three Resistance Factors (fi⁻) in Salmonella panama and Escherichia coli K12. J. gen. Microbiol, *58*, 107.

BAUDENS, J. G. et CHABBERT, Y. A. (1967): Analyse des Facteurs de Résistance transférables isolés en France. Ann. Inst. Pasteur, *112*, *565*.

CHABBERT, Y. A. and ACAR, J. F. (1969): La résistance à la Gentamycine in vitro et in vivo. In: Symposium Gentamycine. Palma de Majorque. pp. 31—37, Editeur Uni labo, Paris, France.

CHRISTOL, D., BURE, A., BOUSSOUGANT, Y. et WITCHITZ, J. L. (1971): Evolution de la résistance à la Gentamycine. In: Presse Médicale No *11*, *79*, pp. 467—470.

SMITH, D. H. (1969): R. factors for aminoglycoside antibiotics. J. Infect. Dis. *119*, 378.

WITCHITZ, J. L., CHABBERT, Y. A. (1971 a): High level transferable resistance to Gentamycin. J. of Antibiotics. Vol. XXIV/2. pp. 137, 139.

WITCHITZ, J. L. and CHABBERT, Y. A. (1971 b): Extension of transferable Gentamycin resistance among Enterobacteria and Pseudomonas in Paris. VII Int. Cong. Chemotherapy, Prague.

PROPERTIES OF AN R FACTOR FROM PSEUDOMONAS AERUGINOSA

DATTA, N., HEDGES, R. W. and SHAW, E. J.

Bacteriology Department, Royal Postgraduate Medical School, Ducane Road
London, W12, England.

Pseudomonas aeruginosa is an organism which is usually resistant to most effective antibiotics and as such posed a great problem in clinical medicine. In 1966 a new semi-synthetic penicillin, carbenicillin, was developed which was active against this organism (KNUDSEN, ROLINSON and SUTHERLAND, 1967). As, after the introduction of any new antibiotic, organisms were carefully monitored for the appearance of resistance, and during the first three years of use, with this particular antibiotic, there was a gradual increase of moderately resistant strains of *Ps. aeruginosa* (LOWBURY, KIDSON, LILLY, AYLIFFE and JONES, 1969). However in March 1969, Lowbury and his colleagues isolated highly resistant strains with a mean inhibitory concentration of 4096 μg/ml from patients in a burns unit in Birmingham. Infecting organisms from the Birmingham patients had been monitored regularly and typed by serological and pyocin methods, it was therefore known that strains of the same type had been present in the same ward, and in some cases infecting the same patient, before showing resistance to carbenicillin. In addition two different types showed this resistance at the same time. It was therefore postulated that the resistance was episomal although at that time transfer was not shown. In the same year other strains, also highly resistant to carbenicillin were isolated in Glasgow (BLACK and GIRDWOOD, 1969); however this does not appear to be a widespread phenomenon and as yet no such strains have been identified in London.

Following the initial suggestion that this resistance was episomal, transfer of resistance to *E. coli* K12 was shown by SYKES and RICHMOND (1970) and FULLBROOK, ELSON and SLOCOMBE (1970). *E. coli* from such transfer experiments was resistant to ampicillin (as well as carbenicillin) and also tetracycline and kanamycin/neomycin. The same resistance pattern was transferable from Pseudomonas strains whether they were from Birmingham or Glasgow. The resistance to penicillins is at the same high level (> 4000 μg/ml) in *E. coli* as in *Ps. aeruginosa* Carbenicillin resistance was mediated by the production of a β-lactamase which was of similar profile to the β-lactamase already found in *E. coli* carrying another R factor (RTEM) of a quite different type from those derived from *Ps. aeruginosa* (SYKES et al., 1970, FULLBROOK et al., 1970).

R factors are classified as either fi^+ or fi^-, fi^+ for fertility inhibition and these inhibit fertility determined by the sex factor F, in *E. coli* K12. fi^- R factors, of course are not fi^+ (WATANABE, NISHIDA, OGATA, ARAI and SATO, 1964). It has sometimes been assumed that the fi^- group is homogenous, but this is not the case. fi^+ R factors determine the production of "sex pili" which are similar to those determined by F, both antigenically and in being receptors for F specific phages. Some fi^- R factors produce pili similar to those encoded by colicin factor I (col I). They can be detected because they act as re-

23

ceptors for I specific phage (If 1). But not all *fi⁻* R factors produce pili which permit absorption and multiplication of this phage (LAWN, MEYNELL, MEYNELL and DATTA, 1967; DATTA and HEDGES, 1971). R factors can also be classified by superinfection immunity. The presence of a plasmid in a bacterial culture leads to the *exclusion* of related plasmids. This seems to be a surface effect (WATANABE, SAKAIZUMI and FURUSE, 1968). Also closely related plasmids cannot co-exist stably in the same cell (MEYNELL and DATTA, 1969). Most *fi⁺* R factors constitute a single compatibility group in that two such cannot stably co-exist. Similarly these R factors which determine the production of I pili cannot co-exist with one another but I-like and F-like can co-exist.

The R factors isolated from *Ps. aeruginosa* in both Birmingham and Glasgow all have the same sensitivity pattern and appear to have the same properties. The one selected for study has been designated RP4.

Table 1

COMPATIBILITY OF RP4 AND OTHER PLASMIDS

Donor	Recipient	R Factor Compatibility Group	Frequency of Transfer
711 (RP4)	J5		1.8×10^{-3}
	J5(F)		2.4×10^{-3}
	J5(R136)	F-like	1.4×10^{-3}
	J5(R64)	I-like	3.0×10^{-3}
	J5(R46)	N	1.4×10^{-3}
	J5(s-a)	W	1.6×10^{-3}

Table 2

STABLE COEXISTENCE OF PAIRS OF PLASMIDS IN **E. COLI** J5

	R Factor Type	Total Colonies Tested	RP4 Lost	Other Factor Lost
J5 (RP4)		217	0	—
(RP4)(F)		50	0	0
(RP4)(538−1)	F-like	248	0	0
(RP4)(R64)	I-like	1356	0	0
(RP4)(R46)	N	281	0	0
(RP4)(s-a)	W	849	0	1

Tables 1 and 2 show that RP4 is not excluded by and can coexist with F-like, I-like and a number of other *fi⁻* R factors which we believe to constitute at least three other compatibility classes (DATTA and HEDGES, 1971; HEDGES and DATTA, 1971). Because RP4 and all the other Pseudomonas-derived R factors confer the same resistance pattern and we have been unable to isolate segregants lacking resistance markers, we have been unable to test whether pairs of such R factors can co-exist with one another.

Despite this compatibility certain patterns of interaction of RP4 and the I-like factor R64 have been observed. Firstly in the presence of R64 or R46 (which belongs to another compatibility group neither F nor I *nor* like RP4) the frequency of transfer is reduced at least 100-fold. This effect is also seen with the derepressed mutant of R64, R64-11 whose own pilus production is constitutive. Secondly *recombination* between R64 (strepto-

Table 3

HOST RANGE OF RP4

			Frequency of Transfer from KI2 - R to			
R Factor	E. coli K12	Ps. aeruginosa	Chromo-bacterium violaceum	Rhizobium melilote	Rhibobium trifolii	Agrobacterium tumefaciens
RP4	10^{-3}	10^{-3}	10^{-5}	10^{-5}	10^{-5}	10^{-8}
R1-19	>1	0	0	0	0	0
R64-11	>1	0	0	0	0	0

mycin R, tetracycline R) or R64-11 and RP4 leads to the production of a plasmid apparently identical with R64 except that it carries the penicillin resistance of RP4. Other recombinants between these two plasmids, including the reciprocal one (a plasmid like RP4 but lacking any penicillinase determinant) have been searched for but not found.

RP4 also differs from the other known R factors in its host range. It is freely transmissible between *E.coli* and *Ps. aeruginosa* and so far all other R factors tried have not been transmissible to Pseudomonas including several F-like and I-like R factors derepressed for pilus synthesis which transfer with 100 percent efficiency between lines of K12.

Table 3 shows that RP4 will also transfer to two strains of Rhizobium — *Rhizobium melilote* and *Rhizobium trifolii*, to *Chromobacterium violaceum* and to *Agrobacterium tumefaciens*, so far no transfer of either an F-like nor an I-like R factor even when depressed for pilus production, to these strains has been obtained.

So RP4 although *fi*$^-$ does not seem to have I-like pili, it does not show superinfection immunity with any known group of R factors and differs in its host range and is therefore proposed to be the first member of another distinct group called P.

REFERENCES

BLACK, W. A. and GIRDWOOD, R. W. A. (1969): Carbenicillin resistance in Pseudomonas aeruginosa. British Medical Journal, *IV*, 234.

DATTA, N. and HEDGES, R. W. (1971): Compatibility groups among *fi*$^-$ R factors. Submitted for publication.

FULLBROOK, P. D., ELSON, S. W. and SLOCOMBE, B. (1970): R Factor mediated β-lactamase in Pseudomonas aeruginosa. Nature, *226*, 1054—6.

HEDGES, R. W. and DATTA, N. (1971): *fi*$^-$ R factors giving chloramphenicol resistance. Submitted for publication.

KNUDSEN, E. T., ROLINSON, G. N. and SUTHERLAND, R. (1967): Carbenicillin: a new semi-synthetic penicillin active against Pseudomonas pyocyanea. British Medical Journal, *III*, 75.

LAWN, A. M., MEYNELL, E., MEYNELL, G. G. and DATTA, N. (1967): Sex pili and the classification of sex factors in the Enterobacteriaceae. Nature, *216*, 343—346.

LOWBURY, E. J. L., KIDSON, A., LILLY, H. A., AYLIFFE, G. A. J. and JONES, R. J. (1969): Sensitivity of Pseudomonas aeruginosa to antibiotics: emergence of strains highly resistant to carbenicillin. Lancet, *II*, 448.

MEYNELL, E. and DATTA, N. (1969): Sex factor activity of drug resistance factors. Bacterial Episomes and Plasmids pp. 120—133. Editors G. E. W. Wolstenholme and M. O'Connor, J. and A. Churchill Ltd., London.

SYKES, R. B. and RICHMOND, M. H. (1970): Intergeneric transfer of a β-lactamase gene between Ps. aeruginosa and E. coli. Nature, *226*, 952.

WATANABE, T., NISHIDA, H., OGATA, C., ARAI, T. and SATO, S. (1964): Episome mediated transfer of drug resistance in enterobacteriaceae. VII two types of naturally occurring R factors. Journal of Bacteriology, *88*, 716.

WATANABE, T., SAKAIZUMI, S. and FURUSE, C. (1968): Superinfection with R factors by transduction in Escherichia coli and Salmonella typhimurium. Journal of Bacteriology, *96* (5), 1796 to 1802.

SOME PROPERTIES OF R-FACTORS ISOLATED FROM PSEUDOMONAS AERUGINOSA

R. B. SYKES, J. GRINSTED, L. INGRAM, J. R. SAUNDERS and
M. H. RICHMOND

Department of Bacteriology, University of Bristol, Medical School, University Walk,
Bristol, England.

Based on a lecture delivered by M. H. Richmond to the Czechoslovak Society of Microbiology
on Friday, 17th September 1971, and published in this volume with the Society's permission.

INTRODUCTION

Although there has been some passing mention of the presence of transferable anti-biotic resistance genes in *Pseudomonas aeruginosa* (LEBEK, 1963; SMITH and ARMOUR, 1966), these reports were brief and rather poorly documented (see HOLLOWAY, 1969). In 1970, however, two papers appeared which definitely established the presence of R-factors in strains of *Ps. aeruginosa* and the ability of these plasmids to specify their own transfer to a wide range of enteric bacteria (SYKES and RICHMOND, 1970; FULL-BROOK, ELSON and SLOCOMBE, 1970). In fact, both these reports referred to a number of strains of *Ps. aeruginosa* isolated from burned patients who had undergone carbeni-cillin therapy in Birmingham (LOWBURY, KIDSON, LILLY, AYLIFFE and JONES, 1969). The carbenicillin resistance of these pseudomonads could be shown to be due to the presence of the β-lactamase specified by an R-factor (β-lactamase Type III; RICHMOND, JACK and SYKES, 1971). Furthermore, the enzyme specified a high level of resistance to all penicillins and cephalosporins when the R-factor concerned was transferred to *Escherichia coli* (SYKES and RICHMOND, 1970).

While this work was in progress, a number of reports appeared that described the detection and isolation of carbenicillin resistant pseudomonads from clinical situations. Examination in our laboratory, with the help of Glaxo Biological Research Department, showed that in one case (BLACK and GIRDWOOD, 1969), the organisms owed their extremely high resistance to the presence of an R-factor, while in the remainder (56 strains in all) the level of resistance — never in fact as high as in R-factor carrying strains — was due not to β-lactamase production but to a high level of 'intrinsic resistance' (SYKES and RICHMOND, 1971). In summary, therefore, R-factor resistance to carbenicillin has, to date, been detected in only two laboratories: the MRC Industrial Injuries and Burns Unit at the Accident Hospital in Birmingham, and the Department of Bacteriology in the University of Glasgow. This is not to say, of course, that such strains do not occur else-where; but they are probably rare — at least at the moment.

We now wish to report on some of the molecular and genetic properties of the two types of R-factor isolated in these strains from these two localities. The first type — found in Strains 1822 and 3425 in Birmingham series (LOWBURY et al, 1969) — has

27

been christened RP1 (i. e. Pseudomonas R-factor Type 1) and the other (from the Glasgow strains) RP4 (DATTA et al, 1972). Although similar in some respects, these two types of R-factor represent two different molecular species of plasmid.

ANTIBIOTIC RESISTANCE MARKES

In view of the high resistance of *Pseudomonas aeruginosa* to many antibiotics, it is difficult to test for the resistance determinants specified by an R-factor in this species. The ability of the strains carrying RP1 and RP4 to break down carbenicillin (LOWBURY, et al, 1969) indicated the presence of a β-lactamase and this was shown to be of Type III (SYKES and RICHMOND, 1970; FULLBROOK, ELSON and SLOCOMBE, 1970; RICHMOND, JACK and SYKES, 1971).

Transfer of both RP1 and RP4 to *E. coli* K12, however, showed that the acquisition of the β-lactamase gene was accompanied by an increase in resistance of the cells to tetracycline, to neomycin and to kanamycin (Table 1). Although the biochemical basis

Table 1

MIC VALUES FOR *E. COLI* K12 RP⁻ COMPARED WITH SIMILAR VALUES FOR *E. COLI* K12 (RP1) OR *E. COLI* K12 (RP4)

Strain	MIC values * (μg/ml.)					
	Ampicillin	Carbenicillin	Cephaloridine	Tetracycline	Kanamycin	Neomycin
E. coli K12 (RP⁻)	<2	<2	<2	<2	<2	<2
E. coli K12 (RP1⁺)	2,500	20,000	100	62	160	160
E. coli K12 (RP4⁺)	5,000	20,000	100	70	320	320

*) MIC values determined as *single cell* resistance in agar plates containing the antibiotic. The value recorded corresponded to the highest concentration at which growth occurs.

of the tetracycline resistance is still unclear, the neomycin/kanamycin resistance was due to the presence of the amino glycoside phosphorylating enzyme — the enzyme normally responsible for the R-factor mediated resistance to these two antibiotics (DAVIES, BRZEZINSKA and BENVENISTE, 1971).

Armed with this knowledge, careful single cell sensitivity tests on the strains of *Pseudomonas aeruginosa* known to be carrying RP1 or RP4 were carried out and the results

Table 2

MIC VALUES FOR *PSEUDOMONAS AERUGINOSA* RP⁻ COMPARED WITH SIMILAR VALUES FOR *PSEUDOMONAS AERUGINOSA* (RP1⁺) AND PSEUDOMONAS AERUGINOSA (RP4⁺).

Strain	MIC values*					
	Ampicillin	Carbenicillin	Cephaloridine	Tetracycline	Kanamycin	Neomycin
Ps. aeruginosa RP⁻	150	40	100	<2	80	80
Ps. aeruginosa RP1⁺	2,500	2,500	5,000	250	2,500	2,500
Ps. aeruginosa RP4⁺	2,500	2,500	5,000	125	1,250	1,250

* MIC values determined as *single cell* resistance on agar plates containing the antibiotic. The value recorded corresponds to the highest concentration at which growth occurs.

compared with those obtained with R⁻ derivatives of the same strains (Table 2). From these experiments we can conclude that both RP1 and RP4 carry the markers *pen-r (Type III): tet-r: neo/kana-r (Phosphorylation)*.

MOLECULAR PROPERTIES OF RP1 AND RP4

A direct examination of DNA prepared from *Pseudomonas aeruginosa* strains carrying RP1 or RP4 showed no satellite bands on CsCl density gradient centrifugation by the method described by SCHILDKRAUT, MARMUR and DOTY (1962). This means either (1) that plasmids exist in the strains but have a density close to that of chromosomal DNA from *Pseudomonas aeruginosa* ($\rho = 1.725$), or (2) that no plasmids exist in the cell, or (3) that plasmids are present but are so small as to be below the limit of detection (in this case the limitations of the method would give a maximum MW of about 10×10^6 if one copy were present per chromosome or correspondingly less if more than one plasmid existed).

Another method has been used to test for plasmids. This was the 'dye/buoyant density' method described by RADLOFF, BAUER and VINOGRAD (1967); it depends on the plasmids existing as covalently closed circular DNA.

Application of this method to strains of *Pseudomonas aeruginosa* carrying RP1 or RP4 showed the presence of covalently closed circular (CCC) DNA in the R⁺ strains but not in R⁻ (Fig. 1). Calculation showed that in strain 1822, RP1 constituted about 1 % of the total cell DNA and RP4 reached 2 %.

Plasmid DNA was prepared by the 'dye/buoyant density method' and was then centrifuged on a neutral sucrose gradient. The S-values of the plasmids were thus determined

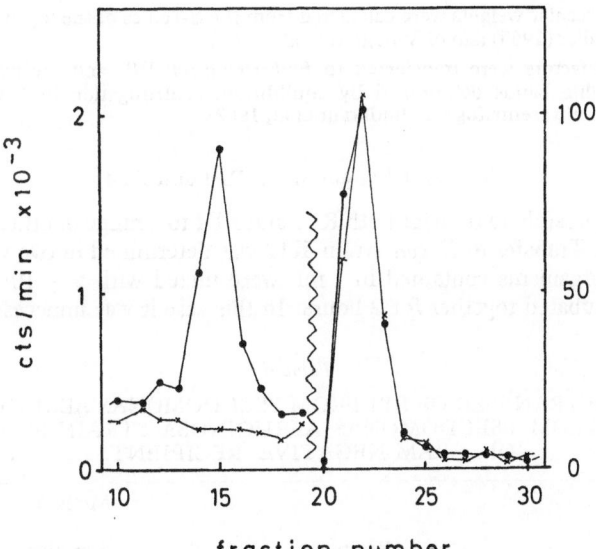

fraction number

Fig. 1. 'Dye/buoyant density' analysis of lysates from RP⁺ and RP⁻ strains of *Pseudomonas aeruginosa* were labelled with ³²PO₄ for about three doubling times and then harvested and lysed. CsCl (to give a density of 1.56 g./cm³) and ethidium bromide (to give a final concentration of about 90 μg./ml.) were added to the lysates and the mixture (total vol. 7.0 ml.) centrifuged at 44,000 rev./min. at 20° for 4 hr. in the 10 × 10 ml. rotor of an MSE SS 50 ultracentrifuge. Forty fractions (9 drops each) were collected and assayed for NaOH insoluble, cold 5% (w/v) trichloroacetic acid insoluble radioactivity. *Pseudomonas aeruginosa* 1822 (RP1⁺), (•); *Pseudomonas aeruginosa* 1822 RP⁻, (x).

and an approximate MW for the molecules were calculated (VINOGRAD et al, 1965; STUDIER, 1965). The densities of the DNA of these two plasmids could be calculated to be about 1.72 — which accounts for the failure to detect their presence in simple CsCl gradient centrifugation (see p. 29). A density of about 1.72 implies that both RP1 and RP4 have a Guanine + Cytosine content of about 60 % (SCHILDKRAUT, MARMUR and DOTY, 1962). Experiments of this type were performed with RP1 and RP4 (Table 3). RP4 (estimated MW: 80×10^6 daltons) proved somewhat larger than RP1 (estimated MW: 40×10^6), despite the similarity of their known marker pattern.

Table 3

PHYSICAL PROPERTIES OF RP1 AND RP4 PLASMID DNA

		Plasmids	
		RP1	RP4
S-value[1]	'open-circular' form	43	54
	'CCC' form	67	88
Molecular weight[2] (Daltons $\times 10^6$)		~40	~80
Buoyant density[3] (g ./cm³)		1.719	1.718

Note 1. R factor DNA was prepared from strains of Pseudomonas aeruginosa by 'dye/buoyant density' centrifugation (see Fig 1). The approximate S-values of the DNA were determined by centrifugation in neutral sucrose gradients.

Note 2. The molecular weights were calculated from the S-values of the 'open-circular' forms by the method of Studier (1965) and of Vinograd et al. (1965).

Note 3. The R-factors were transferred to *Escherichia coli* RP⁻ and the buoyant densities of the resultant satellite bands determined by equilibrium centrifugation in CsCl on a Beckman Model E analytical ultracentrifuge (Schildkraut et al, 1962).

Transfer Properties of RP1 and RP4

It has proved possible to transfer both RP1 and RP4 to a range of other Gram-negative bacterial species. Transfer to *E. coli* strain K12 was determined in two ways. In the first 5×10^7 donor organisms contained in 1 ml. were mixed with 5×10^7 recipients (also in 1 ml.) and incubated together for 2 hours. In this case it was unnecessary to have any

Table 4

FREQUENCY OF TRANSFER OF RP1 FROM PSEUDOMONAS AERUGINOSA STRAIN 1822 AND RP4 FROM PSEUDOMONAS AERUGINOSA STRAIN S8 TO A VARIETY OF GRAM-NEGATIVE RECIPIENTS

Donor	Recipient	Method of Selection	Frequency of Transfer
Ps. aeruginosa 1822 RP1)	*E. coli* W3110 R⁻	Anaerobiosis	5×10^{-4}
Ps. aeruginosa 1822 (RP1)	*E. coli* W3110 R⁻	Rifampicin	7×10^{-4}
Ps. aeruginosa S8 (RP4)	*E. coli* W3110 R⁻	Anaerobiosis	1×10^{-6}
Ps. aeruginosa S8 (RP4)	*E. coli* W3110 R⁻	Rifampicin	7×10^{-5}
Ps. aeruginosa 1822 (RP1)	*Proteus mirabilis*	Rifampicin	1×10^{-5}
Ps. aeruginosa 1822 (RP1)	*Klebsiella aerogenes*	Rifampicin	3×10^{-5}
Ps. aeruginosa 1822 (RP1)	*Aeromonas liquefaciens*	Rifampicin	5×10^{-8}

particular selective markers in the recipient since transfer was detected by plating the mating mixture on agar containing 500 µg carbenicillin/ml. to select the β-lactamase producing cells and incubating the plates anærobically to prevent the donor pseudomonads (which are strict ærobes) from growing. After 24 hours under these conditions the plates were examined and the number of transcipients counted.

In the second type of experiment, transfer to a rifampicin resistant mutant of the recipient was studied using a rifampicin sensitive donor as source of RP1 or RP4. In these experiments the multiplicity of donor to recipient was the same as in the first case and the mating was also continued for 2 hours. In this experiment, however, the transcipients were selected on agar containing 500 µg carbenicillin and 100 µg rifampicin/ml. Table 4 shows the range and frequency of transfer in these two types of experiments (see also DATTA et al, 1972).

Compatibility of RP factors with other plasmids in Enteric Bacteria.

Both RP1 and RP4 were transferred to strains of *Escherichia coli* K12 that already contained other bacterial plasmids. The RP plasmids were able to co-exist in *E. coli* with the Fertility Factor, F, with a range of fi^+ and fi^- F-factors and with the colicinogenic factor I. Furthermore, when RP1 and RP4 were introduced into strains containing plasmids that were derepressed in their ability to initiate conjugation (e. g. F, R1—19, R64—11), the presence of the RP factor had no influence on the frequency of transfer of the derepressed factor, and with one exception, the plasmids had not recombined (Table 5a) (see also DATTA et al, 1972).

Table 5a

Donor	Recipient	Frequency of Transfer			
		Selection	RP1	Selection	Other
W3110(RP1⁺)	J6-2	K★ PY	1×10^{-5}		
W3110(R1-19*drd*)	J6-2			C	3×10^{-2}
W3110(R64)	J6-2			S	4×10^{-4}
W3110(R64-11*drd*)	J6-2			S	5×10^{-1}
W3110(RP1⁺)(R1-19*drd*)	J6-2	K	4×10^{-5}	C	2×10^{-2}
W3110(RP1⁺)(R64)	J6-2	K	5×10^{-5}	S	4×10^{-4}
W3110(RP1⁺)(R64-11*drd*)	J6-2	K	2×10^{-5}	S	7×10^{-1}
J6-2(RP1)(R64-11*drd*) recipient from mating No. 7	W3110	K PY	3×10^{-5} 1×10^{-5}	S	5×10^{-1}
W3110(RP1)(R64-11*drd*) recipient from mating No. 8, selected on K.	J6-2	K PY	2×10^{-5} 5×10^{-4}	S	2×10^{-1}
W3110(Recombinant) recipient from mating No. 8, selected on PY.	J6-2	K	2×10^{-1}	S	3×10^{-1}

```
* K  = Kanamycin
  PY = Carbenicillin
  C  = Chloramphenicol
  S  = Streptomycin
```

31

Recombination between RP factors and other plasmids.

Just because RP factors can co-exist in a cell with another plasmid does not automatically exclude the possibility of recombination between the RP and the other plasmid. In practice, recombination between RP and all other classes of plasmid was uncommon; (Table 5a) the pattern observed was consistent with the independent survival in the cell of the two plasmids concerned. Such independent behaviour of the two plasmids is implicit on the data shown in Table 5b with the exception of RP1 and R64. In this case some co-ordinate transfer of markers derived both from the RP and the R-factor was observed when the transcipients from this cross were subsequently examined (Table 5b) (see also DATTA et al, 1972).

Table 5b

RESISTANCE PATTERNS OF PURIFIED COLONIES FROM SELECTION PLATES
(10 COLONIES TESTED)

Mating	Selection	
	For RP1	For Other
5	5/10 PYKT (RP1 alone) 5/10 PYKTSC (both factors)	10/10 CS (R1-19*drd* alone)
6	10/10 PYKT (RP1 alone) 10/10 PYKTS (both factors)	10/10 ST (R64 alone)
8	*Kanamycin Selection* 10/10 PYTKS (both factors) *Ampicillin Selection* 10/10 PYST, I fi sensitive (recombinant)	10/10 ST (R 64-11*drd* alone)
9	*Kanamycin Selection* 10/10 PYSTK (both factors) *Ampicillin Selection* 10/10 PYST (recombinant)	10/10 ST (R64-11*drd* alone)
10	10/10 PYST (recombinant)	10/10 PYST (recombinant)

Table 6

TRANSFER OF RP1 TO R⁺ AND R⁻ RECIPIENTS

Donor	Recipient	Frequency of transfer
W3110(RP1)	J6-2	1×10^{-5}
	J6-2(R64)	5×10^{-4}
	J6-2(R64-11*drd*)	4×10^{-2}
	J6-2(F'lac)	2×10^{-5}
	J6-2(R1)	4×10^{-5}
	J6-2(R1-19*drd*)	2×10^{-5}
	J6-2(R144)	5×10^{-4}
	J6-2(R144-*drd*)	3×10^{-2}

When W3110(RP4) or W3110(RP1) was mated with J6-2(R64—11) the frequency of transfer of RP4 was much increased. The same result was obtained with other derepressed I-like factors but not with F-like factors (Table 6). The kinetics of transfer suggested that the RP R-factors were being transferred with high efficiency from cells newly infected with R64-11 (Table 7).

Table 7

MATING OF W3110(RP1) WITH J6-2(R64-11*drd*)

Time (mins)	W3110(RP1)	W3110(RP1) (R64-11)	J6-2(R64-11*drd*)	J6-2(R64-11*drd*) (RP1)
0	6.5×10^7		2.5×10^8	
5		4.5×10^6		4×10^5
10	8×10^7	7×10^6	3.0×10^8	5.5×10^5
20		1.6×10^7		1.1×10^6
40	9.5×10^7	2×10^7	4.0×10^8	1.5×10^6
60	1×10^8	2.5×10^7	4.0×10^8	2.4×10^6

Piliation of RP+ strains

The carriage of many types of sex factor is accompanied by the production of sex pili by cells in the population (MEYNELL, MEYNELL and DATTA, 1968). Direct examination of strains of Pseudomonas æruginosa carrying either RP1 or RP4 in the electron microscope for the presence of pili was unsuccessful. Similar studies on *E. coli* (RP1+) and *E. coli* (RP4+) were also unfruitful; but in all cases it is important to stress that both RP1 and RP4 are *repressed* R-factors and that only about $1 : 10^5$ organisms in the cultures would be expected to be piliated.

An alternative method of showing the presence of sex pili (and a preferable method when repressed R-factors are involved) is to propagate one of the so-called sex-specific phages on the cells. Attempts to propagate MS2 phage (specific for F-like pili: STAVIS and AUGUST, 1970) and Ifl phage (specific for I-like pili: LAWN, MEYNELL, MEYNELL and DATTA, 1967) on either *Pseudomonas aeruginosa* or *Escherichia coli* strains carrying RP1 or RP4 failed; and this suggests that cells carrying these plasmids make neither F-like nor I-like pili. Such a conclusion is quite consistent with the compatibility of the plasmids discussed earlier. It must be stressed, however, that the phage propagation is only a really reliable index of pilus type when derepressed R-factors are involved and where, as a consequence, the great majority of the bacteria present will carry pili. At a first approximation, however, it does seem likely that if sex pili are present on cells carrying RP1 or RP4, they have different properties from the F-like and I-like pili encountered so far among R-factor carrying strains.

In conclusion

This lecture is a preliminary report on the properties of two distinct but similar R-factors isolated to date from clinically important strains of *Pseudomonas aeruginosa*. As far as we are aware these are the only two examples of this type of plasmid encountered so far despite a wide survey of strains from a number of Departments in Britain. In all cases, the R-factors have specified a high level of resistance to carbenicillin; although not all carbenicillin-resistant pseudomonads carry the factors (SYKES and RICHMOND, 1971).

By designating the plasmids concerned as RP factors, we do not wish to imply that these elements differ *in principle* from the R-factors so commonly encountered nowadays among enteric bacteria (for example ANDERSON, 1968). Indeed, the RP factors examined in this work seem special only in that they constitute a separate compatibility group of R-factors and can pass the considerable taxonomic boundary between the enteric bacteria and pseudomonads, a property that seem much less widespread among the F-like and I-like plasmids. Indeed, there is circumstantial evidence that certain RP factors may well have reached the pseudomonads in which they were isolated from enteric bacteria cohabiting in the same lesion (ROE, JONES and LOWBURY, 1971).

The detailed molecular characteristics of bacterial proteins are commonly specific to a particular species or biotype (see, for example, the data on bacterial penicillinases: AMBLER and MEADWAY, 1969), but the ability of RP factors to mediate gene transfer between a wide range of distantly related bacterial species would, if widespread, tend to obscure these differences. It seems, therefore, that RP mediated gene transfer between enteric bacteria and pseudomonads cannot be widespread; and among the determinants examined so far seems to be common only with antibiotic resistance genes. This means that their immediate importance is in the field of antibiotic therapy although plasmids such as RP must play an important part in the evolution of bacterial populations in a changing environment.

ACKNOWLEDGMENTS

M. H. Richmond would like to acknowledge with gratitude the kind invitation from the Czechoslovak Microbiology Society to give a lecture in Prague. The work described was supported by Grants for Molecular and Epidemiological research into R-factors and other Plasmids from the Medical Research Council, and for equipment from the Royal Society and ICI Limited. JRS is the recipient of a Scholarship for Training in Research Methods from the MRC and RBS holds a CAPS/SRC Scholarship provided jointly by the Science Research Council and Glaxo Research Limited.

REFERENCES

AMBLER, R. P. and MEADWAY, J. (1969): Chemical structure of bacterial penicillinases. Nature, Lond., *222*, 24.

ANDERSON, E. S. (1963): The ecology of transferable drug resistance in enterobacteria. Ann. rev. Microbiol., *22*, 131.

BLACK, W. A. and GIRDWOOD, R. W. A. (1969): Carbenicillin resistance in Pseudomonas aeruginosa. Brit. med. J., II, 234.

DAVIES, J., BRZEZINSKA, M. and BENVENISTE, R. (1971): R-factors: Biochemical mechanisms of resistance to amino-glycoside antibiotics. Ann. N. Y. Acid. Sci., *182*, 226.

DATTA, N., HEDGES, R., SHAW, J. E., SYKES, R. B. and RICHMOND, M. H. (1972): Properties of an R-factor from Pseudomonas aeruginosa. J. Bact. *108*, 1244.

FULLBROOK, P. D., ELSON, S. W. and SLOCOMBE, B. (1970): R-factor mediated β-lactamase in Pseudomonas aeruginosa. Nature, Lond., *226*, 1054.

HOLLOWAY, B. W. (1969): The genetics of Pseudomonas. Bact. Rev., *33*, 419.

LAWN, A. M., MEYNELL, E. M., MEYNELL, G. G. and DATTA, N. (1967): Sex pili and the classification of sex factors in the Enterobacteriaceae. Nature, Lond., *216*, 343.

LEBEK, G. (1963): Übertragung der Mehrfachresistanz gegen Antibiotika and Chemotherapeutika von E. coli auf andere Species gramnegativer Bakterien. Zentralbl. Bakteriol., *189*, 213.

LOWBURY, E. J. L., KIDSON, A., LILLY, H. A., AYLIFFE, G. A. J. and JONES, R. J. (1969): Sensitivity of Pseudomonas aeruginosa to antibiotics: emergence of strains highly resistant to penicillin. Lancet, *11*, 448.

MEYNELL, E. M., MEYNELL, G. G. and DATTA, N. (1968): Phylogenetic relationships of drug resistance factors and other plasmids. Bact. Rev., *32*, 55.

RADLOFF, R., BAUER, W. and VINOGRAD, J. (1967): A dye-buoyant-density method for the detection and isolation of closed circular duplex DNA: the closed circular DNA of HeLa cells. Proc. nat. Acad. Sci., USA, *57*, 1514.

RICHMOND, M. H., JACK, G. W. and SYKES, R. B. (1971): β-Lactamases of Gram-negative bacteria including Pseudomonads. Ann. N. Y. Acad. Sci., *182*, 243.

ROE, E., JONES, P. J. and LOWBURY, E. J. L. (1971): Transfer of antibiotic resistance between Pseudomonas aeruginosa, Escherichia coli and other Gram-negative bacteria in burns. Lancet, *1*, 149.

SCHILDKRAUT, C. L., MARMUR, J. and DOTY, P. (1962): Determination of the base composition of deoxyribonucleic acid from its buoyant density in CsCl. J. molec. Biol., *4*, 430.

SMITH, D. H. and ARMOUR, S. E. (1966): Transferable R-factors in enteric bacteria infecting the genito-urinary tract. Lancet, *11*, 15.

STAVIS, R. L. and AUGUST, J. T. (1970): The biochemistry of RNA bacteriophage replication. Ann. Rev. Biochem., *39*, 527.

STUDIER, F. W. (1965): Sedimentation studies on the size and shape of DNA. J. molec. Biol., *11*, 373.

SYKES, R. B. and RICHMOND, M. H. (1970): Intergeneric transfer of a β-lactamase gene between Pseudomonas aeruginosa and E. coli. Nature, Lond., *226*, 952.

SYKES, R. B. and RICHMOND, M. H. (1971): R-factors, β-lactamase and carbenicillin resistant Pseudomonas aeruginosa. Lancet, *11*, 342.

VINOGRAD, J., LEBOWITZ, J., RADLOFF, R., WATSON, R. and LAIPIS, P. (1965): The twisted circular form of polyoma virus DNA. Proc. nat. Acad. Sci., USA, *53*, 1104.

IN VITRO AND IN VIVO TRANSFER OF THE R FACTOR TO YERSINIA PSEUDOTUBERCULOSIS CELLS

M. ZAREMBA

Department of Microbiology, University Medical School, Białystok, Poland

The transfer of the R factor has been well documented in a number of Gram-negative bacteria (ANDERSON, 1968; MEYNELL, MEYNELL and DATTA, 1968; MITSUHASHI, 1965; WATANABE, 1967). A few authors only have noticed the fact that organisms of the genus Yersinia may also acquire the R factor from other bacteria of the family *Enterobacteriaceae* during conjugation (GINOZA and MATNEY, 1963; KNAPP and LEBEK, 1967; RUSU, BARON and LĂZĂROAE, 1970).

The present work was designed to prove whether different donor cells belonging to the family *Enterobacteriaceae* would be capable of transferring their R factors to sensitive strains of *Yersinia pseudotuberculosis*.

MATERIAL AND METHODS

The donor strains were selected basing on the results of the minimum inhibitory concentration (MIC) determinations carried out in solid media containing increasing amounts of antibiotics. As donors could serve only the strains displaying a high resistance level to the antibiotics tested (MIC over 400 μg/ml) and being sensitive to nitrofurantoine. The donor strains were isolated from clinical specimens, namely from sputum, bile, feces and urine. They belonged to the genera *Klebsiella* and *Salmonella* as well as to *E. coli* species.

In addition to those of clinical origin the standard E. coli $K_{12}{}^R$ strain was used.

A strain of *Yersinia pseudotuberculosis* Nr 37 (Y. pst. 37) belonging to serotype 1 was employed as the recipient of the R factor. It was isolated from a child's lymph node taken at operation. The recipient strain Y. pst. 37 exhibited a high sensitivity to the antibiotics tested, the MIC values being: A—0,15 μg/ml, C—5μg/ml, S—10 μg/ml, T—2,5 μg/ml, M—3,1 μg/ml (NF—25 μg/ml).

To circumvent the obstacles due to numerous passages on selective media a mutant of Y. pst. 37 resistant to nitrofurantoin (MIC—100 μg/ml) was obtained. The technique employed was that of gradient concentration according to Szybalski.

In order to isolate the Y. pst. 37 cells that having acquired the R factor became resistant to antibiotics, solid media with 30 μg/ml nitrofurantoin, containing one of the below mentioned antibiotics were used: A—25 μg/ml, S—50 μg/ml, C—25 μg/ml, T—50 μg/ml, M—50 μg/ml. Owing to the presence of nitrofurantoin no donor strain could grow on these media.

To follow the transfer of the R factor, 18-hour growths of the donor strains and a similar culture of Y. pst. 37 were blended in 1 : 10 proportions. After addition of an amount of freshly prepared broth the mixed cultures were incubated at 37 °C for 6 hours. Samples were then taken, 10^{-1} to 10^{-8} saline dilutions made and plated on the appropriate media which were incubated at 37 °C for 24 hours and yet for 48 hours at 22 °C. The colonies grown were then read.

In vivo investigations were carried out employing some chosen strains, namely *Klebsiella* 111, *Salmonella enteritidis* 16 and *E. coli* $K_{12}R^+$. White mice "Porton" were given intravenously 0,2 ml of an 18-hour broth culture of the recipient strain Y. pst. 37 incubated at 22 °C. An hour later 0,2 ml amounts of particular donor strains were introduced by the same route. From the mice which died, livers, spleens and kidneys were removed, weighed, homogenized and suspended in physiological saline. The procedure was then as described for the in vitro study.

Similarity of the colonies of Y. pst. grown was confirmed by plate agglutination method employing rabbit immune serum with Y. pst. type 1 antibodies as well as on the basis of the biochemical reactions.

RESULTS

The minimum inhibitory concentrations were determined for 77 strains with the following antibiotics: ampicillin (A), streptomycin (S), chloramphenicol (C), oxytetracycline (T) and monomycine (M).

Because of a high resistance level of the strains to nitrofurantoin (NF) MIC over 25 μg/ml only 23 strains were employed in further investigations and herein: 12-E. coli from urine, 3-*E. coli* — from feces, 3 -*E. coli* $K_{12}R^+$, 2-*Salmonella enteritidis* from feces and 3-*Klebsiella* sp. from feces.

Table 1

INCIDENCE RATE OF Y. PST. 37 CELLS WITH THE R FACTOR ACQUIRED DURING CONJUGATION IN VITRO

Donor	Resistance pattern	Frequency of transfer				
		A	S	C	T	M
Klebsiella 111	ASCT	—	6×10^{-5}	6×10^{-5}	7×10^{-5}	—
E. coli $K_{12}R^+$	ASTM	4×10^{-4}	8×10^{-5}	—	5×10^{-6}	4×10^{-5}
E. coli 8	ACT	1×10^{-3}	—	—	—	—
E. coli 18	ASCT	9×10^{-4}	2×10^{-4}	8×10^{-7}	—	—
E. coli 15	ASCT	3×10^{-6}	4×10^{-6}	1×10^{-6}	4×10^{-7}	—
E. coli 1162	ASCTM	1×10^{-5}	8×10^{-6}	3×10^{-6}	5×10^{-6}	7×10^{-6}
S. enteritidis 16	ASTM	3×10^{-3}	6×10^{-4}	—	3×10^{-7}	5×10^{-4}
S. enteritidis 21	ASCTM	6×10^{-5}	8×10^{-6}	9×10^{-6}	3×10^{-3}	—

Table 1 shows the frequency of occurence of organisms resistant to particular antibiotics in the mixed culture of Y. pst. 37 and the above described strains. Out of the 23 strains tested only 8 transferred their R factors to the sensitive Y. pst. 37 cells.

The Y. pst. 37 cells acquired all the resistance markers or only some of them from the donors. All of them were transferred from the donors: E. coli $K_{12}R^+$, E. coli 18, E. coli 15, E. coli 1162 and S. enteritidis 16. No transfer of resistance to ampicillin was recorded from Klebsiella 111 having the pattern ASCT. E. coli 8 R/ACT/ remitted resistance only to A and the strain of S. enteritidis 21 R(ASCTM) transferred the markers ASC.

The incidence rate of Y. pst. 37 R+ cells differed as to respective antibiotics and was dependent upon the donor strain used. The most numerous were the cells resistant to A, the rate ranging from 10^{-3} to 10^{-6}. Resistances to C and T were being acquired with a similar frequency, namely 10^{-5} to 10^{-7}. The most active donors of the R factor were the strains of S. enteritidis 16, E. coli 8 and E. coli $K_{12}{}^{R+}$. The same frequency of transfer of resistance markers to all the antibiotics tested was noted in the strains of Klebsiella 111 and E. coli 15.

On the basis of the in vitro results 3 strains capable of transferring the R factor to Y. pst. 37 cells were selected to employ in vivo investigations. Resistant Y. pst. 37 strains were searched for in the spleens of the mice infected with Y. pst. 37 and donor cells. The results are depicted in fig. 1.

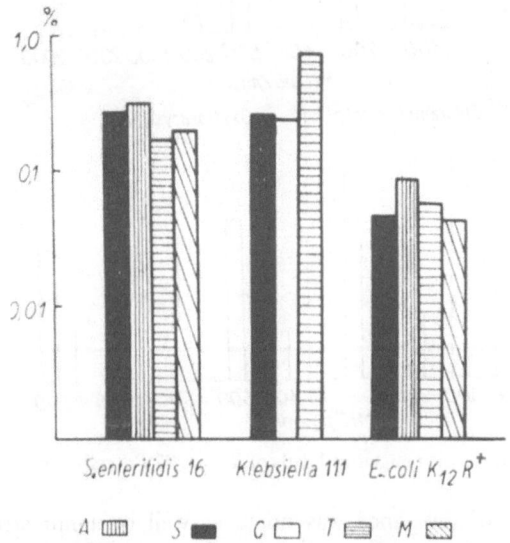

Fig. 1 Percentages of the Y. pst. 37 R+ cells obtained in vivo.

It must be stressed that the percentage of Y. pst. 37 cells having acquired resistance to antibiotics in vivo is high ranging from 0,006 to 0,8. The strain of E. coli $K_{12}{}^{R+}$ appeared to be the least active donor.

Some Y. pst. 37 colonies having acquired the R factor were examined in detail to determine the minimum concentrations of the antibiotics inhibiting their growth.

Fig. 2 shows the results of the examination of 365 colonies of Y. pst. 37 that acquired the R factor from *Klebsiella* 111 cells in vitro and in vivo. The donor strain exhibited the following resistance levels expressed in MIC: A—2000 μg/ml, S—600 μg/ml, C—1000 μg/ml, T—2000 μg/ml. The resistance level of respective Y. pst. 37 R+ cells was recorded to be variable even regarding the same antibiotic. This was the case as well in vitro as in vivo. With streptomycin, a 20-fold difference was noted between the highest and lowest MIC values, more resistant to this antibiotic being the colonies isolated in vitro. Almost all the colonies of Y. pst. 37 resistant to oxytetracycline, isolated in vivo exhibited a high resistance level equal to that of the donor. Resistance of the colonies of Y. pst. 37 isolated in vitro was significantly lower.

Some additional studies were carried out to show that the resistance of Y. pst. 37 R+ cells was associated with the presence of the R factor acquired from enteric bacilli.

It was established indeed since that the Y. pst. 37 R+ cells studied transferred their R factors to sensitive Klebsiella bacilli, the frequency ranging from 10^{-6} to 10^{-4}.

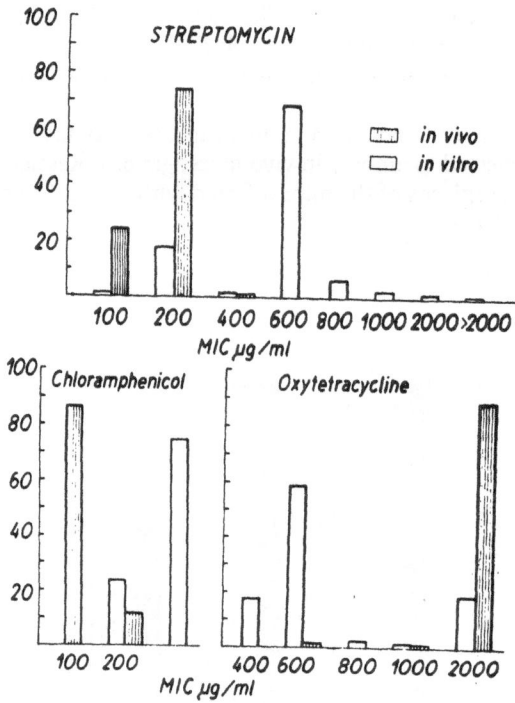

Fig. 2. Distribution of antibiotic resistance levels of Y. pst. 37 R+ cells obtained in vitro and in vivo.

A spontaneous loss of resistance was noted as well in donor strains as in those of Y. pst. 37 R+, in the presence of acridine it being nevertheless much more frequent. Sometimes it amounted to 98% of the cells.

DISCUSSION

Polymorphism is characteristic of human Y. pst. infection (KNAPP, 1959; MOLLARET, 1966). The usual presentation is manifested as mesenteric lymphadenitis and most frequently will be surgically treated since it mimics appendicitis. All the other forms requiring medical treatment with antibiotics.

There have been papers by numerous authors reporting on Y. pst. sensitivity to streptomycin, chloramphenicol, tetracyclines, ampicillin and nalidixic acid and claiming that this organism appears resistant to erythromycin, novobiocin and sulphonamides (KNAPP, 1959; MARTINEWSKIJ and STOGOWA, 1969; MOLLARET, 1965; SOKOLEWICZ and BOROWSKI, 1971).

The strains of Y. pst. isolated, so far from human lymph nodes in Poland were sensitive to most antibiotics (SOKOLEWICZ et al., 1971). The strain Y. pst. 37 employed in this work may be an example. It is of human origin and was isolated during a small epidemy due to Y. pst.

Studies on the possibility of transfer of genetic material on direct contact of Y. pst. and different donor cells, carried out so far, regarded the in vitro conditions only.

The episome F lac+ was transmitted to Y. pestis and Y. pst. cells (LAWTON, MORRIS and BURROWS, 1968; LAWTON and STULL, 1971; MARTIN and JACOB, 1962) as well as was the R factor (GINOZA et al., 1963; KNAPP and LEBEK 1967; RUSU et al., 1970). The standard strains of E. coli always served as donors in all these studies.

RUSU et al. (1970) have demonstrated in their experiments on transfer of the R factor to sensitive Y. enterocolitica cells that the only donors of resistance were the strains of Shigella flexneri. They failed to carry the factor from bacteria of another species. The resistance of Y. enterocolitica acquired was of the same level as that of the donor strain.

It has been well documented in the present work that sensitive Y. pst. cells can acquire the R factor from organisms belonging to different genera of the family Enterobacteriaceae. It appeared that Y. pst. cells could obtain the R factor not only from E. coli cells but from Salmonella and Klebsiella bacilli too.

Not all the in vitro tested strains, resistant to antibiotics could transmit their resistance to Y. pst. cells. It may have been due either to the application of inappropriate media or to the technique employed itself.

The frequency of resistance acquisition recorded in Y. pst. cells, in the present work ranging from 10^{-3} to 10^{-7} remains in good agreement with other authors data (GINOZA, et al., 1963; KNAPP, et al., 1967; RUSU et al., 1970).

The resistance levels, Y. pst. cells exhibited were dependent on the donor strains used as well as on the antibiotic tested.

Attention has been frequently paid to the in vivo transfer of the R factor (ANDERSON, 1968; REED, SIECKMANN and GEORGI, 1969; SMITH, 1969). So far, such studies have not yet been carried out on Y. pst. cells as recipients.

It has however been demonstrated in this study that such transfer may occur during a mixed infection with Y. pst. cells and strains of E. coli, S. enteritidis and Klebsiella in mice. Y. pst. cells resistant to antibiotics were isolated from the spleens of the mice infected. This fact is of great practical value since it suggests the possibility of occurrence of resistant Y. pst. cells in nature. Such strains may be the causative agents of human infections and those in animals.

A high frequency of in vivo occurrence of resistant Y. pst. cells, amounting to 1% suggests that an active multiplication of this organism is not needed the resistance transfer to accomplish. A high rate of multiplication may occur in animals during natural infections.

Studies on the transfer of the R factor to sensitive Y. pst. cells from donors of the family Enterobacteriaceae throw some light on taxonomy of the organism.

Genetic studies of other authors (JONES and SNEATH, 1970; KNAPP et al., 1967; LAWTON et al., 1971) have been suggestive of that the genus Yersinia should be included to the family Enterobacteriaceae.

REFERENCES

ANDERSON, E. S. (1968): The ecology of transferable drug resistance in the enterobacteria. Annual Review of Microbiology, 22, 131.

GINOZA, H. S. and MATNEY, T. S. (1963): Transmission of a resistance transfer factor from Escherichia coli to two species of Pasteurella Journal of Bacteriology, 85, 1177.

JONES, D. and SNEATH, P. H. A. (1970): Genetic transfer and bacterial taxonomy. Bacteriological Reviews, 34, 40.

KNAPP, W. (1959): Pasteurella pseudotuberculosis unter Berücksichtigung ihrer humanmedizinischen Bedeutung. Ergebnisse der Mikrobiologie, 26, 196.

KNAPP, W. and LEBEK, G. (1967): Übertragung der infectiösen Resistenz auf Pasteurellen. Pathologie und Microbiologie, **30**, 103.

LAWTON, W. D., MORRIS, B. C. and BURROWS, T. W. (1968): Gene transfer in strains of Pasteurella pseudotuberculosis. Journal general Microbiology, **52**,, 25.

LAWTON, W. D. and STULL, H. B. (1971): Chromosome mapping of Pasteurella pseudotuberculosis by interrupted mating. Journal of Bacteriology, **105**, 855.

MARTINEWSKIJ, I. L. and STOGOWA, A. G. (1969): Czuwstwitelnost k antibiotikam razlicznych predstawitelej roda Yersinia. Antibiotiki, **1**, 61.

MARTIN, G. and JACOB, F. (1962): Transferet de l'épisome sexuel d'Escherichia coli à Pasteurella pestis. Comptes rendus hebdomadaires des Séances de l'Académie des Sciences, **254/20**, 3589.

MEYNELL, E., MEYNELL, G. G. and DATTA, N. (1968): Phylogenetic relationships of drug-resistance factors and other transmissible bacterial plasmids. Bacteriological Reviews, **32/1**, 55.

MITSUHASHI, S. (1965): Transmissible drug-resistance factor R. The Gunma Journal of Medical Sciences, **14/3**, 169.

MOLLARET, H. H. (1966): Les formes cliniques de l'infection humaine a Bacille de Malassez-Vignal. Pathologie et Biologie, 13, 554.

REED, N. D., SIECKMANN, D. G. and GEORGI, C. E. (1969): Transfer of infections drug resistance in microbially defined mice. Journal of Bacteriology, **100/1**, 22.

RUSU, V., BARON, O. and LĂZĂROAE, D. (1970): Transfert du facteur de résistance (R) des Enterobacteriaceae à Yersinia enterocolitica. Archives Roumaines de Pathologie Expérimentale et de Microbiologie, **29/4**, 571.

SMITH, H. W. (1969): Transfer of antibiotic resistance from animal and human strains of Escherichia coli to resident E. coli in the alimentary tract of man. Lancet, **1/7607**, 1174.

SOKOLEWICZ, E. and BOROWSKI, J. (1971): Charakterystyka szczepów Yersinia pseudotuberculosis wyosobnionych z przypadków chorobowych u ludzi. Medycyna Doświadczalna i Mikrobiologia, **23**, 11.

WATANABE, T. (1967): Infectious drug resistance. Scientific American, **217**, 19.

THE OCCURRENCE OF TRANSFERABLE ANTIBIOTIC RESISTANCE IN ENTERIC BACTERIA ISOLATED IN POLAND

J. BOROWSKI, D. DZIERŻANOWSKA, R. TOMASZEWSKI and
M. BOBROWSKI

Department of Microbiology, University Medical School, Białystok, Poland

The belief is widespread that a considerable number of resistant strains of gram negative bacilli possess in their cytoplasm the so-called resistance factor (R factor). It has been frequently reported, in the world literature, on the incidence rate of the R factor in different bacterial genera (ANDERSON, 1968; MITSUHASHI, 1969; SMITH, 1966; WATANABE, 1963). In Poland, the investigations were initiated on the turn of 1969 resulting in a series of papers on strains of E. coli and Salmonella isolated from animals (TRUSZCZYŃSKI, BORKOWSKA-OPACKA, 1969, 1970) and on those of S. enteritidis and S. typhimurium found in children (LACHMAJER, 1970) all of them harbouring an R factor.

So far, no exhaustive analysis of the epidemiologic situation in this country has been done.

We decided to tackle the problem of the frequency of bacterial strains, having an infectious resistance factor, within the family *Enterobacteriaceae*.

340 at random chosen strains of different *Salmonella, Shigella, E. coli* and *Klebsiella* species were studied.

The strains of *Salmonella* and *Shigella* bacilli were isolated either from carriers or from cases of human typhoid fever and dysentery. Bacteria of the *E. coli* and *Klebsiella* species studied were grown from the urine of patients with urinary tract infections.

Employing the antibiotic dilution technique in a solid medium the minimum inhibitory concentrations were determined against the following antibiotics: ampicillin, streptomycin, chloramphenicol and oxytetracycline.

Strains resistant to four or a smaller number of antibiotics served as donors of the R factor to sensitive organisms. As recipients of the resistance markers the strain *E. coli* K 12 F lac$^+$ met$^-$ and a wild *Klebsiella* 121 strain sensitive to antibiotics were used.

By means of the gradient concentration technique according to Szybalski a mutant resistant to nalidixic acid was obtained from the parental E. coli K 12 strain. Thus this chemotherapeutic agent could be used in selective media to isolate resistant conjugates. When E. coli strains served as donors, the strain Klebsiella 121 was employed as recipient.

The capability of bacteria to transfer the R factor during conjugation was assessed by the classical technique of WATANABE (1963) as well as employing a new, simplified one. To assay this a logarithmic-phase growth of the recipient strain was inoculated on the selective medium. With the aid of a multiinoculator the donor strains, under examination, were plated on the surface of the medium carrying already the recipient and then incubated for 18 h. at 37 °C. In case, a transfer of the resistance determinants to the anti-

43

biotic contained in the selective medium occurred, a growth of the recipient strain was observed on the spot where the donor had been inoculated.

In order to isolate the recipients having acquired the R factor one of the two following media was employed: EMB medium supplemented with nalidixic acid and one of the four examined antibiotics and the citrate medium of SIMMONS with addition of one of the antibiotics.

The results obtained are shown in Table 1.

Table 1

OCCURRENCE OF R-FACTOR STRAINS OF ENTERIC GRAM-NEGATIVE BACTERIA ISOLATED FROM CLINICAL SPECIMENS

Donor strain	Recipient	No strain tested	No strain with transferable R-factor	%
Salmonella sp.	E. coli K_{12}^N	83	18	22
Shigella sp.	E. coli K_{12}^N	40	4	10
E. coli	Klebsiella	130	26	20
Klebsiella sp.	E. coli K_{12}^N	87	33	35
Total		340	81	24

The highest incidence rate of resistant strains possessing the R factor was noted in *Klebsiella* bacilli isolated from patients with urinary tract infections. Among the at random chosen Klebsiella strains 38% were capable of transferring the resistance determinants to four, two or one antibiotic to the sensitive strain *E. coli* K 12. Although one would deem this percentage high enough, it appears however to be twice lower than those reported by other authors. HINSHAW V., PUNCH J., ALLISON M. J. and DALTON H. P. (1969) and ALLISON M. J., PUNCH J. D. and DALTON H. P. (1969) have noted that almost 80 % of the strains of *Klebsiella* isolated from clinical specimens possess the infectious resistance factor. A somewhat higher figure, namely 90 %, was recorded by GARDNER and SMITH (1969). In the latter case the examined strains derived nevertheless from the same source.

A high incidence rate of the R factor was noted in the strains of E. coli. Out of a total of 130 strains examined 26 or 20% transferred the R factor to *Klebsiella* bacilli, this frequency being higher than those recorded by MOORHOUSE (1966) and KABINS and COHEN (1966) but is lower than the figures reported by ALLISON et al. (1969), LEWIS (1968) and HORAK (1969).

Somewhat similar results, to those bearing on the strains of E. coli, were obtained on searching for the R factor within the strains of the genus *Salmonella*. Among them 22% harboured the infectious resistance factor. This figure exceeds the percentages reckoned by American authors (GILL and HOOK, 1966; SCHROEDER, TERRY and BENNETT, 1968; WINSHELL, CHERUBIN, WINTER and NEU, 1969) but is smaller than the percentage stated by KONTAMICHALOU (1967). The smallest number of strains possessing the R factor was recorded in the *Shigella* group. Only 4 out of 40 strains examined were capable of transferring resistance determinants to the sensitive strain of *E. coli*. It should be considered favourable since according to MITSUHASHI (1969) the percentage of the resistant Shigella strains harbouring the R factor is extremely high.

Among 340 examined gram negative bacteria belonging to the genera of *Klebsiella*, *E. coli*, *Shigella* and *Salmonella* 24% possessed the infectious resistance factor.

The resistance patterns of the strains examined are presented in Table 2. The patterns of *Klebsiella* bacilli were of the greatest variety. A simultaneous transfer of resistance markers to all the four antibiotics examined was frequently recorded in these bacilli. It should be emphasized that as many as 24 out of 33 strains of *Klebsiella* transferred their resistance determinants to ampicillin.

Table 2

RESISTANCE PATTERNS IN THE STRAINS OF THE ENTERIC BACTERIA TESTED

Organism	Resistance patterns in the donor strain	No of resistant isolares	Resistance patterns transferred*)
Salmonella sp.	T	39	T(18)
Shigella sp.	ASCT	4	ACT(2), CT(1), T(1)
E. coli	ASCT	22	ASCT(3), SCT(12), ST(3), AS(3), SC(1)
	AST	2	ST(1), S(1)
	AT	1	T(1)
	S	1	S(1)
Klebsiella sp.	ASCT	20	ASCT(7), SCT(4), ACT(2), AC(2), CT(1) A(2), C(1), S(1)
	AST	4	AST(2), A(2)
	SCT	2	SCT(2)
	AT	3	AT(2), A(1)
	A	4	A(4)

*) Number of strains with R-factors are indicated in parentheses

Resistance markers to streptomycin, chloramphenicol and oxytetracycline were noted to be most frequently transferred simoultaneously in the strains of *E. coli* (42%), but only 12% of the 26 strains studied did transfer their determinants to all the four antibiotics i. e. ampicillin, streptomycin, chloramphenicol and oxytetracycline. Other strains of *E. coli* remitted resistance markers to two or one antibiotic.

Concerning the 4 strains of *Shigella* resistant to ampicillin, streptomycin, chloramphenicol and oxytetracycline, two transferred their resistance to ampicillin, chloramphenicol and oxytetracycline, one to chloramphenicol and oxytetracycline and one only to oxytetracycline. In no case the transfer of resistance to streptomycin was recorded.

It was surprising that all the *Salmonella* bacilli tested were resistant only to oxytetracycline.

Occasionally and first of all in *Klebsiella* bacilli segregation of resistance markers was noted.

A particular emphasis should be placed on the fact that the strains of *E. coli* and *Klebsiella* tested were isolated from patients with significant bacteriuria. Moreover while taking into account the serological examination of the strains of *E. coli* and the results of the determination of their sensitivity to the standard colicin sets of FREDERICQ and ABBOTT-SHANNON as well as bacteriophage type examination of *Klebsiella* bacilli, the conclusion will be drawn that all the strains are typical of our milieu being the cause of nosocomial infections in this region (BOROWSKI, DZIERZANOWSKA, ZAREMBA, 1970; DZIERZANOWSKA et al. unpublished data). Thus, these strains play an unequivocal role in the spread of infections among patients in urological wards. It may be assumed that the failure in the management of patients with urinary tract infections encountered during hospitalisation would be due to an intensive use of antibiotics resulting in a prompt selection of the strains with the R factors.

The epidemiologic role of the strains of *Shigella* and *Salmonella* tested in this study remains to be explored. Nevertheless there is some evidence suggesting that at least in the case of bacteria of the genus *Salmonella*, the way of the spread of antibiotic resistant strains may be somewhat similar.

Based on the data presented here it must be concluded that more detailed studies on the epidemiology of strains with extrachromosomal resistance factor would be advocated. Some more efforts will be needed until new simple methods of screening for strains with R factors have been devised. It seems that the method applied to this work can partly fulfil this task. The results are however reliable when the frequency of transfer of the R factor is high, being within the range of 10^{-4} or over.

This work was supported by the Microbiological Committee of the Polish Academy of Sciences.

REFERENCES

ALLISON, M.|J., PUNCH, J. D. and DALTON, H. P. (1969): Frequency of transferable drug resistance in clinical isolates of Klebsiella, Aerobacter and Escherichia. Antimicrobial Agents and Chemotherapy 94.

ANDERSON, E. S. (1968): The ecology of transferable drug resistance in the enterobacteria. Annual Review of Microbiology, **22,** 131.

BOROWSKI, J., DZIERZANOWSKA, D. and ZAREMBA, M. (1970): The diagnostic and epidemiologic significance of nephropathogenic Escherichia coli serotypes. Archivum Immunologiae et Therapiae Experimentalis, **18,** 332.

GARDNER, P. and SMITH, D. H. (1969): Studies on the epidemiology of resistence (R) factors. I Analysis of Klebsiella isolates in a general hospital. Annals of Internal Medicine, **71,** 1.

GILL, F. A. and HOOK, E. W. (1966): Salmonella strains with transferable antimicrobial resistance. Journal of the American Medical Association, **198,,** 129.

HINSHAW, V., PUNCH, J., ALLISON, M. J. and DALTON, H. P. (1969): Frequency of R factor-mediated multiple drug resistance in Klebsiella and Aerobacter. Applied Microbiology, **17,** 214.

HORAK, V. (1969): Frequency of occurrence of E. coli strains capable of transferring their multiple drug resistance in genito-urinary tract infections and some pecularities of their R factors. Journal of Hygiene, Epidemiology, Microbiology and Immunology, **13,** 230. (in Russian.)

KABINS, S. A. and COHEN, S. (1966): Resistance transfer factor in Enterobacteriaceae. New England Journal of Medicine, **275,** 248.

KONTOMICHALOU, P. (1967): Studies of resistance transfer factors. Pathologia et Microbiologia, **30,** 71.

LACHMAJER, M. (1970): Studies on the infectious drug resistance factors in Salmonella straine isolated in Poland. Experimental Medicine and Microbiology, **22,** 21.

LEWIS, M. J. (1968): Transferable drug resistance and other transferable agents in strains of Escherichia coli from two human populations. Lancet, **1,** 1389.

MITSUHASHI, S. (1969): The R-factors. Journal of infectious Diseases **119,** 89.

MOORHOUSE, E. C. (1966): E. coli antibiotic resistance transfer. Irish Journal of Medical Sciences, **2,** 375.

SCHROEDER, S. A., TERRY, P. M., and BENNETT, J. V. (1968): Antibiotic resistance and transfer factor in Salmonella, United States 1967. The Journal of the American Medical Association, **205,** 903.

SMITH, D. H. (1966): Drug resistance of enteric bacteria mediated by R factors. Antimicrobial Agents and Chemotherapy — 1966, pp. 274.

TRUSZCZYŃSKI, M. and BORKOWSKA-OPACKA B. (1969): Studies on infective drug resistance of E. coli strains isolated from pathologic cases in pigs. Medycyna Doświadczalna i Mikrobiologia, **21,,** 357 (in Polish).

TRUSZCZYŃSKI, M. and BORKOWSKA-OPACKA, B. (1970): The infective drug resistance of Salmonella strains isolated from animals. Medycyna Doświadczalna i Mikrobiologia, **22,** 111.

WATANABE, T. (1963): Infective heredity of multiple drug resistance in bacteria. Bacteriological Review, **27,** 87.

WINSHELL, E. B., CHERUBIN, C., WINTER, J. and NEU, H. C. (1970): Antibiotic resistance of Salmonella in the Eastern United States. Antimicrobial Agents and Chemotherapy — 1969, p. 86.

EPIDEMIOLOGICAL INVESTIGATIONS OF R-FACTORS IN MAN AND ANIMALS IN SWITZERLAND

G. LEBEK

Institute of Hygiene and Microbiology, University of Bern, Switzerland

It is known that R-factors have gained a strong distribution among a number of Enterobacteriaceae species, for instance in E. coli and Shigella, and that the proportion of cells carrying R-factors has increased from year to year.

I have the impression that this development has come to a standstill in the last two years. Therefore it is useful to get an overall impression of the distribution of R-factor carrying bacteria in patients, healthy persons and domestic animals. This will permit conclusions as to antibacterial therapy. The proportion of R-factor carrying cells does not depend only on selection by antibacterial drugs, but also on hygienic circumstances because of the infectivity of the R-factors. Therefore information about these hygienic circumstances will be useful too. Last but certainly not least the composition of the R-factors is of genetic interest.

Table 1

DISTRIBUTION OF R FACTORS AMONG STRAINS OF ENTEROBACTERIACEAE ISOLATED 1970 FROM PATIENTS IN SWITZERLAND

Strains	Number of strains examined	Number of strains carrying R factors	%
Salmonella	348	74	21,0
Shigella	37	32	86,5
Enteric coli	183	124	67,7
E. coli	840	529	63,0
Klebsiella	349	145	41,5
Aerobacter	152	63	41,4
Proteus	330	87	26,4
Total	2239	1054	47,1

Table 1 shows a compilation of the *Enterobacteriaceae* isolated from patient material in 1970. The proportion of R-factor carrying cells is highest in *Shigella* species. These are followed by *E. coli, Klebsiella, Aerobacter* and *Proteus*. The smallest proportion is shown by *Salmonellae*.

However, our most recent results indicate that these figures are not entirely accurate.

When conventional culture methods are used for the isolation of *Salmonellae* from feces, F-like R-factors may be lost, because these factors are not stable in *Salmonellae*. The situation is different for not-F-like R-factors, which are stable also in *Salmonellae*.

If the first isolation from feces is made on culture media containing antibiotics, F-like R-factors are preserved. By this procedure the proportion of R-factor carriers in *Salmonellae* is seen to increase. Table 2 contains the pattern of R-factors in *E. coli*. The infectious resistance against Nalidixic acid and Furadantin was not examined. 51 different spectra of determinants could be distinguished. Some of them were particularly frequent. For instance — in the order of frequency — TSSu, T, A, TSu, TCSASu, TCSSu and TCASu.

In Table 3 the strains have been arranged according to the frequency of the individual resistances. Resistance against Sulfonamides has the highest frequency. Then follow T, S

Table 2

DISTRIBUTION OF R FACTORS AMONG E. COLI ISOLATED 1970 FROM PATIENTS IN SWITZERLAND

R⁻	311	TCSu	7	CKASu	1
T	52	TASu	9	CSSuTrim	1
S	4	TKA	1	CASuTrim	1
A	44	TCA	2	SASuTrim	3
Su	17	SASu	3	TCSASu	34
TS	13	TSuTrim	5	TCSKSu	2
TA	9	CSuTrim	2	TSKASu	3
TC	1	CSSu	9	TKASuTrim	3
TSu	35	CASu	1	TSASuTrim	4
CSu	6	SSuTrim	17	TCSSuTrim	5
SSu	25	TCSSu	26	TSKSuTrim	1
ASu	5	TCASu	20	TCASuTrim	5
CA	4	TKASu	1	CSKASu	11
SA	2	TSKSu	1	CSASuTrim	5
KA	1	TSKA	2	TCSKASu	19
TSSu	78	TSASu	17	CSKASuTrim	1
TSA	2	CSASu	6	TCSKASuTrim	3

Legend: T = Tetracycline, C = Chloramphenicol, S = Streptomycin, K = Kanamycin, A = = Ampicillin, Su = Sulfanilamide, Trim = Trimethoprim

Table 3

ISOLATION FREQUENCY OF RESISTANCE TO T, C, S, K, A, Su, Trim IN E. COLI STRAINS FROM PATIENTS CARRYING R FACTORS

resistant to	number of strains	%
—	319	37,0
T	360	42,9
C	172	20,5
S	297	35,4
K	50	5,9
A	222	26,4
Su	392	46,7
Trim	56	6,7
single resistance	117	14,0
double resistance	101	12,0
triple resistance	136	16,2
quadruple resistance	79	9,4
fivefold resistance	73	8,7
sixfold resistance	20	2,4
sevenfold resistance	3	0,4

and A. The other resistances are rare. Resistance determinants against Gentamycin could not be found, but resistance against Trimetoprim was found.

Determinants for Trimetoprim-resistance could not be separated from those making for Sulfonamide-resistance. It is possible, that two groups of Su-determinants occur in nature. One group which combines Su-resistance and Trim-resistance and another group, which codes for Su-resistance only.

Table 4

DISTRIBUTION OF R FACTORS AMONG KLEBSIELLA ISOLATED 1970 FROM PATIENTS IN SWITZERLAND

Resistance pattern of R factors	Number	Resistance pattern of R factors	Number
R⁻	204	CSASu	9
T	7	CASuTrim	3
CA	3	TCSKA	1
KA	4	TCSASu	36
TCA	8	TCASuTrim	5
TASu	3	TSASuTrim	3
TSA	12	CSASuTrim	4
SASu	3	TCSASuTrim	20
TCSA	3	TCSKASu	2
TSKA	2	CSKASuTrim	6
TSASu	3	TCSKASuTrim	7
TCASu	1		

In Table 4 R-factor carrying *Klebsiella* strains are grouped according to the pattern of R-determinants. If compared to *E. coli*, *Klebsiella* strains show considerably less variation in their patterns. There are only 23. Also the frequency distribution of the individual spectra is different.

The most frequent spectrum in *Klebsiella* is TCSASu, followed by TCSASuTrim and TSA. The reason of this difference is not yet known. In any case, a different mode of selection is not a causal factor, because the patients from whom both species were isolated received the same antibiotic treatment.

Table 5

DISTRIBUTION OF R FACTORS AMONG AEROBACTER ISOLATED 1970 FROM PATIENTS IN SWITZERLAND

Resistance pattern of R factors	Number	Resistance pattern of R factors	Number
R⁻	89	TCSSu	1
T	4	CSASu	3
TA	18	CASuTrim	1
CA	4	TCSASu	8
ASu	1	TCKASu	1
TSA	2	TCSSuTrim	1
TCA	7	TCASuTrim	1
TASu	3	CSKASu	1
CSSu	1	TCSASuTrim	2
CASu	1	TCKASuTrim	1
SKA	1	TCSKASuTrim	1

Table 5 contains the results for *Aerobacter*. As only 152 strains were examined, the results are perhaps not representative enough. We found about the same spectra as in *Klebsiella*. The proportion of R-factor carrying cells is almost equal in the two species, so that one gets the impression that the same kinds of R-factors occur in both species.

In Table 6 you will find the resistance spectra in *Proteus* strains. Most of them belong to the species *Proteus* mirabilis. Of the other three *Proteus* species only a few strains could be examined.

Nevertheless we see noteworthy differences. While two thirds of the *Proteus vulgaris* strains and in *Proteus morganii* even three quarters of the strains carry R-factors, are such factors rare in our *Proteus mirabilis* strains. Only 14.3% of them contain R-factors, and

Table 6

DISTRIBUTION OF R FACTORS AMONG PROTEUS STRAINS ISOLATED 1970 FROM PATIENTS IN SWITZERLAND

Resistance pattern of R factors	Number of strains of the following Proteus species				Total
	mirabilis	vulgaris	morganii	rettgeri	
R⁻	209	22	11	1	243
TC	3				3
TA	2	1	3	1	7
ASu			25		25
CA			1		1
TCS	4				4
TASu	14	6	2		22
TCA		1	2	1	4
TSSu	6				6
TCSA		1			1
TSASu	3		1		4
TCSK			1		1
TCASu		3	2		5
TCSSu	2				2
TCKASu	2				2
Total	245	34	48	3	330

these can be transmitted only in rare instances to the acceptor strains used for the other species. Swarming *Proteus mirabilis* strains lose their flagellae after R-infection and regain them after loss of the R-factor. For this reason one should not use cells from swarming cultures for resistance tests. The number of different resistance spectra is very small. *Proteus mirabilis* has only 9, *Proteus vulgaris* only 6 and *Proteus morganii* only 9.

Table 7 shows the results for *Salmonellae*. I have already mentioned a source of error when isolating R-factor carrying *Salmonellae*. This is valid for this table too. Also here we see only 11 different resistance spectra.

The following investigations were carried out in part with the cooperation of SCHEURER, ANAGNOSTIS, TARCHINI and CASAL.

They concern R-factors in the intestinal flora of patients, healthy persons and domestic animals. It could be shown that R-factors occur preponderantly in *E. coli*, rarely in *Citrobacter* and only in a few humans in *Klebsiella*, *Aerobacter* and *Proteus* strains. The *Pseudomonas* group was not included in this investigation.

Table 7

DISTRIBUTION OF R FACTORS AMONG SALMONELLA ISOLATED 1970 FROM PATIENTS IN SWITZERLAND

	R⁻	T	SSu	KS	TSu	TSSu	SKSu	TSASu	CSASu	TCSSu	TCSKASu
S. paratyphi B	12					2	1				
S. abony	2										
S. typhimurium	94		9	15	15				2		
S. brandenburg	9	2				1		1			
S. heidelberg	6		4								
S. thompson	2										
S. tenessee	22		2			4					
S. newport	9										
S. kottbus	2										1
S. blockley	2										
S. miami	1										
S. typhi	6		1	1							
S. enteritidis	88		6							2	
S. panama	12	3	2								
S. anatum	7										
	274	5	24	16	15	7	1	1	2	2	1

There are great differences in the proportion of R-factor carrying E. coli in the intestinal flora. The differences range from 100% to 10^{-4}%, which is the limit of our method of detection.

Table 8 contains the results for hospital patients, healthy nurses of a large hospital, healthy soldiers, healthy school children and a group of vegetarians. Of 88 hospital patients 84.1% had R-factors in their intestinal flora. A few patients harbored several different R-factors. The distribution of individual resistance spectra is similar to that of *E. coli* isolated from general patient material. T, TSSu and TCSSu were the most frequent ones.

Of 100 nurses 88% carried R-factors in their intestinal Coli bacteria. The investigated nurses worked in different departments. There was no difference in the frequency of a positive finding of R-factors between nurses of different hospital departments, but there were differences in the spectrum of determinants. The nurses working in urological and pediatric departments had more complex R-factors than nurses from the other departments. The resistance spectra obtained from the nurses were similar to those of their patients.

Among 51 healthy soldiers, 26 were carriers of R-factors. In smears from rooms and objects of daily use of the soldiers, we could often demonstrate E. coli with the same resistance spectrum as in the bacteria isolated directly from the soldiers.

However, these resistances were not transmissible.

Out of 101 children of the three lower classes of a primary school in Berne, we found 66 with R-factors in their fecal flora. The parents of the examined children stated that the children had not received antibacterial drugs in the last two years preceding the investigation. As a last group we examined 28 persons belonging to a religious community, which takes no drugs and lives on a vegetarian diet. In 16 persons we found R-factors in the intestinal flora, in one case in *Salmonella typhimurium*. It should be noted that we could demonstrate in this group R-factors with 4 and even 5 resistance determinants. There is a rather great similarity in the resistance spectra in these persons. Preferential combinations are: TSSu, T, CSSu and TCSSu.

Table 8

DISTRIBUTION OF R FACTORS AMONG E. COLI ISOLATED FROM FAECES OF HEALTHY AND ILL HUMAN SUBJECTS IN SWITZERLAND

Resistance pattern of R factors	Number of ill persons	Number of healthy nurses	Number of healthy soldiers	Number of healthy 6−9 years old pupils	Number of healthy vegetarian persons
Total	88	100	51	101	28
R⁻	14 = 15,9 %	18 = 18 %	25 = 49 %	35 = 34,6 %	12 = 42,9 %
T	22		2	7	
S		1	1	2	
TSu	3				
TS	1	2	1	12	3
CS				1	
SSu	4	8	7	5	1
CSu	2				
KSu				1	
TCSu	4	1		1	
TCS				1	
TSSu	21	38	10	21	7
TKSu					1
CSSu	19		3	5	
CSA	2	1			
TCSA		3			
TCSSu	32	8	10	12	
TSASu	5	3			
TKASu					1
TCASu	2	1			1
TSKSu		1	1	2	
SKASu		1			
CSASu	1				
TCSKSu				1	
TCSASu		11			2
TCSKASu		3			

Our results show that R-factors are widely distributed in the intestinal flora of healthy persons. Everything taken together, more than 50% of the population carries R-factors.

The results obtained from vegetarians refusing drugs proves that this distribution is not only a consequence of selection by antibacterial therapy. Also the application of antibacterial drugs outside of human and veterinarian medicine contributes to the spreading of R-factors in nature.

In the whole world antibiotics are added to the food of chickens, pigs, sheep and calves in order to increase the productivity. Food of a high quality and the costly maintainance of good hygienic housing conditions are circumvented by this practise.

In order to study the selection pressure exerted by this feeding with antibiotics, we examined the feces of pigs, calves, cows and horses. The results are seen in Table 9.

Table 9

DISTRIBUTION OF R FACTORS AMONG E. COLI ISOLATED FROM FAECES OF DOMESTIC ANIMALS (SEVERAL FARMS WITH TETRACYCLINE APPLIED TO THE ANIMALS)

Resistance pattern	R factors in E. coli strains from			
	Pig	Calf	Cow	Horse
T	49	3	5	1
TSu	87	5	2	
SSu	17	6		
TSSu	92	19	14	
CSSu	9	11	6	
TCSSu	12	13	3	
CSASu	8	3		
TSASu	23	5	4	
TSKSu	6	4	2	
TSKASu	12	1	1	
TCSKSu	5	1	8	
TCSKASu	7	1		
Number of investigated animals	112	23	47	9
Number of animals with R factors	112	23	22	1
Number of animals without R factors	0	0	25	8

Of 112 pigs and 23 calves all were carriers of R-factors in their intestinal bacteria. In every fecal specimen several different R-factors could be demonstrated. The calves acquired the R-factors already in the first days of their lives, even before the administration of antibiotics with solid food. R-factor carrying E. coli were found abundantly in the stables. For instance in the excrements, on the walls, on the clothing and on the hands of the stable attendants, so that there was ample possibility for contamination. It was astonishing that at first only a few *Coli* with R-factors were isolated from the feces, but that only a short time afterwards all *Coli* bacteria contained R-factors, before the animals themselves received antibiotics.

For feeding purposes, only Tetracycline was used in the investigated stables. Therefore it was easy to understand that all animals with positive findings carried determinants for Tetracycline resistance. But also R-factors with C-, K-, S- and Su-determinants were

53

found. The presence of K-, S- and Su-resistance determinants can be explained by therapy of sick animals.

C-determinants might have been introduced together with R-factors carrying them and might have been selected afterwards together with the other determinants.

It is striking that all new-borne calves acquired abundant *E. coli* with R-factors without having received antibiotics.

We shall continue to study this question. (It can be assumed that bacterial contamination from the environment is involved.)

Table 10

DISTRIBUTION OF R FACTORS AMONG E. COLI ISOLATED FROM FAECES OF DOMESTIC ANIMALS (ON FARM WITHOUT ANTIBIOTICS APPLIED IN THE FEED TO THE ANIMALS)

Resistance pattern	R factors in E. coli strains from	
	Calf	Cow
S	1	
SSu	1	
Number of investigated animals	5	19
Number of animals with R factors	1*	
Number of animals without R factors	4	19

* treated with Streptomycin and Penicillin

Table 10 proves that the occurrence of R-factors in calves is connected with antibiotic feeding.

This table shows results from 2 stables in a mountain region, where antibiotic feeding is not used. All 19 cows and 3 of 4 calves were free of R-factors. One calf had bacteria with R-factors containing determinants for S and SSu resistance respectively. This calf had been treated with Streptomycine and Penicilline for a diarrhaea.

This investigation was supported by Schweizerischer Nationalfonds. I thank Miss U. NYDEGGER and Miss Ch. HOIDA for careful technical assistance.

REFERENCES

ANAGNOSTIS, D. (1969): Die Verbreitung von R-Faktoren in der Darmflora gesunder Schulkinder Berns. Inauguraldissertation, Bern.
ANDERSON, E. S. (1969): Ecology and Epidemiology of transferable drug resistance. In: Bacterial Episomes and Plasmids, pp. 102—115. Editors G. E. W. Wolstenholme and Maeve O'Connor, J. and A. Churchill Ltd., London.
CASAL, E. (1971): R-Faktoren in den Faeces von Kühen und Kälbern. Inauguraldissertation, Bern.
LEBEK, G. (1969): Die infektiöse bakterielle Antibiotikaresistenz. Hans Huber, Bern und Stuttgart.
MITSUHASHI, S. (1971): Transferable drug resistance factor R. University Park Press, Baltimore, London, Tokyo.
SCHEURER, U. Ch. (1968): Ueber das Vorkommen antibiotikaresistenter Darmkeime bei gesunden Rekruten. Inauguraldissertation, Bern.
TARCHINI, J. C. (1971): Die Verbreitung von R-Faktoren im Krankenhaus. Inaugural dissertation, in Vorbereitung.
WATANABE, T. (1969): Transferable drug resistance: The nature of the problem. In: Bacterial Episomes and Plasmids, pp. 81—97. Editors G. E. W. Wolstenholme and Maeve O'Connor, J. and A. Churchill Ltd., London.

MULTIPLE DRUG RESISTANCE OF PATHOGENS
IN PURULENT SURGICAL INFECTIONS

S. M. NAVAŠIN and I. P. FOMINA

National Institute of Antibiotics, Moscow, USSR

Clinical aspects of infective resistance discussed here are closely connected with other problems and especially genetic and molecular biological ones. At the same time clinical material as a source of R-factors of pathogenic organisms not only raises questions but also answers them. The present state of drug resistance under conditions of clinics is to some extent a criterion of the validity of the theoretical postulates providing a definition as for a rule or an exception.

This paper presents data on the state of sensitivity of main "problem" pathogens in two surgical clinics of Moscow in 1965 and 1969—1970.

Comparative analysis of the isolation rate of various species of microorganisms causing purulent infections showed no significant shifts in the ratio of different bacterial species within the period of observation. In both periods, i. e. 1970 and 1965 staphylococci in pure cultures (59.5 per cent) or in associations with other microorganisms, such as *E. coli*, *Proteus spp*, *Enterococceae* (20 per cent) were isolated from surgical cases with purulent infections, the numbers of *E. coli*, *Proteus spp* and *Ps. aeruginosa* being 13.4, 4.7 and 1.7 per cent respectively. *Staph. albus* as a causative agent of severe purulent infections, such as pneumonia, peritonitis, etc. especially in children was often isolated, the number of which among all staphylococcal isolates ranged from 25 to 70 per cent.

Antibiograms of the above organisms isolated in 1965 and 1969—1970 (365 and 570

Table 1

COMPARATIVE SENSITIVITY TO ANTIBIOTICS OF CLINICAL STRAINS OF
STAPHYLOCOCCUS ISOLATED FROM PATIENTS IN 1965 AND 1969—1970

Antibiotic	Resistant strains (per cent)	
	1965	1969—1970
Benzylpenicillin	78.3	54.4
Methicillin	11.3	15.9
Ampicillin	—	50.0
Erythromycin	48.4	37.3
Streptomycin	68.9	69.1
Tetracycline	74.5	71.3
Chloramphenicol	59.7	49.3
Kamamycin	4	17.3
Vancomycin	0.5	0
Fusidin	0.9	1.9

strains respectively) showed no tendency for increased occurrence of resistant strains to the antibiotics most widely used in clinics and what is more the number of *Staphylococcus* sensitive to benzylpenicillin increased from 21.7 to 45.6 per cent, the number of staphylococci sensitive to erythromycin also increased, but to a lesser extent (Table 1). Among resistant cultures isolated in 1969—1970, the same as in previous periods strains characterized by the following resistance spectra, i. e. benzylpenicillin (P); erythromycin (E); PE, tetracycline (T), streptomycin (S); kanamycin (K), chloramphenicol (Ch); P, T, S, were most often isolated.

Because of high rates of mixed infections in surgical clinics, broad spectrum antibiotics and parenteral tetracycline in particular, as well as various antibiotic combinations are of primary use. However, the average percentage of staphylococci resistant to tetracycline, chloramphenicol or streptomycin practically did not change within 1965—1970. Simultaneously the number of isolates with multiple drug resistance decreased (Table 2).

Table 2

DYNAMICS OF MULTIPLE DRUG RESISTANCE IN *STAPHYLOCOCCUS* ISOLATED FROM PATIENTS IN 1965 AND 1969—1970

Resistance determinants	Resistant strain (per cent)	
	1965	1969—1970
No (sensitive)	12.3	19.6
P (T) (S)	18.4	10.2
P, E, PS, TS	6.1	11.4
PES, PET, STCh, PST, PSTCh, PETCh	36.8	22.8
PESTK, PESTCh, PSTChK	24.4	36.0

At present, as well as long before the wide use of semi-synthetic penicillins, staphylococci resistant to methicillin are being isolated from clinical cases. In 1970 their number amounted to 15.9 per cent. As a rule, they were simultaneously resistant to most other antibiotics, including all penicillin but dicloxacillin. Multiple resistance of staphylococci to antibiotics was not usually observed with respect to vancomycin and fusidin. Strains resistants to the latter two antibiotics were seldom isolated; 0.5 and 0.9 per cent in 1965 or 0 and 1.9 per cent in 1970 respectively. In connection with increased severity of staphylococcal infections possibly due not only to decreased rate or level of antibiotic sensitive staphylococci, but also to the changed host reactivity because of previous therapy with antibiotics, hormones and other biologically active substances, a complex of pathogenic properties in staphylococci with multiple antibiotic resistance was studied. Comparison of the findings with antibiograms for *Staph. albus* usually classified as facultative pathogenic organisms was of special interest.

Not trying to identify the antibiotic resistance determinants with the features defining the pathogenic properties of the microbe, in spite of the fact that such a relation was obvious in some instances, i. e. conversion of non-toxigenic cultures of *Staph. aureus* to toxigenic ones on their lysogenization with moderate phages, isolated from toxigenic cultures (FREEMAN (1951), DORUBUSH et al (1969)) they should be considered in a complex as factors promoting the survival of the selected cells. Among the strains characterized by antibiotic sensitivity or multiple drug resistance, pathogenic staphylococci were isolated at the same rate (Table 3). No preferable distribution of epidemic staphylococci was observed within one clinic. Both sensitive and resistant strains belong mainly to phage groups I and II. However, 56.1 per cent of resistant staphylococci and

26.5 per cent of sensitive ones could not by typed with the International set of 22 phages. Similar findings of other authors are available (SIGIMOTO and YOSHIOKA (1970)).

Antibiotic sensitivity in gramnegative organisms was relatively stable within the observation period of 5 years, with a tendency of the resistance lowering by 1970. In

Table 3

SOME FEATURES OF ANTIBIOTIC RESISTANT *STAPHYLOCOCCUS*

Resistance determinants	Strains (per cent)					
	Pigments			Hemolysis	Virulence for mice	Betalacta-mase production
	White	Yellow	Golden			
No (sensitive)	64.3	14.3	21.4	71.4	50.0	50.0
P (T) (S)	35.7	—	64.3	35.7	35.7	42.9
PS, TS, PE	83.3	—	16.7	66.6	46.7	66.6
PES, PET, STCh, PST, PSTCh, PETCh	70.5	5.9	18.6	55.3	39.0	35.3
PESTK, PESTCh, PSTChK	100	—	—	68.4	66.6	66.6

1969—1970 the numbers of *E. coli* resistant to streptomycin, tetracycline and chloramphenicol amounted to 53.3, 54.7 and 38.6 respectively, in 1965 the respective values being 62.6, 67.8 and 53.9 per cent (Table 4).

Table 4

COMPARATIVE ANTIBIOTIC SENSITIVITY OF *E. COLI* ISOLATED FROM PATIENT IN 1965 AND 1969—1970

Antibiotic	Resistant strains (per cent)	
	1965	1969—1970
Streptomycin	62.6	53.3
Tetracycline	67.8	54.7
Chloramphenicol	53.9	38.6
Kanamycin	27.0	29.9
Ampicillin	35.6	46.1
Carbenicillin	—	43.1
Cephaloridine	—	37.7

In 1970 the most typical sets of the resistance markers among strains with multiple resistance were the following: STCh, STChK, STChK A (ampicillin), C (cephaloridine), Ca (carbenicillin). The numbers of *E. coli* resistant to kanamycin were practically the same in 1965 and 1969—1970, while the number of strains with moderate resistance to the antibiotic increased at the MIC within 6.2—12.5 mcg/ml from 21 per cent in 1965 to 45 per cent in 1970.

In the practice of general surgery in the clinics under observation, ampicillin was not used for the treatment of post-operative purulent complications, whereas a significant number of *E. coli* resistant to the antibiotic was isolated in both 1965 and 1969—1970, i. e. 46.1 and 35.6 per cent respectively, the number of moderately resistant strains being 60 per cent at the MIC of 12.5—25 mcg/ml.

In most instances strains resistant to ampicillin were simultaneously resistant to carbenicillin and cephaloridine. Strains resistant to the latter two antibiotics amounted to 43.1 and 37.7 per cent respectively. Some decrease in the number of E. coli with multiple resistance to 3—6 or more antibiotics was observed. If in 1965 the number of such strains was 69.7 per cent of the total number of the isolates, in 1969—1970 the value decreased approximately by 13 per cent and was 57 per cent (Table 5).

Table 5

DYNAMICS OF MULTIPLE DRUG RESISTANCE IN E. COLI ISOLATED FROM PATIENTS IN 1965 AND 1969—1970

Resistance determinants	Resistant strains (per cent)	
	1965	1969—1970
No (sensitive)	17.4	12.3
T (S), (K)	12.9	20.5
TS, TCh, TK	8.7	19.1
TSCh, TKCh, TKA	31.3	24.2
TSChKAC, TSChKA	29.7	13.7

The mechanism of the initial high resistance of E. coli to carbenicillin and cephaloridine not connected with the wide use of the antibiotics requires special discussion and is possibly due to the natural cross resistance of the microbe to the group of antibiotics with the same type of the mechanism of action. One of the courses of the resistance of E. coli to broad spectrum semi-synthetic penicillins is the synthesis of specific enzymes coded by R-factor, which destroy the antibiotics.

Studies on betalactamase production in the strains of E. coli resistant to ampicillin, carbenicillin and cephaloridine showed that in most instances the strains had multiple resistance with the following set of the resistance markers: T Ch S K A Ca C. It was found that strains producing betalactamase among penicillin resistant isolates amounted to 57.9 per cent, the resistance of the other strains was not associated with enzyme production. Out of 10 strains of the above group with simultaneous resistance to kanamycin, 3 strains inactivated the antibiotic by phosphorylation. No pronounced relation between multiple drug resistance of the microbe and other features, such as colicinogenic capacity, hemolytic activity and other properties controlled by episomes was shown (SMITH (1967)).

Colicinogenic properties were found in 66.3 per cent of sensitive strains and 48—50 per

Table 6

SOME PROPERTIES OF ANTIBIOTIC RESISTANCE CLINICAL STRAINS OF E. COLI ISOLATED FROM PATIENTS DURING THE OBSERVATION PERIOD

Resistance determinants	Strains (per cent)			
	Betalactamase production	Colicino-genicity	Hemolysis	Virulence for mice
No (sensitive)	22.2	66.3	Some strains	83.8
T (S)	33.3	33.3	,,	66.6
TK, TS, TCh	23.4	28.6	,,	71.4
TSCh, TKCh, TKA	56.0	48.0	,,	96.0
TSChKAC, TSChKACa	40.0	50.0	,,	90.0

cent of strains with multiple resistance. Strains virulent for mice were isolated practically at the same rate among both sensitive strains and strains with multiple resistance (Table 6).

Close phenomena with respect to the isolation rate of antibiotic resistant strains were also found in *Proteus spp* (Table 7). The isolation rate of the strains resistant to

Table 7

ANTIBIOTIC SENSITIVITY OF *PROTEUS SPP* STRAINS ISOLATED
FROM PATIENTS IN 1965 AND 1969−1970

Antibiotic	Resistant strains (per cent)	
	1965	1969−1970
Tetracycline	100	98
Streptomycin	75.4	75.9
Kanamycin	34.9	57.6
Chloramphenicol	42.1	42.4
Ampicillin	23.2	22.7

streptomycin, chloramphenicol, tetracycline and ampicillin was practically the same within the observation period of 5 years, the most often set of R-factors being S Ch K A (resistance of *Proteus* spp to tetracycline and cephaloridine is primary). However, a definite shift in the structure of *Proteus spp* sensitivity to ampicillin and kanamycin was observed. The number of strains with moderate sensitivity to the antibiotics somewhat increased and the ranges of the MIC of them approached the utmost blood levels in patients treated with high doses of the antibiotics. At the same time a definite tendency for decreased isolation of *Proteus spp* with multiple resistance was observed. Thus, in 1965 strains of *Proteus spp* resistant to 3 or more antibiotics amounted to 85.4 per cent, the respective figure in 1969−1970 being 68.3 per cent (Table 8).

Table 8

DYNAMICS OF MULTIPLE RESISTANCE IN *PROTEUS SPP* STRAINS
ISOLATED FROM PATIENTS IN 1965 AND 1969−1970

Resistance determinants	Resistant strains (per cent)	
	1965	1969−1970
No (sensitive)	—	—
T (S), (K)	14.6	21.7
TS, TCh, TK	17.4 ⎫	13.3 ⎫
K Ch A, SK ChA	36.3 ⎬ 85.4	26.5 ⎬ 68.3
S Ch K A	31.7 ⎭	28.5 ⎭

Therefore some decrease in the isolation of antibiotic resistant strains in clinics showed in our studies and described earlier (SIGIMOTO and YOSHIOCA (1970), BULGER and SHERRIS (1968), BULGER and LARSON (1970), SMITH (1967)) as well as definite correlation between occurrence of multiple drug resistance and efficiency of antibiotic therapy is indicative of the presence of some mechanisms controlling the „balance constancy" preventing epidemic distribution of resistance. The diversity of antibiotic resistance characteristics, wide ranges of the MIC of benzylpenicillin and isolation of significant number of staphylococci with the resistance mechanisms not connected with betalactamase production, constant high levels of resistance in staphylococci to erythromycin, tetracycline and streptomycin are indirect evidences of a double mechanism of the resistance control, i. e. chromosomic and episomic. Recently it was proved experimentally (NOVICK (1967)).

Absence of seldom occurrence of bacterial resistance to some antibiotics, such vancomycin or polymyxin or on the contrary a high level of initial natural resistance in microbial strains, for instance primary resistant to semisynthetic penicillins must be indicative of the fact that development and rapid distribution of resistance are defined by both the antibiotic and the microbe.

At present a significant success has been achieved in mapping of genes controlling the synthesis of individual proteins of 30S and 50S subunits reconstruction of ribosomes devoided of proteins responsible for resistance to some antibiotics inhibiting the protein synthesis (MIZUSHIMA and NOMURA (1970), MASUKAWA (1969)).

The studies on episome controlled enzymatic inactivation of some groups of antibiotics have stimulated synthesis of antibiotic derivates with substituted functional groups stable to enzymatic transformation. Fruitfulness of this line of work is evident from synthesis of semi-synthetic derivatives of aminoglycosides resistant to specific enzymes (UMEZAWA et al (1971)).

From this point of view revision of some antibiotics, considered at present to be of low clinical value, such as mannosidostreptomycin, kanamycin B and C, etc. seems expedient with the purpose of studying the mechanisms of their resistance to enzymatic transformations.

All of us dealing with the practical problems of antibiotic therapy are much interested in the possibility of creating a genetic basis for rapid distribution of multiple drug resistance among evolutionally not connected groups of microorganisms.

However, inspite of widespread strains with episomic antibiotic resistance is taken as the main mechanism of multiple resistance, many of the experimental findings remain to be explored from this position. These are first of all:

— Prolonged maintenance of constant ratios in sensitive and resistant microorganisms and in particular during the observation period under conditions of the common antibiotic therapy policy.

— Decreased isolation of antibiotic resistant strains and strains with multiple resistance especially among staphylococci found in our studies and described earlier.

— As for this country, the peak of R-factor distribution should be attributed to 1965 to 1966. At present, at least with respect to pathogenes of purulent infections the "balance constancy" between distribution of the microbes carrying R-factor and efficiency of antibiotic therapy may be considered to be established.

— Inspite of the capacity of the recipient cell for modifying and limiting the functions of heterologous DNA on recombination, resulting on transfers of R-factor in its qualitative and quantitative alterations, most of the strains isolated in our studies were characterized by homogenous resistance levels and practically all strains with multiple resistance of staphylococci and gramnegative organisms were highly sensitive to all antibiotics of the set at a MIC of 250 to 1000 mcg/ml.

— Among betalactamase producing staphylococci resistant to benzylpenicillin 22.2 per cent of the isolates were in our studies sensitive to erythromycin. However, it is known that determinants of resistance to these antibiotics controlling betalactamase are transfered from strains to strain by phage transduction "en block" and such different markers are seldom transfered alone. Inspite of a great diversity of benzylpenicillin resistance levels at the MIC for the resistant staphylococcal strains ranging from 2—3 to

100 units/ml or more, the resistance to erythromycin was homogenous and the MIC for all strains resistant to erythromycin and isolated in 1969—1970 was 250—500 mcg/ml more.

— Contradictions between isolation of strains with multiple resistence and real efficacy of antibiotic therapy, which is especially evident with respect to benzylpenicillin. In this country in clinical practice benzylpenicillin is not widely used in "mega" doses. Still even in 1965—1966, at the period of the highest levels of staphylococcal resistance to this antibiotic (90 per cent or more in some clinics), penicillin therapy was effective by no means in more than 10 per cent of the cases.

— Multiformity of multiple drug resistance with different sets of the resistance markers, including and employing for its explanation the possibility of phenotypic suppression by the host cell and segregation of single genes, sex incompatibility preventing bacterial conjugation, etc., rather strict specificity of particular mechanisms of its realization (enzymatic inactivation of penicillin, aminoglycosides, chloramphenicol; changes in permeability of cell walls as one of possible mechanisms of resistance to tetracyclines).

Speculativeness of this arguments at the present stage is obvious. However, a necessity for elucidating ratios and practical importance of episomal and chromosomal determinants of resistance for every antibiotic is obvious as well. During the decade of rapid distribution of R-factors among pathogenic organisms, as well as in minds of scientists, we get accustomed to extrachromosomal localization of the determinants of resistance to benzyl-penicillin. However, now we are certain in a possibility of controlling betalactamase production at both the episomal and the chromosomal levels of the bacterial cell. This possibly explains the diversity of antibiotic resistance levels in staphylococcal isolates. Analogous findings are now available with respect to aminoglycosides.

At the beginning we tried to approve the expediency of a common conception for the mechanisms of multiple drug resistance. However, analysis of clinical data may be indicative of a diversity of such mechanisms and possible significance of at least two of them, the main ones, that is chromosomal and extrachromosomal. Evaluation of the role of every of the mechanisms and their interactions will be of help in establishing the tactics controlling the distribution of resistant microorganisms.

REFERENCES

BULGER, R. J. and SHERRIS, J. C. (1968): Decreased incidence of antibiotic resistance among Staph. aureus. Annals of Internal Medicine, 69, 1099.

BULGER, R. J. and LARSON, E. (1970): Decreased incidences of resistance to antimicrobial agents among E. coli and Klebsiella-Aerobacter. Annals of Internal Medicine, 66, 72/I, 65.

DORNBUSCH, K. et al (1969): Extrachromosomal control of methicillin resistance and toxin production in Staph. aureus. Journal of Bacteriology, 98/2, 351.

FREEMAN, V. J. (1951): Studies on the virulence of bacterophageinfected strains of Corinobacterium diphteriae. Journal of Bacteriology, 1951, 61, 675.

MASUKAWA, H. (1969): Localisation of sensitivity of kanamycin and streptomycin in 30 S ribosomal proteins of E. coli. Journal of Antibiotics, ser. A 22/12, 612.

MIZUSHIMA, S. and NOMURA, M. (1970): Assembly mapping of 30 ribosomal proteins of E. coli Nature, 226/5252, 1214.

NOVICK, R. P. (1967): Penicillinase plasmids of Staph. aureus. Federation Proceedings, 26/I, 29.

SIGIMOTO, N. and YOSHIOKA, H. (1970): Trends of antibiotics resistance of Staphylococci in Hokkaido district in 1968. Chemotherapy (Tokyo), 18/6, 850.

SMITH, H. W. (1967): The transmissible nature of the genetic factor in E. coli that controls haemolysin production. Journal of General Microbiology, 47/, 153.

SMITH, R. (1967): The current status of R-factors. Editorial Annals of Internal Medicine, 67/6, 1337.

UMEZAWA, H. et al. (1971): Synthesis of 3-deoxykanamycin effective against kanamycin-resistant E. coli and Ps. aeruginosa. Journal of Antibiotics ser. A, 24/4, 274.

STUDIES ON THE DRUG RESISTANCE OF STAPHYLOCOCCI AND ESCHERICHIA COLI AGAINST ANTIBIOTICS

GENERAL TENDENCY OF RESISTANT STRAINS AND MULTIPLE-DRUG RESISTANCES

H. OTAYA, S. OKAMOTO, E. INOUE*, Y. ADACHI, S. MACHIHARA
and M. YOSHIMURA

Shionogi & Co., Ltd., Doshomachi, Osaka, Japan

We have been investigating the drug resistance of clinical strains of *Staphylococcus aureus* and *Escherichia coli*, isolated in main hospitals all over Japan, annually since 1965. Our objective was to investigate the annual trends of bacterial resistance to antibiotics and sulfonamides frequently used in hospitals in Japan. In this paper, we will report firstly on the general tendency of drug-resistant strains, and secondly on the multiple-drug-resistant strains of these species of bacteria.

I. MATERIALS AND METHODS

1. Bacterial strains

Bacterial isolates and hospitals were selected by a statistical sampling method and bacterial isolates which were sampled in the central clinical laboratories or other equivalent laboratories of hospitals were examined. Isolated strains were *S. aureus* and *E. coli*.

Testing method: Isolated strains were propagated in a modified Müller-Hinton broth medium (37 °C, 18 hr). A loopful from each culture was suspended in 5 ml of saline with a 1 mm standard platinum loop. Modified Müller-Hinton's medium was mainly used except for the sulfonamide testing *E. coli* isolates where Sauton medium (modified Krüger-Thiemer) was employed. Drug-sensitivity tests were performed using the two-fold agar dilution method with the same media. One mm platinum loop. Agar streak method. (about 10^4 cells and $3 \sim 4 \times 10^6$ cells, respectively, 37 °C, 18 hr).

Standard strains for the control: S. aureus FDA 209-P and *E. coli* mutaflor were used.

2. Chemotherapeutic agents tested

S. aureus: Erythromycin (EM), penicillin-G (PC-G), streptomycin (SM), chloramphenicol (CP), tetracycline (TC), kanamycin (KM), cephalothin (CET), cephaloridine (CER), sulfamethoxazole (SIM) and aminobenzyl-penicillin (AB-PC) were used.

E. coli: CP, TC, SM, KM, CET, CER, SIM and AB-PC were used.

In addition to these drugs, we have been testing cephalexin, cephaloglycin, cephazolin, carbenicillin and some other drugs since 1970, of which the results are not shown in this paper yet.

* Present address: Gracia Hospital, Osaka, Japan

3. Period of study (June, 1965 ~ May, 1969)

Each year was divided into two parts in the annual investigation; and each annual period of investigation started in June and ended in May the following year, as stated:

1965   June, 1965 ~ May, 1966
1966   June, 1966 ~ May, 1967
1967   June, 1967 ~ May, 1968
1968   June, 1968 ~ May, 1969

II. GENERAL TENDENCY OF RESISTANT STRAINS

Fig. 1 shows the geographical distribution of our sampling hospitals. We have chosen about 300 hospitals each year. This number is equivalent to about 10% of the main hospitals in Japan. The correlation analysis of the hospital numbers, population sizes and numbers of isolated strains indicated positive correlation among these factors with the level of significance of $P = 0.01$. Thus the results of our investigation should reflect the general tendency of drug resistances of *S. aureus* and *E. coli* in main Japanese hospitals.

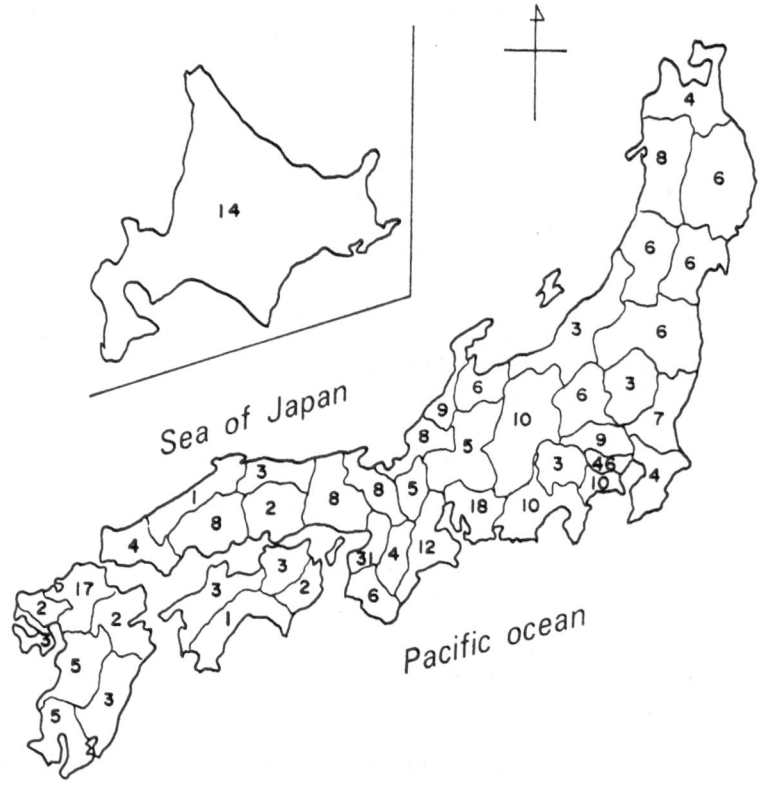

Fig. 1 Distribution map of sampling hospitals. Figures in the map show number of sampling hospitals in individual prefectures.

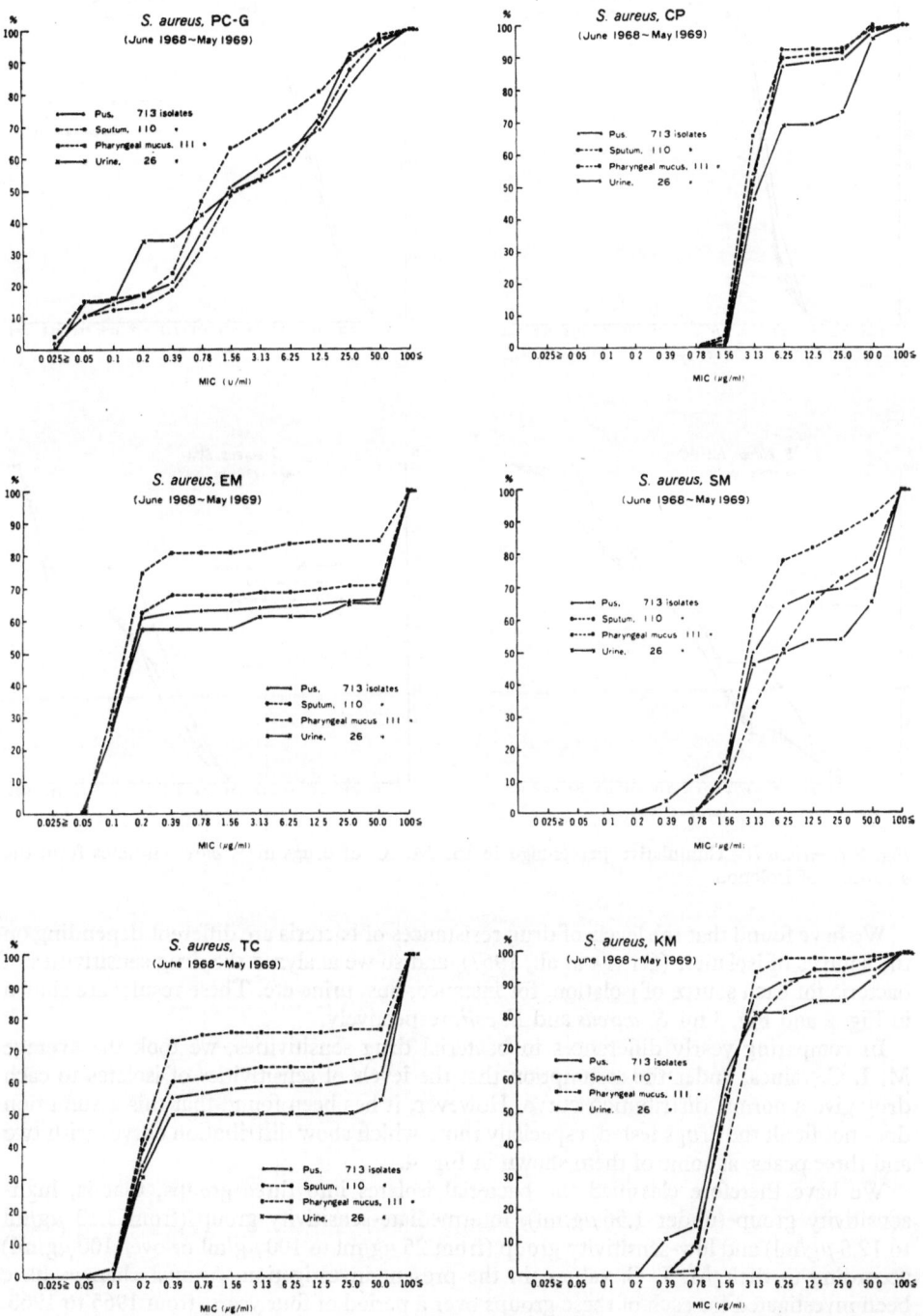

Fig. 2

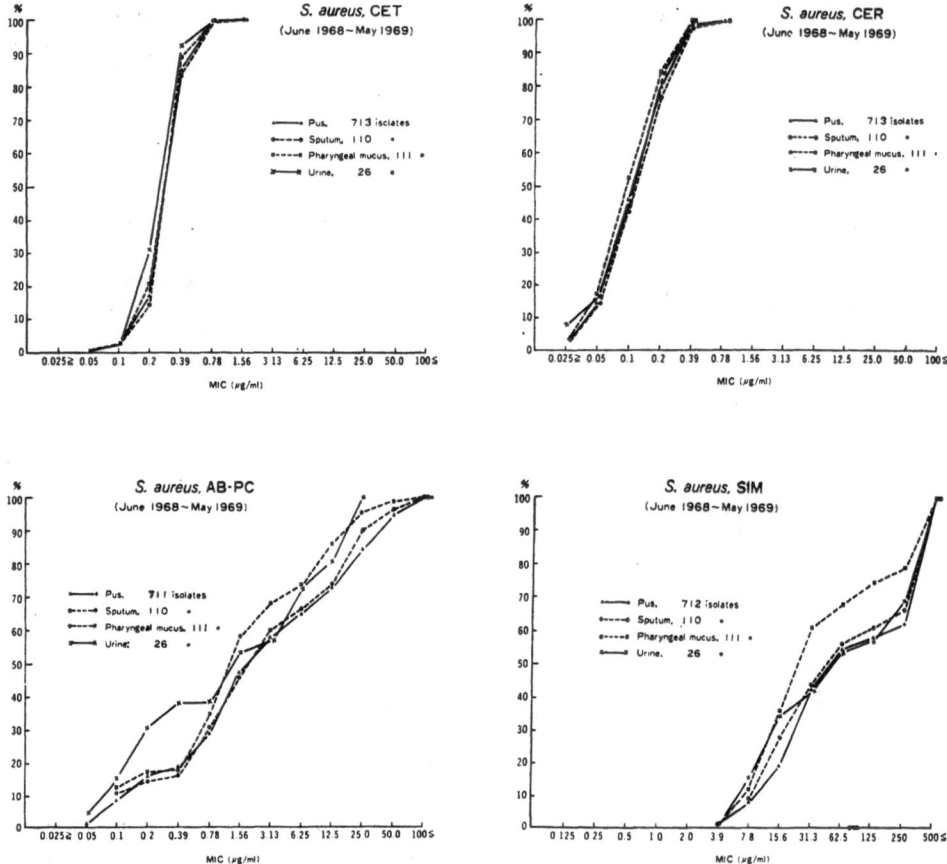

Fig. 2 (continued) Cumulative percentage in the M.I.C. of drugs in *S. aureus* isolates from the 4 sources of isolation.

We have found that the levels of drug resistances of bacteria are different depending on the sources of isolation (OTAYA at al., 1967), and so we analyzed the drug sensitivities of bacteria for each source of isolation, for instance, pus, urine etc. These results are shown in Fig. 2 and Fig. 3 for *S. aureus* and *E. coli*, respectively.

In comparing yearly differences in bacterial drug sensitivities, we took the average M. I. C. values, under the assumption that the levels of sensitivities of isolates to each drug give a normal distribution curve. However, it has been found that this assumption does not fit all the drugs tested, especially those which show distribution curves with two and three peaks, as some of them shown in Fig. 4.

We have therefore classified the bacterial isolates into three groups, that is, high-sensitivity group (under 1.56 μg/ml), intermediate-sensitivity group (from 3.13 μg/ml to 12.5 μg/ml) and low-sensitivity group (from 25 μg/ml to 100 μg/ml or over 100 μg/ml) according to their M. I. C. values, in the present investigation. Annual changes have been investigated for each of these groups over a period of four years, from 1965 to 1968.

The following changes have been found for each drug by this method. These data can be summarized as in Table 1.

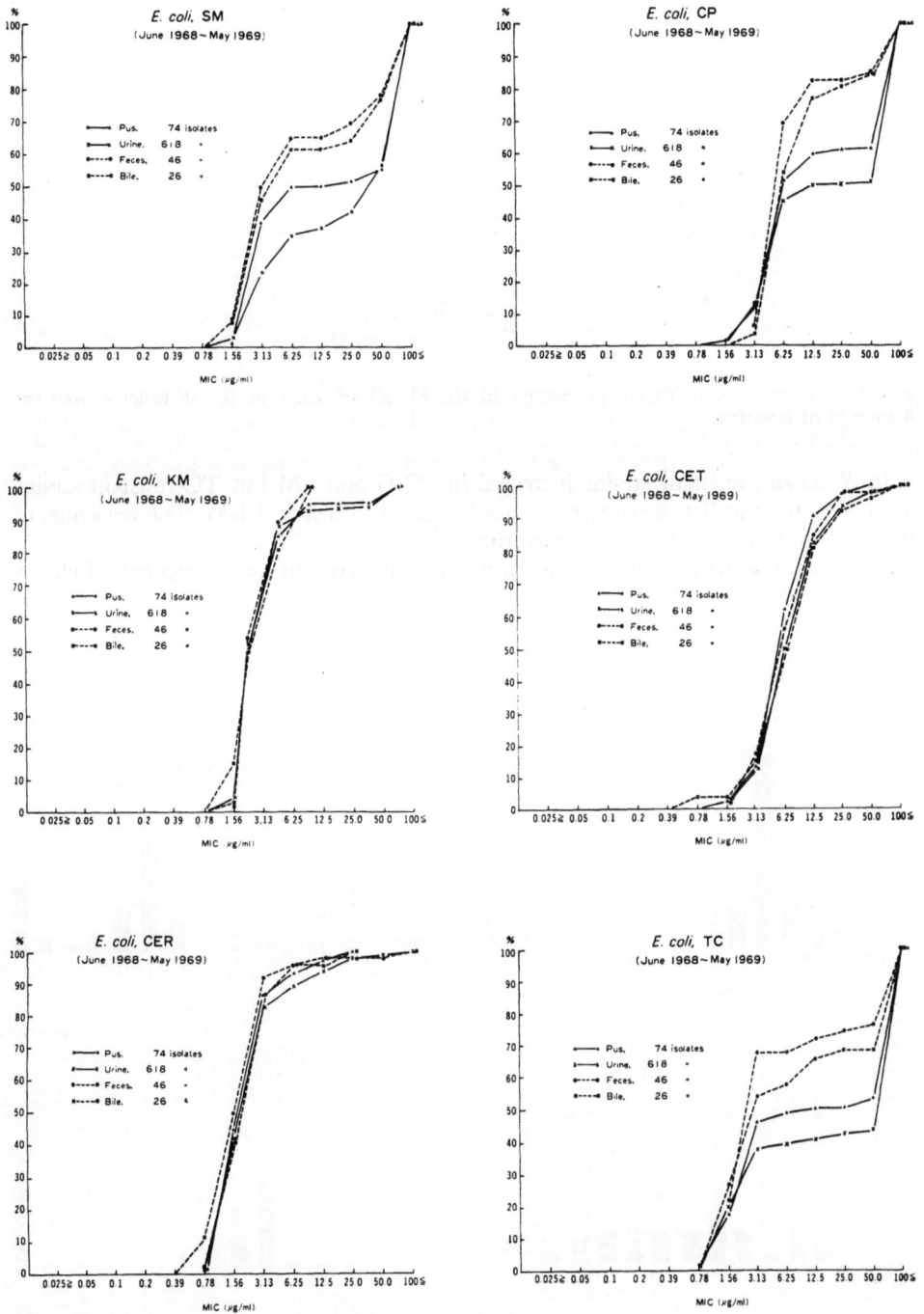

Fig. 3

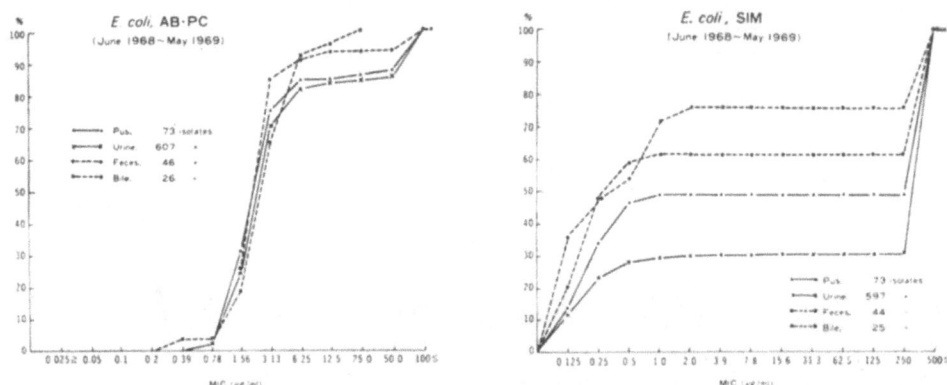

Fig. 3 (continued) Cumulative percentage in the M.I.C. of drugs in E. coli isolates from the 4 sources of isolation.

In *S. aureus,* resistant strains increased in PC-G and EM but TC-resistant strains decreased. Intermediate-sensitivity groups increased in SM and KM. The behaviors of these groups in future should be interesting.

In *E. coli,* it is remarkable that no change was observed in the frequencies of all the

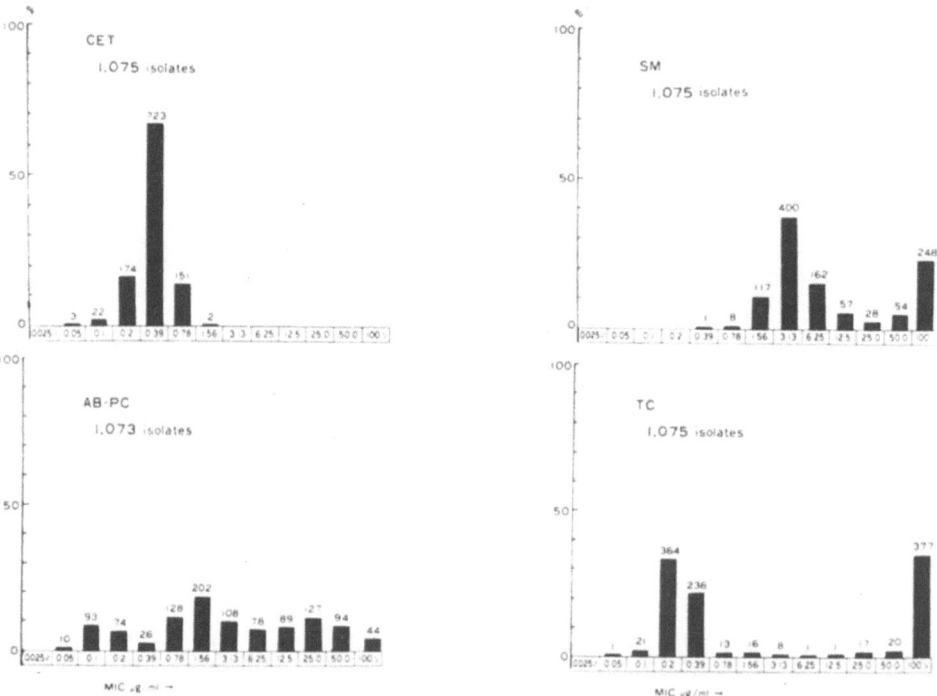

Fig. 4 Distribution of the M.I.C. of some antibiotics having 2 or 3 peaks (*S. aureus;* June 1968 to May, 1969).

three groups. Marked increase was found in the TC-high-sensitivity group in *E. coli* similarly as with *S. aureus*. It seems particularly interesting that both high-sensitivity group and low-sensitivity group increased in KM and AB-PC. Further detail of these findings has been published elsewhere (OTAYA et al., 1970).

Table 1

GENERAL TENDENCY OF THE CHANGES IN ANTIBIOTIC-SUSCEPTIBILITY OF *S. AUREUS* AND *E. COLI* (1965−1968). (OTAYA ET AL, 1970.)

	Group	PC-G	AB-PC*	SM	CP	TC	KM	EM	CET	CER**
	High-sensitivity group	↓	→	↓	↓	↑	↓	↓	→	→
S. aureus	Intermediate-sensitivity group	↓	→	↑	↑	↓	↑	↓	→	→
	Low-sensitivity group	↑	→	→	↘	↓	↑	↑	→	→
	High-sensitivity group	↑	→	↓	↑	↑			↑	↓
E. coli	Intermediate sensitivity group	↓	→	↑	↓	↓			→	↑
	Low-sensitivity group	↑	→	→	→	↑			→	↑

↑, increase; ↓, decrease; →, no change; ↘, slight decrease.
* 1967∼1968. ** 1966∼1968.

Conclusion: From the above mentioned results, we have been able to learn more accurately the general tendency and annual trends of the drug resistances of *S. aureus* and *E. coli* in the main hospitals in Japan by grouping the bacterial isolates into three, and comparing the annual change of each of these groups.

III. MULTIPLE-DRUG RESISTANCES

As mentioned before, we have found that the levels of drug resistances of bacteria are different depending on the sources of their isolation. Therefore, we have studied *S. aureus* strains isolated only from pus and *E. coli* strains isolated only from urine.

Table 2

DIFFERENTIATION BETWEEN SENSITIVE AND RESISTANT STRAINS (OTAYA ET AL, 1971)

Drug	M.I.C. (μg/ml) regarded as resistant	
	S. aureus	*E. coli*
PC-G	3.13 $\leq$ (μ/ml)	−
CP	25 $\leq$	25 $\leq$
EM	3.13 $\leq$	−
SM	25 $\leq$	25 $\leq$
TC	25 $\leq$	25 $\leq$
KM	25 $\leq$	25 $\leq$
CET	25 $\leq$	25 $\leq$
CER*	25 $\leq$	25 $\leq$
AB-PC*	3.13 $\leq$	25 $\leq$
SIM	125 $\leq$	125 $\leq$

* A description of these two (CER in *E. coli* and AB-PC in *S. aureus* and *E. coli*) is not shown in this paper because of shortness of test period.

69

Table 3

MAIN TYPES OF COMBINATIONS OF DRUG RESISTANCES AND THEIR FREQUENCIES IN *S. AUREUS* ISOLATES FROM PUS SPECIMENS   (OTAYA et al, 1971)

Type resistant to	Order	Combination	1965 No.	1965 %	1966 No.	1966 %	1967 No.	1967 %	1968 No.	1968 %	Total No. (B)	Total %	(B)/(A) %
		All	51	100	59	100	61	100	31	100	202	100	10.20
2 drugs	1	SIM, PC—G	14	27.5	35	59.3	26	42.6	11	35.5	86	42.6	4.34
	2	SIM, TC	17	33.3	10	16.9	9	14.8	4	12.9	40	19.8	2.02
	3	SM, PC—G	1	2.0	4	6.8	9	14.8	6	19.4	20	99.9	1.01
		All	90	100	59	100	79	100	57	100	285	100	14.39
3 drugs	1	SIM, TC, PC—G	39	43.3	36	61.0	38	48.1	27	47.4	140	49.1	7.07
	2	SIM, SM, PC—G	12	13.3	6	10.2	7	8.9	6	10.5	31	10.9	1.57
	3	SIM, TC, SM	19	21.1	5	8.5	3	3.8	3	5.3	30	10.5	1.52
		All	97	100	71	100	110	100	98	100	376	100	18.99
4 drugs	1	SIM, TC, SM, PC—G	65	67.0	31	43.7	39	35.5	21	21.4	156	41.5	7.88
	2	SIM, EM, TC, PC—G	13	13.4	18	25.4	44	40.0	42	42.9	117	31.1	5.91
	3	SIM, EM, SM, PC—G	1	1.0	5	7.0	7	6.4	6	6.1	19	5.1	0.96
	3	SIM, EM, TC, SM	5	5.2	2	2.8	5	4.5	7	7.1	19	5.1	0.96
		All	65	100	103	100	100	100	112	100	380	100	19.19
5 drugs	1	SIM, EM, TC, SM, PC—G	32	49.2	69	67.0	62	62.0	80	71.4	243	63.9	12.27
	2	SIM, EM, TC, CP, PC—G	12	18.5	8	7.8	16	16.0	17	15.2	53	13.9	2.68
	3	SIM, EM, TC, CP, SM	11	16.9	9	8.7	2	2.0	5	4.5	27	7.1	1.36
		All	26	100	42	100	43	100	34	100	145	100	7.32
6 drugs	1	SIM, EM, TC, CP, SM, PC—G	21	80.8	21	50.0	23	53.5	12	35.3	77	53.1	3.89
	2	SIM, KM, EM, TC, SM, PC—G	0	0	16	38.1	13	30.2	19	55.9	48	33.1	2.42
	3	SIM, KM, EM, TC, CP, SM	5	19.2	4	9.5	2	4.7	0	0	11	7.6	0.56
7 drugs		SIM, EM, TC, CP, SM, KM, PC—G	4		15		21		13		53		2.68
Total strains resistant to from 1 to 7 drugs											1980	(A)	100

None of the strains was resistant to CET or CER.

Table 4

MAIN TYPES OF COMBINATIONS OF DRUG RESISTANCES AND THEIR FREQUENCIES IN *E. COLI* ISOLATES FROM URINE SPECIMENS (OTAYA et al., 1971)

Type resistant to	Order	Combination	1966 No.	1966 %	1967 No.	1967 %	1968 No.	1968 %	Total No.(B)	Total %	(B)/(A) %
2 drugs		All	32	100	57	100	65	100	154	100	13.02
	1	SM, SIM	15	46.9	26	45.6	35	53.8	76	49.4	6.42
	2	TC, SIM	9	28.1	17	29.8	14	21.5	40	26.0	3.38
	3	TC, SM	4	12.5	6	10.5	7	10.8	17	11.0	1.44
3 drugs		All	26	100	55	100	70	100	151	100	12.76
	1	TC, SM, SIM	17	65.4	35	63.6	36	51.4	88	58.3	7.44
	2	SM, CP, SIM	4	15.4	12	21.8	17	24.3	33	21.9	2.79
	3	SM, CET, SIM	4	15.4	2	3.6	2	2.9	8	5.3	0.68
	3	TC, CP, SIM	0	0	3	5.5	5	7.1	8	5.3	0.68
4 drugs		All	129	100	185	100	187	100	501	100	42.35
	1	TC, SM, CP, SIM	121	93.8	165	89.2	170	90.9	456	91.0	38.55
	2	TC, SM, CET, SIM	4	3.1	11	5.9	5	2.7	20	4.0	1.69
	3	SM, CET, CP, SIM	3	2.3	5	2.7	8	4.3	16	3.2	1.35
5 drugs		All	33	100	67	100	69	100	169	100	14.29
	1	TC, SM, CET, CP, SIM	26	78.8	53	79.1	51	73.9	130	76.9	10.99
	2	TC, SM, KM, CP, SIM	7	21.2	13	19.4	17	24.6	37	21.9	3.13
	3	TC, SM, KM, CET, SIM	0	0	1	1.5	0	0	1	0.6	0.08
6 drugs		TC, SM, CET, CP, KM, SIM	5		9		14		28		2.37
Total strains resistant to from 1 to 6 drugs									1183	(A)	100

71

In classifying sensitivity and resistance, we have followed the criteria of M. I. C. shown in Table 2. These criteria are generally used in diagnostic laboratories in Japan.

Table 3 shows the data of *S. aureus*. The most frequent three combinations of drug resistances are shown for each type. Annual changes are not marked, but it draws our attention that four-drug-resistant and five-drug-resistant strains are most frequent. The data for each single drug are shown in our papers (OTAYA et al., 1971)

Table 4 shows the data of *E. coli*. Some special types of multiple-drug-resistant strains are particularly frequent as compared with *S. aureus*. This finding may suggest that these frequent types are due to R factors.

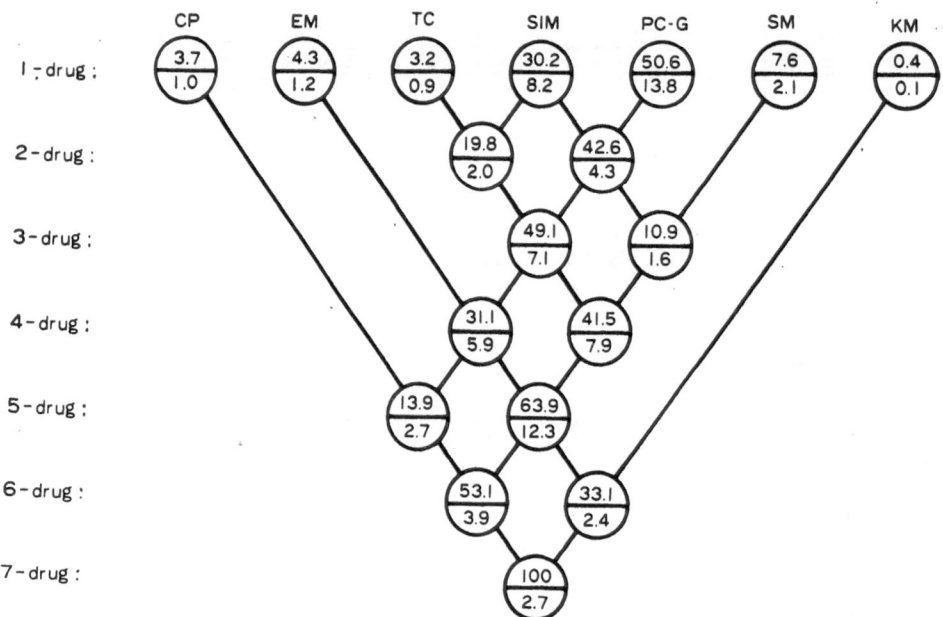

Fig. 5 A model of the main processes for development of multiple-drugresistant strains of *S. aureus* (1980 resistant strains). (Otaya et al., 1971.)
The figures over the line in the circles represent the frequencies (in %) among the strains resistant to each corresponding number of drugs, and the figures under the line are the frequencies (in %) among the total resistant strains.

Fig. 5 shows a model of the main process for the development of multiple-drug-resistant strains of *S. aureus* based on the relative frequency.

The model indicates that the basic markers of the multiple-drug-resistant strains of *S. aureus* are sulfonamide, PC-G and TC, and that three-drug-resistant, four-drug-resistant strains and so on, develop by the addition of other-drug-resistance markers. It is interesting that four-drug-resistant and five-drug-resistant strains are most frequent, and that six-drug-resistant and seven-drug-resistant strains are less frequent.

A similar model for *E. coli* is shown in Fig. 6 on a similar basis. Sulfonamide, SM and TC are basic markers and multiple-drug-resistant strains are assumed to develop as a result of addition of other drug-resistance markers. These might be in the forms of R factors. Otherwise this finding might indicate that four-drug-resistance R factors are predominant, in view of the fact that four-drug-resistant strains are most frequent.

The presence of R factors with all the drug-resistance markers except CET and CER is

72

already known. We assumed that CET resistance of our strains may be also related to R factors and in fact Watanabe (personal communication) has recently shown that the resistance to CET as well as to AB-PC is controlled by R factors employing some of our multiple-drug-resistant strains reported in the present paper.

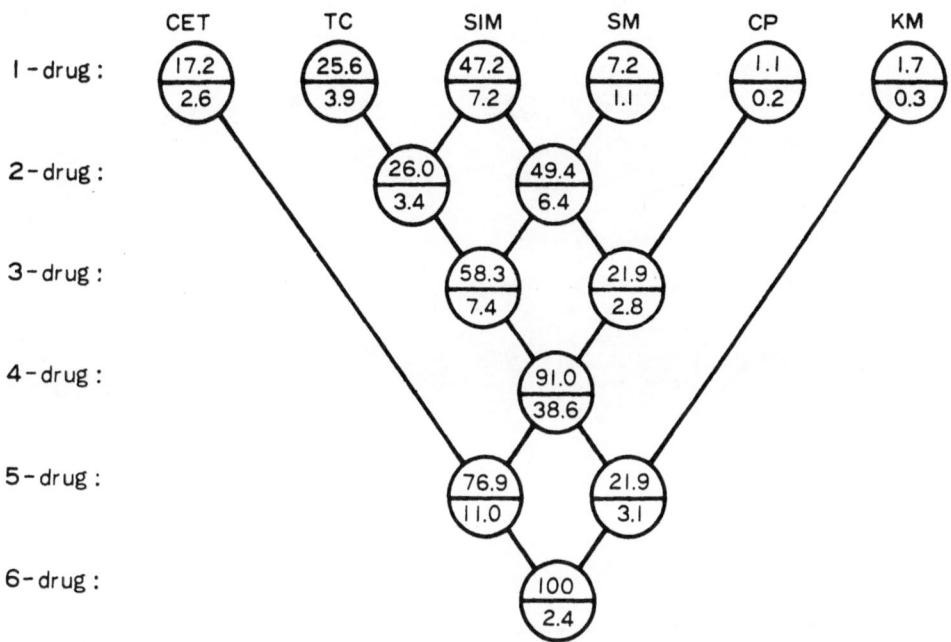

Fig. 6 A model of the main processes for development of multipledrugresistant strains of *E coli*. (1183 resistant strains). (Otaya et al., 1971.) As in Fig. 5.

Conclusion: We have reported on the frequencies of representative types of multiple-drug-resistant strains of *S. aureus* and *E. coli* and have presented a hypothesis of the process for their development on the basis of relative frequency.

REFERENCES

OTAYA, H and INOUE, E. (1967): Report on the drug resistance of *Staphylococci* and *Escherichia coli* against antibiotics and sulphonamide I. (in Japanese). Modern Medicine, **22/11,** 2544.

OTAYA, H., OKAMOTO, S., INOUE, E., ADACHI, Y., MACHIHARA, S. and YOSHIMURA, M. (1970): Studies on the drug resistance of *Staphylococci* and *Escherichia coli* against antibiotics. II. General tendency of resistant strains. The Journal of Antibiotics, **23/7,** 324.

OTAYA, H., OKAMOTO S., INOUE, E., ADACHI, Y., MACHIHARA, S. and YOSHIMURA, M. (1971): Studies on the drug resistance of *Staphylococci* and *Escherichia coli* against antibiotics. III. Multiple-drug resistances. The Journal of Antibiotics, **24/3,** 155.

RESISTANCE TRANSFER IN VIVO AND ITS INHIBITION

B. WIEDEMANN

Institute of Hygiene, University of Frankfurt, G. F. R.

The *Enterobacteriaceae*, which are able to cause various infections in men and animals are able to resist the chemotherapeutic procedures when carrying R-factors. As we cannot assume that the antibiotic-resistance occurs in the time of therapy at the area of infection, we can rather refer to the diseases of the draining urinary passage, so that an increase of resistance is very often a fresh infection (LINCOLN et al. 1971). These resistant strains of enterobacteriaceae in general have their origin in the intestinal-flora of men or animals, which here occurs by continual selection in the time of therapy and prophylaxis, so a special attention has to be paid to the arising of resistant microorganisms in this field. After we had realized this, it was possible to consider the distribution of pathogenic enterobacteriaceae having resistance properties. In addition to the selection, which was done by therapy, the transmission of R-factors in the intestinal-flora is of essential importance, as both mechanisms, acting together, lead to an increase of spreading.

For a long time the results of the selection are known by experiments, which were already done before the R-factors occured (SCHRÖTER et al. 1970). In addition to this, some other points of view have to be considered. Therefore the transmission of resistance-features in vivo has to be eludicated clearly.

The results which we know up till now indicate, that it is more difficult to demonstrate the resistance-transmission in vivo than in vitro (WATANABE 1963). Apart from the selective application, this transmission was obtained in vivo by an alteration of the normal flora in the intestine. KASUYA (1964) and GUINEE (1965), for instance, obtained a good R-factor transmission in mice, which had been fed with antibiotics before in order to reduce their intestinal-flora. Also positive results were found in sterile mice (KASUYA 1964; SALZMANN a. KLEMM 1968). WALTON (1966), obtained the same results by feeding chicken with R-factor-bearing strains of *E. coli*, directly after they were born and their intestinal tract was sterile. The recipient strains had been administered 6 hours later, before giving them food and water. With this technique R-factors of E. coli to E. coli and of E. coli to Salmonella in vivo could be transferred. A much more complicated way chose SMITH (1969), who settled the intestine of voluntary test persons with nalidixic-acid-resistant *E. coli*, and after this they had to take a donor-strain in high concentration orally. By this method he also could identify transmission in vivo.

In our own experiments it was important to imitate the normal conditions. At first we examined a natural contamination with R-factor-bearing strains. (Tab. 1) and stated, that a serological not typable *E. coli*-strain with a transmissionable multiple-resistance in a concentration of 10 000/g appeared, and after 10 days it was not demonstrable any more. A second contamination with a low bacterial count was not demonstrable already after

Table 1

NATURAL CONTAMINATION OF THE INTESTINAL FLORA WITH R-FACTOR
BEARING ENTEROBACTERIACEAE

Bacteria	Days	1	10	13	15
E. coli O 1		7.3	—	—	—
E. coli O 55		—	6.7	—	—
E. coli O 76		—	6.2	—	—
E. coli u ACKST	R+	4.0	—	—	—
E. coli u AST	R+	—	—	3.0	—
E. coli u AST	R−	—	—	3.0	3.0
E. coli u AKS	R−	—	—	3.0	—
E. coli u K	R−	—	6.2	—	—
E. coli u		7.0	7.1	7.2	6.8
Enterobacter S	R−	—	—	—	4.0

two days. This indicates that firstly no transmission to the permanent flora takes place, and secondly the R-factor-bearing strain is eliminated relatively fast. To prove this, we contaminated three test persons with a R-factor-bearing wild-type of *E. coli* 0 87, which carried a R-factor with a fivefold-resistance. We obtained following results (Fig. 1).

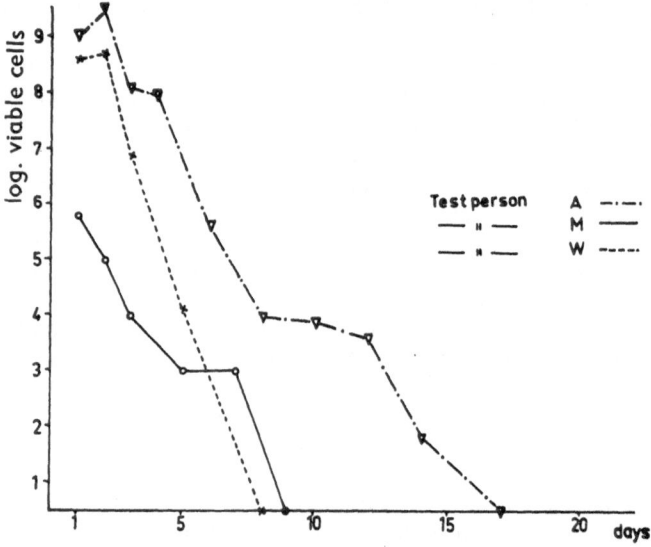

Fig. 1 Elimination of E. Coli 0 87 R+ after Oral Contamination

After a sharp initial increase and the herewith related growth and settlement of the contaminating bacteria the viable cell count in the stool rapidly decreased. After 8 to 19 days finally the infection was over. The bacteria together with the R-factor were eliminated from the intestinal-flora.

The transmission of the R-factor to the resident flora is shown in Tab. 2, 3 and 4.

In all three test-persons, reported here, no transmission has been stated, only in the test-person "W" occurs the same R-factor of *E. coli* 0 89 for one day. The conditions are seen much clearer in their graphical description (Fig. 2).

Table 2

ENTEROBACTERIAL FLORA OF TESTPERSON A. ORAL CONTAMINATION WITH E. COLI O 87 R (ACKST) ON 52nd DAY

Bacteria	time (days)			1	3	21	49	50	53	54	55	56	58	60	62	64	66	69	73	77
E. coli	13	CST	R−														3,8			
E. coli	18					5,1														
E. coli	19a				6,7															
E. coli	21	C	R−	5,0																
E. coli	25			6,2	7,5	5,7										5,4				
E. coli	30			5,9		5,5											6,9			
E. coli	40						7,5							6,3						
E. coli	44	T	R−					6,3							5,7			5,5		
E. coli	57						3,3													
E. coli	73				6,7															
E. coli	86					5,9														
E. coli	87	ACKST	R−						8,7	9,5	7,4	7,1	5,3	3,8						
E. coli	87	CKST	R+							7,4	7,4	7,6	5,3							
E. coli	87	CKS	R+						9,0	9,4	8,1	8,0	5,6	4,0	4,9	3,6	1,8	2,8		
E. coli	92	CKST	R−										5,3		5,8					
E. coli	92	CST	R+																	
E. coli	92	CST	R−											5,5	5,5	3,4	4,7			
E. coli	92	CS	R−												5,2			3,1	5,0	
E. coli	92	CT	R−															2,8	4,6	
E. coli	102			5,5	5,3	4,8	3,0	3,0												
E. coli	106			6,2	7,0			6,7												
E. coli	116	T	R−	4,6	7,0															4,7
E. coli	125ac			5,5	7,0															
E. coli	129			6,2	7,6	5,9	8,4	6,9												
E. coli	u	ACKS	R+									7,4	6,5	6,1	6,9	6,4	7,9	6,8	7,4	5,2
E. coli	u	CKS	R+														3,0			
E. coli	u	CST	R+														3,3			
E. coli	u	CST	R−											5,4	4,3	5,3	3,8	2,8		
E. coli	u	KT	R−		4,4															
E. coli	u	S	R−	3,8																
E. coli	u	T	R+		5,2															
E. coli	u	T	R−		5,0	4,5		5,0												
Enterobacter		CT	R+														3,8		4,8	
Enterobacter		T	R+														4,4			
Enterobacter		SC	R−	3,9													4,7			
Klebsiella		S	R−		3,0															

u = untypable. The figures indicate the log of viable cells.

77

Table 3

ENTEROBACTERIAL FLORA OF TESTPERSON M. ORAL CONTAMINATION WITH E. COLI 0 87 R (ACKST) on 32nd DAY

Bacteria	time (days)			1	19	27	33	34	35m	35a	37	39	41	44
E. coli	O 1	AT	R+			6,3					6,4			
E. coli	O 12	CKS	R+									5,3		
E. coli	O 25	T	R-		7,2		6,4							
E. coli	O 25	CT	R-									<3,0	<3,0	
E. coli	O 40	AST	R+									3,8	3,6	
E. coli	O 40	AST	R-											3,3
E. coli	O 40													
E. coli	O 57	AKS	R-			6,4				6,0	<3,0			
E. coli	O 57													
E. coli	O 73	AKS	R-				7,6	6,1	3,5		5,7	6,4	7,2	7,4
E. coli	O 81							5,4						
E. coli	O 87	ACKST	R+				4,4	3,3	5,0					
E. coli	O 87	ACKS	R+				5,8	5,0	<3,0					
E. coli	O 87	CKS	R+						4,0					
E. coli	O 87	AST	R+							<3,0				
E. coli	O 104	AST	R+							3,3				
E. coli	u	AST	R+	6,6		6,5	7,0	5,6	6,7	6,1	6,8	6,3	6,9	6,8
E. coli	u	AK	R-					5,1	3,3					
E. coli	u	AKS	R-						3,8	5,4				
E. coli	u	ST	R-						3,6		<3,0			
Enterobacter		S	R-	3,3							3,9			
Enterobacter						3,3								
Citrobacter		ST	R-						7,1	4,3				<3,0
Citrobacter		KST	R+							3,3				<3,0

u = untypable. The figures indicate the log of viable cells.

Table 4

ENTEROBACTERIAL FLORA OF TESTPERSON W. ORAL CONTAMINATION WITH E. COLI O 87 R(ACKST) ON 63rd DAY

Bacteria / time (days)	1	20	61	62	63	64	65m	65a	66	68	71	75	85	96	118
E. coli O 2	—	—	5,5	—	—	—	—	—	—	—	—	—	—	—	—
E. coli O 4	—	—	5,5	4,7	—	—	—	—	—	—	—	—	—	—	—
E. coli O 6	—	—	—	—	—	—	—	—	—	—	—	—	—	—	4,5
E. coli O 8	6,7	—	5,5	—	—	—	—	—	—	—	—	—	—	—	—
E. coli O 8 T R+	6,0	—	—	—	—	—	—	—	—	—	—	—	—	—	—
E. coli O 39	—	—	—	—	—	—	—	—	—	—	—	—	6,8	5,2	—
E. coli O 41	5,9	—	—	—	—	—	—	—	—	—	—	—	—	—	—
E. coli O 57	—	—	6,0	—	—	—	—	—	7,0	—	5,8	—	—	6,5	—
E. coli O 57 ST R+	—	—	6,5	—	—	—	—	—	—	—	—	—	—	—	5,5
E. coli O 73	—	—	—	—	—	—	—	—	—	4,3	—	—	—	—	—
E. coli O 73 AT R+	—	—	—	—	—	—	—	—	—	—	—	—	3,9	—	5,4
E. coli O 75	—	—	—	—	—	—	—	—	—	—	—	—	—	—	4,5
E. coli O 82	—	—	—	—	4,8	—	—	—	—	—	—	—	—	—	—
E. coli O 87 S R-	—	—	—	—	—	—	—	5,4	—	—	—	—	—	—	—
E. coli O 87 ACKST R+	—	—	—	—	—	8,6	8,7	6,6	6,8	4,1	—	—	—	—	—
E. coli O 87 ACKS R+	—	—	—	—	—	7,8	8,3	6,3	6,2	1,4	—	—	—	—	—
E. coli O 87 CKS R+	—	—	—	—	—	8,1	8,4	6,7	6,9	3,4	—	—	—	—	—
E. coli O 89 ACKST R+	—	—	5,8	5,4	—	—	—	6,1	—	—	—	—	—	—	—
E. coli O 89 KST R+	—	—	—	4,8	5,3	—	—	—	—	3,8	—	—	—	—	—
E. coli O 89 ST R+	—	—	6,6	5,1	5,1	—	—	—	—	<3,0	—	4,3	—	4,1	—
E. coli O 141	7,0	8,0	6,5	5,2	6,0	—	7,9	5,7	7,3	5,9	5,3	6,2	6,0	5,5	—
E. coli u AST R+	—	—	—	—	—	—	—	—	—	—	—	—	4,2	—	—
E. coli u AT R+	—	—	—	—	—	—	—	—	—	—	—	—	3,7	—	—
Enterobacter	4,1	—	—	—	4,4	—	—	—	—	—	—	—	—	—	—

u = untypable. The figures indicate the log of viable cells.

79

If we compare the results with the transmission in vitro, in which already after one hour much higher transmission was achieved, with such a high bacterial count at the same R-factor (Fig. 3), we have to suppose a strong inhibition in vivo.

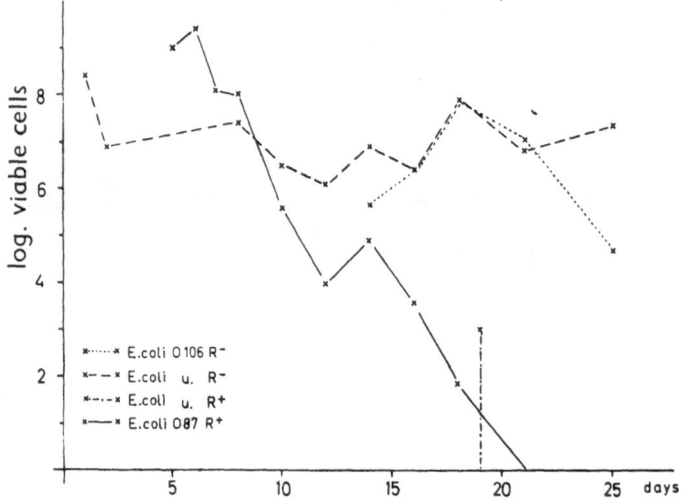

Fig. 2 R-Factor Transmission in Vivo (Human Being)

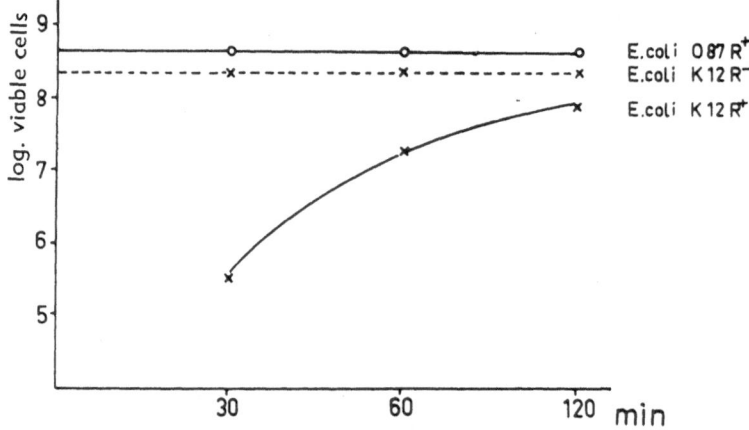

Fig. 3. R-Factor Transmission in Vitro: Cross: E. Coli 087 (ACKST) $R^+ \times$ K 12 R^-

As the in vivo-transmission in sterile raised mice was known, we tried the same transmission in sterile piglets (Fig. 4).

Here it is obvious that the transfer in vivo is only little inhibited under these conditions.

Relating to these experiments and the basic data of literature we realize, that the inhibition-mechanism of the low transmission is as following:

1. The anaerobic conditions in the intestinal tract.
2. The influence of the bile salts.
3. The effect of the metabolic products of accompanying bacteria.

4. Growth-period of the donor and recipient strains.
5. The cell-wall characteristics of the acceptor bacteria.

The promoting influence of oxygen on the transmission of a resistance plasmid is well known (LEBEK, 1969, MITSUHASHI 1971). The results in sterile animals show that

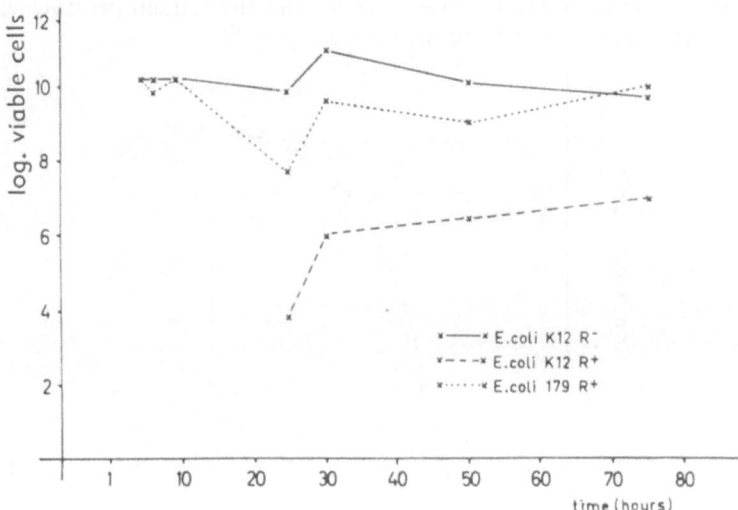

Fig. 4   R-Factor Transmission in Vivo (Gnotobiotic Pig)

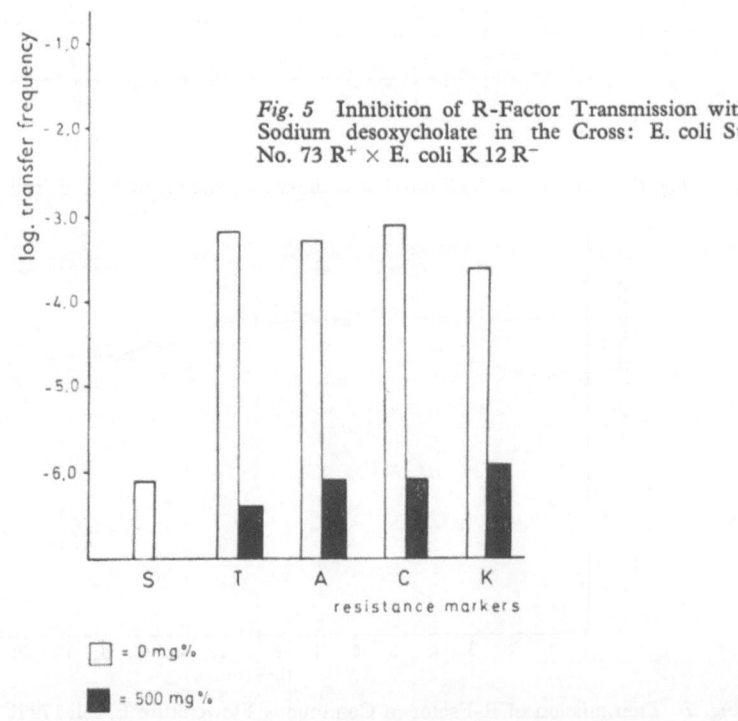

Fig. 5   Inhibition of R-Factor Transmission with Sodium desoxycholate in the Cross: E. coli St. No. 73 R⁺ × E. coli K 12 R⁻

these conditions do not inhibit the transmission in vivo at all. Quite similarly, a low influence is known of the bile salts. Here also several studies have been done recently. However it is impossible to come to a final conclusion. Therefore, we examined cholic acid, desoxy-cholic acid, sodium cholate, sodium-desoxycholate, sodium-taurocholate and sodium-glycocholate. In every case the minimum and maximum concentration was applied, refering to its true physiological extent. Here only the sodium desoxycholate showed an intense decrease of the resistance transmission (Fig. 5).

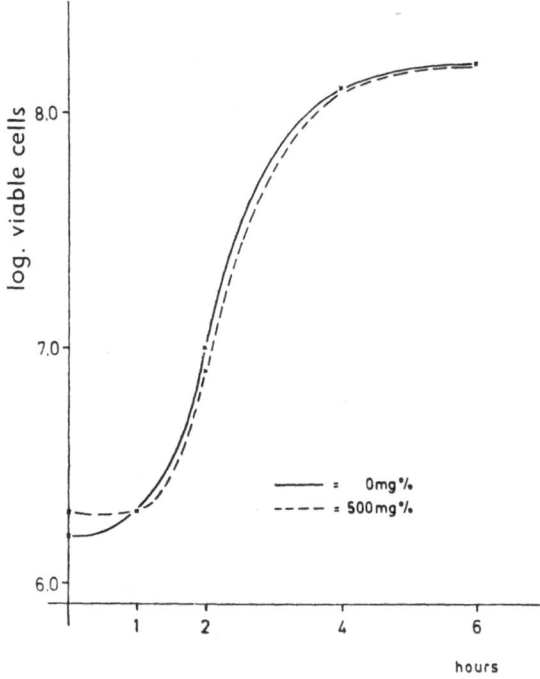

Fig. 6 Influence of Sodium-Desoxycholate on the Growth of E. coli St. No. 73 R⁺

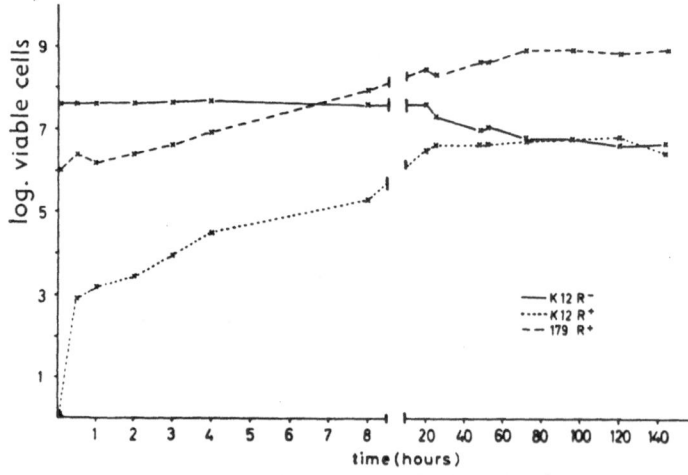

Fig. 7 Transmission of R-Factor in Continuous Flowculture E. coli 179 R⁺ × E. coli K 12 R⁻

The following growth-curve (Fig. 6) shows that an influence on the growth is not responsible for the inhibition.

All other bile salts, which were examined, did not show any essential influence even in a concentration of 500 mg %. Mostly the decrease was in the extent of 10 per cent.

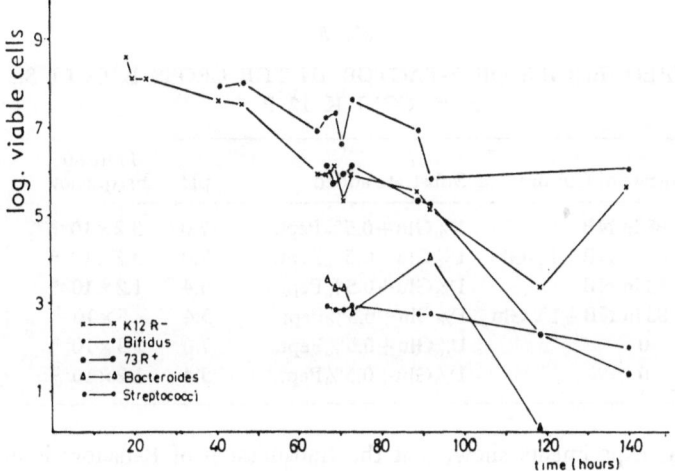

Fig. 8   Transmission of R-Factor in Continuous Flowculture in Contact with other Intestinal Bacteria E. coli 179 R+ × E. coli K 12 R−

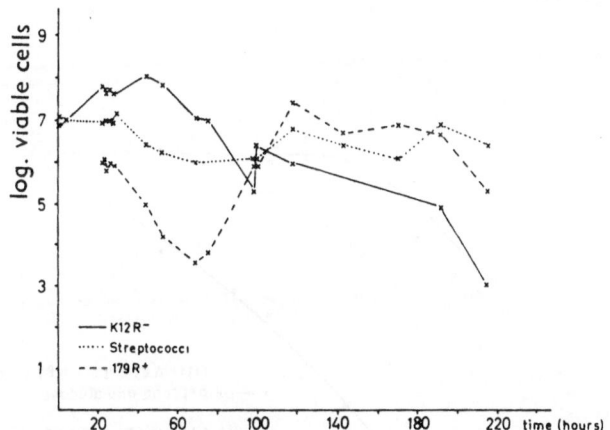

Fig. 9   Transmission of R-Factor in Continuous Flowculture in Contact with Streptococci E. coli St. No. 179 R+ × E. coli K 12 R−

When we carried out our in vitro-studies, not in the applied batch-culture, but in the continuous flowculture, we received an experimental model, which was proportionally well related to natural conditions. We used this model for proving the influence of foreign bacteria in the transmission of R-factors. By inoculation of the chemostat with donor- and recepient-bacteria at a flow-rate of 0,075 per hour, we got the following: (Fig. 7).

Already after one hour of common growth, 1000 R+ recipient bacteria occured, after 8 additional hours about 10⁵. By addition of 2 ml stool suspension in the dilution of

1 : 100, before inoculation with the donor-strain, we received no transmission to the acceptor-strain *E. coli* K 12 (Fig. 8).

Better reproducible conditions will be obtained in the chemostate, if defined individual cultures have been used for inoculation. In Fig. 9 the inhibition of the R-factor transmission by streptococcus faecalis is shown.

Table 5

TRANSFER FREQUENCIES OF R-FACTOR IN THE CROSS E. COLI St. No. 179 R+
X E. COLI K 12 R-

Filtrate of Culture	Substrate added	pH	Transfer Frequency
K 88 in NB	1% Glu+0.5% Pept.	7.0	3.2×10^{-3}
K 88 in NB+1% Glu	1% Glu+0.5% Pept.	7.0	3.2×10^{-3}
K 88 in NB	1% Glu+0.5% Pept.	5.4	1.2×10^{-3}
K 88 in NB+1% Glu	1% Glu+0.5% Pept.	5.4	5×10^{-8}
0	1% Glu+0.5% Pept.	7.0	2.5×10^{-3}
0	1% Glu+0.5% Pept.	5.4	1.2×10^{-3}

The previous experiments show, that the transmission of R-factors is inhibited by simultaneous growth of other enterobacteria. This inhibition may be the result of the formation of certain metabolic products. Therefore it must be possible to obtain the same inhibition in culture-filtrate.

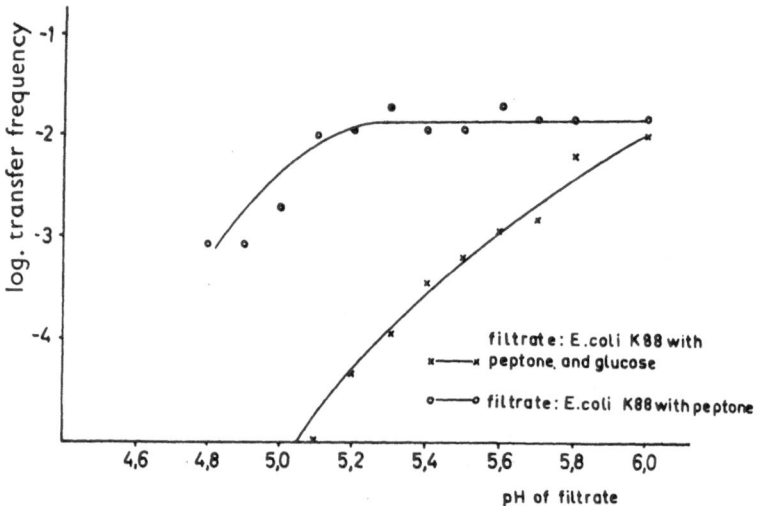

Fig. 10   Influence of pH on R-Factor Transmission

Tab. 5 shows clearly, that the transmission of the R-factor R(ACKST) from *E. coli* St. No. 179 to E. coli K 12 at a pH of 5,4 is inhibited by the culture filtrate of E. coli 0 141:K 85B, 88L: H 4.

The mentioned filtrates are each enriched with glucose and peptone.

Two reproducible results are seen here:

1. The inhibition only occurs in a pH within the acid level

2. If E. coli 0 141: K 85B, 88L: H 4 grows without glucose, no inhibition will occur.

In Fig. 10 the interdependence of the transmission-frequency from the pH-value is shown, in Fig. 11 the interdependence of the concentration of the filtrates.

The previous studies in the chemostate are all carried out in the same speed of multiplication, which is controled by the flow-rate.

The mean generation-time is here about 7 hours. Even this size may have an influence on the transmission-frequency. Therefore we studied together with BERGMANN the

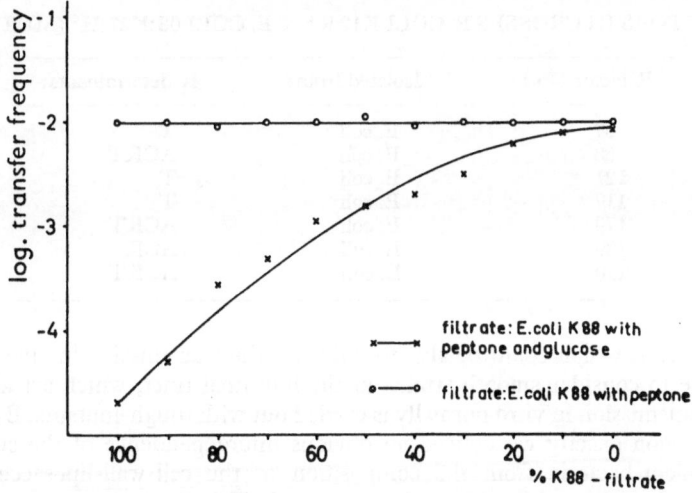

Fig. 11 Influence of Filtrate Concentration on R-Factor Transmission

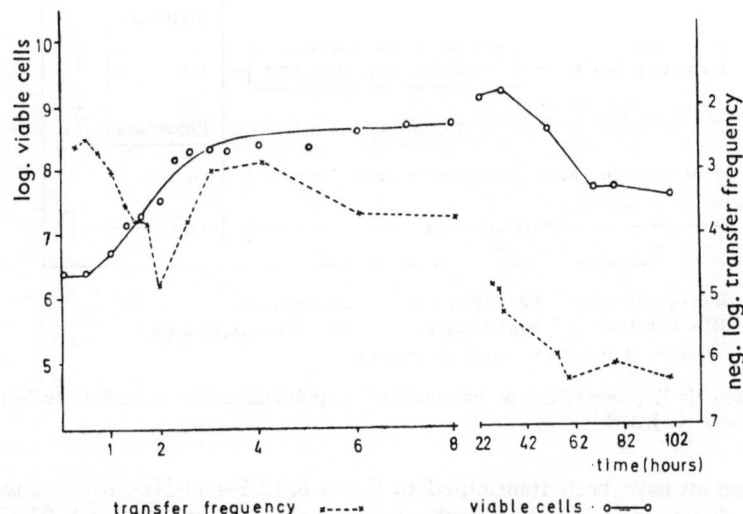

Fig. 12 Transfer Frequency: E. coli St. No. 179 R⁺ × E. coli K 12 R⁻

       Growth Phase: E. coli St. No. 179 R⁺

interdependence of the transmission frequency from the growth period of the donor-cultures (Fig. 12).

The curve shows exactly the alteration of the transmission frequency, in the different growth-periods, whereby an obvious decrease in the transmission ability is proved as well in the lag-phase as in a great part in the logarithmic growth period; while at the end of the logarithmic phase, as well as at the beginning of the stationary, a maximum was obtained. After waiting a while, the value of the batch-culture decreased within 6 to 100 hours, just to the value below the limit of identification.

Table 6

R-FACTORS IN CROSSES E. COLI K12 R+ × E. COLI 08:K27:H⁻ (MUTANTS)

R-factor No.:	Isolated from:	R-determinants:
67	E. coli	T
68	E. coli	ACKT
121	E. coli	T
117	E. coli	T
179	E. coli	ACKT
189	E. coli	ACK
190	E. coli	ACKT

Another factor, which could be able to influence the transmission in vivo, is the fact, that we have to consider smooth strains in the intestinal tract, which act as acceptors, whereas a transmission in vitro normally is carried out with rough-mutants. By examining this phenomenon exactly we noticed an obvious interdependence of the susceptibility of the recipient-bacteria from the composition of the cell-wall-liposaccharide. The R-factors which were used for this study are set up in Tab. 6.

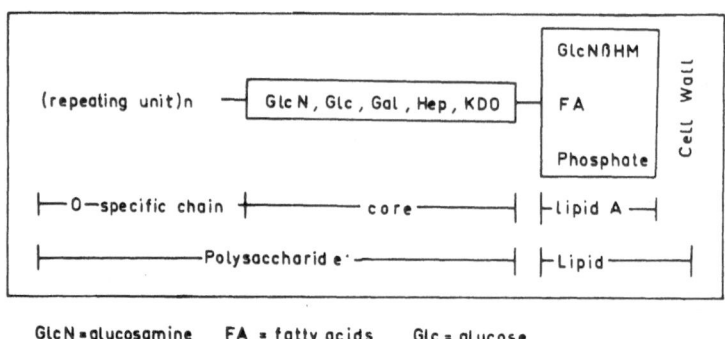

GlcN = glucosamine   FA = fatty acids   Glc = glucose
Gal = galactose   Hep = heptose   KDO = ketodeoxyoctonate
GlcNßHM = N-ß-hydroxymyristyglucosamine

Fig. 13 Schematic Representation of Salmonella-Lipopolysaccharides according to SCHMIDT, G., B. JANN and K. JANN

These plasmids have been transmitted to *E. coli* K 12 F-met-Nx-, which afterwards was used as donor strain. As the acceptor we used the mutants of E. coli 08:K27:H⁻ (provided by SCHMIDT), which had streptomycin resistance selective-marker. The diagram of the cell wall polysaccharide composition is shown in Fig. 13.

Some of the mutants are defect, which were found in the 0-specific part, as well as in the core-polysaccharide. Their characteristics are shown in Fig. 14.

The results of these transmission-experiments are nearly identical (Fig. 15).

If the capsule is missing (F 294) no remarkable alteration will arise. A high increase of the transmission-frequency, however, will be found, if the 0-specific part (F 464) is

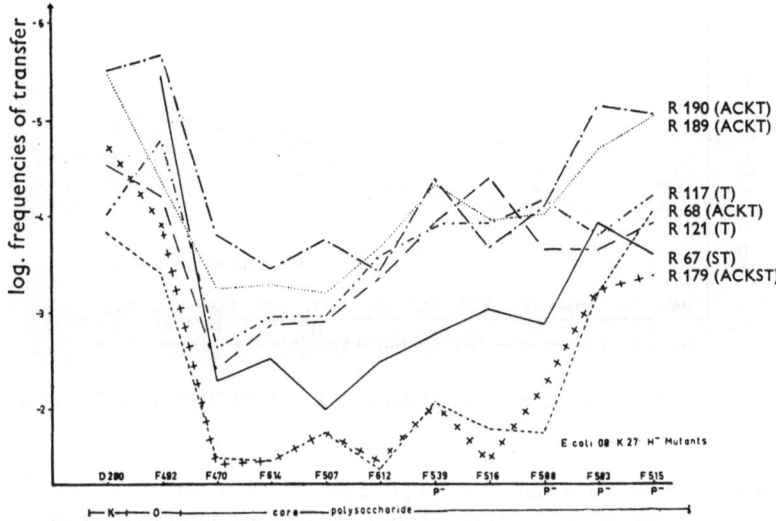

Fig. 14 Transfer of R-Factors to Mutants of E. Coli

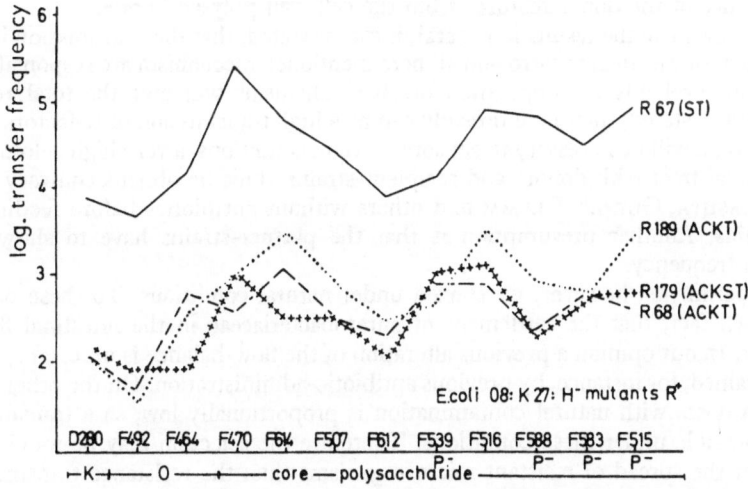

Fig. 15 Transfer of R-Factors from Mutants of E. coli 08:K 27:H⁻ to E. coli K 12

missing. For example the transmission frequency of R-68 shows an increase from —log 5,5 to —log 1,3. In the following decomposition of the core polysaccharide, a decrease in the recipient characteristics occurs, here it is obvious, that the mutants, in which the phosphate in the polysaccharide-part is missing, are especially bad recipients for the R-factors. The figures of the individual R-factors may well be different, but on principle all of them show the same tendency. In order to study the influence of the cell wall polysaccharide upon the donor-quality, we applied the R-factor bearing strains of *E. coli* 08:K27:H⁻ and their mutants as donor, which we received from the above mentioned experiments. The recipient was here *E. coli* K 12 (W 1876), which is

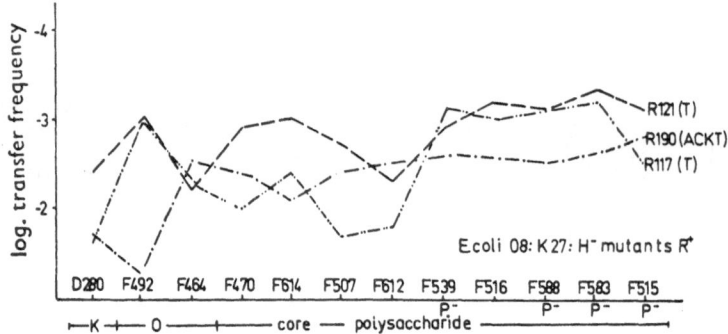

Fig. 16 Transfer of R-Factors from Mutants of E. coli 08:K 27:H⁻ to E. coli K 12

nalidixic-acid resistant. This marker we applied for selection out of the mixed culture. In Fig. 16 the donor features (F 492, F 612, F 588) are improved homogeneously, whereas some other strains give homogeneously bad transmission.

If we consider the results, represented in Fig. 16, we cannot conclude a homogeneous interdependence of the donor features from the cell wall polysaccharide.

If we try to evaluate the results in general, it can be stated, that the transmission in vivo proceeds much slower than in vitro and all here mentioned mechanism are responsible for the inhibition. Probably a co-operation of all mechanisms will give the total results. If SMITH (1969) stated, that there possibly can be a high transmission of R-factors in the intestinal-flora, it will be necessary to get some certain conditions, a very high colonisation of the intestinal tract with donor- and recipient-strains. This he obtains contrary to the authors as KASUYA, GUINEE, KLEMM and others without antibiotics before feeding the bacteria-strains. Another presumption is that the partner-strains have to show high transmission frequency.

In our experiments, however, we started under natural conditions. To these belongs the wellknown fact, that the settlement of enterobacteriaceae in the intestinal-flora is very difficult. In our opinion a previous alteration of the flow-balance is necessary, which could be obtained, for instance, by previous antibiotic-administration. On the other hand, the infection doses with natural contamination is proportionally low, so a transmission is likely impossible under these conditions. Therefore the selection may be much more important for the spread of resistant micro-organisms than the resistance transmission. In addition to it the resulting selective enrichment of the donor-strain facilitates the transfer.

Since the increasing spread of the R-factors in the last years, since 1960, the situation has changed considerably, because of the selected resistant germs, which not only show a resistance-determinant against the applied antibiotics, but in addition also against other, mostly the important antibiotics in use. Besides a fast elimination of resistant strains of the intestine follows after stopping the therapy, as the chromosomal-resistant bacteria are defect mutants, whose metabolic activity, compared with the wild-type, is reduced. Whereas R-factors-carrying enterobacteriaceae have an unchanged chromosome, and they carry the resistance determinants as an additional activity (WATANABE 1963), they have the same chance to settle in the intestine as the resident wild-type has.

We have to consider, that very often there can be a combination of R-factors with other plasmids, especially with the col-factors, by which these strains perhaps have an additional advantage in selection. With FREDERICQ and KRCMERY we could demonstrate, that Col-factors very often can be transferred together with R-factors. By *Salmonella*-strains we could demonstrate, that R-factor-bearing strains more often carry Col-factors, than sensitive salmonella types.

An important point of view is the fact, that R-factors can be transferred more easily to rough-mutants than to intact wild-types. As JAROLMEN and KEMP (1969) showed, in this way it is possible to select R-factor-bearing rough forms, which are non-pathogenic, with simultaneous application of antibiotics. If we follow this concept consequently, we could suppose, that the R-factors and their transmission in vivo, with simultaneous antibiotic-selection could be a resource to isolate resistant, but non-pathogenic strains. This knowledge, however, is disproved by the fact, that by culturing of R-factor-carrying strains from material of patients, always pathogenic wild-types had been grown and not the non-pathogenic rough-mutants.

In summary we can state, that the R-factor-transmission in vivo under natural conditions is inhibited to such an extend, that it proceeds very slowly. If there wouldn't be the different inhibition-mechanisms with the existing selection, there probably would be nearly only multiple-resistant enterobacteriaceae. If it is possible to make one of the described mechanisms useful for therapeutic purpose, in blocking up the R-factor transmission entirely, that will be uncertain for the next time, this, however would be only partial help. In simultaneous selection by antibiotic therapy and prophylaxis nevertheless a dangereous side-effect of the antibiotic treatment arises, by leading the R-factor carrying strains, selected in the intestinal-flora to relapse, which then cannot be treated any more.

This is an undesired side-effect of antibiotics, which can be demonstrated in experiments, but until now it was impossible to judge the efficiency of a medicament with it.

This paper was intended to be a demonstration of the fact, that "in vivo-transmission" only apparently are of no importance. The real effects are shown by selection, which within the intestinal-flora of man and animals, after the appearance of transferable resistance-plasmid have obtained a completely different signification.

REFERENCES

GUINEE, P. A. M. (1965): Transfer of Multiple Drug Resistance from E. coli to Salmonella typhi murium in the Mouse intestine. Antonie Leeuwenhoek **31**, 314–322.

JAROLMEN, H. and KEMP, G. (1969): R-Factor Transmission in Vivo. J. Bact. **99**, 487–490.

KASUYA, M. (1964): Transfer of Drug Resistance between Enteritic Bacteria in the Mouse. J. Bact. **88**, 322–328.

LEBEK, G. (1969): Die infektiöse bakterielle Antibiotikaresistenz. Verlag Hans Huber, Bern und Stuttgart.

LINCOLN, K. (1970): Resistant Urinary Infections Resulting from Changes in Resistance Pattern of Faecal Flora Induced by Sulphonamide and Hospital Environment. Brit. Med. J. 305–309.

MITSUHASHI, S. (1971): Transferable Drug Resistance Factor R. University Park Press.

SALZMAN, C. T. and KLEMM, L. (1968): Transfer of Antibiotic Resistance (R-Factor) in the Mouse Intestine. Proc. Soc. exp. Biol **128**/2 392–394.

SMITH, H. W. (1969): Transfer of Antibiotic Resistance from Animal and Human Strains of Escherichia Coli to Resident E. coli in the Alimentary-Tract of Man. Lancet 1, 1174—1176.

SCHRÖTER, G., H. P. R. SEELIGER a. H. KNOTHE(1970): Der Einfluß der Antibiotika auf die Darmflora des Menschen. Zbl. Bakt. I. Ref. **219**, 363—406.

WALTON, J. R. (1966): In Vivo Transfer of Infectious Drug Resistance. Nature **211**, 312—313.

WATANABE, T. (1963): Infective Heredity of Multiple Drug Resistance in Bacteria. Bact. rev. **27**, 87—115.

Parts of this lecture are published in:

WIEDEMANN, B., H. KNOTHE, and E. DOLL: Übertragung von R-Faktoren in der Darmflora des Menschen. Zbl. Bakt. I. Orig. **213**, 183—193.

WIEDEMANN, B., H. KNOTHE, I. FISCHER and K. DE BARY (1970): Die Hemmung der R-Faktor-Übertragung in vivo. Drug Research **20**, 1147—1149.

WIEDEMANN, B., G. SCHMIDT: Die Bedeutung der Lipopolysaccharid-Struktur von E. coli für die Übertragung von R-Faktoren. Zbl. Bakt. (in press).

ANTIBIOTICS, ANIMALS AND R FACTORS IN MAN

J. R. WALTON

University of Liverpool, Department of Veterinary Preventive Medicine, Veterinary Field Station, Leahurst, Neston, Wirral, Cheshire, England

One of the major food requirements for contemporary civilization is an adequate supply of animal protein. In order to provide this, many countries have used intensive animal rearing and fattening systems. The introduction of the intensive system has produced specific problems with regard to the maintenance of animal health. This does not mean that the basic concept of the intensive system is at fault; on the contrary, when correctly applied, intensive methods are both humane and highly efficient. The maintenance of animal health under high density stocking is basically an exercise in herd management rather than being concerned with the problems of the individual. More care has to be taken in recognising early signs of disease and in understanding the environmental and nutritional conditions necessary for optimal physical health and food conversion. Community health and preventive medicine can be utilized to their fullest extent and due to the lack of emotional factors these two concepts can be more vigorously applied on intensive units than in the human field.

Antibiotics have an important part to play in farm animal husbandry. Unfortunately, with the commencement of intensive rearing antibiotics were used on a few farms as an attempted panacea for poor hygiene and bad management but this was soon recognised to be false economy. Many of the problems related to the use of antibiotics would be more readily controlled if these drugs were not obtainable through unofficial sources or by illegal purchase and if the medical and veterinary professions made greater efforts to ensure that all their members were fully aware of the theoretical and practical problems associated with antibiotic therapy.

In 1967 in the United Kingdom the overall use of antibiotics in human medicine was four times that in animal husbandry and veterinary medicine; the actual quantities of antibiotics used by both populations can be seen from Table 1 (SWANN, 1969). DURING 1969 more than one million prescriptions were issued to humans for chloramphenicol

Table 1

TOTAL ANTIBIOTIC USEAGE IN MAN AND ANIMALS IN UK DURING 1967

use	amount used (tons)	population (millions)
Medical	240	55
Veterinary	168	335

reference: Swann, 1969

91

alone; this represents about 650 kilograms, of which about 405 kilograms (89 thousand prescriptions) were for oral use, the remaining 245 kilograms (1 ¼ million prescriptions) for skin, eye and ear infections. Considering the warnings issued by numerous authorities about the use of this drug, these figures indicate that chloramphenicol is not being handled in a prudent manner in the medical field. It is too early yet for any results to be evident in agriculture from the antibiotic control measures suggested by Swann. It is clear, however, that users of antibiotics in the veterinary field are much more critical than are doctors of their methods of antibiotic prescribing.

Ample evidence is now available that a wide variety of R factors are present in both human and animal intestinal bacteria but there are conflicting reports about the origins of these R. factors. In order to resolve part of this problem I have looked for the presence of enteric bacteria carrying R factors in live animals, on freshly killed carcases and in retail butcher's meats (WALTON, 1966; WALTON, 1970; WALTON and LEWIS, 1971), Table 2.

Table 2

R+ BACTERIA FOUND IN LIVE PIGS, PIG CARCASSES, PROCESSED PIG MEAT AND MAN

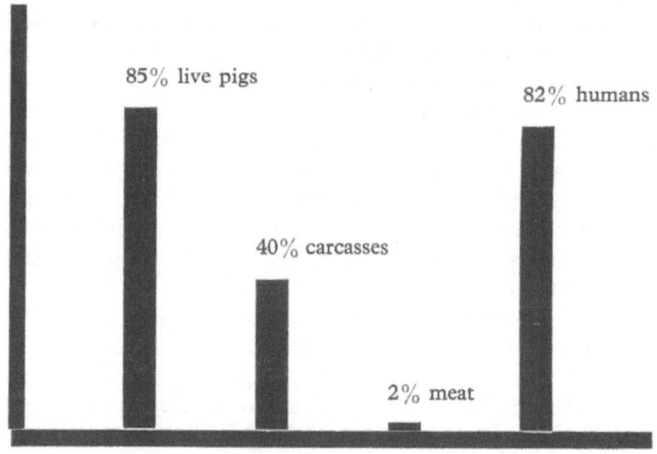

Cattle and pigs from farms in North-west England were examined for multiply resistant *Escherichia coli* and an attempt was made to relate the use of antibiotics on these farms with the appearance of resistance determinants in the bacteria. Good correlation was found between antibiotics that were being used and the resistance determinants present in the strains of *E. coli*. Secondly, freshly killed beef and pig carcases were screened for surface contamination by drug-resistant faecal *E. coli*. Both the inside and outside carcase surfaces were examined for drug-resistant bacteria which were able to transfer resistance. As expected, the pig carcases were more heavily contaminated than the beef carcases, but in general only about 40% of contaminated carcases yielded faecal *E. coli* with transferable resistance. Thirdly, raw and cooked meats were purchased from butchers' shops and examined for contamination by drug-resistant coliforms. Samples of each meat were shaken in sterile buffer solution and the resulting suspension examined for bacterial content. In general all samples tested were contaminated with numerous types of bacteria. However, many of the bacteria possessed an optimal growth temperature of less than 37 °C. but the few enteric bacteria present produced normal sized colonies at this temperature after overnight incubation. This finding indicated that most of the bacteria originated from sources other than human or animal intestinal contents and were probably associated with unclean water or contaminated utensils.

Of special interest are the raw and cooked meats (Table 3). Of 25 samples of each meat examined, only 1 mince and 1 sausage sample yielded R$^+$ *E. coli*. All four types of meat were contaminated and the coliform and total bacterial counts shown in Table 3 represent the highest viable count obtained for the particular meat product. In some cases the main contaminating organism was a proteus but in no case was faecal *E. coli* found on the cooked

Table 3
BACTERIAL CONTAMINATION OF MEATS

	Raw mince	Raw sausage	Cooked ham	Cooked pork
Samples	25	25	25	25
R$^+$ E. coli	1	1	0	0
Coliforms/gm	4×10^2	1×10^3	5×10^2	1×10^3
Bacteria/gm	8×10^7	6×10^5	1×10^6	1×10^5

meats. Clearly these figures indicate a gross pollution of cooked meat products by human handlers. The general lack of enteric *E. coli* on the raw meats possibly indicates a dilution effect from jointing the meat and possibly a reduction in *E. coli* count on the carcase surface during the cooling and holding period. The very small number of samples yielding R$^+$ *E. coli* (2%) and the infrequency of multiple resistance determinants is an indication either that these determinants are unstable or that drug-resistant faecal *E. coli* have very little opportunity of contaminating even suspect meats like sausage meat or mince beef. A recent report from Canada indicates that a similar situation exists in that country in respect of food contamination (ALEXANDER and TITTIGER, 1971). The authors of this report also found a high contamination rate with non-faecal coliforms (81.6%) which had a lowered temperature optimum and they considered that the presence of any coliforms in cooked meat products is a true indication of recontamination. Finally, the need for strict plant sanitation was stressed and for the education of employees in personal hygiene and proper work methods.

In comparison with the farm animal figures, the frequency of R$^+$ bacteria in humans is remarkably similar (Table 2). Figures of 70—80% of humans carrying R$^+$ enteric bacteria are often quoted (MOORHOUSE and McKAY, 1968). Also the recent work on the contamination of British river waters with drug-resistant *E. coli*, especially of human origin and resistant to chloramphenicol, sheds further doubt on the animal being the prime source of multiple drug resistance factors for man (SMITH, 1970). It must also be remembered that many humans are receiving oral antibiotics daily for twenty or thirty years and this situation does not exist in farm animal medicine. In conclusion, I consider that it is totally wrong to assume that man acquired his R factors from animal bacteria, especially as we know that at least 70% of field strains of enteric bacteria, both human and animal, possess transfer factors.

REFERENCES

ALEXANDER, D. C. and TITTIGER, F. (1971): Bacteriological studies on meat pies and frozen prepared dinners. Canadian Journal of Comparative Medicine, **35**, 5.
MOORHOUSE, E. C. and McKAY, L. (1968): Hospital study of transferable drug resistance. British Medical Journal, **2**, 741.

Report of the Joint Committee on the Use of Antibiotics in Animal Husbandry and Veterinary Medicine. H. M. Stationery Office, 1969.

SMITH, H. W. (1970): Incidence in river water of *Escherichia coli* containing R factors. Nature, **228**, 1286.

WALTON, J. R. (1966): Infectious drug resistance in *Escherichia coli* isolated from healthy farm animals. The Lancet, **11**, 1300.

WALTON, J. R. (1970): Contamination of meat carcasses by antibioticresistant coliform bacteria The Lancet, **11**, 561.

WALTON, J. R. and LEWIS, L. E. (1971): Contamination of fresh and cooked meats by antibiotic-resistant coliforms. The Lancet, **11**, 255.

BACTERIAL DRUG RESISTANCE IN ANIMALS

P. A. M. GUINÉE

National Institute of Public Health, Bilthoven, The Netherlands

Problems of antibiotic resistance in animal pathogens are largely confined to the Enterobacteriaceae and Staphylococci (SMITH, 1967).

This paper is restricted to resistance in those *Enterobacteriaceae* which have specific significance for animals, e. g. *Salmonella* and *E. coli*. It should be emphasised *a priori* that emergence of resistant strains in animals is not necessarily associated with the therapeutic use of drugs, because at least equal amounts of antibiotics are added to animal feeds in nutritional levels (10—20 ppm) for growth promotion, or in prophylactic levels to protect the animals against disease during critical stages in their life.

In most countries, there is a strict legislation on the use of drugs for nutritional and prophylactic purposes.

Resistance in Salmonella

One should distinguish between clinical Salmonellosis in animals on one hand and healthy carriers on the other. Since the latter do not show any symptoms, they will not be recognized as *Salmonella* carriers during inspection after slaughter and will be used for human consumption.

Three serotypes of *Salmonella* are particularly important in clinical Salmonellosis in animals: *S. dublin*, *S. cholerae-suis* and *S. typhimurium*. *S. dublin* causes systemic infections in calves and to a lesser degree in adult cattle. The disease is commonly treated with chloramphenicol. For calves, a combination of chloramphenicol (per injectionem) and furazolidone (per os) is usually employed.

During the period 1959—1969 we tested 8812 *S. dublin* strains isolated from cattle and calves for resistance to tetracycline and chloramphenicol.

As shown in Table 1 (MANTEN, GUINEE, KAMPELMACHER, 1970), there is no increase of the percentage of resistant strains. The rate of resistance in *S. cholerae suis* is even lower; of 500 strains tested during 1959—1969, 3 were tetracycline resistant; the remainder were fully sensitive.

The situation in S. typhimurium is entirely different. Particularly in intensively-reared calves, *S. typhimurium* is by far the most frequently encountered serotype. *S. typhimurium* as an animal pathogen behaves slightly different from the two aforementioned serotypes. On one hand *S. typhimurium* causes gastro-enteritis and death in intensively-reared calves and, to a lesser degree, in pigs. On the other hand, we have observed *S. typhimurium* infections in herds of intensively-reared calves which progressed with hardly any symptoms at all. (GUINEE, EDEL, KAMPELMACHER, 1967). Also *S. typhimurium* can be regularly isolated from normal pigs (KAMPELMACHER, GUINEE, HOFSTRA, VAN KEULEN, 1963) These animals cannot be identified during inspection after slaughter. Consequently, many Salmonella contaminated foods will reach the human consumer. Meat and meatproducts are considered as the main source of *Salmonella* infection in man in The

Table 1

RESISTANCE OF S. DUBLIN FROM CATTLE AND CALVES, TO TETRACYCLINE AND CHLORAMPHENICOL 1959–1969

Year	Number of strains tested	Percentage of resistant strains	T	C	T+C
1959	1367	1.4%	16	1	2
1960	1234	0.6%	7	–	1
1961	511	1.2%	6	–	–
1962	389	0.3%	1	–	–
1963	394	1.5%	6	–	–
1964	541	4.4%	22	1	1
1965/66	1056	0.7%	5	1	1
1967	1425	3.6%	49	2	1
1968	844	4.5%	35	2	1
1969	1051	4.1%	43	–	–
Total	8812	2.3%	190	7	6

T = tetracycline
C = Chloramphenicol

Netherlands (VAN SCHOTHORST, EDEL, KAMPELMACHER, 1970). Between 50–60% of all human isolates are *S. typhimurium* (GUINEE, KAMPELMACHER, VALKENBURG, 1967).

We also tested during 1959–1969 8467 *S. typhimurium* isolates from animals for resistance. The results are summarized in Figure 1. The strains were isolated from diseased animals as well as from healthy slaughter animals. Ampicillin-resistance screening was started in 1966. There is an increase of the percentage of tetracycline-resistant

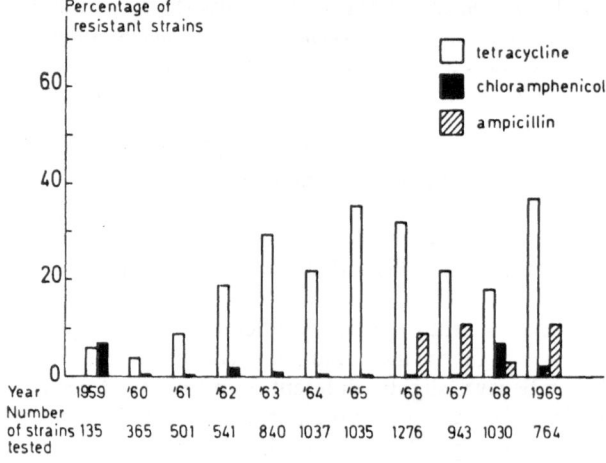

Fig. 1. Resistance to tetracycline, chloramphenicol and ampicillin in S. typhi murium, isolated from animals (cattle, calves, pigs and poultry) during 1959–1969.

strains from 1959 onwards to 1965. No explanation can be given for the variation in the percentage of resistant strains during later years. The percentage of chloramphenicol-resistant strains remained at a more or less constant level during this period.

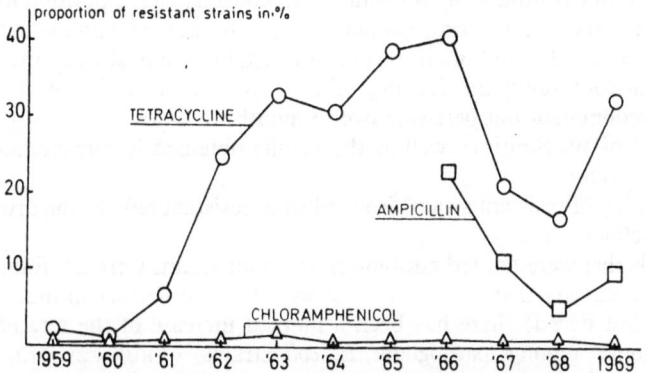

Fig. 2. *Salmonella typhimurium* — Incidence of resistance among human strains with regard to tetracycline, ampicillin and chloramphenicol over the period 1959—1969

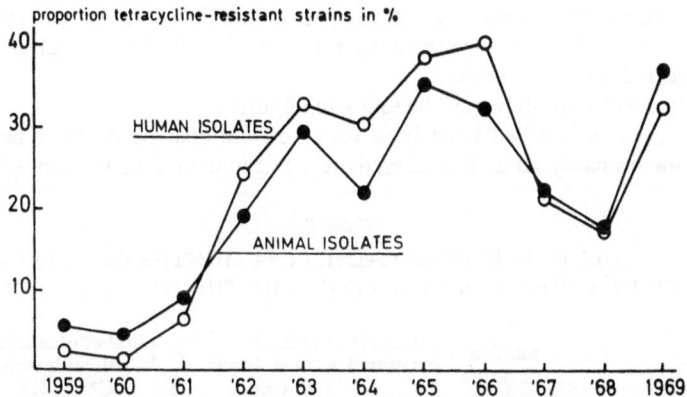

Fig. 3. *Salmonella typhimurium* — Increase of proportion of tetracycline — resistant strains in the period 1959—1969

Figure 2 presents the rates of resistant *S. typhimurium* strains of human origin in the same period.

Figure 3 shows the paralellism between the rates of resistance in human and animal isolates of *S. typhimurium*.

Resistance in E. coli.

Certain serologically-defined *E. coli* strains are associated with pathological conditions in animals, such as neonatal diarrhea in piglets, bowel oedema in pigs, enteritis in pigs and calves and certain conditions in poultry (SOJKA, 1957). The morbidity and mortality of these infections is very high and antibiotics are indispensable for treatment and prevention.

E. coli is also a normal inhabitant of the intestinal tract and forms the bulk of the gramnegative aerobic intestinal flora in most species of animals.

Already in 1957 it was pointed out by W. Smith that the antibiotics used even in low levels caused an alteration in the intestinal flora from sensitive to resistant. Tetracycline-resistant *E. coli* strains appeared to predominate in the intestinal flora of pigs which had been fed tetracycline continuously for some time, contrary to the position in pigs that had not been fed tetracycline (SMITH, CRABB, 1957). The phenomenon could be explained as an alteration in the *E. coli* flora in favour of resistant strains already present (GUINEE, 1963). After discontinuing the feeding of tetracycline, the resistant strains gradually became less predominant but persisted over 5 months.

The findings of W. Smith as well as the results obtained in our laboratory indicated two relevant aspects:

1. The majority of resistant strains isolated were resistant only to the drug used, in this case to tetracyclines

2. in animals that were not fed antibiotics, resistant strains were not found, or found in much lower percentages than in animals that were fed antibiotics continuously.

During the last decade there has been a marked increase of the rate of resistance to several antibiotics among pathogenic *E. coli* strains. (TRUSZCZYNSKI, BORKOWSKA, CIOSEK, 1966; KONDRACKI, 1967; GREENFIELD, BANKIER, 1969; ADEN, REED, UNDERDAHL, MEBUS, 1969; OVERGOOR, 1966, 1967 and 1971). There has been an increase of the resistance to streptomycin, sulfonamide and tetracycline and chloramphenicol.

The changing pattern of drug resistance in pathogenic E. coli has led us to re-investigate the drug resistance of the non-pathogenic intestinal *E. coli* flora of calves which were intensively-reared on a calf station.

Some of the results are shown in the following figures.

The animals examined had been born on a conventional farm. They acquired their intestinal flora probably from the immediate environment i. e. the cow-shed or their

Table 2

RESISTANT E. COLI IN BREEDING-CALVES (>4 MONTHS OF AGE) ON VARIOUS
FARMS IN 4 DIFFERENT PROVINCES IN THE NETHERLANDS

Province	number of farms	number of animals examined with resistant E. coli	number of animals yielding E. coli with resistance to				
			T*	C*	K*	A*	F*
Friesland	6	55	42	39	27	19	22	13
Overijssel	3	14	7	7	6	5	4	2
Utrecht	5	54	52	52	40	31	29	18
Gelderland	4	20	12	12	8	11	10	—
Total	18	143	113(79%)	110	81	66	65	33

*T = tetracyclin; C = chloramphenicol; K = kanamycin;
A = ampicillin; F = Furazolidone

dams. The calves remained for about 1 week with the dams and were then transported to the calf station. On the calf station, they were fed milk substitutes containing various antibiotics.

In view of this we expected the first specimens of faeces which were collected on the first day at the calf station, to be free or nearly free of resistant *E. coli* bacteria.

However, this was not the case. Nearly all specimens were found to yield resistant E. coli.

Because of the high incidence of resistant *E. coli* in one-week old calves to be fattened, we also studied the incidence of resistant *E. coli* in breeding calves. These calves are not fattened by means of milk replacers containing antibiotics, but are reared for milkproduction by means of other feeds which do not contain antibiotics.

Resistant *E. coli* was found in nearly 80% of the calves (Table 2).

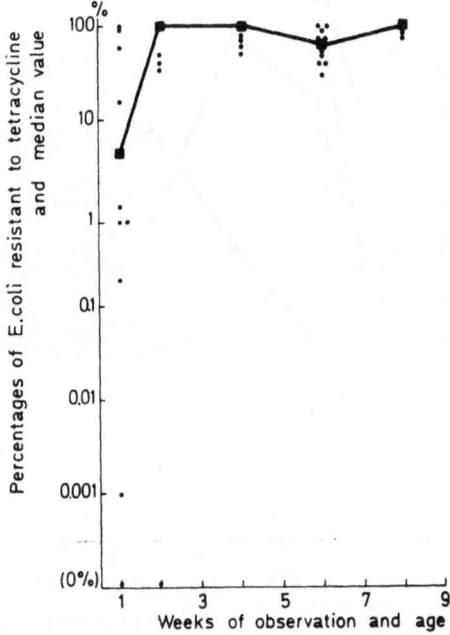

Fig. 4. Tetracycline-resistant E. coli in 11 calves fed 75 ppm oxytetracycline and 50 ppm furazolidone continuously.

In Figure 4 a summary is given of the observations on a group of 11 calves on the calf station which were fed continuously on 75 parts per million (ppm) of oxytetracycline and 50 ppm of furazolidone from the first week of life. The percentage of tetracycline-resistant *E. coli* in individual specimens was determined. The values as well as the median value are given in the figure. Only one specimen in the first week harboured no tetracycline-resistant E. coli; the other 10 specimens yielded varying percentages of tetracycline-resistant *E. coli*. From the second week, all specimens yielded more than 30% tetracycline-resistant *E. coli*.

The percentages of E. coli with resistance to chloramphenicol, kanamycin and ampicillin in individual specimens were estimated in a similar way.

In Figure 5 the median value of the percentages of *E. coli* with resistance to tetracycline, chloramphenicol, ampicillin and the neomycin/kanamycin group are presented. The values in the individual specimens have been omitted for clarity. The increase in incidence of kanamycin-resistant strains is probably associated with the fact that 4 animals were treated once with neomycin during the first or second week of observation. There is also some increase of ampicillin- and chloramphenicol-resistance although these drugs were not employed at all.

During the investigation, a number of resistant strains was collected and the transferability of the resistance markers to a nalidixic acid-resistant mutant of *E. coli*

K12 F⁻(Nal^r) tested; 66% of the strains transferred part or whole of their resistance markers, depending on the method of selection. Kanamycin-resistance-determinants were most frequently transferred.

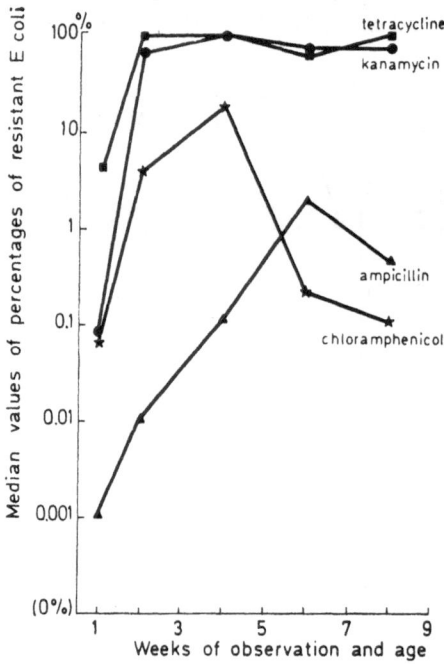

Fig. 5. Tetracycline-resistant E. coli in 11 calves fed 75 ppm oxytetracycline and 50 ppm furazolidone continuously.

RESISTANCE MARKERS, TRANSFERABLE TO E. COLI $K_{12}F$⁻NAL^r, IN 349 E. COLI STRAINS FROM 11 CALVES FED 75 PPM OXYTETRACYCLINE AND 50 PPM FURAZOLIDONE CONTINUOUSLY

Number of resistant strains		Number of strains with transferable resistance	
Total	349	229	(66%)
Tetracycline	325	141	(43%)
Chloramphenicol	221	116	(53%)
Furazolidone	201	0	
Kanamycin.	161	132	(80%)
Ampicillin	180	28	(16%)

Similar results as shown in the previous figures were obtained in groups of calves that were fed either chlortetracycline or penicillin and streptomycin: tetracycline and kanamycin-resistant strains emerged rapidly and plentifully; chloramphenicol and ampicillin-resistant strains emerged less plentifully.

The changes in patterns of bacterial resistance in *Salmonella* and *E. coli* in animals during the last decade may be summarized as follows:

1. There is no significant emergence of resistance in animal pathogens like *S. dublin* and *S. cholerae-suis*.

2. In *S. typhimurium*, the most frequently found serotype, resistance to tetracycline has increased sharply during the last ten years; chloramphenicol-resistance has remained on a constant level of 1—2%.

3. The resistance of pathogenic strains of E. coli to streptomycin, sulfonamide, tetracycline, chloramphenicol and neomycin has increased greatly.

4. E. coli strains in the intestinal tract of intensively-reared animals that are fed antibiotics continuously are now predominantly multi-resistant. Resistant, frequently multi-resistant E. coli can now also be found in animals on an antibiotic-free diet and even in newly born animals.

The treatment and prevention of E. coli infections is becoming invalidated by the increasing number of multiresistant strains of pathogenic E. coli as well as "normal" E. coli.

Several investigators have also reported an increased prevalence of resistant E. coli in human beings (LEBEK, 1967; LEWIS, 1968; WIEDEMANN, KNOTHE, HÖLZER, 1969; GUINÉE, UGUETO, VAN LEEUWEN, 1970). Is there reason to believe in a connection between the animal reservoir of resistant E. coli on one hand and the increasing prevalence in man on the other?

Table 3

INCIDENCE OF RESISTANT AND R+ E. COLI IN NON-VEGETARIANS, VEGETARIANS AND BABIES BELOW THE AGE OF 6 MONTHS

	Number of people investigated	Technique A 1 specimen		Technique A and B 1 specimen	
		% with resistant E. coli	% with R-factor	% with resistant E. coli	% with R-factor
Military kitchen personnel 1960—1961	100			19	
1.A Military kitchen personnel 1968—1969	400	38	25(18)*	45	28(21)
1.B Office employees 1968—1969	86	23	9(8)	31	16(16)
11.B vegetarians 1968—1969	77	36	24(9)	44	26(10)
11.B Babies below the age of 6 months living at home	87	32	18(8)		

*) 25% yielded one or more E. coli strains which transferred their resistance to E. coli K12 F⁻ W 3110 Nal^R. — 18% yielded strains which transferred their resistance also to S. typhimurium and/or S. panama

It must be stated that contamination with intestinal microorganisms of the carcasses during the slaughtering proces of animals cannot be prevented. In this way, meat and meatproducts can be contaminated with resistant E. coli (MOORHOUSE, GRADY, O'CONNOR, 1969) and resistant E. coli can be transported from animals through meat and meatproducts to the human consumer. If this mechanism was the most important source of infection with resistant E. coli for man, one might expect that resistant E. coli would occur in meat-eating individuals more frequently than in non-meat-eating individuals. We examined the prevalence of resistant E. coli in meat-consuming adults, vegetarians and babies below the age of 6 months who had been born and were living at home. None of these people had been treated with antibiotics or had been hospitalized during the three previous months. In table 3 the most relevant results have been summarized. To enable comparison, the Table has been divided according to the number of specimens tested per person and the techniques employed, because these were different in the various groups. The results of an investigation of 100 military personnel carried out in 1961 are also given in this table.

Technique A consisted of rubbing a cotton swab soiled with feaces over the surface of a plate of culture medium on which discs containing several antibiotics were placed. In technique B, the proportions of tetracycline-resistant E. coli in the faecal specimens were estimated.

The percentage of persons with resistant E. coli was larger in the vegetarians than in the office employees. The percentage with resistant E. coli in the babies was about equal to that in the vegetarians and higher than in the office employees.

I would not conclude from these data that meat and meat-products do not play any part in the infection of human beings with resistant E. coli. Meat should be considered as a source of E. coli as well as of Salmonellae, but in our studies other factors were apparently more important than meat or meatproducts. One of these factors might have been vegetables or uncooked salads that had been in contact with contaminated surface waters. In many places, surface waters are contaminated with Salmonella and E. coli strains, many of them carrying R-factors (STURTEVANT, FEARY, 1969) as a consequence of the continuous voidance of effluent water from water purification plants where the number of Entero-bacteria is reduced only with a factor 10–100.

One must assume that resistant E. coli is cycling from animals to man and from man through the environment to animals.

In the Report of the Swann Committee (Swann report) it is advocated to distinguish and separate antibiotics for use as feed additives from antibiotics for therapeutic purposes. Antibiotics to be used as feed additives (feed antibiotics) should fulfill the conditions that they have no therapeutic value for human therapy and show no cross-resistance with therapeutic antibiotics.

LEGISLATION ON THE ADDITION OF DRUGS TO FEEDS IN THE NETHERLANDS
(ABSTRACT)

I. Permitted drugs: penicillin
penicillin and streptomycin (3 : 7)
oxytetracycline
bacitracin
tylosin
spiramycin
oleandomycin
furazolidone (only calves)

II. Feeds   Mixed feeds (pigs and broilers)   10 ppm
milk replacer for piglets   50 ppm
artificial milk for fattening calves   100 ppm

The recommendations of the Swann Committee were based mainly on public health implications.

The results of the investigations mentioned before, lead to similar recommendations, however based on the complications in veterinary therapy rather than on public health implications. Not only should the use of low levels of antibiotics be reconsidered according to these recommendations, also the employment of drugs like chloramphenicol and neomycin-kanamycin in veterinary medicine should be restricted as much as possible to preserve their therapeutic value for as long as possible.

¡ABSTRACT

The emergence of drug-resistance among animal pathogens is largely confined to the Enterobacteriaceae, in particular *Salmonella* and *E. coli*.

In *S. dublin,* causing systemic infections in calves and cattle, and *S. cholerae suis* (var. kunzendorf) associated with enteric disease in pigs no significant development of resistance has been observed, despite the fact that chloramphenicol has been generally used to treat *S. dublin* infections.

In *S. typhimurium* resistance to tetracycline has increased roughly from 2% in 1959 to 40% in 1965 and has since then remained on about the same level. Chloramphenicol-resistance has constantly been on a relatively low level (1—2%).

In pathogenic E. coli there has been a trend towards multiresistance during recent years. More than 50% of the strains are resistant to streptomycin, sulfonamide and tetracycline; the resistance to chloramphenicol and neomycin, although on a lower level, is increasing.

This is also true for non-pathogenic *E. coli* strains. Already more than 10 years ago it was reported that tetracycline-resistant strains of E. coli predominated in herds fed tetracycline continuously. At that time most of the strains were mono-resistant. In animals which were not fet continuously with antibiotic-containing feed, resistant E. coli strains were found only sporadically.

This situation has changed during the last decade:

1. many of the *E. coli* strains isolated from intensively reared animals are now multi-resistant; about 60% of these strains are able to transfer part or whole of their resistance patterns to E. coli K12;

2. resistant strains are now also found in animals which are not fed antibiotics continuously (horses, cattle).

REFERENCES

ADEN, D. P., N. D. REED, N. R. UNDERDAHL, C. A. MEBUS (1969): Transferable drug resistance among Enterobacteriaceae isolated from cases of neonatal diarrhea in calves and piglets. Applied Microbiology **18**, 961—964.

GREENFIELD, J., J. C. BANKIER (1969): Sensitivity of freshly isolated bacterial pathogens to certain antibiotics and nitrofurazone. Canadian Journal of Comparative Medicine **33**, 39—43.

GUINEE, P. A. M. (1963): Experimental studies on the origin and significance of antibiotic-resistant Escherichia coli in animals and man. Proefschrift Utrecht.

GUINEE, P. A. M., E. H. KAMPELMACHER, J. J. VALKENBURG (1967): Salmonella isolations in the Netherlands, 1961—1965. Zentralblatt für Bakteriologie I. Orig. **204**, 476—484.

GUINEE, P. A. M., WEDEL, E. H. KAMPELMACHER (1967): Studies on Salmonella infection in fattening calves. Zentralblatt für Veterinärmedizin **14**, 163—169.

GUINEE, P. A. M., N. UGUETO, N. van LEEUWEN (1970): Escherichia coli with resistance factors in vegetarians, babies and nonvegetarians. Applied Microbiology 531—535.

KAMPELMACHER, E. H., P. A. M. GUINEE, K. HOFSTRA, A. van KEULEN (1963): Further studies on Salmonella in slaughterhouses and in normal slaughter pigs. Zentralblatt für Veterinärmedizin **10**, 1—27.

KONDRACKI, M. (1967): Badania wrażliwości szczegow E. coli wyosobnionych z terenowych przypadków kolibakteriozy cielat na antybiotyki i preparaty nitrofuranowe. I. Wrażliwośc na antybiotyhi in vitro. Medycyna Weterynaryjna **24**, 355—356.

LEBEK, G. (1967): Medizinische Aspekte der infektiosen Antibiotika-Resistenz gram-negatives Darmbakterien. Pathologia et Microbiologia **30**, 1015—1036.

LEWIS, M. J. (1968): Transferable drug resistance and other transferable agents in strains of Escherichia coli from two human populations. Lancet 1968[1], 1389—1393.

MANTEN, A., P. A. M. GUINEE, E. H. KAMPELMACHER, C. E. VOOGD (1971): An eleven years study of drugresistance in Salmonella in the Netherlands. WHO Bull (in press).

MOORHOUSE, E. C., M. F. O. GRADY, H. O'CONNOR (1969): Isolation from sausages of antibiotic-resistant Escherichia with R factors. Lancet 1969[II] **50**, 50—52.

OVERGOOR, G. H. A. (1966): Gevoeligheid van uit praktijkmateriaal geïsoleerde bacterien ten opzichte van de meest gebruikelijke antibiotica en chemotherapeutica. Tijdschrift voor Diergeneeskunde **91**, 1760—1766.

OVERGOOR, G. H. A. (1967): Gevoeligheid van uit praktijkmateriaal geïsoleerde bacterien ten opzichte van de meest gebruiekelijke antibiotica en chemotherapeutica. Tijdschrift voor Diergeneeskunde **92**, 515.

OVERGOOR, G. H. A. (1971): Voortgezette onderzoekingen met betrekking tot de gevoeligheid van uit praktijkmateriaal geïsoleerde bacterien ten opzichte van de meest gebruikelijke antibiotica en chemotherapeutica. Tijdschrift voor Diergeneeskunde **96**, 685—692.

SMITH, H. W. (1967): The effect of the use of antibacterial drugs, particularly as food additives, on the emergence of drug-resistent strains of bacteria in animals. New Zeeland Veterinary Journal **15**, 153—166.

SMITH, H. W., W. E. CRABB (1957): The effect of the continuous administration of diets containing low levels of tetracyclines on the incidence of drug-resistant Bacterium coli in the faeces of pigs and chickens: the sensitivity of the Bact. coli to other chemotherapeutic agents band. Veterinary Record **69**, 24—30.

SOJKA, W. J. (1965): Escherichia coli in animals. Farhnam Royal, Common. Agricultural Bureau (Review Series no. 7 of the Commonwealth Bureau of Animal Health, Weybridge).

STURTEVANT, A. B., T. W. FEARY (1969): Incidence of infectious drug resistance among lactose-fermenting bacteria isolated from raw and treated sewage. Applied Microbiology **18**, 918.

SWANN report. Joint Committee on the use of Antibiotics in Animal Husbandry and Veterinary medicine. Report. London H. M. S. O. 1969. 83 pp.

TRUSZCZYNSKI, M., B. BORKOWSKA, D. CIOSEK (1966): Wrażliwośe na antybiotyki serotypów paleczki okreznicy wyosobnionych z przypadków chorobowych u świń. Medycyna Weterynaryjna **22**, 264.

VAN SCHOTHORST, M., W. EDEL, E. H. KAMPELMACHER (1970): Voortgezette onderzoekingen over het voorkomen van Salmonella in gehakt in de maand juli, 1965—1969. Tejdschrift voor Diergenneeskunde **95**, 279—282.

WIEDEMANN, B., H. KNOTHE, P. HÖLZER (1969): Untersuchungen über die Verbreitung von R-Faktoren. Zentralblatt für Bakteriologie I Orig. **212**, 97—103.

INCREASE OF FLAVOMYCIN SENSITIVITY OF BACTERIA
BY R FACTORS

TSUTOMU WATANABE, YASUKO OGATA, KATOMI SUGAWARA
and KAZUYO ODA

Department of Microbiology, Keio University School of Medicine, Tokyo, Japan

Various antibiotics and synthetic chemotherapeutic agents have been used as feed additives for livestock and poultry for the purpose of growth promotion (see STOKSTAD, 1954; JUKES, 1955) in many countries. Consequently, drug-resistant bacteria have considerably increased among the enteric bacteria of these animals, and a majority of these bacteria have been found resistant to multiple drugs due to the presence of R factors (transferable drug resistance factors) (SMITH and HALLS, 1966; ANDERSON, 1968). Multiple-drug-resistant bacteria of common pathogenicity to man and animals, such as *Salmonella* species, can be transmitted to man from animals, and besides this, R factors can be transferred to human pathogens via non-pathogenic bacteria such as *Escherichia coli*. The potential dangers of the increase of R factor-carrying bacteria in animals were systematically discussed in the so-called Swann Report (1969) and it was pointed out that the increase of R factor-carrying bacteria in animals is really causing a problem of public health. Thus the development of effective antibiotics as feed additives which do not cause an increase of R factor-carrying bacteria in animals has been strongly expected.

Flavomycin (also called flavophospholipol and moenomycin) (WALLHAUSER, NESEMANN, PRAVE, and STEIGLER, 1966; HUBER, SCHACHT, WEIDENMÜLLER, SCHMIDT-THOME, DUPHORN, and TSCHESCHE, 1966; Von WASIELEWSKI, MUSCHA-WECK, and SCHÜTZE, 1966) is an antibiotic which is being specifically used as a feed additive for livestock and poultry (BAUER, and DOST, 1966; TUREK, LETTNER, and STEINACKER, 1967) in many countries. We have recently found that R factors give increased flavomycin sensitivity to their host bacteria. Bacteria carrying a sex factor F and colicin agent Ib also showed increased sensitivity to this antibiotic. The mechanism of the increased flavomycin sensitivity of bacteria carrying R factors and other episomal elements is apparently due to the presence of sex pili. We have also shown that the mutations of R factor-carrying bacteria to flavomycin resistance are not mediated by R factors. These results will be reported in the present paper, and their implications to the public health problem of antibiotic feeding will be discussed.

MATERIALS AND METHODS

Various substrains of *E. coli* K-12 were used. They were CSH-2 (*met⁻ pro⁻*) F⁻ and F⁺, W3110/I (*gal⁻ λ⁻ colI-r*) F⁻, W3110/I (Col Ib) (carrying colicin agent Ib), W3110/I (Col Ib *drd*) (carrying a derepressed mutant of Col Ib), W677/PTS (*pro⁻ thr⁻ leu⁻ thi⁻ man⁻ xyl⁻ mal⁻ gal⁻ lac⁻ str-r tsx-r*) F⁻, W2252 (*met⁻ λ⁻* Hfr), W2252 *def*F (strain with defective, integrated F mutant derived from W2252 and unable to mate) (Watanabe and Okada, 1965), AB312 (*lac⁻ thr⁻ leu⁻ thi⁻ λ⁻* Hfr), AB313 (*lac⁻ thr⁻ leu⁻ thi⁻ str-r* Hfr), H3000 (*thi⁻* Hfr), JE2217 (*pil⁻ str-r*) F⁻, JE2571 (*thr⁻ leu⁻ gal⁻ lac⁻ xyl⁻ mal⁻ attλ⁻ fla⁻ pil⁻ str-r*) F⁻ and B380 (*his⁻ gal⁻ pil⁻*) F⁻. The last three strains do not form type 1 pili (common pili not associated with sex factors) (Brinton, 1965) and were supplied to us by Y. NISHIMURA (JE2217 and JE2571) and C. C. BRINTON, Jr. (B380). Besides these K-12 substrains, *Salmonella typhimurium* LT-2 wild type was also used.

Table 1

STRAINS OF R FACTORS USED IN THIS STUDY

Strain number	Drug resistance marker*	*fi* type **
222	Su, Sm, Cm, Tc	+
222—R₃	Su, Sm, Cm	+
222—Tc	Tc	+
K	Su, Sm, Cm, Tc	+
S—b	Su, Sm, Cm, Tc	+
N—6	Su, Sm, Tc	+
N—9	Su, Sm, Tc	+
R₆	Su, Sm, Cm, Tc, Km	+
R1	Su, Sm, Cm, Ap	+
R1—19	Su, Sm, Cm, Ap	—
N—1	Su, Sm, Tc	—
N—3	Su, Sm, Tc	—
R—15	Su, Sm	—
S—a	Su, Sm, Cm, Km	—
R64	Sm, Tc	—
R64—11	Sm, Tc	—

* Su: sulphonamide, Sm: streptomycin, Cm: chloramphenicol, Km: kanamycin, Tc: tetracycline Ap: aminobenzyl penicillin.
**fi: fertility inhibition. *fi*⁺ R factors inhibit the formation of F pili when they are in male strains, while *fi*⁻ R factors do not have this inhibitory function (Watanabe, Fukasawa, and Takano, 1962; Watanabe, Nishida, Ogata, Arai, and Sato, 1964).

Strains of R factors used in this study are listed in Table 1. *fi*⁺ R factors induce the formation of sex pili similar or identical to F pili, while *fi*⁻ R factors form sex pili similar or identical to I pili (see MEYNELL, MEYNELL, and DATTA, 1968). These R factors are, therefore, also called F-like R factors or R(F) and I-like R factors or R(I), respectively (MEYNELL et al., 1968; NOVICK, 1969). R factors 222-R₃ and 222-Tc are spontaneous deletion mutants derived from 222 (WATANABE and LYANG, 1962). R1—19 and R64—11 are derepressed (*drd*) mutants derived from R1 and R64, respectively (MEYNELL and DATTA, 1967). These *drd* mutants do not produce cytoplasmic repressors which inhibit the formation of sex pili. Accordingly, they fully develop sex pili and exhibit high conjugal transferability. R1—19 behaves as *fi*⁻ phenotypically, because it does not produce a repressor for the formation of F pili by the sex factor F in the same cells, although some other *drd* mutants are known which do produce repressors but are insensitive to the repressors (MEYNELL and COOKE, 1969). The strains with a *drd* mutant of Col Ib, described above, were isolated and supplied to us by Ohki and Ozeki (1968) but similar mutants were also isolated by EDWARDS and MEYNELL (1968).

Bacteria were cultured on nutrient agar medium (pH 7.3) containing Polypeptone (Takeda) 1%, Meat-extract (Kyokuto) 1%, NaCl 0.3% and Bacto-agar (Difco) 1.5%, or in Penassay broth (Difco) (pH 7.0) at 37 °C with gentle shaking in L-shaped tubes.

Growth of bacteria in broth was followed by determining optical densities (O. D.) at 530 mμ using a photoelectric colorimeter (Erma). Flavomycin used was a pure sample supplied by Farbwerke Hoechst AG, Germany. Flavomycin was dissolved and diluted in distilled water. Each bacterial strain was grown in broth to O. D. 0.4 (containing approximately 5×10^8 cells per ml) and diluted to 10^{-4} with physiological saline. A standard loopful of this dilution was streaked on nutrient agar containing varying concentrations (in two-fold dilutions) of flavomycin. The inoculated plates were incubated at 37° C overnight and the colonies developed were roughly scored. The concentration of flavomycin two times higher than that on the maximal drug concentration on which the number of colonies was about equal to that on a drug-free control plate was taken as the minimal inhibitory concentration (M. I. C.) of the antibiotic for this strain. Flavomycin sensitivity of each strain was also studied in broth: Bacteria were grown in Penassay broth containing varying concentrations of flavomycin and their growth curves were followed turbidimetrically. At the end of 10 hours observation, surviving bactria were plated on drug-free nutrient agar and their sensitivity to various drugs was studied by replica plating. In order to isolate mutants of R$^+$ bacteria of higher flavomycin resistance, R$^+$ bacteria were subcultured on nutrient agar containing increasingly higher concentrations of flavomycin.

Table 2

MINIMAL INHIBITORY CONCENTRATIONS OF FLAVOMYCIN FOR VARIOUS SUBSTRAINS OF *ESCHERICHIA COLI* K12

Strain	Minimal inhibitory concentration of flavomycin (μg/ml.)
CSH$-$2 F$^-$	20
CSH$-$2 (222)	5
CSH$-$2 (222$-$R^3)	2.5
CSH$-$2 (222$-$Tc)	1.25
CSH$-$2 (K)	5
CSH$-$2 (S$-$b)	10
CSH$-$2 (N$-$6)	1.25
CSH$-$2 (N$-$9)	2.5
CSH$-$2 (R$_6$)	10
CSH$-$2 (R1)	10
SCH$-$2 (R1$-$19)	5
CSH$-$2 (N$-$1)	5
CSH$-$2 (N$-$3)	10
CSH$-$2 (R$-$15)	5
CSH$-$2 (S$-$a)	2.5
CSH$-$2 (R64)	5
CSH$-$2 (R64$-$11)	1.25
CSH$-$2 F$^+$	1.25
W2252 (Hfr)	1.25
W2252 *def*F	20
AB312 (Hfr)	1.25
AB313 (Hfr)	1.25
H3000 (Hfr)	2.5
W3110/I F$^-$	20
W3110/I (Col Ib)	5
W3110/I (col Ib *drd*)	1.25
JE2217 F$^-$	20
JE2571 F$^-$	20
B380 F$^-$	5

For studying the frequency of R transfer, CSH-2 F⁻ R⁺ was used as a donor and W677/PTS as a recipient. Each strain was grown to O. D. 0.4 in broth, and 1 ml of a donor culture was mixed with 9 ml of a recipient culture in a 200 ml Erlenmeyer flask, which was then incubated in a 37° C water-bath for 60 min without aeration. The mixed culture was then diluted properly and plated on BTB-lactose-nutrient agar (nutrient agar containing 0,0045% bromothymolblue and 1% lactose) containing 1,000 μg/ml of dihydrostreptomycin sulfate (Sankyo) plus 25 μg/ml of chloramphenicol (Sankyo) or tetracycline hydrochloride (Lederle), or 500 μg/ml of sulfathiazole (Takeda). The recipient clones which received R factors formed lactose-nonfermenting colonies on these selective media. When the effect of flavomycin was to be tested on the frequency of R transfer, 0.5 ml of varying concentrations of flavomycin solution was added to 8.5 ml of a recipient culture immediately before 1 ml of a donor culture was added to the recipient. Subsequent procedure for determining the frequency of R transfer was identical to that described above.

RESULTS

As the results are shown in Table 2, many of the *E. coli* strains carrying R factors or other episomal elements showed increased sensitivity to flavomycin as expressed by the M. I. C. values. It seems of particular interest that the strains with non-repressed type episomes are, as a rule, more sensitive to flavomycin than those with self-repressed type episomes.

Typical growth curves of CSH-2 strains with and without R factors are shown in Figures 1 to 6. These figures and similar data with other strains, not shown here, indicate

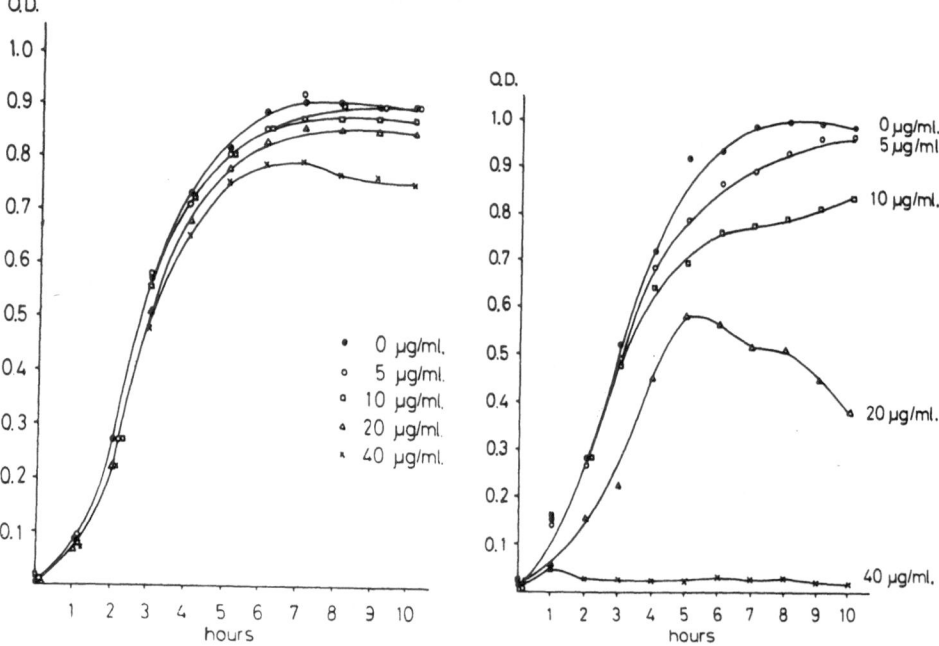

Fig. 1 Growth curves of *Escherichia coli* CSH−2 F⁻ R⁻ in broth containing varying concentrations of flavomycin.

Fig. 2 Growth curves of *Escherichia coli* CSH−2 (222) in broth containing varying concentrations of flavomycin.

108

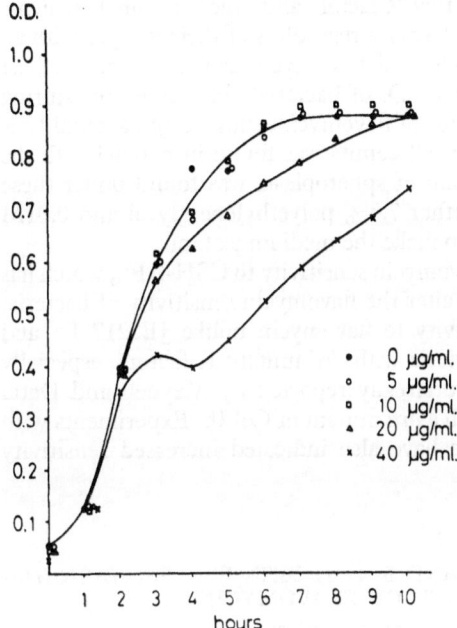

Fig. 3 Growth curves of *Escherichia coli* CSH−2 (R1) in broth containing varying concentrations of flavomycin.

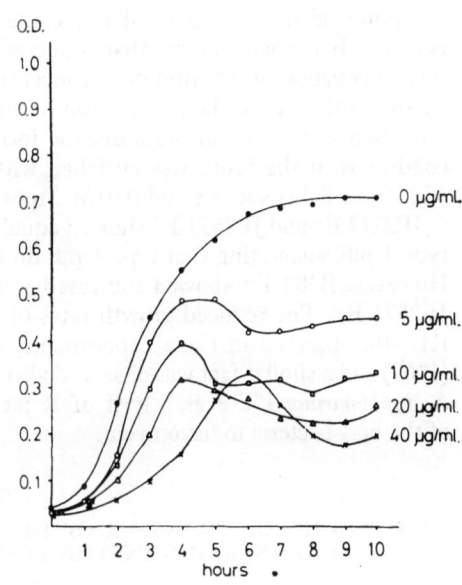

Fig. 4 Growth curves of *Escherichia coli* CSH−2 (R1−19) in broth containing varying concentrations of flavomycin.

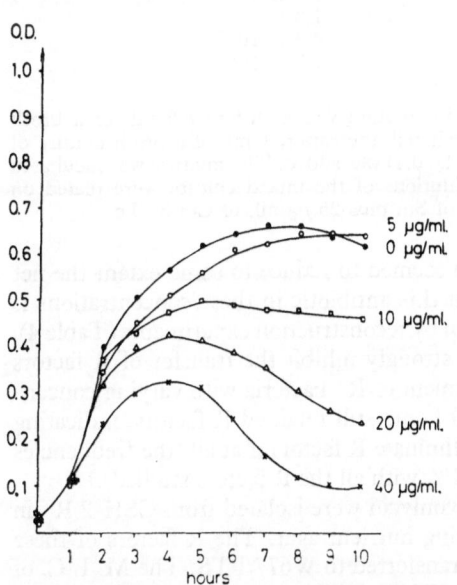

Fig. 5 Growth curves of *Escherichia coli* CSH−2 (R64) in broth containing varying concentrations of flavomycin.

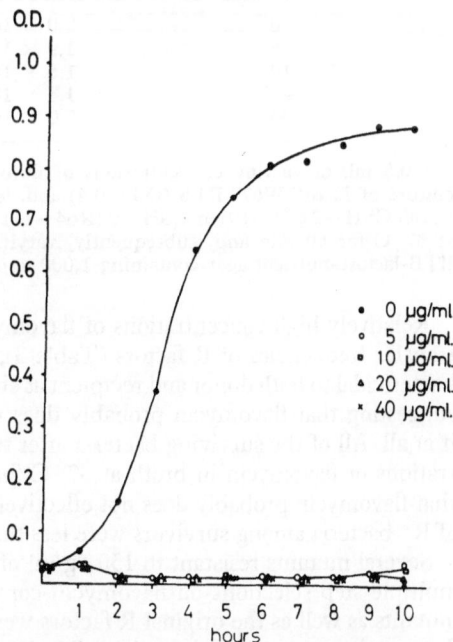

Fig. 6 Growth curves of *Escherichia coli* CSH−2 (R64−11) in broth containing varying concentrations of flavomycin.

109

more clearly than the M. I. C. determination that R factors and other episomal elements increase the flavomycin sensitivity of the host bacteria regardless of their *fi* types with an exception od *def*F, which did not confer increased flavomycin sensitivity on its host bacteria. It is characteristic that reduction in O. D. of bacterial cultures occurs during their incubation in the inhibitory concentrations of flavomycin, suggesting bacterial lysis by this antibiotic. In fact, reduction of viable cell counts was found in parallel with the reduction in O. D. Furthermore, the formation of spheroplasts was found under these conditions, if the broth was enriched with either 7.5% polyethylene glycol and 0.01M $MgSO_4$ or 0.3M sucrose and 0.01M $MgSO_4$ to make the medium isotonic.

JE2217 F⁻ and JE2571 F⁻ showed equal flavomycin sensitivity to CSH-2 F⁻, which has type 1 pili, suggesting that type 1 pili do not alter the flavomycin sensitivity of bacteria. However, B380 F⁻ showed increased sensitivity to flavomycin unlike JE2217 F⁻ and JE2571 F⁻. The reduced growth rates of bacteria with *drd* mutant R factors, especially R1−19, observed in these experiments, were already reported by Meynell and Datta (1967) and a similar fact was observed also with a *drd* mutant of Col Ib. Experiments with *S. typhimurium* LT-2 as a host of R factors have also indicated increased sensitivity of the host bacteria to flavomycin.

Table 3

FREQUENCIES OF TRANSFER OF R1−19 AND R64−11 BETWEEN *ESCHERICHIA COLI* STRAINS IN THE PRESENCE OF FLAVOMYCIN

Flavomycin concentration (μg/ml.)	Frequency of transfer (per introduced donor cell) ⋆	
	R1−19	R64−11
0	2.0×10^{-1}	9.3×10^{-1}
5	1.9×10^{-1}	6.9×10^{-1}
10	1.6×10^{-1}	1.3×10^{-1}
20	1.3×10^{-1}	4.3×10^{-2}
40	5.0×10^{-2}	1.5×10^{-2}

⋆ 0.5 ml. of varying concentrations of flavomycin solution was added to 8.5 ml. of a broth culture of *E. coli* W677/PTS (O.D. 0.4) and, immediately thereafter, 1 ml. of a broth culture of *E. coli* CSH−2 (R1−19) or CSH−2 (R64−11) (O. D. 0.4) was added. The mixture was incubated at 37° C for 60 min and, subsequently, varying dilutions of the mixed culture were plated on BTB-lactose-nutrient agar containing 1,000 μg/ml. of Sm plus 25 μg/ml. of Cm or Tc.

Relatively high concentrations of flavomycin seemed to reduce to some extent the net transfer frequencies of R factors (Table 3), but this antibiotic in these concentrations is bactericidal to both donor and recipient as shown by reconstruction experiments (Table 4), suggesting that flavomycin probably does not strongly inhibit the transfer of R factors if at all. All of the surviving bacteria after treatment of R⁺ bacteria with varying concentrations of flavomycin in broth at 37° C for 10 hours still retained R factors, indicating that flavomycin probably does not effectively eliminate R factors if at all (the frequencies of R⁻ bacteria among survivors were less than 1% with all the R factors studied).

Several mutants resistant to 150 μg/ml of flavomycin were isolated from CSH-2 R⁺ in multiple-step selections on flavomycin-containing nutrient agar. The R factors of these mutants as well as the original R factors were transferred to W677/PTS. The M. I. C. of flavomycin was compared for these R⁺ clones of W677/PTS but no difference was found among them, indicating that the mutations of R⁺ bacteria to flavomycin resistance are not mediated by R factors.

Table 4

KILLING EFFECT OF FLAVOMYCIN ON *ESCHERICHIA COLI* STRAINS WITH
AND WITHOUT R FACTORS

Flavomycin concentration (μg/ml.)	Surviving bacteria/ml.*		
	CSH$-$2 (R1$-$19)	CSH$-$2 (R64$-$11)	W677/PTS
0	5.3×10^8	7.9×10^8	2.3×10^8
5	4.9×10^7	3.7×10^6	2.5×10^8
10	3.2×10^7	1.9×10^6	2.3×10^8
20	9.8×10^6	9.0×10^5	1.5×10^8
40	9.2×10^6	8.0×10^5	4.0×10^7

* 8.5 ml. of a broth culture of *E. coli* W677/PTS (O. D. 0.4), 1 ml. of broth and 0.5 ml. of varying concentrations of flavomycin solution were mixed and incubated at 37° C for 60 min. In the series with CSH$-$2 (R1$-$19) and CSH$-$2 (R64$-$11), 1 ml. of a broth culture (O. D. 0.4), 8.5 ml. of broth and 0.5 ml. of varying concentrations of flavomycin solution were mixed and incubated at 37° C for 60 min.

DISCUSSION AND CONCLUSIONS

It has been described above that R factors, F and colicin agent Ib in *E. coli* and R factors in *S. typhimurium* increase the flavomycin sensitivity of the host bacteria. The fact that non-repressed type episomes give more marked flavomycin sensitivity to their host bacteria than self-repressed types suggests that the presence of sex pili may be responsible for the increased flavomycin sensitivity of bacteria. The finding that *def*F without fertility does not change the flavomycin sensitivity of the host bacteria also supports this view. Type 1 pili apparently have no connection with the flavomycin sensitivity of bacteria. The increased flavomycin sensitivity of B380 F$^-$ may be due to an unknown, additional mutation. Prophage λ also seems to have no effect on the flavomycin sensitivity of the host bacteria in view of the data shown in Table 2. It is interesting to note that MITSUHASHI et al. (1970), independently of our work, found that macarbomycin, an antibiotic which is chemically related to but definitely distinct from flavomycin (TAKAHASHI, OKANISHI, UTAHARA, NITTA, MAEDA, and UMEZAWA, 1970), has a similar action on episome-carrying *E. coli*. Our comparative studies of flavomycin and macarbomycin (supplied by Meiji Seika Co., Tokyo) have disclosed that flavomycin has anti-bacterial activity twice stronger than macarbomycin and that cross resistance occurs between these two antibiotics in both CSH-2 R$^-$ and R$^+$ strains. These findings will be reported later.

The mechanism of action of flavomycin on *Staphylococcus aureus* was found to be due to the inhibition of cell wall synthesis (HUBER and NESEMANN, 1968). Lysis of bacteria in a hypotonic medium by a similar mechanism may probably be occurring also in *E. coli* and *S. typhimurium* assuming from the reduction in turbidity of bacterial cultures during their growth in flavomycin-containing broth and from the spheroplast formation in isotonic media containing flavomycin. The presence of sex pili may probably facilitate the permeation of flavomycin into the cells. An alternative possibility is that the presence of episomal elements (particularly those in non-repressed states) may induce some other mechanism of increased sensitivity of the cells to flavomycin simultaneously with the formation of sex pili.

The fact that bacteria with R factors are more sensitive to flavomycin than R$^-$ bacteria seems to offer a great advantage to this antibiotic as a feed additive together with its low toxicity and its extremely low absorbability through intestines (BAUER and DOST, 1966).

It draws our particular attention that R+ bacteria with sex pili (and therefore with conjugal donor ability) have more marked sensitivity to flavomycin. Bacteria with R factors can mutate to flavomycin resistance, but this resistance is not mediated by R factors and is likely to be due to chromosomal gene mutations. Thus flavomycin seems to satisfy the requirements of the Swann Report and to have an additional advantage that it probably does not increase R+ bacteria in animals as well as *in vitro*. Furthermore, flavomycin is likely to reduce R+ bacteria in animal intestines, although *in vivo* studies should be performed before we can draw a definitive conclusion on this point.

We acknowledge the receipt of bacterial strains, flavomycin and macarbomycin. This investigation was supported by U. S. Public Health Service research grant AI-08078 from the National Institute of Allergy and Infectious Diseases. A part of the content of this paper has been reported at the VIIth International Congress of Chemotherapy in August, 1971 in Prague.

REFERENCES

ANDERSON, E. S. (1968): The ecology of transferable drug resistence in the enterobacteria. Ann. Rev. Microbiol., **22**: 131–180.

BAUER, F. and DOST, G. (1966): Moenomycin in animal nutrition. Antimicrob. Agents & Chemother. – 1965, 749–752.

BRINTON, C. C., Jr. (1965): The structure, function, synthesis and genetic control of bacterial pili and a molecular model for DNA and RNA transport in gram negative bacteria. Trans. N. Y. Acad. Sci., **27**: 1003–1054.

EDWARDS, S. and MEYNELL, G. G. (1968): A general method for isolating derepressed bacterial sex factors. Nature, **219**: 869–870.

HUBER, G. and NESEMANN, G. (1968): Moenomycin, an inhibitor of cell wall synthesis. Biochem. Biophys. Res. Commun., **30**: 7–13.

HUBER, G., SCHACHT, U., WEIDENMÜLLER, H. L., SCHMIDT-THOME, J., DUPHORN, J. and TSCHESCHE, R. (1966): Moenomycin, a new antibiotic. II. Characterization and chemistry. Antimicrob. Agents & Chemother. – 1965, 737–742.

JUKES, T. H. (1955): *Antibiotics in Nutrition*. Medical Encyklopedia Inc., New York.

MEYNELL, E. and COOKE, M. (1969): Repressor-minus and operatorconstitutive, derepressed mutants of F-like R factors. Genet. Res., Camb., **14**: 309–313.

MEYNELL, E. and DATTA, N. (1967): Mutant drug resistance factors of high transmissibility. Nature, **214**: 885–887.

MEYNELL, E., MEYNELL, G. G. and DATTA, N. (1968): Phylogenetic relationships of drug-resistance factors and other transmissible bacterial plasmids. Bacteriol. Rev., **32**: 55–83.

MITSUHASHI, S., IYOBE, S., HASHIMOTO, H. and UMEZAWA, H. (1970): Preferential inhibition of the growth of *Escherichia coli* strains carrying episomes. J. Antibiot., **23**: 319–323.

NOVICK, R. P. (1969): Extrachromosomal inheritance in bacteria. Bacteriol. Rev., **33**: 210–235.

OHKI, M. and OZEKI, H. (1968): Isolation of conjugation-constitutive mutants of colicin factor Ib. Molec. Gen. Genet., **103**: 37–41.

SMITH, H. W. and HALLS, S. (1966): Observations on infective drug resistance in Britain. Brit. Med. J., **1**: 266–269.

STOKSTAD, E. L. R. (1954): Antibiotics in animal nutrition. Physiol. Rev., **34**: 25–51.

Swann Report: *Report of Joint Committee on the Use of Antibiotics in Animal Husbandary and Veterinary Medicine*, Her Majesty's Stationery Office, London (1969).

TAKAHASHI, S., OKANISHI, A., UTAHARA, R. NITTA, K., MAEDA, K. and UMEZAWA, H. (1970): Macarbomycin, a new antibiotic containing phosphorus. J. Antibiot., **23**: 48–50.

TUREK, F., LETTNER, F. and STEINACKER, G. (1967): Kückenmastversuch mit dem Antibiotikum Flavomycin. Die Bodenkultur, **18**: 147–151.

WALLHAUSER, K. H., NESEMANN, G., PRAVE, P. and STEIGLER, A. (1966): Moenomycin, a new antibiotic. I. Fermentation and isolation. Antimicrob. Agents & Chemother. – 1965, 734=736.

Von WASIELEWSKI, E., MUSCHAWECK, R. and SCHÜTZB, E. (1966): Moenomycin, a new antibiotic. III. Biological properties. Antimicrob. Agents & Chemother. – 1965, 743–748.

WATANABE, T., FUKASAWA, T. and TAKANO, T. (1962): Conversion of male bacteria of *Escherichia coli* K12 to resistance to phages by infection with the episome „resistance transfer factor." Virology, **17**: 218–219.

WATANABE, T. & LYANG, K. W. (1962): Episome-mediated transfer of drug resistance in *Enterobacteriaceae*. V. Spontaneous segregation and recombination of resistance factors in *Salmonella typhimurium*. J. Bacteriol., **83**: 422—430.

WATANABE, T., NISHIDA, H., OGATA, C., ARAI, T. and SATO, S. (1964): Episome-mediated transfer of drug resistance in *Enterobacteriaceae*. VII. Two types of naturally occuring R factors. J. Bacteriol., **88**: 716—726.

WATANABE, T. and OKADA, M. (1965): Mating induced by colicinogenic factor B in an F⁻ strain of *Escherichia coli* K12. Symp. Biol. Hung., **6**: 97—99.

AN IMPROVED TECHNIQUE FOR QUANTITATIVE DETECTION OF FECAL COLIFORMS AND PSEUDOMONAS AERUGINOSA ON SURFACES AND IN AIR

N. J. PETERSEN, M. S. FAVERO, W. BOND, L. A. CARSON, J. H. MARSHALL, and D. E. COLLINS

Biophysic Unit, Public Health Service, Phoenix, Arizona, U. S. A.

The changing character of nosocomial infections has been clearly evident in recent years. The emergence of Gram-negative bacilli as prominent pathogens in hospital acquired infections has been documented in the United States by KESSNER and LEPPER (1967) as well as EICKHOFF, BRACHMAN, BENNETT, and BROWN (1969). The work of ISENBERG (1971), among others, suggests that factors associated with the hospital environment may play a role in the evolving pattern of nosocomial infections. However, there are few studies relating the prevalence of such infections to the levels of Gram-negative bacilli associated with the hospital environment. Quantitative determinations of antibiotic resistance patterns among the Gram-negative flora of hospitals also are lacking. One reason for the dearth of data in this area has been the difficulty in making meaningful quantitative measurements of potentially pathogenic Gram-negative bacilli on surfaces and in air.

Techniques are available for assessing the total level of microorganisms on surfaces and in air using relatively rich primary recovery media. Similarly, selective media are available for the isolation of specific Gram-negative bacilli from clinical specimens. The need for a system to quantitatively determine the levels of specific Gram-negative bacilli on surfaces and in air prompted the studies reported here. It was reasoned that such a system could be used to identify reservoirs, transmission routes and antibiotic resistance patterns of Gram-negative pathogens in the hospital environment.

Initial efforts concentrated on the detection and enumeration of fecal coliform bacteria associated with the intramural hospital environment. This group of Gram-negative microorganisms was selected because it is composed of members such as *Escherichia* spp. and *Klebsiella* spp. which not only are part of the indigenous flora of humans, but are frequently incriminated in nosocomial infections. In addition, the group can be easily identified. Studies by HAJNA and PERRY (1943) showed that the use of E. C. broth at elevated incubation temperatures (*i. e.*, 44.5° C) provided a more valid estimation of coliform bacteria of fecal origin than the standard presumptive (production of gas in lactose broth at 37° C) and confirmed (production of gas in brilliant green lactose bile broth at 37 °C) tests for coliform bacteria. GELDREICH, CLARK, HUFF, and BEST (1965) furthered this basic concept by using elevated temperature and a selective-differential medium, subsequently designated FC medium, which was used in conjunction with the membrane filter procedure. GELDREICH (1967) showed that there was a positive correlation between coliform colonies detected with this procedure and their fecal origin. The elevated temperature, which is the primary selective factor, was responsible for the detection of not only *Escherichia coli*, but also other coliform types which were derived

115

from feces of warm blooded animals. Further tests demonstrated that 93 per cent of typical colonies developing on the membrane filter after incubation at 44.5° C confirmed as fecal coliform bacteria in E. C. broth.

In our study, fecal coliform bacteria are defined according to the criteria listed in Standard Methods for the Examination of WATER and WASTEWATER (1965), i. e., those bacteria that produce gas in E. C. broth when incubated at 44.5° C for 24 hours. Bacteria which produce gas in lactose broth and brilliant green lactose bile broth (37° C) but do not produce gas in E. C. broth are designated as non-fecal coliforms.

A variety of sampling procedures and culture media was used during the evolution of an assay procedure for the rapid detection and identification of fecal coliform bacteria. A series of surveys of environmental microbial contamination in pediatric and surgical wards of six hospitals provided the data for the evaluation of these procedures. In a typical enrironmental survey, airborne microbial contamination was measured in each room and in hallways using two slit samplers operated for 30 min at 28.3 LPM at each sampling site. One sampler contained a plate of Trypticase Soy Agar (TSA; BBL[1] [Trypticase peptone 1.5%, Phytone peptone 0.5%, NaCl 0.5%, and Agar 1.5%]) and the other a plate of MacConkey's Agar (MAC; Difco [Peptone 1.7%, Proteose peptone 0.3%, Lactose 1.0%, Bile Salts No. 3, 0.15%, NaCl 0.5%, Agar 1.35%, Neutral Red 0.003%, and Crystal Violet 0,0001%]). Surface contamination was measured by pressing TSA Rodac (Falcon Plastics, Division of Becton — Dickinson Co.) plates and MAC Rodac plates against the floor near each bed and in the hallways. This sampling technique described by HALL and HARTNETT (1964) utilizes a disposable agar contact plate to which viable surface particles adhere and on which they can be cultured.

Air sampling and TSA Rodac plates were incubated at 37° C and colonies counted at 48 hr to measure total microbial contamination in terms of viable particles per unit volume and area, respectively. Air sampling and MAC Rodac plates were incubated for 48 hr at 37° C. Typical coliform-like colonies were picked from MAC plates and inoculated into lactose broth (Difco [Beef Extract 0.3%, Peptone 0.5%, and Lactose 0.5%]). Isolates which were gas positive in lactose broth after incubation at 37° C were confirmed as coliform bacteria in brilliant green lactose bile broth (BGLB; Difco [Peptone 1.0%, Lactose 1.0%, Oxgall 2.0%, and Brilliant Green 0.00133%]). In both instances incubation was at 37° C for 48 hours. Of 269 coliform-like colonies picked from MAC plates in the first survey, only 55 colonies or 20 percent confirmed as coliforms.

In view of the relatively inefficient detection of coliform organisms in environmental samples collected on MAC plates, efforts were made to find a more discriminating medium for sampling. Accordingly, Bacto-m-FC agar (Difco [Tryptose 1.0%, Proteose Peptone No. 3, 0.5%, Yeast Extract 0.3%, Lactose 1.25%, Bile Salts No. 3, 0.15%, NaCl 0.5%, Aniline Blue 0.01%, Agar 1.5%, and Rosalic Acid (in 0.2N NaOH) 0.0001%]) was evaluated for this purpose. Since this medium had been used predominantly in the broth form with the membrane filter technique for testing the microbiological quality of water, it was necessary to determine whether or not the solid agar medium could be employed directly without altering the reliability originally reported by GELDREICH, et. al. (1965).

Using rectal swabs as a source of fecal coliform bacteria, streaks for isolated colonies were made on FC agar plates which were incubated at 44.5° C for 24 hr. A total of 82 colonies were picked from these plates and inoculated into lactose broth. The isolates represented a variety of colony types ranging in color from dark blue through green and tan to clear. Sixty of the selected colonies were blue or green in color and were considered

---

[1] Use of trade names are for identification only and does not constitute endorsement by the Public Health Service or by the U.S. Department of Health, Education, and Welfare.

typical. The remaining 22 colonies were considered atypical. Isolates in gas positive lactose tubes were confirmed for coliform and fecal coliform bacteria in brilliant green lactose bile broth and E. C. broth (BBL [Trypticase Peptone 2.0%, Lactose 0.5%, Bile Salts Mixture 0.15%, K_2HPO_4 0.4%, KH_2PO_4 0.15%, and NaCl 0.5%]), respectively. Tubes containing E. C. broth were incubated in a circulating water bath at 44.5° C ±0.2° C for 24 hours.

It was found that 92 per cent of all typical colonies isolated confirmed as fecal coliforms. This was in good agreement with the results of investigators who used this medium in water microbiology. Of considerable interest was the finding that 68% of the 22 atypical colonies also confirmed as fecal coliforms.

Assured of the reliability of FC agar when used in other than membrane filter techniques, an attempt was made to use this medium in both air and surface sampling of the environment during the third hospital survey. However, FC agar appeared to be a poor primary sampling medium because no typical colonies and only three atypical colonies were detected from 90 samples. None of the three atypical colonies confirmed as fecal coliforms. Subsequent comparison of FC agar as the sole sampling medium with bacteria initially cultured on TSA and then replicated onto FC agar substantiated the conclusion that it does not perform well as a primary recovery medium for fecal coliforms in the environment.

Accurate enumeration of environmentally stressed enteric bacteria from air and surface samples is often hampered when selective media are employed. Based on the rationale that environmentally stressed bacteria would be more apt to grow out initially on a relatively rich medium such as TSA than on one that is selective in nature, several laboratory experiments were conducted to develop a rapid method of quantitatively transferring colonies growing on TSA air sampling and Rodac plates to FC agar so that fecal coliform bacteria could be enumerated. Several replicate plating techniques were investigated for this purpose. The technique which produced the best results utilized sterile velvet as the transferring surface. Air sampling and TSA Rodac plates were incubated at 37°·C for 24 hr and colonies were counted. A piece of sterile velvet (46 cm × 97 cm) was taped to a flat work surface in a laminar flow clean bench. The clean bench protected the velvet from extraneous contamination and has been described by Favero and Berquist (1968). Each TSA Rodac plate was pressed lightly against the velvet surface in a position marked by a circle on the velvet. An FC agar Rodac plate was then lightly touched to the velvet in the same position and subsequently incubated at 44.5° C for 24 hours. This procedure permitted replication of colonies from 50 Rodac plates in approximately 15 minutes. The reliability of the technique was tested by replicating 10 TSA Rodac plates, each having 10 colonies of a known fecal coliform. All 100 colonies were reproduced as typical fecal coliform colonies on FC agar plates.

Colonies on large (150 mm diam.) plates of TSA used for air sampling were similarly replicated onto 150 mm plates of FC agar using by a 23 cm × 23 cm piece of sterile velvet tightened over a circular form having an outside diameter just slightly smaller than the inside diameter of the plate. After incubation, typical colonies appearing on the FC agar were counted and picked for confirmation as fecal coliform bacteria. This technique was used in 15 surveys in which each replicated TSA air sample or Rodac sample was matched with a MAC sample from a contiguous site. This permitted compilation of data comparing the recovery of fecal coliform bacteria replicated on FC agar with the recovery of fecal coliforms collected directly on MAC agar.

Table 1 presents data from 15 pediatric and surgical ward surveys. Based on 170 matched air samples, fecal coliforms were detected on 22 per cent of replicated FC agar plates compared with 2 per cent of the MAC plates. The FC agar also produced superior

117

results on Rodac samples although the difference was not as marked. Seventy of 1017 FC agar Rodac plates were positive for fecal coliforms compared with 41 of 1017 MAC plates, or 7 and 4 per cent, respectively. The two media did equally well in recovering non-fecal coliforms. The efficiency of FC agar in detecting fecal coliforms was found to be

Table 1

ENVIRONMENTAL AIR AND SURFACE SAMPLES POSITIVE FOR COLIFORMS ON FC AGAR AND MACCONKEY'S AGAR

Sample Type	Number Samples Tested	Samples Positive for Fecal Coliforms		Samples Positive for Non-fecal Coliforms	
		Number	Percent	Number	Percent
TSA Air Samples Replicated on FC Agar	170	38	22	36	21
MacConkey's Agar Air Samples	170	4	2	34	18
TSA Surface Samples Replicated on FC Agar	1017	70	7	106	10
MacConkey's Agar Surface Samples	1017	41	4	121	12

considerably higher than that for MAC as shown in Table 2. Thirty-five per cent of all typical colonies picked from FC agar confirmed as fecal coliforms, while only eight per cent of coliform-like colonies picked from MAC plates confirmed as fecal coliforms.

Table 2

DETECTION ON FC AGAR AND MACCONKEY'S AGAR OF COLIFORM BACTERIA BASED ON SELECTION OF TYPICAL COLONIES FROM ENVIRONMENTAL SAMPLES

Medium	Number Colonies Picked	Fecal Coliforms		Non-fecal Coliforms		Total Colifroms	
		Number	Percent	Number	Percent	Number	Percent
TSA Replicated onto FC Agar	416	144	35	161	39	305	73
MacConkey's Agar	322	26	8	113	35	139	43

It was obvious that typical colonies picked from environmental samples on FC agar did not confirm as fecal coliforms with the efficiency found for both water and rectal swab samples (92 to 93 per cent). No explanation can be offered for this difference. HOWEVER, GELDREICH (1969) noted that the relatively heavy inocula of actively growing cells involved in the replicating technique differed greatly from the inocula for which the medium was designed. It was observed that the use of heavy inocula reduced the selectivity of the medium resulting in a greater frequency of false positive colonies.

Both fecal coliforms and non-fecal coliforms isolated from pediatric and surgical wards during 24 surveys were identified to genus. The distribution of these isolates by genus is presented in Table 3. It was found that the genera *Escherichia* and *Klebsiella* accounted for

118

92 per cent of the fecal coliforms, while the genus *Enterobacter* was predominant in the non-fecal coliform group. Because the source of non-fecal coliforms is ordinarily not a warm blooded animal, the frequency with which these microorganisms were found in the hospital environment was surprising. More surprising was that 11 per cent of non-fecal coliforms were *Escherichia*. These findings suggest that the standard tests used in water microbiology to differentiate fecal and non-fecal coliforms may be inappropriate for coliforms isolated from the hospital environment.

Table 3

DISTRIBUTION BY GENUS OF FECAL AND NON-FECAL COLIFORMS FROM ENVIRONMENTAL SAMPLES

Coliform Type	Number Identified	GENUS					
		Escherichia		*Klebsiella*		*Enterobacter*	
		Number	Percent	Number	Percent	Number	Percent
Fecal	144	53	37	80	55	11	8
Non-fecal	158	17	11	35	22	106	67

Typical colonies appearing on an FC agar replicate plate can be enumerated and an estimate of airborne or surface contamination can be made based on this number. In 24 surveys of eight different pediatric and surgical wards, it was found that the concentrations ranged from 0 to 2.1 fecal coliform particles per cubic meter of air with a mean value of 0.7. The mean value for surface contamination was 87 fecal coliform particles per square meter with a range of 28 to 194. The relatively infrequent occurrence of these microorganisms among the total microbial population in the hospital environment can be appreciated by noting that in these wards approximately one out of every 1000 viable airborne particles and five out of every 1000 viable surface particles was a fecal coliform. However, no data are available indicating how accurately this system measures the actual level of environmental contamination with organisms of fecal origin. In an effort to estimate the efficiency of the technique described here for enumerating airborne fecal coliforms, a comparison was made with a three-stage glass impinger described by MAY (1966). This impinger was reported to have a high sampling efficiency for aerosolized *E. coli*. Twenty-four paired samples were collected in a pediatric ward by operating the impinger and slit sampler simultaneously, side by side. The impinger was operated in accordance with the instructions of its developer and the replication technique was used with the slit sampler. In 21 of 24 paired samples, the slit sampler detected equal or greater numbers of airborne microorganisms than did the impinger. A fecal coliform was never recovered using the liquid impinger, while 10 out of 24 replicated samples from the slit sampler were positive for fecal coliforms. Although it was concluded that the replication technique was superior to the impinger in detecting airborne fecal coliforms in the hospital environment, the true sampling efficiency of the technique is still not known.

The key feature of this system is that a relative quantitation of specific Gram-negative bacilli in environmental samples is achieved. PETERSEN, BRIGHAM, MARSHALL, VENICE, BOND and FAVERO (1970) demonstrated the possible value of quantitating environmental fecal coliforms by conducting two surveys in a pediatric ward in which both epidemiological data and microbiological culture data on the patients were collected. A concomitant decrease in the prevalence of gastrointestinal illness, throat swabs positive for *E. coli*, and environmental samples positive for microorganisms of fecal origin from the first survey to the second survey suggested a direct relationship between environmental contamination and gastrointestinal illness. In addition, an airborne route of transmission was suggested.

The replication technique was also used to detect and enumerate other microorganisms, particularly *Pseudomonas aeruginosa*. After inoculating an FC agar plate from the velvet, a Pseudosel Agar (BBL [Gelysate Peptone 2.0%, $MgCl_2$ 0.14%, K_2SO_4 1.0%, Agar 1.36%, and Cetrimide[2] 0.03%]) plate was pressed against the same surface. In this manner, a single survey provided quantitative and qualitative data concerning several types of organisms of medical significance. Pseudosel Agar plates were incubated at 37° C for 24 hours and examined for green fluorescing colonies typical of *P. aeruginosa*. All suspicious colonies were picked and inoculated into Asparagine broth (K_2HPO_4 0.1%, $MgSO_4$ 0.05%, Asparagine 0.3%). The tubes were incubated at 37° C and observed for fluorescence under UV light (long wave) after 24 and 48 hours. Tubes showing fluorescence were selected, and 0.1 ml from each inoculated into Acetamide broth (NaCl 0.5%, K_2HPO_4 0.14%, KH_2PO_4 0.07%, $MgSO_4$ 0.05%, Acetamide 0.1%, and Phenol red 0.001%). The presence of *P. aeruginosa* was confirmed by strong alkaline reaction in Acetamide broth in 24 hours. Pseudosel Agar was shown to replicate *P. aeruginosa* colonies from TSA with 100 per cent efficiency and approximately 70 per cent of all suspicious colonies isolated from Pseudosel Agar replicates of environmental samples confirmed as *P. aeruginosa*.

P. aeruginosa was frequently found in inhalation therapy equipment in the wards surveyed in this study, demonstrating the ability to grow rapidly in distilled water as described by FAVERO, CARSON, BOND, and PETERSEN (1971). Using the replication technique, *P. aeruginosa* was detected in environmental samples from all but one of the eight wards routinely surveyed. However, in spite of the high numbers of these microorganisms present in various water reservoirs, the levels of *P. aeruginosa* in air and on surfaces were about a log lower than those determined for fecal coliforms.

While the replication procedures described here have yet to be applied to a comprehensive epidemiological study of nosocomial infections, it is felt than an improved technique now exists for detecting and enumerating specific Gram-negative bacilli present in the hospital environment. Hopefully, this tool will provide a means of better defining the role of the environment in nosocomial infections, including effects on the antibiotic resistance patterns in the hospital microflora.

REFERENCES

EICKHOFF, T. C., BRACHMAN, P. S., BENNETT, J. V., and BROWN, J. F. (1967): Surveillance nosocomial infections in community hospitals. I. Surveillance methods, effectiveness, and of initial results. Journal of Infectious Diseases, 120/3, 305.

FAVERO, M. S., and BERQUIST, K. R. (1968): Use of laminar air-flow equipment in microbiology. Applied Microbiology, 16/1[2] 182.

FAVERO, M. S., CARSON, L. A., BOND, W. W., and PETERSEN, N. J. (1967): Crowth of *Pseudomonas aeruginosa* in distilled water from hospitals. Science, 173/3999.

GELDREICH, E. E., CLARK, H. F., HUFF, C. B., and BEST, L. C. (1965): Fecal-coliform-organism medium for the membrane filter technique. Journal of American Water Works Association, 57/208, 214.

GELDREICH, E. E. (1967): Fecal coliform concepts in stream pollution. Water and Sewage Works, 1967 Edition.

GELDREICH, E. E. (1969): Personal communication.

HAJNA, A. A., and PERRY, C. A. (1943): Comparative study of presumptive and confirmative

[2] Trade name for Cetyl trimethyl ammonium bromide.

media for bacteria of the coliform group and for fecal streptococci. American Journal of Public Health, **33**, 550.

HALL, L. B., and HARTNETT, M. J. (1964): Measurement of the bacterial contamination on surfaces in hospitals. Public Health Reports, **79**, 1021.

ISENBERG, H. D., and BERKMAN, J. I. (1971): The role of drug-resistant and drug-selected bacteria in nosocomial disease. Annals of the New York Academy of Science, **182**, 42.

KESSNER, D. M., and LEPPER, M. H. (1967): Epidemiologic studies of Gram-negative bacilli in the hospital and community. American Journal of Epidemiology, **85**, 45.

MAY, K. R. (1966): Multistage liquid impinger. Bacteriological Reviews, **30/3**, 559.

PETERSEN, N. J., BRIGHAM, K. L., MARSHALL, J. H., VENICE, L. A., BOND, W. W., and FAVERO, M. S. (1970): Relationships between the prevalence of gastrointestinal disease and environmental contamination on a pediatric ward, Arizona Medicine, **27/10**, 5.

Standard Methods for the Examination of Water and Wastewater, 12th Edition. American Public Health Association. New York. (1965.)

DEVELOPMENT OF RESISTANCE AND ITS SUPPRESSION UNDER THE INFLUENCE OF VARIOUS PENICILLINS

W. RITZERFELD

Institute of Hygiene, University of Münster, G. F. R.

The resistance of pathogenically important microorganisms against antibiotics — caused either by selection or by chromosomal and especially extrachromosomal mechanisms — is of interest to the physician as well as to the medical microbiologist. Our own research work was performed on the resistance of more than 6000 bacterial strains collected from urine specimens in 1970. The antibacterial substances used were those that are commonly employed in the plate diffusion test, which is conducted on DST-agar with discs supplied by the manufacturer; abbreviations of the drugs: Peni = Penicillin G,

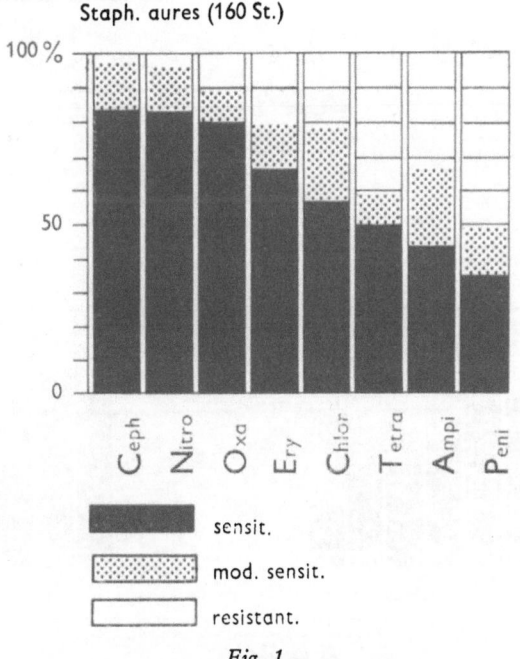

Fig. 1.

Ampi = Ampicillin, Oxa = Oxacillin, Carb = Carbenicillin, Ce = Cephalosporin, Ery = Erythromycin, Chlor — Chloramphenicol, Tetra = Tetracycline, Novo = Novobiocin, Kan = Kanamycin, Coli = Colistin, Gent = Gentamicin, Nitro =

Nitrofurantoin, Nali = Nalidixic acid. A controlled strain of known susceptibility was included in each test series. According to the results of the sensitivity testing, the bacterial strains were called "sensitive", "moderately sensitive" or "resistant". In the following discussion of the test results, particular emphasis was put on the individual types of Penicillin.

Fig. 1 shows the sensitivities of the Staphylococcus strains (n = 160). Some of the Penicillins yield quite favourable results. Cephalosporin and Oxacillin are highly effective whereas Ampicillin and Penicillin G are of little effect only. As to the former agents, however, strains of lesser susceptibilities than those tested here must be expected.

Fig. 2 reflects the situation of the *Enterococci* (n = 1440) in comparison to *Streptococcus viridans* (n = 510). Here it is quite evident that Ampicillin is superior to the other types

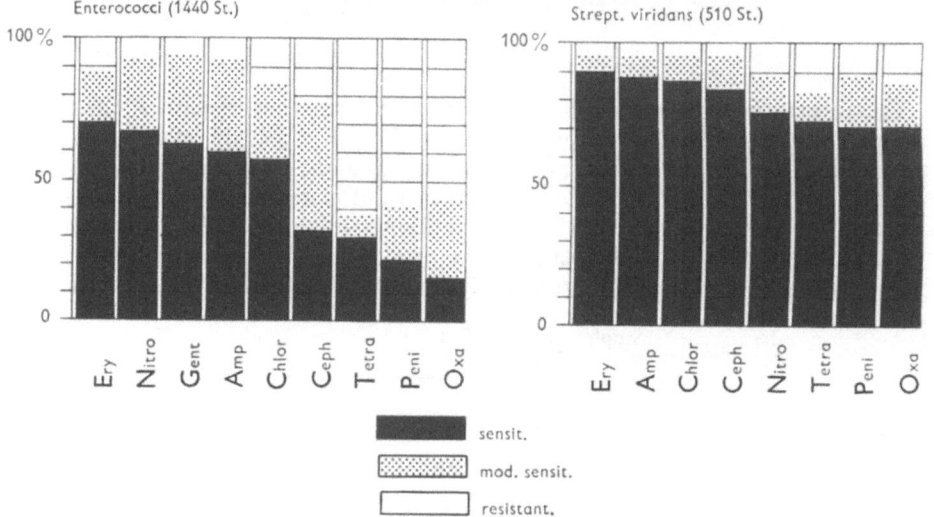

Fig. 2.

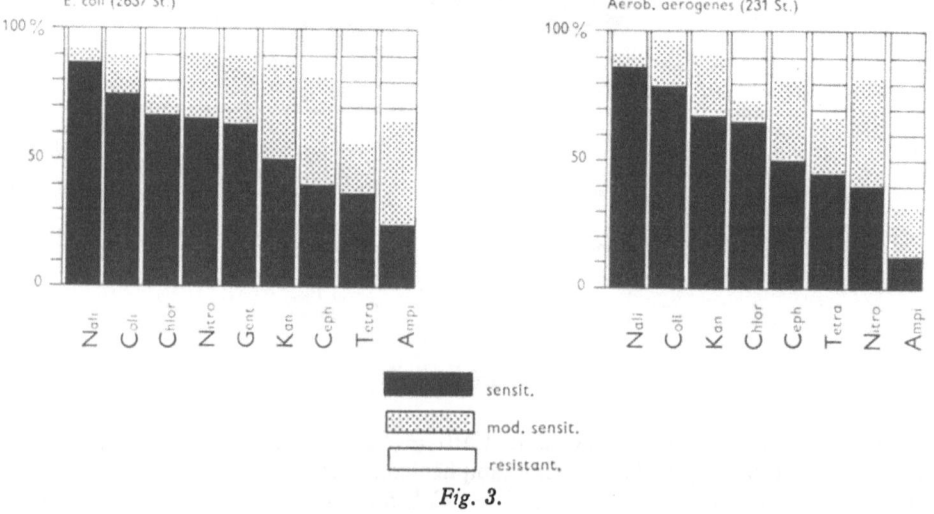

Fig. 3.

of Penicillin and yields the best effect. Penicillin G and Oxacillin appear at the far end of the graph.

Fig. 3 shows that E. coli (n = 2637) and Aerobacter aerogenes (n = 231) are fairly sensitive to Cephalosporin but not to Ampicillin.

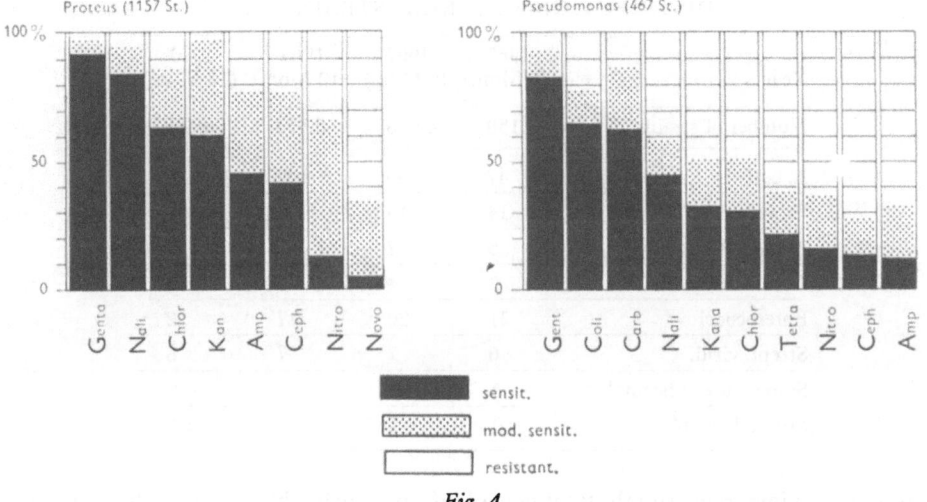

Fig. 4.

The resistance characteristics of *Proteus* (n = 1157) and *Pseudomonas* (n = 467) are shown in fig. 4. *Proteus* is moderately sensitive to Ampicillin and Cephalosporin, whereas *Pseudomonas appears* to be resistant against both of these drugs. *Pseudomonas* is sensitive to Carbenicillin, but some strains are observed to be moderately sensitive and resistant.

The results show that some types of Penicillin have a good effect, but resistant strains are to be expected frequently. Primarily this is true for the so-called problem bacteria: *Pseudomonas*, *Proteus* and *Enterococci* which are not only poorly sensitive but also have an increased rate of appearance.

Table 1

PROBLEM BACTERIA FROM SWABS
(18124 specimens)

Species	1959–1961 (n = 9754)	1968 (n = 4247)	1970 (n = 4123)
Pseudomonas	4%	11%	12%
Proteus	3%	8%	10%
Staph. a ureus	21%	16%	16%
Enterococci	5%	5%	7%

The increased rate of appearance in the periods 1959 to 1961, 1968 and in 1970 is shown in table 1 listing the proportional distribution of microorganisms including *Staph. aureus* which were collected from the swabs (n = 18124) sent mainly from hospitals of our district. The increase of *Pseudomonas* and *Proteus* is obvious within the past 10 years, while *Staph. aureus* is diminishing.

The distribution (%) of the strains (n = 19387), isolated in 1965, 1967, 1969 and 1970 from fresh urine specimens, is demonstrated in table 2. The significance of *Proteus*, *Pseudomonas* and *Enterococci* is evident.

Table 2

DISTRIBUTION OF URINE STRAINS (%)

Year	1965 (8 Mon.)	1967 (9 Mon.)	1969 (12 Mon.)	1970 (12 Mon.)
Number of strains	2.150	4.038	6.553	6.646
E. coli	47	46	42	40
Proteus	14	13	17	17
Pseudomonas	5	7	7	7
Aerob. aerogenes	2	4	6	3
Enterococci	21	20	17	22
Strept. virid.	6	7	7	8
Staph. aureus haemol.	5	3	3	2
Strept. haemol.	<1	<1	<1	<1

It is of great importance for the treatment of infections to be able to control these problem bacteria. In addition to new antibiotics, combinations of antibacterial agents are proposed to lead to an addition of the effect of one agent to the other or to an enhancement of the antibacterial effect of one of the agents only. It is also under discussion, whether the application of a combination of substances can prevent or diminish the development of resistant microorganisms. Pertinent studies were performed by us with Penicillin V and Oxacillin some time ago. We found that in vitro relatively small doses of Oxacillin made Penicillin V effective against bacterial strains which had been resistant to Penicillin V alone. Oxacillin probably inactivates penicillinase.

In this paper we report on our in vitro studies of Carbenicillin, Oxacillin and Flucloxacillin. We tried to answer the question whether the effect of Carbenicillin on bacteria could be influenced by adding Oxacillin or Flucloxacillin.

First, the effect of Oxacillin on the amount of Carbenicillin required to inhibit bacterial growth, was studied on each of 22 strains of *Enterococci* and *Pseudomonas*, and on 20 strains of Proteus. All of the strains were sensitive to Carbenicillin and resistant to Oxacillin at the beginning. In order to get resistant strains, they were repeatedly passed over DST-agar with Carbenicillin test discs (100 mcg). After 18 hrs. of incubation the inhibition zone was measured and material of this zone was picked up and spread on another agar plate. The strains were spread in a radial fashion around the test discs. Changes of the MIC-values were established by the use of tube dilution tests.

At the same time tests were done in a similar way for the inhibition of the development of bacterial resistance to Carbenicillin. In this test an Oxacillin test disc (100 mcg) was placed on the Carbenicillin test disc (100 mcg). Oxacillin by itself did not inhibit any growth of the strains studied. Again bacteria were taken from the inhibition zone and passed over agar plates about ten times. The tube dilution test was used to check for resistance to Carbenicillin.

The results of these studies are shown in fig. 5. Of 22 strains of *Pseudomonas* 14 were significantly more sensitive to Carbenicillin after treatment with a combination of

Carbenicillin and Oxacillin than after treatment with Carbenicillin alone which made them resistant. For 6 strains no differences were seen between those treated with a combination of Carbenicillin and Oxacillin and those treated with Carbenicillin alone. Only two strains were more resistant to Carbenicillin after treatment with the combination than after treatment with Carbenicillin alone.

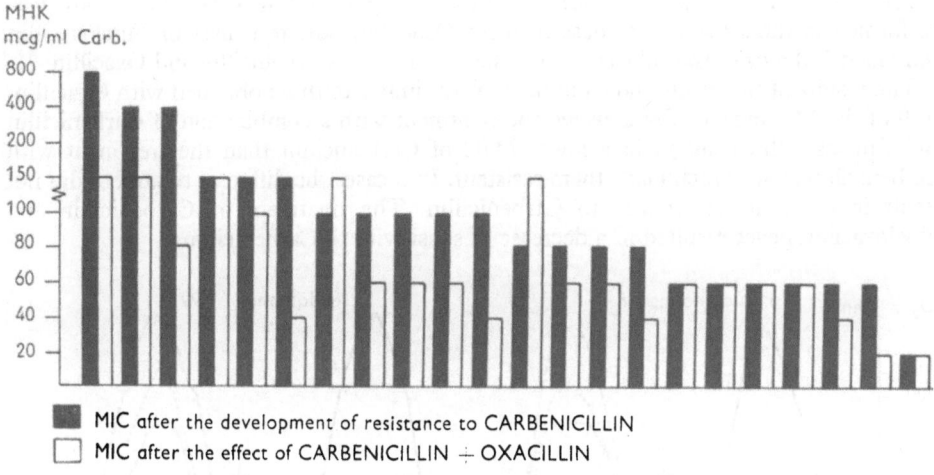

■ MIC after the development of resistance to CARBENICILLIN
☐ MIC after the effect of CARBENICILLIN + OXACILLIN

Fig. 5 MIC values of 22 pseudomonas strains.

The results obtained with *Enterococci* were similar. For 16 strains the MIC of Carbenicillin was lower in the group treated with a combination of Carbenicillin and Oxacillin than in the Carbenicillin treated controlled group. For 6 strains no differences were found.

No positive effect of the combination of Carbenicillin with Oxacillin was found for

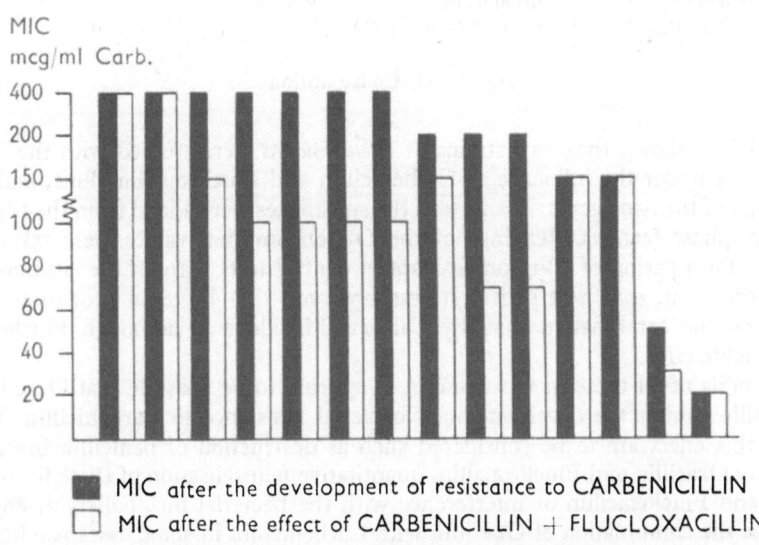

■ MIC after the development of resistance to CARBENICILLIN
☐ MIC after the effect of CARBENICILLIN + FLUCLOXACILLIN

Fig. 6 MIC values of 14 pseudomonas strains.

Proteus. Of the 20 strains 16 were equally sensitive to Carbenicillin after treatment with the combination and with Carbenicillin alone. 4 strains were less sensitive after treatment with Carbenicillin and Oxacillin.

Following these investigations, the effect of a combination of Carbenicillin with Flucloxacillin was studied in the same way. All of the 14 strains of *Pseudomonas* tested in this study, were resistant to Flucloxacillin (MIC more than 400 mcg/ml), and moderately sensitive to Carbenicillin with MIC's between 10 and 150 mcg/ml. The study was performed in the same way as described for Oxacillin. The test discs of Flucloxacillin contained 100 mcg of the substance, like the test discs of Carbenicillin and Oxacillin.

The results of this study shown in fig. 6 were similar to those obtained with Oxacillin. In 9 of the 14 strains of *Pseudomonas* the treatment with a combination of Carbenicillin and Flucloxacillin resulted in a lower MIC of Carbenicillin than the treatment with Carbenicillin alone which made them resistant. In 5 cases the different treatment did not result in different sensitivities to Carbenicillin. The treatment of Carbenicillin and Flucloxacillin never resulted in a decrease of sensitivity to Carbenicillin.

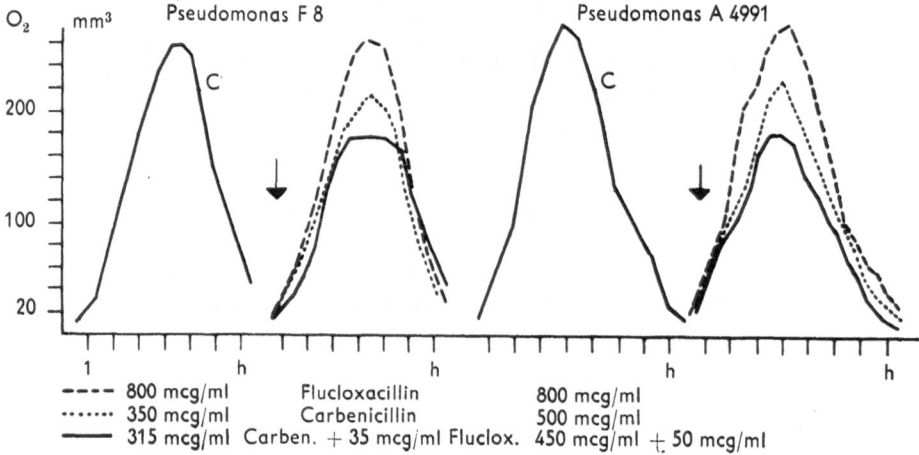

Fig. 7 O₂-Consumption

In fig. 7 it is shown that, two strains of *Pseudomonas* were studied with the O₂-consumption test under the influence of Carbenicillin and Flucloxacillin alone, and of the combination of the two agents. In this test, the substances were added from the beginning of the log. phase (arrow). Readings of the O₂-consumption values were taken every 25 minutes for a period of 20-minutes. Parallel control tests without the substances (C) were performed in each test series. It was observed that bacterial growth was more inhibited by the combination than by Carbenicillin alone — although Flucloxacillin alone was ineffective.

On the basis of all these in vitro results, it appears to be possible that Oxacillin and Flucloxacillin inhibit the development of bacterial resistance to Carbenicillin. Various causes of this effect are to be considered such as destruction of penicillin inactivating ferments by Oxacillin and Flucloxacillin, quantitative neutralisation of these ferments by Oxacillin and Flucloxacillin or interference with the bacterial metabolism at any other level. Since the combination of Oxacillin with Carbenicillin in some cases resulted in an elevation of the MIC of Carbenicillin it must be considered that formation of penicillinase can also be induced by Oxacillin. In vivo protein binding of Penicillins and other mechanisms might be important for the effectiveness of Penicillins and their combinations too.

We can support the concept of the colloque of the French association of microbiologists in December 1970 at the Institut Pasteur, concerning these problems of combination. Further research work is required to arrive at valid conclusions which possibly could be of significance for the therapist.

FISH CULTURING AND R FACTORS

TSUTOMU WATANABE*, TAKASHI AOKI**, CHIYO YADA*,
YASUKO OGATA*, KATOMI SUGAWARA*, TATSUO SAITO*,
and SYUZO EGUSA**

ABSTRACT

The results of our investigation of R factors related to fish culturing are summarized: Considerable fractions of *Aeromonas liquefaciens* and *Aeromonas salmonicida* strains isolated from diseased cultured fish have been found to carry R factors. These fish included eel (*Anguilla japonica*), carp (*Cyprinus carpio*), ayu (*Plecoglossus altivelis*), amago (*Oncorhynchus rhodurus* f. *macrostomus*) and brook trout (*Salvelinus fontinalis*). It has also been shown that gram-negative bacilli isolated from the intestines of normal-looking cultured fish as well as from the water of fish ponds carry R factors at high frequencies. A new finding reported here is the detection of R factors in *Vibrio* strains isolated from the intestines of normal-looking cultured yellowtails (*Seriola quinqueradiata*). R factors detected in *Aeromonas* strains exhibited some specificities; all of the R factors from *Aeromonas* strains so far studied belonged to the *fi⁻* type and yet they did not cause restriction of bacteriophages. A majority of them had the markers of resistance to sulfonamides and tetracyclines. The possible implication to public health of the R factors related to fish culturing is discussed.

INTRODUCTION

Fish culturing is an important industry in countries such as Japan, where fish meat serves as a major source of animal protein in food. Eel (*Anguilla japonica*), carp (*Cyprinus carpio*), rainbow trout (*Salmo gairdneri* f. *irideus*), ayu (*Plecoglossus altivelis*), amago (*Oncorhynchus rhodurus* f. *macrostomus*), yellowtail (*Seriola quinqueradiata*) and several other species of fish are cultured in Japan. Rainbow trout and some other species of fresh-water salmonid fish are cultured in many countries. Carp is cultured on relatively large scales in Germany, Israel and Eastern European countries, and channel catfish is cultured in the Mississippi delta area in the United States. France has recently started culturing eel and some salt-water fish. The techniques of fish culturing may differ depending on the species of fish and also from country to country. Figures 1 to 4 show some typical fish culturing farms in Japan.

It is usual in fish culturing to keep as many fish as possible in a limited space in order to increase productivity per unit space. Overcrowding tends to cause unfavourable conditions for the health of cultured fish, and bacterial infections of cultured fish occur frequently, sometimes giving tremendous losses to the fish culturists. Some typical bacterial infections of cultured fish are shown in Figures 5 to 10.

* Department of Microbiology, Kei o University School of Medicine, Tokyo, Japan
** Department of Fisheries, Faculty of Agriculture, The University of Tokyo, Tokyo, Japan

For the purpose of preventing and treating bacterial infections of cultured fish, various antibiotics and synthetic chemotherapeutic agents have been used as feed additives for fish in many countries like in livestock and poultry (SCHÄPERCLAUS, 1955, 1956, 1958; SNIESZKO, 1957, 1959; HOSHINA, 1962; WOLF and SNIESZKO, 1963). However, the growth promotion effect of these drugs is obscure in fish unlike in livestock and poultry (SNIESZKO, 1957, 1959). Chemotherapeutic agents are sometimes administered directly into fish ponds for drug bathing of fish to treat and prevent bacterial infections (MUROGA and EGUSA, 1968). The chemotherapeutic agents most widely used for fish culturing are sulfonamides (Su), nitrofuran derivatives, tetracyclines (Tc) and chloramphenicol (Cm).

We had suspected that the use of antibiotics and other chemotherapeutic agents for fish culturing may have caused an increase of drug-resistant strains of fish-pathogenic bacteria in view of the reported effects of antibiotic feeding on animal enteric bacteria (see ANDERSON, 1968; SMITH, 1969; the so-called Swann Report, 1969) and also from our experiences that the use of drugs to infected fish has sometimes been ineffective in treating the infections in recent years. We have in fact shown that a considerable fraction of *Aeromonas liquefaciens* strains isolated from cultured fish are resistant to several drugs (AOKI and EGUSA, 1971). The patterns of drug resistances of some of the drug-resistant *A. liquefaciens* strains suggested to us that their drug resistances might be due to R factors. Our preliminary study with two of such strains has shown that their drug resistances are indeed due to R factors (WATANABE, OGATA, AOKI, and EGUSA, 1969). In other words, their drug resistance markers were found transferable *en bloc* to *Escherichia coli* K-12 by mixed cultivation but cell-free culture filtrates of these drug-resistant *A. liquefaciens* strains could not convert *E. coli* K-12 to drug resistance, indicating that the drug resistances of these *A. liquefaciens* strains were controlled by R factors.

Then, a more extensive investigation has been carried out on the drug-resistant strains of *A. liquefaciens* isolated from diseased as well as healthy cultured fish and soft-shelled turtles (*Trionyx sinensis japonicus*), and a considerable fraction of them were found to carry R factors (AOKI, EGUSA, OGATA, and WATANABE, 1971). A majority of these R factors had the markers of resistance to Su and Tc and all of them were found to belong to the *fi⁻* type (see WATANABE, FUKASAWA, and TAKANO, 1962; WATANABE, NISHIDA, OGATA, ARAI and SATO, 1964 for *fi* type). R factor-carrying strains have been found also in *A. salmonicida*, which is known to cause infections in salmonid fish living in cold fresh water (AOKI, EGUSA, KIMURA, and WATANABE, 1971).

We have become interested in the origin of R factors of these drug-resistant *Aeromonas* strains and have suspected that they might have come from the bacteria in the water of fish ponds. We have investigated the gram-negative bacilli isolated from the water of fish ponds as well as from the intestines of normal-looking cultured fish to see the presence or absence and incidence of R factors, if present, in these bacteria. We have found that these bacteria carry R factors at high frequencies (WATANABE, AOKI, OGATA, and EGUSA, 1971).

Our current investigation has shown that *Vibrio* strains isolated from cultured salt-water fish yellowtails carry R factors at high frequencies. These results will be reported here together with the summaries of our already published data.

MATERIALS AND METHODS

Culture media used. Nutrient agar medium with 0.5% sodium chloride was used for isolating bacteria from fresh-water fish and from the intestines of fresh-water fish, and nutrient agar medium containing 3% sodium chloride was used for isolating bacteria from the intestines of yellowtails. BTB-lactose-nutrient agar medium containing 0.0045%

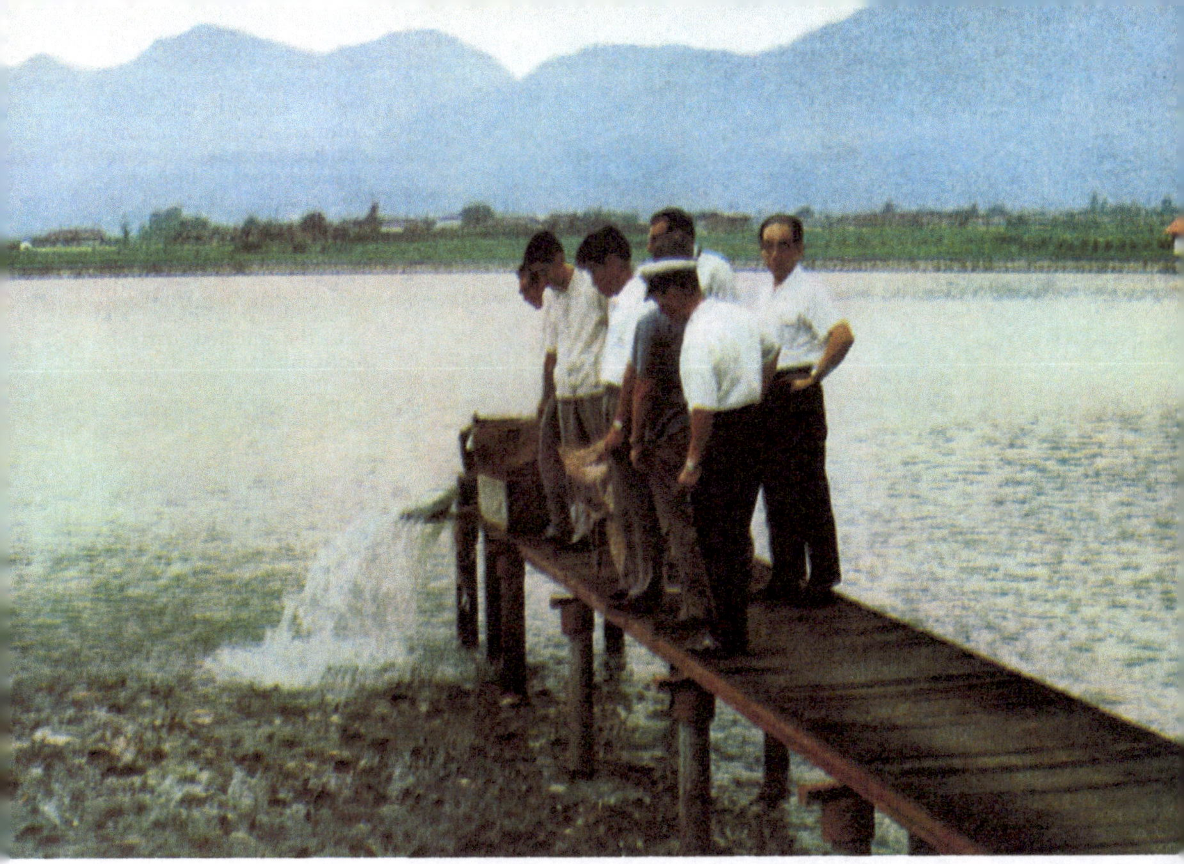

Fig. 1. A pond for culturing carp in Nagano Prefecture. The people are feeding carp.

Fig. 2. Ponds for culturing ayu in Shiga Prefecture. Ayu is cultured in running water. The water is either derived from rivers or lakes or pumped up from underground. Amago is cultured in more or less similar types of ponds but the water for culturing amago must be colder than that for ayu.

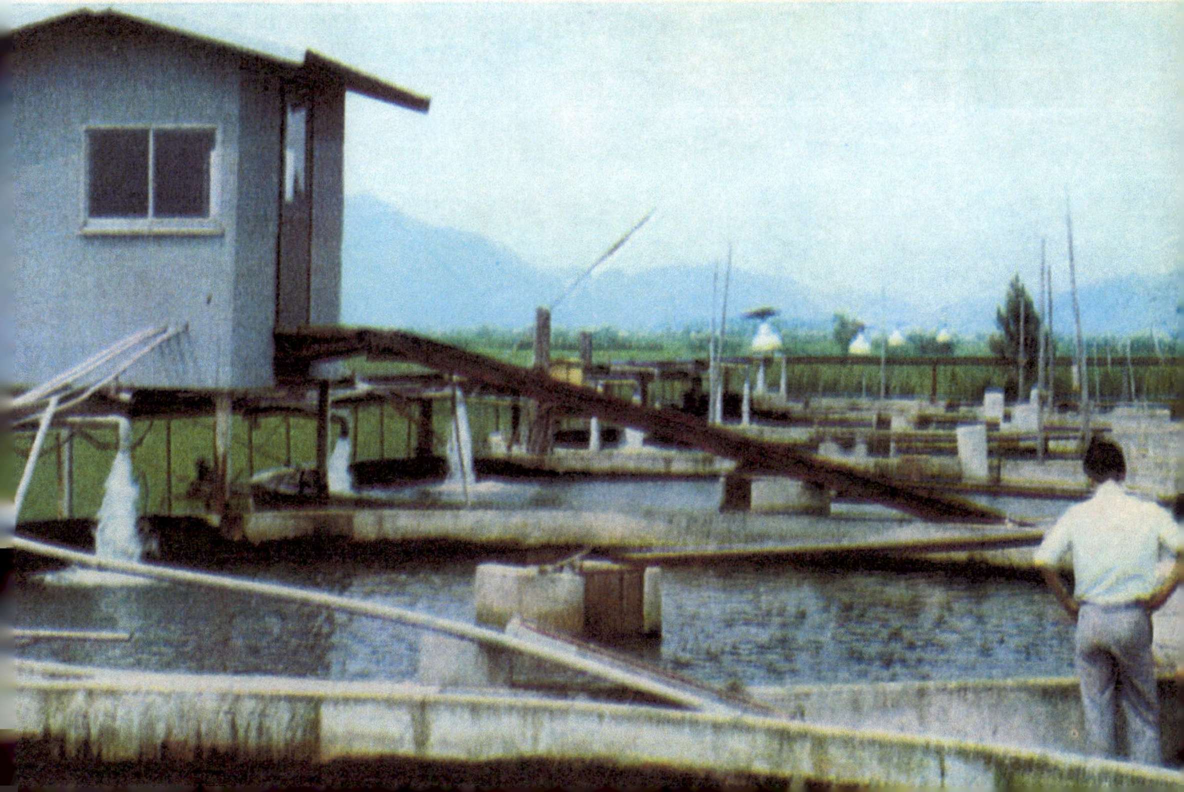

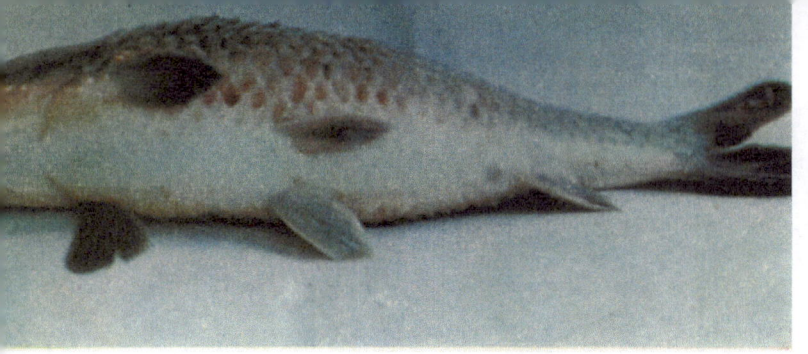

Fig. 5. Red-fin disease of cultured carp. Hyperemia and haemorrhage start from fins and spread throughout the entire surface of the body. Hyperemia and haemorrhage are observed also in various visceral organs. Red-fin disease is caused by *Aeromonas liquefaciens* and kills the infected carp by septicemia.

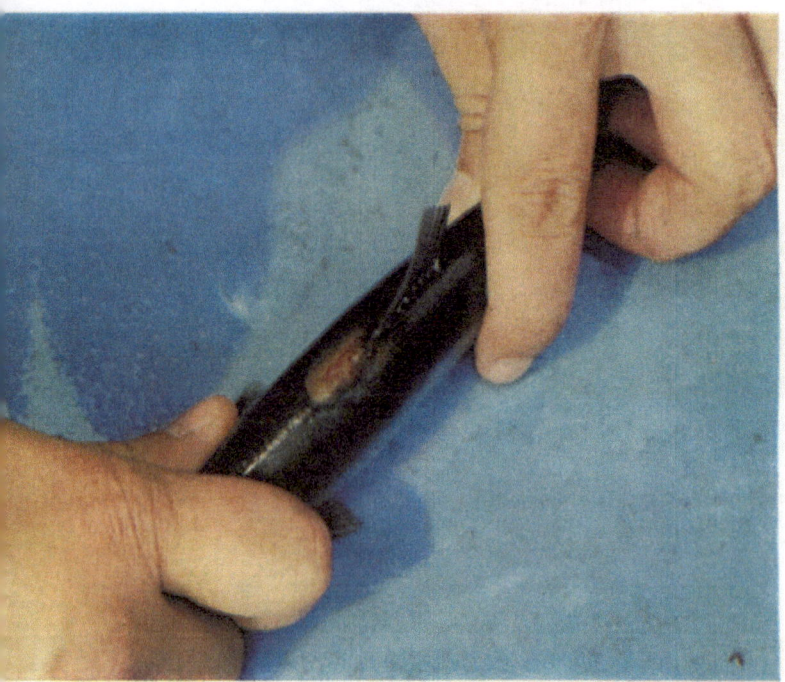

Fig. 6. Ulcer of ayu with "lantern disease". Infection with *Aeromonas liquefaciens* apparently has already occurred in the ulcer.

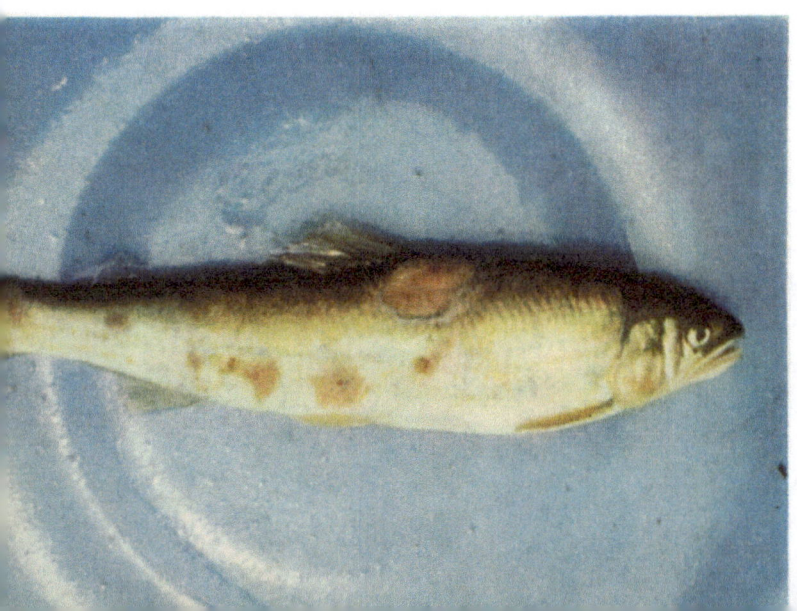

Fig. 7. Ayu with "lantern disease" and severe infection with *Aeromonas liquefaciens*. This ayu is still alive but almost dying. It has a big ulcer on the back and many haemorrhagic areas on the surface of the body.

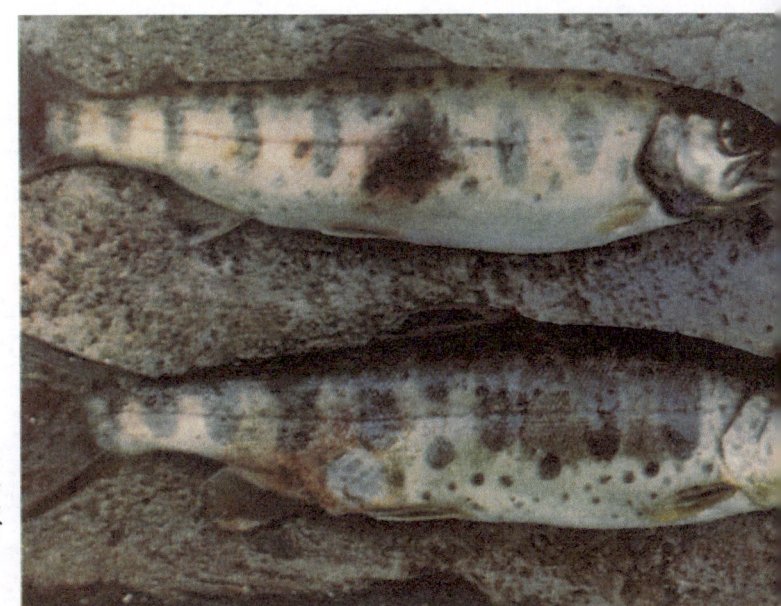

Fig. 8. Amago suffering from furunculosis. Large haemorrhagic abscesses are observed. Furunculosis of amago is caused by *Aeromonas salmonicida*.

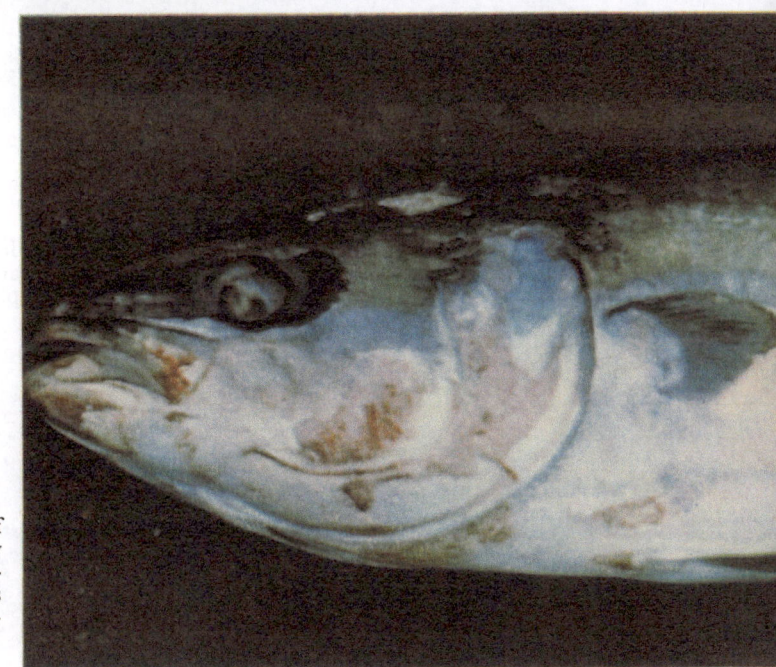

Fig. 9. Tuberculoidosis of cultured yellowtail. Many haemorrhagic spots are observed on the skin. This disease is caused by *Pasteurella* species.

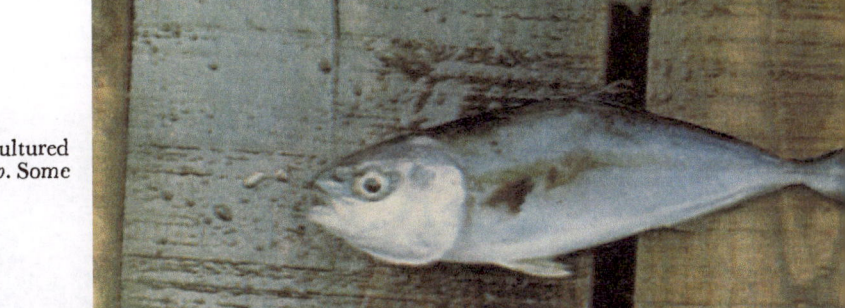

Fig. 10. Infection of cultured yellowtail with *Vibrio*. Some ulcers are observed.

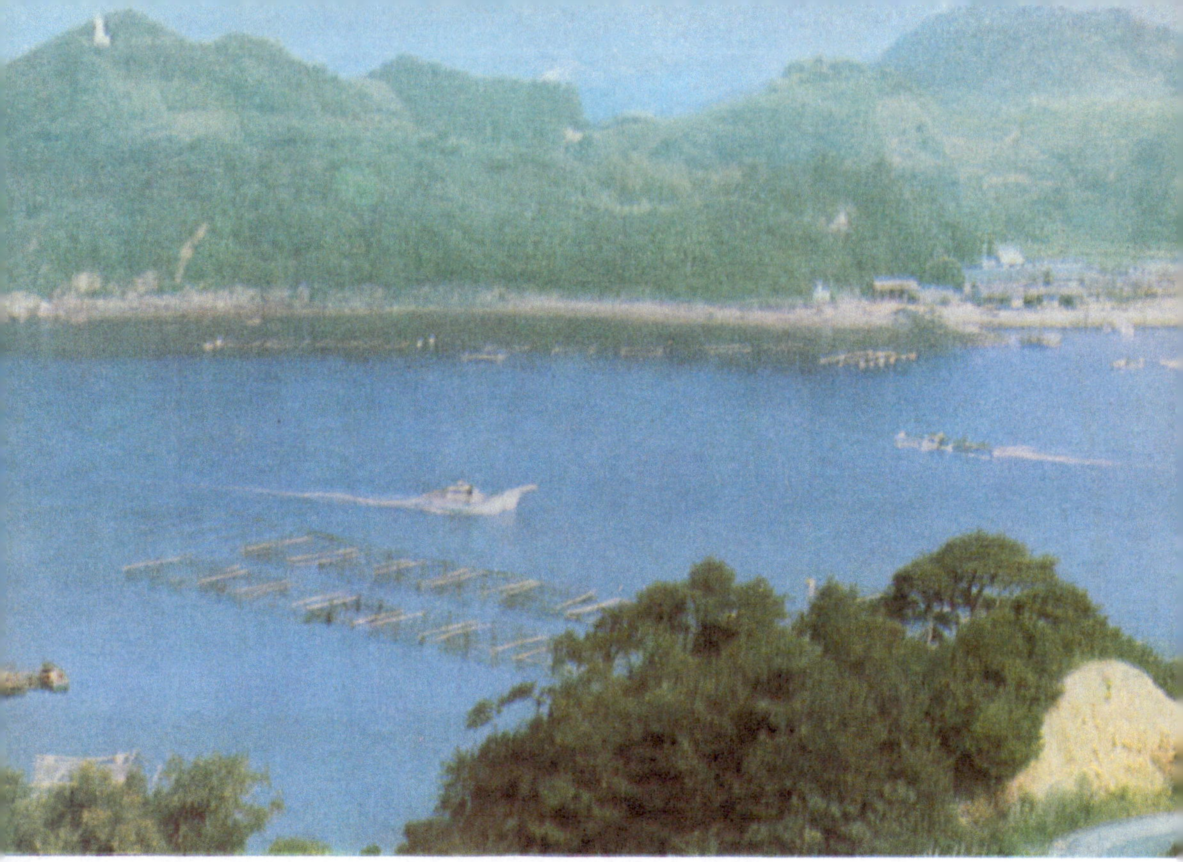

Fig. 3. Bird's-eye-view of a bay where yellowtails are cultured in net-cages. Net-cages for culturing yellowtails are usually kept in bays close to the coast, so that they are not taken away by high tides.

Fig. 4. Frozen fish used as feed for cultured yellowtails. Non-delicious, inexpensive small fish are used as feed for cultured yellowtails. For feeding chemotherapeutic agents to them, these small fish are ground to paste to which the drugs are added in proper concentrations.

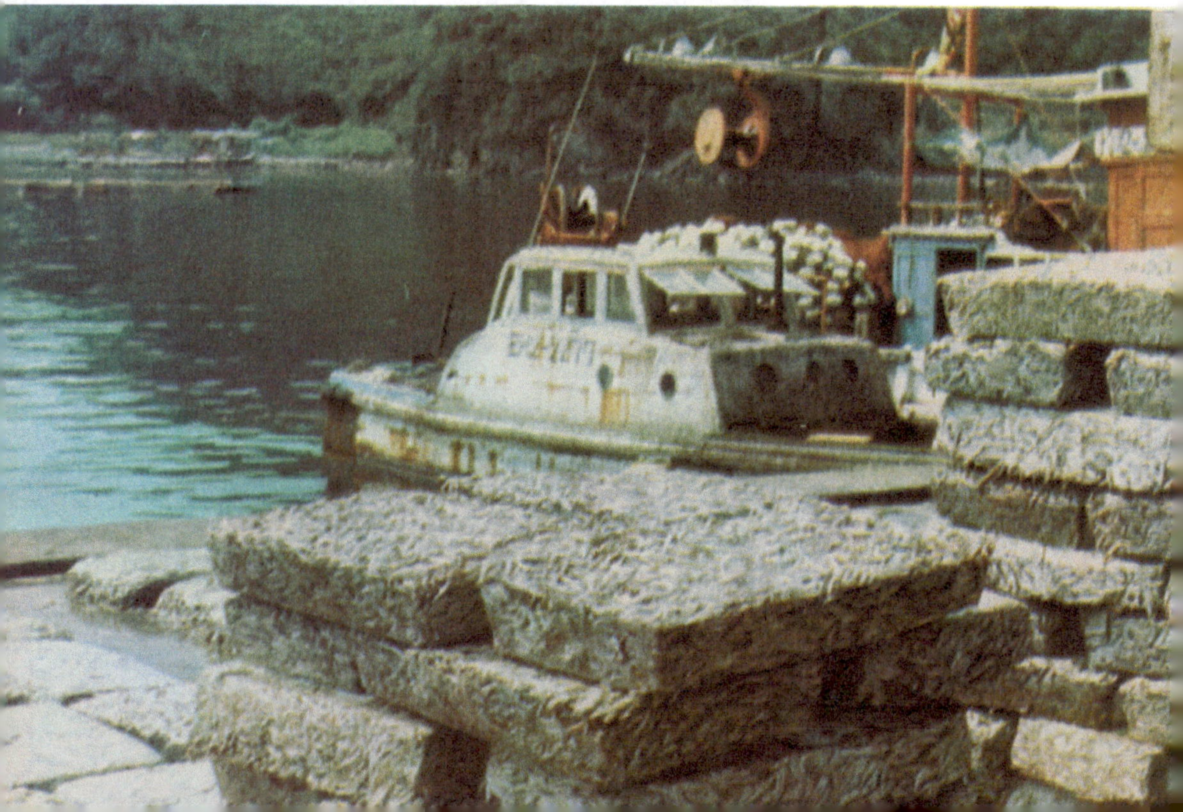

bromothymolblue and 1% lactose in addition to the ingredients of nutrient agar medium was used as a differentiation medium for lactose-fermenting and -non-fermenting strains. These media were enriched with 25 μg/ml of chloramphenicol (Parke, Davis and Co.) or tetracycline hydrochloride (Lederle) to facilitate the isolation of drug-resistant strains. Drug-free medium was used in parallel for quantitative assay of viable bacterial counts in the samples. A liquid medium used was Pennassay broth (Difco).

Procedure for isolation of gram-negative bacilli. Cultured as well as wild fish were caught with either nets or baites, immediately put into an ice box and brought back to laboratories within one hour. They were then dissected and their intestinal tracts were quickly and aseptically removed, and the intestinal tracts of five fish from the same pond or net-cage were pooled and weighed. An equal weight of physiological saline (pH 7.2) was added to these intestinal tracts and they were homogenized in a homogenizer (Nippon Seiki Co.) at 2,000 rpm for three minutes. The homogenates were properly diluted with physiological saline and varying dilutions were plated on nutrient agar with and without antibiotics. Water samples from fish ponds were also properly diluted with physiological saline and plated on similar media. The inoculated plates were incubated at 28 to 30° C for isolating *A. liquefaciens* and salt-water *Vibrio* strains and at 25° C for isolating *A. salmonicida* strains from overnight to three days. Three to four of the developed colonies on each plate were picked up at random and each of them was used for identification, drug sensitivity test and detection of R factor.

Procedure for identification of gram-negative bacilli. The isolated gram-negative bacilli were identified mainly following Bergey's Manual of Determinative Bacteriology (1957). *A. liquefaciens* was identified with the procedure of Bullock (1964).

Procedure for determination of drug sensitivities of gram-negative bacilli. The drug sensitivities of the gram-negative bacilli isolated were studied with Sensitivity Disks (Showa Co.) and the drug sensitivity levels were classified into four classes, very sensitive, fairly sensitive, slightly sensitive and resistant, from the diameters of the inhibition zones following the instructions of the Showa Disks. Slightly sensitive and resistant classes were used as drug-resistant strains for further studies. This classification of drug resistance was found reasonable by comparing it with the levels of minimal inhibitory concentrations determined with the ordinary agar dilution method using several bacterial strains carrying various R factors.

Table 1

GRAM-NEGATIVE BACILLI ISOLATED FROM INTESTINES OF CULTURED EELS IN SHIZUOKA PREFECTURE IN AUGUST, 1969

Selected by *	Species or genus	R+ strains / Studied strains	Resistance marker of R factor *	Number of R factor strain
Cm	*Enterobacter cloacae*	4/4	Su, Tc	4
Tc	*Enterobacter cloacae*	3/3	Su, Tc	2
			Su, Sm, Cm, Tc	1
	Citrobacter	3/3	Su, Sm, Tc	2
			Tc	1
	Aeromonas liquefaciens	2/2	Su, Tc	2
None	*Aeromonas liquefaciens*	3/3	Su, Tc	3
	Escherichia coli	1/1	Tc	1

* Su = sulfonamide; Sm = streptomycin; Cm = chloramphenicol; Tc = tetracycline.
Quantitative viable cell counts were not carried out with these eels, but later studies with other specimens have shown that intestines of eels contain about 10^7 gram-negative bacilli/g.

Procedure for detection of R factors. The procedure used for detecting R factors in isolated *Aeromonas* strains has been described in detail elsewhere (AOKI et al., 1971b; WATANABE et al., 1971). In order to detect R factors in salt-water *Vibrio* strains, the *Vibrio* strains were grown in Penassay broth containing 3% sodium chloride at 28 to 30° C with aeration to a cell density of about 5×10^8/ml, and it was mixed with an equal volume of *E. coli* CSH-2 (methionine- and proline-requiring F⁻ substrain of K-12) which had been grown in ordinary Penassay broth at 37° C with aeration. The mixed culture was incubated at 37° C overnight without aeration and a loopful of the mixed culture was isolated on BTB-lactose-nutrient agar containing a single drug to which the *Vibrio* strain was resistant. If lactose-fermenting colonies developed, they were regarded as the clones of *E. coli* CSH-2 which received R factor, because *Vibrio* strains do not ferment lactose.

Procedure for determination of fi type of R factors. If the drug resistances of the isolated *Aeromonas* or *Vibrio* strains were found transferable to *E. coli* CSH-2 by mixed cultivation, the R factors were then transferred from *Aeromonas* or *Vibrio* to *E. coli* W2252

Table 2

GRAM-NEGATIVE BACILLI ISOLATED FROM EEL POND WATER IN SHIZUOKA PREFECTURE IN AUGUST, 1969

Selected by *	Species or genus	R⁺ strains /	Studied strains	Resistance marker of R factor *	Number of R factor strain
Cm	*Enterobacter cloacae*	11/12		Su, Tc	8
				Su, Sm, Cm, Tc	2
				Tc	1
	Citrobacter	1/5		Su, Tc	1
	Klebsiella	0/4			
	Pseudomonas	0/3			
	Alcaligenes	0/3			
Tc	*Aeromonas liquefaciens*	7/13		Su, Tc	7
	Vibrio	1/10		Su, Tc	1
	Citrobacter	3/8		Tc	1
				Su, Tc	1
				Su, Sm, Tc	1
	Escherichia coli	1/6		Su, Tc	1
	Enterobacter cloacae	4/5		Su, Tc	4
	Klebsiella	0/1			
	Hafnia	0/1			
	Enterobacteriaceae (unidentified)	1/2		Tc	1
None	*Alcaligenes*	0/20			
	Pseudomonas	0/11			
	Vibrio	1/8		Su, Sm, Tc, Km, Nm	1
	Escherichia coli	1/5		Su, Sm, Cm	1
	Aeromonas liquefaciens	0/5			
	Citrobacter	2/4		Tc	2
	Achromobacter	0/3			
	Enterobacter cloacae	0/1			
	Enterobacteriaceae (unidentified)	1/2		Tc	1

* Su = sulfonamide; Sm = streptomycin; Cm = chloramphenicol; Tc = tetracycline; Km = kanamycin; Nm = neomycin.

The viable counts of gram-negative bacilli recovered from the water samples were 3.5×10^4 — 5.6×10^5/ml. The number of colonies developed on nutrient agar with Cm or Tc was about one-fourth of those on drug-free nutrient agar (rough estimate).

(methionine-requiring stable Hfr derivative of K-12), and the clones of W2252 which received the R factors were studied for their sensitivity to male-specific bacteriophages f1 and f2. If W2252 (R+) was found sensitive to these bacteriophages, the R factor was regarded as *fi−* and otherwise as *fi+* (WATANABE et al., 1962, 1964).

RESULTS

Investigation of gram-negative bacilli isolated from intestines of normal-looking cultured fresh-water fish and from the water of their ponds. The summaries of the results are shown in Tables 1 to 8. As seen in these tables, the gram-negative bacilli isolated from both the

Table 3

GRAM-NEGATIVE BACILLI ISOLATED FROM INTESTINES OF CULTURED CARP IN NAGANO PREFECTURE IN MAY, 1970

Selected by *	Species or genus	R+ strains /	Studied strains	Resistance marker of R factor *	Number of R factor strain
Cm	*Pseudomonas*	0/16			
	Aeromonas liquefaciens	0/1			
Tc	*Aeromonas liquefaciens*	10/17		Su, Tc	10
	Enterobacter aerogenes	0/1			
	Enterobacteriaceae (unidentified)	0/1			
None	*Aeromonas liquefaciens*	0/15			
	Pseudomonas	0/5			

* Su = sulfonamide; Cm = chloramphenicol; Tc = tetracycline.
The viable counts of gram-negative bacilli recovered from the intestines were $3.2 \times 10^7 -$ $- 5.6 \times 10^7/g$. The viable counts of Cm-resistant and Tc-resistant gram-negative bacilli from the same samples were $7.2 \times 10^3 - 3.7 \times 10^4/g$ and $1.5 \times 10^6 - 2.1 \times 10^6/g$, respectively.

Table 4

GRAM-NEGATIVE BACILLI ISOLATED FROM CARP POND WATER IN NAGANO PREFECTURE IN MAY, 1970

Selected by *	Species or genus	R+ strains /	Studied strains	Resistance marker of R factor *	Number of R factor strain
Cm	*Pseudomonas*	0/12			
Tc	*Aeromonas liquefaciens*	5/8		Su, Tc	5
	Pseudomonas	0/4			
None	*Aeromonas liquefaciens*	0/11			
	Pseudomonas	0/6			

* Su = Sulfonamide; Cm = chloramphenicol; Tc = tetracycline.
The viable counts of gram-negative bacilli recovered from the water samples were $1.9 \times 10^2 -$ $- 6.0 \times 10^3/ml$. The viable counts of Cm-resistant and Tc-resistant gram-negative bacilli from the same samples were $3.0 \times 10^1 - 9.0 \times 10^1/ml$ and $1.9 \times 10^2 - 6.0 \times 10^3/ml$, respectively.

intestines of normal-looking cultured fish and the water of fish ponds had R factors at high frequencies. The results shown in Table 7 include exceptionally the data with some diseased amago (suffering from furunculosis), because one of our purposes of investigating amago was to isolate *A. salmonicida* strains, which are not found in healthy amago. The

Table 5

GRAM-NEGATIVE BACILLI ISOLATED FROM INTESTINES OF CULTURED AYU IN SHIGA PREFECTURE IN AUGUST, 1970

Selected by *	Species or genus	R+ strains / Studied strains	Resistance marker of R factor *	Number of R factor strain
Cm	Citrobacter	3/11	Su, Sm, Cm, Tc	3
	Aeromonas liquefaciens	4/9	Su, Sm, Cm	4
	Hafnia	3/3	Su, Sm, Cm	3
	Enterobacter cloacae	0/1		
	Pseudomonas	0/1		
	Achromobacter	0/1		
	Enterobacteriaceae (unidentified)	0/2		
Tc	Aeromonas liquefaciens	0/24		
	Hafnia	0/2		
	Citrobacter	1/1	Su, Tc	1
	Enterobacteruiaceae (unidentified)	0/1		
None	Aeromonas liquefaciens	3/19	Su	1
			Su, Tc	1
			Su, Sm, Cm	1
	Citrobacter	1/3	Su, Sm, Cm, Tc	1
	Hafnla	1/1	Su, Sm, Cm	1
	Enterobacter aerogenes	0/1		
	Enterobacter cloacae	0/1		
	Enterobacteriaceae (unidentified)	0/2		

* Su = sulfonamide; Sm = streptomycin; Cm = chloramphenicol; Tc = tetracycline.
The viable counts of gram-negative bacilli recovered from the intestines were $1.1 \times 10^6 - 2.4 \times 10^7$/g. The viable counts of Cm-resistant and Tc-resistant gram-negative bacilli from the same samples were $1.5 \times 10^4 - 1.8 \times 10^6$/g and $3.5 \times 10^5 - 4.6 \times 10^7$/g, respectively.

Table 6

GRAM-NEGATIVE BACILLI ISOLATED FROM AYU POND WATER IN SHIGA PREFECTURE IN AUGUST, 1970

Selected by *	Species or genus	R+ strains / Studied strains
Cm	Citrobacter	0/3
Tc	Aeromonas liquefaciens	0/11
	Pseudomonas	0/2
	Citrobacter	0/1
	Escherichia coli	0/1
	Hafnia	0/1
	Enterobacteriaceae (unidentified)	0/1
None	Aeromonas liquefaciens	0,12
	Pseudomonas	0/4
	Citrobacter	0/1
	Enterobacter aerogenes	0/1

* Cm = chloramphenicol; Tc = tetracycline.
The viable counts of gram-negative bacilli recovered from the water samples were $9.0 \times 10^1 - 2.6 \times 10^3$/ml. The viable counts of Cm-resistant and Tc-resistant gram-negative bacilli from the same samples were $< 1.0 \times 10^1 - 9.0 \times 10^1$ and $1.0 \times 10^1 - 8.4 \times 10^2$/ml, respectively.

136

Table 7

GRAM-NEGATIVE BACILLI ISOLATED FROM INTESTINES OF CULTURED AMAGO IN GIFU AND SHIGA PREFECTURES IN JUNE, 1971

Selected by *	Species or genus	R+ strains/	Studied strains	Resistance marker of R factor *	Number of R factor strain
Cm	*Aeromonas salmonicida*	15/15		Su, Sm, Cm	15
	Pseudomonas	0/5			
	Aeromonas liquefaciens	0/5			
Tc	*Aeromonas liquefaciens*	3/19		Su, Tc	3
	Hafnia	0/8			
None	*Aeromonas liquefaciens*	4/17		Su, Sm, Cm	4
	Aeromonas salmonicida	2/12		Su, Sm, Cm	2
	Hafnia	0/2			
	Enterobacteriaceae (unidentified)	0/3			

* Su = sulfonamide; Sm = streptomycin; Cm = chloramphenicol; Tc = tetracycline.
  The viable counts of gram-negative bacilli recovered from the intestines were 1.0×10^4 —
— 8.1×10^7/g. The viable counts of Cm-resistant and Tc-resistant gram-negative bacilli from the same samples were $< 1.0 \times 10^2 - 2.0 \times 10^6$/g and $< 1.0 \times 10^2 - 3.6 \times 10^5$/g, respectively. The results in this table include the data with some diseased amago (suffering from furunculosis).

Table 8

GRAM-NEGATIVE BACILLI ISOLATED FROM AMAGO POND WATER IN GIFU PREFECTURE IN JUNE, 1971

Selected by *	Species or genus	R+ strains/	Studied strains	Resistance marker of R factor *	Number of R factor strain
Cm	*Pseudomonas*	0/1			
Tc	*Aeromonas liquefaciens*	0/4			
None	*Pseudomonas*	0/2			
	Aeromonas salmonicida	1/1		Su, Sm, Cm	1

* Su = sulfonamide; Sm = streptomycin; Cm = chloramphenicol; Tc = tetracycline.
  The viable counts of gram-negative bacilli recovered from the water sample were 4.3×10^2/ml in an amago pond. The viable counts of Cm-resistant and Tc-resistant gram-negative bacilli from the same sample were 10/ml and 7/ml, respectively.

Table 9

PROPERTIES OF SOME R FACTORS FROM AEROMONAS STRAINS

Aeromonas species carrying R factor	Resistance marker of R factor *	Number of strains	*fi***	Restriction of phage				
				T1	T7	W−31	λ	P1
A. liquefaciens	Su, Tc	39	−	−	−	−	−	−
	Su, Sm, Cm	6	−	−	−	−	−	−
	Su	2	−	−	−	−	−	−
	Su, Cm, Tc	1	−	−	−	−	−	−
	Su, Sm, Cm, Tc	1	−	−	−	−	−	−
A. salmonicida	Su, Sm, Cm	2	−	−	−	−	−	−
	Su, Tc	1	−	−	−	−	−	−

* Su = sulfonamide; Sm = streptomycin; Cm = chloramphenicol; Tc = tetracycline.
** *fi*-fertility inhibition (see Watanabe *et al.*, 1962, 1964).

most frequent types of R factors related to fish culturing had Su and Tc resistance markers, and as far as studied, all of them belonged to the fi^- type (Table 9). As we have reported previously (WATANABE et al., 1964), most fi^- R factors from *Shigella* strains cause restriction and modification of bacteriophages and other deoxyribonucleic acids, whereas fi^+ R factors do not have these capacities, although some exceptional R factors have later been found (WATANABE, 1967; BANNISTER and GLOVER, 1968). It is interesting to note that all the R factors from *Aeromonas* strains lacked the capacity of restriction despite the fact that they belonged to the fi^- type (Table 9). The fi type of the R factors isolated from *A. salmonicida* in amago has not yet been studied. Gram-negative bacilli isolated from rainbow trouts and their ponds are under current investigation. The results of these studies will be reported later.

Table 10

VIBRIO STRAINS ISOLATED FROM INTESTINES OF CULTURED
YELLOWTAILS IN SHIKOKU IN JULY AND AUGUST, 1971

Selected by *	R^+ strains / strains	Resistance marker of R factor *	Number of R factor strain
Cm	4/21	Su, Cm	2
		Sm, Cm, Ap	2
Tc	25/46	Su, Sm, Cm, Tc	25

* Su = sulfonamide; Sm = streptomycin; Cm = chloramphenicol; Tc = tetracycline; Ap = aminobenzyl penicillin.

The viable counts of gram-negative bacilli recovered were $1.0 \times 10^2 - 4.6 \times 10^6$/g. The viable counts of Cm-resistant and Tc-resistant gram-negative bacilli recovered from the same samples were $< 1.0 \times 10^2 - 5.3 \times 10^3$/g and $< 1.0 \times 10^2 - 9.9 \times 10^5$/g, respectively. The study of the frequencies of R^+ strains among the isolates on drug-free medium and the resistance markers of their R factors has not yet been completed.

Investigation of Vibrio strains isolated from intestines of normal-looking cultured yellowtails. We have carried out a rather extensive investigation of cultured yellowtails on the coasts of Shikoku Island of Japan in July and August, 1971. We have chosen 20 culturists of yellowtails in these areas which are reasonably apart from each other so that the chance of cross infections among them is very small. According to the records of the fish culturists, Su, Cm and/or Tc have been heavily used in all of these areas for the purpose of controlling bacterial infections. Table 10 shows the data with *Vibrio* strains isolated from normal-looking yellowtails. As seen in this table, the frequencies of R factor-carrying *Vibrio* strains were relatively high. Further identification of these *Vibrio* strains and the determination of the fi type of their R factors are now in progress and the results of these studies will be reported later.

DISCUSSION

Considerable fractions of *A. liquefaciens* and *A. salmonicida* strains isolated from diseased and healthy cultured fish have been found to carry R factors. These fish included eel, carp, ayu, amago and brook trout. It has also been shown that gram-negative bacilli isolated from the intestines of normal-looking cultured fish as well as from the water of fish ponds carry R factors at high frequencies. A new finding reported in the present paper is the detection of R factor-carrying *Vibrio* strains from cultured yellowtails. This is the first report of the isolation of R-factor-carrying bacteria from salt-water fish. We have previously studied the intestinal bacteria of wild eels but no R factor-carrying strains have been found among them, indicating that the high incidence of R factor-carrying bacteria in cultured fish is due to selection by antibiotics and other chemotherapeutic agents used for fish culturing (AOKI et al., 1971b; WATANABE et al., 1971). The origin of the R factors in *Vibrio* strains is obscure like in the R factor-carrying bacteria detected in fresh-water fish. Contamination of fish feed with human bacteria carrying R factors at the time of handling the fish feed is quite possible. Another possibility may be the contamination of sea water with sewage water, which may well contain R factor-carrying bacteria, although this possibility has not yet been investigated. We are planning to investigate the intestinal bacteria of wild yellowtails to see the presence or absence and incidence of R factors, if present, in them. This investigation is expected to give us a clue to solving this problem.

At any rate, there is no doubt that the pool of R factors in our environment has been amplified by the use of chemotherapeutic agents for fish culturing. The increase of the pool of R factors in our environment is undesirable, because it will increase the possibility of R factor transfer to human pathogens. Especially in Japan, where the meat of yellowtails and some other cultured fish is often eaten raw, the high incidence of R factor-carrying bacteria in them may be hazardous to public health by the transfer of the R factors to human pathogens indirectly.

Antibiotics and other chemotherapeutic agents have been used for fish culturing too freely or too carelessly. We should restrict the use of at least the drugs that select for R factor-carrying bacteria. Similar drugs are also being used for culturing ornamental fish such as goldfish and tropical fish and we have found R factors in *A. liquefaciens* strains isolated from diseased goldfish (WATANABE et al., 1969; AOKI et. al., 1971b). But the scales of culturing these ornamental fish are generally small and these fish are not for eating and therefore the presence of R factor-carrying bacteria in them may not create a serious public health problem.

An important and often overlooked point in the use of drugs for fish culturing is the antibiotic residue, which is already known to cause hypersensitive reactions in particular persons in the case of milk contaminated with penicillins and some other antibiotics. The check of the withdrawal period, when drugs are not given to fish, must be strictly performed.

Although no workers other than ourselves have yet undertaken the investigation of R factors related to fish culturing, it is most likely that R factors may be present in bacteria related to fish culturing also in other countries. In fact we have already found that a strain of *A. salmonicida*, which was isolated by S. F. SNIESZKO from a diseased brook trout in the United States as early as 1959 and which has been maintained in laboratories as an international standard strain for a number of years, still carries R factor (AOKI et al., 1971a).

R factors found in *Aeromonas* strains exhibit some specific properties; a majority of them have Su and Tc resistance markers. R factors with Cm resistance marker are rather exceptional in spite of the fact that Cm has been often used for fish culturing in large amounts. We have recently found that the Cm marker of R factors is genetically unstable in *Aeromonas* strains and is spontaneously lost at high frequencies (unpublished data). This fact may account for the rarity of Cm resistance R factors in *Aeromonas* strains. Another peculiarity with R factors in *Aeromonas* strains is that all of the R factors detected in *Aeromonas* strains belonged to the fi^- type. This fact may be also explainable by our recent finding that fi^+ R factors are all genetically unstable in *Aeromonas* strains (unpublished data). The third specificity with the *Aeromonas* R factors is that they do not cause restriction of bacteriophages although they belong to the fi^- type. The reason for this interesting finding is not known at the present moment. NAOMI DATTA (personal communication) has recently found that the R factors of our *A. liquefaciens* strains form a new class of incompatibility group W (W for WATANABE) among various fi^- R factors. The properties of the *Vibrio* R factors are now under investigation in our laboratories.

Acknowledgments

We acknowledge the cooperation of many people in collecting the fish samples used for this investigation.

This investigation was supported in part by United States Public Health Service research grant AI-08078 from the Institute of Allergy and Infectious Diseases.

REFERENCES

ANDERSON, E. S. (1968): The ecology of transferable drug resistance in the Enterobacteria. Annual Review of Microbiology, **22**, 131—180.

AOKI, T. and EGUSA, S. (1971): Drug sensitivity of *Aeromonas liquefaciens* isolated from freshwater fishes. Bulletin of the Japanese Society of Scientific Fisheries, **37**, 176—185.

AOKI, T., EGUSA, S., KIMURA, T. and WATANABE, T. (1971a.) Detection of R factors in naturally occurring *Aeromonas salmonicida* strains. Applied Microbiology (in press).

AOKI, T., EGUSA, S., OGATA, Y. and WATANABE, T. (1971b.): Detection of resistance factors in fish pathogen *Aeromonas liquefaciens*. Journal of General Microbiology, **65**, 343—349.

BANNISTER, D. and GLOVER, S. W. (1968): Restriction and modification of bacteriophages by R$^+$ strains of *E. coli* K12. Biochemical and Biophysical Research Communications, **30**, 735—738.

Bergey's Manual of Determinative Bacteriology (7th edition). (1957): Waverly Press, Baltimore, Maryland.

BULLOCK, G. L. (1964): *Pseudomonᵈdales* as fish pathogens. Industrial Microbiology, **5**, 101—108.

HOSHINA T. (1962): Studies of red-fin disease of eel. Journal of the Tokyo University of Fisheries, **6**, 1—105.

MUROGA, K. and EGUSA, S. (1968): Chlortetracycline bath as a treatment of bacterial diseases of fish. I. Fish Pathology, **2**, 141—147.

SCHÄPERCLAUS, W. (1955): Aufsehenerregende Heilungs- und Bekämpfungserfolge bei der infektiösen Bauchwassersucht des Karpfens durch antibiotische Mittel. Deutsche Fischereizeitung, **2**, 330—334.

SCHÄPERCLAUS, W. (1956): Bekämpfung der infektiösen Bauchwassersucht durch Antibiotika. Zeitschrift für Fischerei, **7**, 599—628.

SCHÄPERCLAUS, W. (1958): Bewährung des Chlornitrins in der teichwirtschaftlichen Praxis und neue Versuche über die Anwendbarkeit weiterer Breitspektrum-Antibiotica bei der Bekämpfung der infektiösen Bauchwassersucht des Karpfens. Zeitschrift für Fischerei, **7**, 599—628.

SMITH, H. W. (1969): Veterinary implications of transfer activity. Ciba Foundation Symposium on Bacterial Episomes and Plasmids, pp. 213—223. Edited by G. E. W. Wolstenholme and M. O'Connor. J. and A. Churchill, London.

SNIESZKO, S. F. (1957): Use of antibiotics in the diet of salmonid fishes. Progressive Fish Culturists, **19**, 81—84.

SNIESZKO, S. F. (1959): Antibiotics in fish diseases and fish nutrition. Antibiotics and Chemotherapy, **9**, 541—545.

Swann Report. (1969): Report of Joint Committee on the Use of Antibiotics in Animal Husbandary and Veterinary Medicine. Her Majesty's Stationery Office, London.

WATANABE, T. (1967). The concept of R factors. Symposium on Infectious Multiple Drug Resistance, pp. 5—16. Edited by S. Falkow. U. S. Government Printing Office, Washington, D.C.

WATANABE, T., AOKI, T., OGATA, Y. and EGUSA, S. (1971): R factors related to fish culturing Annals of the New York Academy of Sciences, **182**, 383—410.

WATANABE, T., FUKASAWA, T. and TAKANO, T. (1962): Conversion of male bacteria of *Escherichia coli* K12 to resistance to f phages by infection with the episome ‚resistance transfer factor'. Virology, **17**, 218—219.

WATANABE, T., NISHIDA, H., OGATA, C., ARAI, T. and SATO, S. (1964): Episome-mediate transfer of drug resistance in Enterobacteriaceae. VII. Two types of naturally occurring R factors. Journal of Bacteriology, **88**, 716—726.

WATANABE, T., OGATA, Y., AOKI, T. and EGUSA, S. (1969): Studies on the drug resistance of fish-pathogenic bacteria. I. Detection of R factors. Japanese Journal of Bacteriology, **25**, 42—43.

WOLF, K. and SNIESZKO, S. F. (1963): Uses of antibiotics and other antimicrobials in therapy of diseases of fishes. Antimicrobial Agents and Chemotherapy, **1**, 597—603.

EPIDEMIOLOGICAL SURVEYS OF DRUG RESISTANCE

F. VÝMOLA

Institute of Hygiene and Epidemiology, Prague

The development of drug resistance is a natural characteristic of most bacterial genera, but it is accelerated by the extensive use of chemotherapeutics in medical practice, particularly in hospitals both in therapy and as prophylactic agents under various circumstances and the abuse of some antibiotics in the agriculture and the food industry. Chemotherapeutics cannot only continually change the original status of sensitivity of numerous microbes, but to a considerable degree also influence their ecology and biological activity, including their antigenic abilities, thereby obviously affecting immunity in the individuals and in the whole populations. The widespread use of the different preparations has altered the picture of many diseases and changed patterns of medical regime.

Systematic observation of the development of drug resistance in bacterial agents of diseases is an important element in the surveillance of bacterial infections. The gradually analyses and the evaluation of the statistical data would utilize in outlining and implementing the general concept of strategy in employment of antibiotics particularly in chemotherapy.

The surveillance of drug resistance should follow:

Uniform methodology for determinating antibiotic sensitivity in bactera. Uniform measurement of sensitivity in vitro is an important condition for evaluating results in any laboratory. Only in this way it will be possible to evaluate results obtained everywhere.

Standard forms of documentation of the bacterial strains isolated to be tested for sensitivity should comprise; among other epidemiologically important items, data relating to:

the spectrum of antibiotics used (with reference to time and place) in the treatment of the infections caused by the species concerned, the form of administration, the size of the daily and total doses and the types of antibiotic preparations employed.

The exact taxonomy of the bacterial population isolated. It is necessary to define which value expresses sensitivity or resistance to specific antibiotics in different bacterial species. The definition of sensitivity is based on the value of minimal inhibition concentration (MIC) and minimal bactericidal concentration (MBC). For clinical purposes MIC, respectively MBC are determined in relation to the attainable concentrations in body fluids and tissues after optimal dosage and form of administration.

Epidemiological surveys of drug resistance follow the dynamics of changing sensitivity and should reveal all causes of resistance, multi- and polyresistance development in all important bacterial populations. In this sphere there is still much to be done in order to come to an agreement on uniform criteria.

Strains must be selected at random to ensure valid conclusions. The method of random selection of strains for sensitivity measurements depends on the character of disease, epidemiological situation, number of illnesses and number of positive isolations of pathogens. It is recommended that in hospital-infections the sensitivity should be tested in all the pathogens isolated, as there usually are different types of resistance within the same isolated bacterial species.

Information should be collected on: The circulation and biological properties of the most important etiologic agents of human and animal diseases. The changing antibiotic sensitivity and resistance patterns in most bacterial species are not only influenced by the abuse of antibacterial drugs, but also, to a considerable degree, depend on the prevallence of individual bacterial infections in the human and animal populations. The higher the development of resistance in an aetiological agent, the more favourable are the conditions of its spread (hospital infections, infections in domestic animals in big fattening stations).

The consumption of individual chemotherapeutics in individual medical establishments and health districts. These data are indispensable for the worker whose task is to outline the general strategy of the selection and employment of antibiotics. It would seem logical that this role should be played by the specialists who work in the surveys of drug resistance. Lack of control of the consumption of individual chemotherapeutics or the regimen for their use and particularly disregard for the present state of resistance to some antibiotics in massive use is one of the main causes of the unfavourable trends in drug resistance in many countries of the world.

The consumption of some antibiotics in fattening cattle and in the food industry provide valuable information on the extent to which resistant variants of animal strains are segregated as a result of the continuous selective pressure exterted by the widespread use of some antibiotic. These animal strains can colonize the human population and transmit resistance to human population via different mechanisms.

Records of bacterial infections in relation to the aetiological agent and antibiotic therapy are a valuable complementary aid to the epidemiologist and therapeutist. They enable them to form a certain idea of the rationality of the chemotherapy as it is practised and the total consumption of those antibiotics which are "favoured" by clinicians. Different antibiotics are prescribed by paediatricians, urologists, dermatologists, otorhinolaryngologists, surgeons, infectionists, in treating burns, etc., against the same agents (staphylococci, pseudomonades, coli bacilli, Proteus and other organisms) since the results of in vitro sensitivity tests permit these indications. It seems that the aim of epidemiological surveillance of drug resistance is to convince clinicians and general practioners to introduce more rational regimens of chemotherapy with regard to contemporary position of individual antibiotics in particular cases.

Surveys of resistance in individual bacterial species in relation to the: type of resistance and to the phenomenon of transmissible (infectious) resistance.

The follow-up of type resistance in different bacteria with respect to single antibiotics provides information on the extend to which such preparations can influence the increase of resistance in the respective bacterial species not only against the particular antibiotic used, but also other especially those of a similar chemical structure.

If the phenomenon of transmissible resistance (infectious resistance by plasmidal or episomal transference) appears in hospitals infections, respectively in any bacterial epidemy, it is necessary to ascertain a frequence of resistance transfer factor (RFT) not only among pathogenic bacteria, but also in saprophytes. It is necessary to follow simultaneously a frequency of donor and recipient bacterial strains containing RTF in many different bacterial species.

Priority should be given to surveillance of drug resistance in:

1. *Pseudomonas aeruginosa* in relation particularly to gentamicin, carbenicillin and colistin.
2. *Esch. coli* with reference to sulphonamides, chloramphenicol, tetracyclines, ampicillin etc.
3. *Salmonellae*, particularly *S. typhosa*, with reference to chloramphenicol and ampicillin
4. *Shigellae* in relation to sulphonamides, tetracyclines and chloramphenicol
5. *Staphylococcus aureus* in relation to all preparations with antistaphylococcal activity, especially macrolides, lincomycin, gentamicin and "resistant" penicillins
6. *Proteus*, particularly *Proteus mirabilis* in relation to cephalosporines, gentamicin, ampicillin and its combination with dicloxacillin.

Attention should furthermore be paid to *Bordetella, Yersinia, Serratia* etc.

The objective of surveillance of drug resistance is to detect all factors which influence resistance trends and changes in the biological properties of pathogens. This enables to determine the position of individual antibiotics in relation to different aetiological agents and infections. Furthermore, in order to elaborate an effective antibiotic policy of the use of antibiotics both in medicine and other purposes and of their production on a contemporary basis and long-term perspective.

REFERENCES

ALEXANDER, M., ALDAG, V., HENZE, B. (1970): Progress in antimicrobial and anticancer chemotherapy, vol. I., p. 453. Proceedings of the 6th Int. Congr. of Chemotherapy in Tokyo, 1969. University of Tokyo Press.

GARROD, L. P., O. GRADY, F. (1971): Antibiotic and Chemotherapy, 3rd Edition, Livingstone, Edinbourgh, London.

GUMP, D. W., WHITCOMB, C. C. (1970): Progress in antimicrobial and anticancer chemotherapy, vol. I., p. 449. Proceedings of the 6th Int. Congr. of Chemotherapy in Tokyo 1969. University of Tokyo Press.

ERICSSON, H. M., SHERRIS, J. G. (1971): Acta Pathologica Scandinavica, Sect. B, Suppl. No 217.

VÝMOLA, F. (1970): Progress in antimicrobial and anticancer chemotherapy, vol. I., p. 458. Proceedings of the 6th Int. Congr. of Chemotherapy in Tokyo, 1969. University Tokyo Press.

FREQUENCY OF COLICINE PRODUCTION AND OCCURRENCE OF TRANSMISSIBLE RESISTANCE IN HAEMOLYTIC STRAINS OF E. COLI, ISOLATED FROM DIARRHOEATIC PIGS

F. FEDERIČ, A. SOKOL and Z. KOPPEL

Department of Microbiology, University of Veterinary Medicine, Košice, Czechoslovakia

INTRODUCTION

It is a known fact that haemolytic strains of E. coli are often isolated from swine, sheep, cattle and sometimes from fowl and freely living animals. The isolation of haemolytic E. coli in humans, especially in babies is not a rarity. Relatively the biggest losses are caused by those strains in swine at which the disease in dependence on age is demonstrated either by diarrhoea, or by oedema disease. The problem of coli infections in the sense of the latest knowledge in bacterial genetics comes to the fore in the veterinary medicine.

It has been proved that a full series of properties of E. coli may be determined by plasmids that are transmissible to other microorganisms from Enterobacteriaceae. In this way, for example, the drug-resistance, colicine production as well as haemolytic activity, are conditioned. One can suppose that in the population of animals fed with "nutritional" levels of antibiotics are the strains of E. coli exposed to selective pressure, favourising microorganisms resistant to the antibiotics employed.

However in the conditions of intensive breeding the dominant strain is a result of many selective pressures. Such a strain is simultaneously a picture of vivid genetic interactions in intestinal tract and should represent microorganism by its genetical equipment best suitable for the present conditions. Strains of E. coli that are isolated from different breedings should contain a large scale of microorganisms that are equipped, besides others also with different plasmids.

MATERIAL AND METHOD

For experiments there have been used strains of E. coli that were isolated from pigs with diarrhoea as well as from pigs that showed symptoms of oedema disease.

From the series of strains isolated at the same time and from the same breeding only one strain was chosen which produced haemolysis on the blood agar, made from defibrinated sheep blood. The examined strains were derived from diseased cases in 1969—1970. By such selection of strains the largest possible genetic heterogenity of examined strains was insured.

E. coli 185 Nx was used as a recipient strain, obtained by kindness of V. KRČMÉRY, from the Institute of Hygiene in Bratislava. As indicator strains for establishment of colicine production there were used strains of E. coli ROW and E. coli Bl, obtained from J. ŠMARDA from Department of Biology UJEP in Brno.

For crosses were used MacConkey Agar DIFCO, as bouillon Nutrion broth DIFCO.

We received nalidixic acid as a substance from Slovakofarma of Hlohovec, the rest antibiotics we have used as preparations for injection from SPOFA. The sensitivity of strains to 7 antibiotics (streptomycin — S, chloramphenicol — C, tetracycline — T, oxytetracycline — O, neomycin, furadantin and nalidixic acid — Nx) was established by method employing antibiotic discs SPOLANA on blood agar.

For crossing there were used strains of 6 hours bouillon cultures, shaken at 37° C. Mixed cultures of the donor (2 ml) and the recipient (2ml) were incubated for 2 hrs., and the mixture was spread onto selective media (partly with two antibiotics, partly with each antibiotic separately). By analogous way was performed a resistance determinant mobilization test: 2 ml culture of donor has been mixed with 2 ml culture of intermediate recipient and was incubated for 2 hrs. without shaking at 37° C. Afterwards to that mixture was added culture of final recipient (2 ml). As a donor was used strain *E. coli 284*, as intermediate recipients all strains, that have not resistance determinants transmissible by simple crossing and as final recipient strain E. coli 185 Nx.

To the results are included only crossings with higher frequency of transmission as 10^{-4}. Hybrids from selective media were tested for simultaneous transmission of Col or Hly factor.

RESULTS

All studied strains were tested by simple conjugational test with E. coli 185 Nx. Mixed cultures were spread on media with T, Nx and T + Nx. From 44 tetracycline resistant strains, 26 strains transmitted resistance determinant to tetracycline, that is 59%. From 31 colicine producing strains Col factor was transferred by 11 strains, that is 35%. From all 50 haemolytic strains haemolytic activity was transferred by 9 strains, that is 18%. (Table 1.)

Table 1

TRANSMISSIBILITY OF SINGLE MARKERS OF FIFTY HAEMOLYTIC STRAINS OF E. COLI ISOLATED FROM SWINE FOR E. COLI 185 Nx IN CONJUGATIONAL TESTS

Marker	No of Strains Marker		Transmissibility in %
	Possessed	Transmissible	
Resistance to Tetracycline	44	26	59
Production of Colicine	31	11	35
Haemolytic Activity	50	9	18

Streptomycin resistant strains (4) were submitted to conjugational tests with strain E. coli 185 Nx. Mixed cultures were inoculated into media with T, Nx, S, T + Nx, S + Nx and T + S + Nx. Only 2 strains were able to transfer resistance determinant to streptomycin. Resistance determinant to streptomycin was transferred in one occassion by itself (strain no. 7562), in second case together with resistance determinant to chloramphenicol (strain No. 284). In no case tested marker was transferred simultaneously. From streptomycin resistant strains (resistant simultaneously to tetracycline), 3 transferred resistance determinant to tetracycline as seen on selective media with T + Nx. In all three cases also Col factor was simultaneously transferred. In one case (strain No. 3) transferred also resistance determinant to chloramphenicol. In no case transmission of haemolytic activity appeared (Table 2).

148

Table 2

RESULTS OF CONJUGATIONAL TESTS STREPTOMYCIN-RESISTANT
HAEMOLYTIC STRAINS OF E. COLI WITH E. COLI 185 Nx

| | Donor | | | | Recipient | | | | Hybrid | | |
| | Tested Markers | | | | Tested Markers | | | | Tested Markers | | |
Marks	Resistance to	Production of Colicine	Haemolysis	Mark	Resistance to	Production of Colicine	Haemolysis	Selective Markers	Resistance to	Production of Colicine	Haemolysis
112	TOS	+	+					S, Nx	0	0	0
	TOS	+	+					T, Nx	TONx	+	−
3	TOSC	+	+					S, Nx	0	0	0
	TOSC	+	+	185	Nx	−	−	T, Nx	TOCNx	+	−
7562	TOS	+	+					S, Nx	SNx	−	−
	TOS	+	+					T, Nx	TONx	+	−
284	SC	−	+					S, Nx	SCNx	−	−

From 44 tetracycline resistant strains 9 strains transferred haemolytic activity to *E. coli* *185* Nx in simple conjugational test. In three strains it was only haemolytic activity, in 5 strains the haemolytic activity was transferred simultaneously with resistance determinant to tetracycline and in one case haemolytic activity was transferred simultaneously with resistance determinant to tetracycline and with Col factor. (Table 3).

Table 3

RESULTS OF CONJUGATIONAL TESTS TETRACYCLINE-RESISTANT
HAEMOLYTIC STRAINS OF E. COLI TRANSMISSIBLE HAEMOLYTIC ACTIVITY
TO E. COLI 185 Nx

DONOR		RECIPIENT	HYBRID	
95/70	T, Col⁻, Hly⁺		185 Nx,	Col⁻, Hly⁺
99	T, Col⁻, Hly⁺		185 Nx,	Col⁻, Hly⁺
1618	T, Col⁻, Hly⁺		185 Nx,	Col⁻, Hly⁺
S-41	T, Col⁻, Hly⁺		185 TNx,	Col⁻, Hly⁺
S-48	T, Col⁻, Hly⁺	185 Nx, Col⁻, Hly⁻	185 TNx,	Col⁻, Hly⁺
179	T, Col⁻, Hly⁺		185 TNx,	Col⁻, Hly⁺
5	T, Col⁺, Hly⁺		185 TNx,	Col⁻, Hly⁺
7171	T, Col⁺, Hly⁺		185 TNx,	Col⁻, Hly⁺
1730	T, Col⁺, Hly⁺		185 TNx,	Col⁺, Hly⁺

18 tetracycline resistant strains unable of the independent transmission of resistance determinant to tetracycline were submitted to resistance determinant mobilization test employing noncolicinogene, tetracycline sensitive and streptomycin resistant (mobile resistance) strain of *E. coli 284* as donor of transfer factor. Transfer factor obtained from

that donor has mobilized always only one studied genetic determinant. Mobilization occured in 5 strains: in three strains mobilized resistance determinant to tetracycline, in one strain Col factor and in one strain Hly. (Table 4).

Table 4

TESTS RESULTS OF MOBILIZATION OF EXTRACHROMOSOMAL GENETIC DETERMINANTS AT HAEMOLYTIC STRAINS OF E. COLI ISOLATED FROM SWINE

Donor $\times$ Intermediate Recipient $\times$ Final Recipient $=$ Hybrid
284 SC, Col⁻, Hly⁺ 185 Nx, Col⁻, Hly⁻

Intermediate Recipient	Hybrid	Determinants		
		Mobile	Mobiled	Immobiled
7 T, Col⁺, Hly⁺	185 SCNx, Col⁺, Hly⁺	Col	Hly	T
1618 T, Col⁺, Hly⁺	185 SCNx, Col⁺, Hly⁺	Hly	Col	T
101 T, Col⁺, Hly⁺	185 TSCNx, Col⁺, Hly⁻	Col	T	Hly
186 T, Col⁺, Hly⁺	185 TSCNx, Col⁺, Hly⁻	Col	T	Hly
4847 T, Col⁺, Hly⁺	185 TSCNx, Col⁺, Hly⁻	Col	T	Hly

CONCLUSION

The first study concerning occurrence of some plasmids at *E. coli* performed on this workplace has more-less informative and qualitative character.

It had to prove first of all considerable differences in the equipment of individual studied strains by three examined groups of markers, that is resistance determinants, Col factors and transmissible haemolytic activity (*Hly*). The second part of the experiment showed which plasmids are independently able to be transferred for the suitable recipient. Greater attention was paid to streptomycin resistant strains which were examined for the possibility of simultaneous transfer of different markers by aid of hybrid selection on two kinds of selective media. In this part of experiment a strain that could be a good donor in extrachromosomal genetic determinants mobilization tests on the ground of its high frequency of transfer resistance determinant to streptomycin was chosen.

In tetracycline resistant strains we studied the ability of transfering the haemolytic activity as well as possibilities of simultaneous transferring of some other markers.

Results of extrachromosomal genetic determinants mobilization tests showed the possibility of all studied markers mobilization.

TRANSMISSIBLE RESISTANCE IN ROUTINE LABORATORY PRACTICE

J. BOHUŠ

Department of Microbiology, District Station of Hygiene, Liptovský Mikuláš,
Czechoslovakia

This report is the summary of my study of the transmissible resistance in routine laboratory practice. The partial results of this work were recently published during last years (BOHUŠ, J. and BALÁŽ, M. 1968, BOHUŠ, J. 1971, BOHUŠ, J. and BALÁŽ, M. 1971).

Numerous data on transmissible resistance accumulated by research workers are not fully applicated in the practice. In many diagnostic laboratories the methods of sensitivity tests are used, which do not take into consideration the principles of transmissible resistance. I want here to point out briefly some of these methods and to propose procedures which are in an accordance with transmissible resistance and which should be accepted by all diagnostic laboratories.

1. In most cases only one colony is picked up for sensitivity test from one isolated strain. If the transfer, segregation and recombination of R factors is considered, many colonies from one strain should be tested.

2. Sensitivity tests of pathogenic strains or these with supposed etiological significance are very often preferred to the sensitivity tests of commensal strains. It is known that some nonpathogenic strains can serve as stable sources of R factors. It is necessary, therefore, to take into consideration results of sensitivity tests of all strains without regard to their ethiological importance.

3. To avoid the transfer of R factors from commensal to pathogenic strains, bacteriologists should not recommend such a drug for the therapy, which is included in the transmissible resistance of commensal strains.

4. From the view point of prevention it is necessary to search for R factors in the persons exposed to an increased risk of infection by pathogenic intestinal strains as are microbiologists, epidemiologists and infectologists. This is valid also in the case of premature babies, newborn children and sucklings babies where the occurence of pathogenic strains might have a serious consequence.

5. The results of sensitivity tests of the strains isolated in the beginning of epidemic are very often extended to the strains which are isolated during the next course of the epidemic. If we presume transfer of R factors from commensal intestinal microflora to pathogenic strains, then every strain isolated in epidemic should be tested for sensitivity.

6. According to our experience, doctors in hospitals are not acquainted sufficiently with principles and practical importance of transmissible resistance. All bacteriologists working in hospitals should spread these informations among workers from various medical branches.

7. All diagnostic laboratories should make records on polyresistance of strains during

the long time intervals. These data when statistically evaluated can serve as criteria for consumption planning of antibacterial drugs in a given district.

We have observed the dynamics and the types of resistance of strains belonging to some genera of *Enterobacteriaceae* for the period from 1966 to 1970. According to their origin and species the strains were divided up into five groups. Sensitivity or resistance to one or

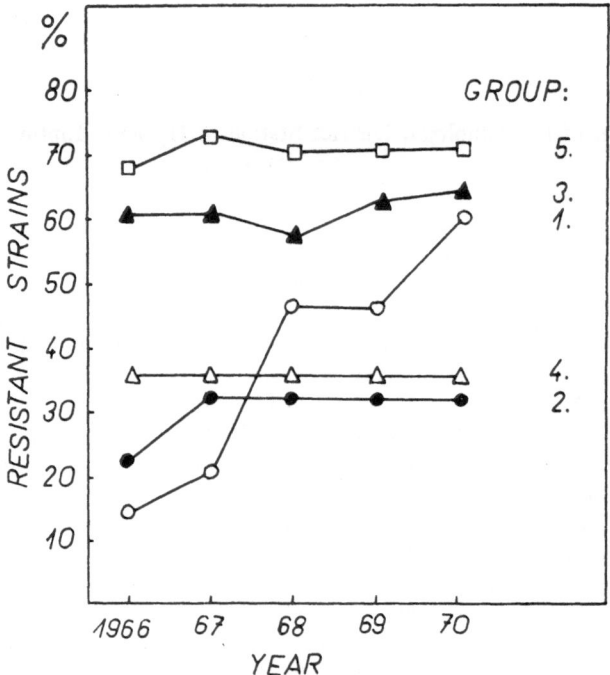

Fig. 1 The resistance of Enterobacteriaceae strains isolated from 1966 to 1970. Groups 1. to 5.: see text for explanation.

more drugs related to R-6 factor was recorded (Tc-Sm-Su-Kn-Ne-Cm, see footnotes to table).

Resistance of *Shigella* strains (1. group) rised from 15 per cent in 1966 to 60 per cent in 1970. Resistance of salmonella strains (2. group) has retained at the level of 33 per cent after initial increase. This could be conditioned by the rapid segregation of R factors in these microorganisms. The resistance of *coli — aerobacter* strains isolated from childrens' stools up to two years of age (3. group) has not changed and has retained at 60 per cent level. Similarly stable was the resistance of these microbes isolated from clinical specimens such as sputum, pus and so on (4. group) and from urine (5. group) and has retained on 35 or 70 per cent level respectively.

The data on the occurence of various types of resistance in the above mentioned groups of strains are summarized in the table. The type of resistance corresponding to R-6 factor (Tc-Sm-Su-Kn-Ne-Cm) was prevalent in 2., 3., and 4. groups. In 1. and 5. groups the prevailing type of resistance was corresponding to R-4 factor (Tc-Sm-Su-Cm). Other types of resistance corresponded to segregational products of original R-6 and R-4 factors. Resistance types such as Tc, Tc-Sm-Su, Sm-Su and Tc-Cm were comparatively more frequent. We arranged all these types by such a manner, that they have formed complementary pairs giving together original R-6 factor. They really seem to be segregants of R-6 factor as we have observed most of them in segregation of R-6 factor in experimental conditions. On the other hand the possibility exists, that these segregants can recombine and give original R-6 factor.

Table

THE RESISTANCE TYPES OF ENTEROBACTERIACEAE STRAINS ISOLATED FROM 1966 TO 1970

Type of resistance (drugs)[1]	Group of strains[2]				
	1.	2.	3.	4.	5.
Tc Sm Su Kn Ne Cm	31	24	1228	219	277
Tc Sm Su – – – Cm	209	11	734	120	458
– – – Kn Ne – –		1		3	3
Tc – – – – –	21	29	347	143	209
– Sm Su Kn Ne Cm	1		10	1	3
– – – – – Cm	6		50	21	13
Tc Sm Su Kn Ne –	2	2	46	4	3
Tc Sm Su – – – –	11	3	155	116	76
– – – – Kn Ne Cm		3	2		3
Tc – – Kn Ne Cm		11	10		
– Sm Su – – –	2		85	119	47
Tc – – Kn Ne – –	2		20	1	
– Sm Su – – Cm	8		52	23	37
Tc – – – – Cm	14	1	108	26	39
– Sm Su Kn Ne –				4	2
Total:					
resistant	307	85	2847	800	1170
sensitive	568	216	1821	1528	510
examined	875	301	4668	2328	1680

[1] Tc, Tetracycline; Sm, Streptomycine; Su, Sulphonamides; Kn, Kanamycine; Ne, Neomycine; Cm, Chloramphenicol

[2] See text fo further explanation

REFERENCES

BOHUŠ, J., BALÁŽ, M. (1968): Role of some members of Enterobacteriaceae family in maintaining and spreading of the transferable polyresistance. Folia Microbiologica, **13**, 275.

BOHUŠ, J. (1971): Acceptance of R factor by a Shigella sonnei strain from commensal Escherichia coli strains during dysentery. Journal of Hygiene, Epidemiology, Microbiology and Immunology, **15**, 225.

BOHUŠ, J. and BALÁŽ, M. (1971): Study of transmissible polyresistance in routine laboratory practice. Journal of Hygiene, Epidemiology, Microbiology and Immunology (In press).

II.

GENETIC
AND MOLECULAR-BIOLOGIC ASPECTS
OF RESISTANCE FACTORS

Moderators:

S. GLOVER (Edinburgh)
P. FREDERICQ (Liège)
T. WATANABE (Tokyo)
D. SMITH (Boston)

ANTIBIOTICS AS TOOLS IN CELL RESEARCH

V. BETINA

Department of Technical Microbiology and Biochemistry, Faculty of Chemistry,
Bratislava, Czechoslovakia

Microbiologists are tempted to consider antibiotics as chemical weapons of micro-organisms in their struggle for survival. Physicians might admire them as, in terms of Paul Ehrlich, "magical bullets" and powerful drugs. Biochemists include antibiotics among secondary metabolites with almost unknown raison d'ètre for microorganism which produce them. But together with molecular biologists, they find some antibiotics to be useful tools in studying various aspects of cell structure and function.

The use of antibiotics as metabolic inhibitors in cell research has greeatly increased our understanding of the following processes: (i) biosynthesis of nucleic acids and proteins, (ii) intermediary metabolism, (iii) cell wall synthesis, (iv) functions of cell membranes, (v) energy metabolism, and (vi) morphogenesis and differentiation.

Antibiotics and the central dogma of molecular biology

In 1970 the "central dogma" of molecular biology was intensively discussed in the light of findings that, in special cases, DNA molecules are synthesized by an RNA-dependent DNA polymerase. The "central dogma" was re-formulated by its father CRICK (1970) and illustrated with a triangle which represents the so-called general and special transfers of information.

In the central part of Figure 1 Crick's triangel is presented. Its solid arrows show general transfers, dotted arrows show special transfers of information. On the same figure effects of some antibiotics on the biochemical machinery of the transfers of information are indicated. Several antibiotics are known to inhibit DNA replication. Others interfere in the processes of transcription, i. e., synthesis of RNA catalyzed by DNA-dependent RNA polymerase. Protein synthesis — the translation process is inhibited by many antibiotics and only some of them are given on the picture. The natural message for the translation processes is RNA, but in a special transfer *in vitro* single-stranded DNA was translated directly in the presence of neomycin B (McCARTHY and HOLLAND, 1965). The translation occured in a special cell-free system, though it could probably be made to happen, using neomycin B, in an intact bacterial cell (CRICK, 1970).

Inhibitors of DNA and RNA synthesis

How do antibiotics affect DNA synthesis? In most cases inhibitors of DNA replication form complexes with DNA molecules which prevents their replication (Figure 2). For instance, mitomycin C induces cross-linking of complementary DNA, a proces which

157

facilitates renaturation after heat treatment but which tends to block progress of the replicative enzyme along the DNA molecule *in vivo* (SZYBALSKI and IYER, 1967).

Antibiotics interfering with RNA synthesis can be divided into two groups. The first one includes inhibitors which form complexes with DNA templates and prevent RNA synthesis by preventing progress of the "reading" enzyme, DNA-dependent RNA polymerase, along the template. Actinomycin D is a classical example of such inhibitors

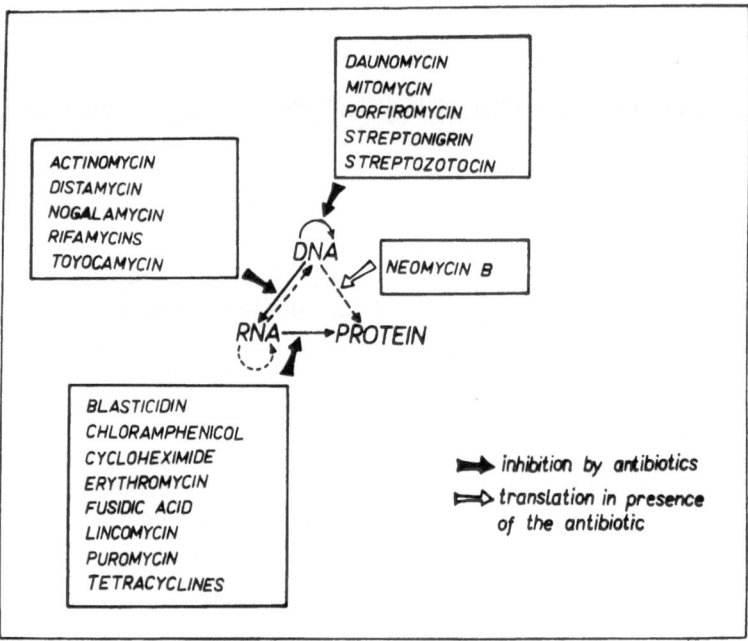

Figure 1 Effects of antibiotics on transfers of information. DNA replication is inhibited by daunomycin and other antibiotics. Actinomycin and others inhibit transcription. Translation is inhibited by blasticidin and other drugs. Neomycin B is necessary for a direct translation from DNA to protein. See text for details.

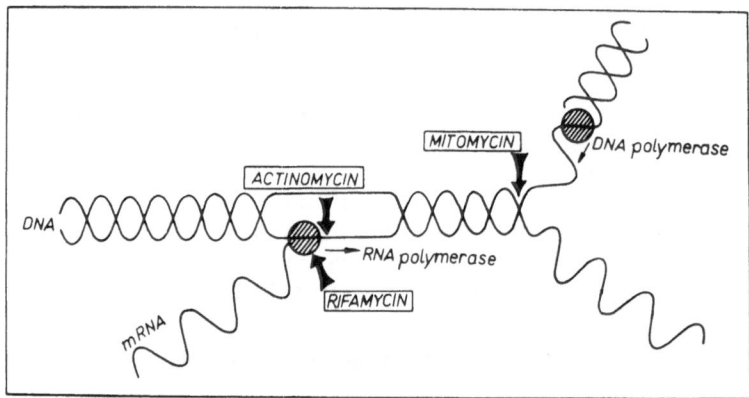

Figure 2 Inhibitors of DNA and RNA synthesis. Mitomycin C inhibits DNA replication by forming complexes with DNA. Actinomycin D binds to DNA and prevents RNA synthesis. Rifamycin inhibits transcription by interacting with RNA polymerase.

158

(REICH, CERAMI and WARD, 1967) which also include distamycin A (PUSCHENDORF and GRUNICKE, 1969; CHANDRA, ZIMMER and THRUM, 1970; PUSCHENDORF, PETERSON, WOLF, WERCHAU and GRUNICKE, 1971), chromomycin A₃ (SAKAI and TAKEBE, 1970), nogalamycin (ELLEM and RHODE, 1970) and streptonigrin MIZUNO and GILBOE, 1970).

To the second group of inhibitors of RNA synthesis belong those that interact with DNA-dependent RNA polymerase and prevent its functioning. MARINO, BALDI and TOCCHINI-VALENTI (1968) have demonstrated that rifampicin, a member of the rifamycin antibiotics, blocks RNA synthesis in vivo by acting directly on the RNA polymerase. Tirandamycin seems to have similar effects (REUSSER, 1970).

Antibiotics belonging to the first group of inhibitors of transcription might also inhibit, at least at higher concentrations, DNA synthesis which antibiotics of the second group do not. It was found recently by McDONNELL, GARAPIN, LEVINSON, QUINTRELL, FANSHIER and BISHOP (1970) that actinomycin D at high concentrations delineates two enzymatic activities present in Rous sarcoma virus (an RNA tumor virus): synthesis of DNA from an RNA template, with the formation of an RNA:DNA hybrid, and subsequent synthesis of double-stranded DNA. Only the latter process is inhibited by actinomycin D.

Transcription is done by the enzyme RNA polymerase. Escherichia coli has a polymerase which consists of a core enzyme catalysing the polymerization of nucleotides into long strands of RNA and a sigma factor which programmes to the core enzyme which individual genes of the DNA molecule should be transcribed. The sigma factor temporarily combines with the core enzyme and this complex is able to recognize initiation sequences of genes. After an initiation of a transcription the sigma factor dissociates and becomes free for another molecule of core enzyme. On the other hand, the core enzyme after having finished a transcription is free for forming another complex with a different sigma factor (CHAMBERLIN, McGRATH and WASKELL, 1970).

The functioning of bacterial DNA-dependent RNA polymerase is sensitive to rifamycin antibiotics. In special situations new types of RNA polymerase can occure in a bacterial cell. A rifampicin-resistant mutant of E. coli posesses an altered RNA polymerase. The mutant enzyme is markedly more resistant to the drug than the enzyme derived from the wild type (MARINO et al., 1968). Structural alterations of RNA polymerase were observed during sporulation of Bacillus subtilis (SONENSHEIM and LOSICK, 1970; LOSICK, SHORENSTEIN and SONENSHEIM, 1970). After an infection of E. coli cells by bacteriophage T7 a new RNA polymerase was observed which was insensitive to rifamycin because it was a transcription product of T7 gene and was physically and biochemically distinct from the host cell RNA polymerase (CHAMBERLIN et al., 1970). Thus rifamycins are tools which help to distinguish different types of RNA polymerase. In general, rifamycin antibiotics are active on procaryotic types of RNA polymerases that are present in bacteria, mitochondria and chloroplasts but do not act on RNA polymerases from eucaryotic cell nuclei (MODRIGUEZ-LOPEZ and MUNOZ, 1970; DEZELÉE, SENTENAC and FROMAGEOT, 1970). However, mitochondrial RNA polymerase from rat liver was sensitive to rifampicin only in a cell-free system (GADALETA, GRECO and SACCONE, 1970). The lack of inhibition in the presence of intact mitochondria from rat liver and from yeast (WINTERSBERGER and WINTERSBERGER, 1970) indicates that mitochondrial membrane is impermeable to the antibiotic and suggests that probably mitochondrial polymerase in vivo may not be affected by rifamycin antibiotics. On the other hand, these antibiotics do not affect directly growth of the green algae Chlorella pyrenoidosa, but cause bleaching most probably due to a direct effect on the chloroplast RNA polymerase (MODRIGUEZ-LOPEZ and MUNOZ, 1970). In blue-green algae RNA polymerase is possibly the main target of the rifamycin antibiotics which has in common with the enzymes of bacteria, mitochondria and chloroplasts in their sensitivity to the rifamycins.

Antibiotics and translation of the genetic message

Processes of translation, i. e. synthesis of protein molecules in the cell can be affected by several antibiotics. Protein synthesis will be discussed only briefly here but details can be found elsewhere (e. g. OCHOA, 1968).

Besides of a genetic message transcribed in a molecule of messenger RNA (mRNA) representing a program of synthesis, raw materials in form of amino acids, some "machinery" and energy are necessary for translation. The machinery consists of amino acid transfer RNAs (tRNA), ribosomes, several enzymes and of special regulating factors.

Amino acids must be, firstly, activated and then bound to specific tRNA molecules which transfer them to ribosomes. The antibiotic borrelidin is known to interfere in binding of activated amino acids to tRNA which results in inhibition of protein synthesis in *E. coli* and in *Saccharomyces cerevisiae* (HÜTTER, PORALLA, ZACHAU and ZÄHNER, 1966; NASS, PORALLA and ZÄHNER, 1969; NASS and HASENBANK, 1970).

Ribosomes are characterized by their sedimentation constants. A 70S unit of bacterial, mitochondrial or chloroplast ribosome consists of two subunits: 30S and 50S. Eucaryotic cytoplasmic 80S ribosomes are heavier, their subunits being 40S and 60S. During translation ribosomes combine with mRNA the codones of which temporarily combine with anticodones of tRNAs bringing activated amino acids to ribosomes and synthesis of a peptide chain proceeds. The synthesis of the peptide chain has three main stages: initiation, elongation and termination, each of them consisting of several steps (Figure 3).

Initiation begins when a 30S ribosome subunit combines with mRNA at the site of the initiation codon to which the anticodon of a tRNA transferring formylated methionine is attached. This step requires special initiation factors, Mg ions and GTP. N-formyl-methionine is the first amino acid in the peptide chain to be synthesized. The first step is followed by attachment of a 50S subunit. Next step, the binding of the second complex aminoacyl-tRNA requires GTP and a chain elongation factor. Aminoacyl-tRNAs other than Fmet-tRNA are bound at the 50S aminoacyl binding site (site A).

Step 3 is catalyzed by an enzyme in the 50S subunit which combines formylmethionine with the second amino acid by a peptide bond. This leads to a liberation of the first tRNA.

The so-called translocation is the following step. The ribosome shifts to the right on our scheme (Figure 3), whereby the growing peptidyl-tRNA shifts from the 50S amino-acyl (A-site) to the peptidyl binding site (P-site) and the A-site falls in line with the next codon. Another aminoacyl-tRNA complex is attached to the ribosome and, by its anticodon, to the codon of the mRNA. These processes repeat and lead to elongation of the peptide chain. Chain termination, the last stage of the translation occurs when a 70S ribosomal couple with its peptidyl-tRNA reaches a termination codon in its progress along the messenger. Chain termination leads to the release of free polypeptide and tRNA and to dissociation of the 70S ribosome couple to its components — 30S and 50S subunits.

Numbered arrows on Figure 3 indicate possibilities of intervention by antibiotics into translation processes as follows.

(1) Streptomycin and some other structurally related antibiotics combine with 30S subunits and so prevent protein synthesis (SCHLESSINGER, 1969). Conflicting results were obtained when binding of tetracyclines to ribosomes and ribosomal subunits was studied. Some authors report specific binding to the 30S subunit, others emphasize an association

with the 50S subunit (for references see LASKIN, 1967). Some more recent findings will be discussed by KERSTEN and FEY (1971) at this Symposium.

(2) Chloramphenicol inhibits peptide bond formation (GURGO, APIRION and SCHLESSINGER, 1969). Its other effects will be mentioned later.

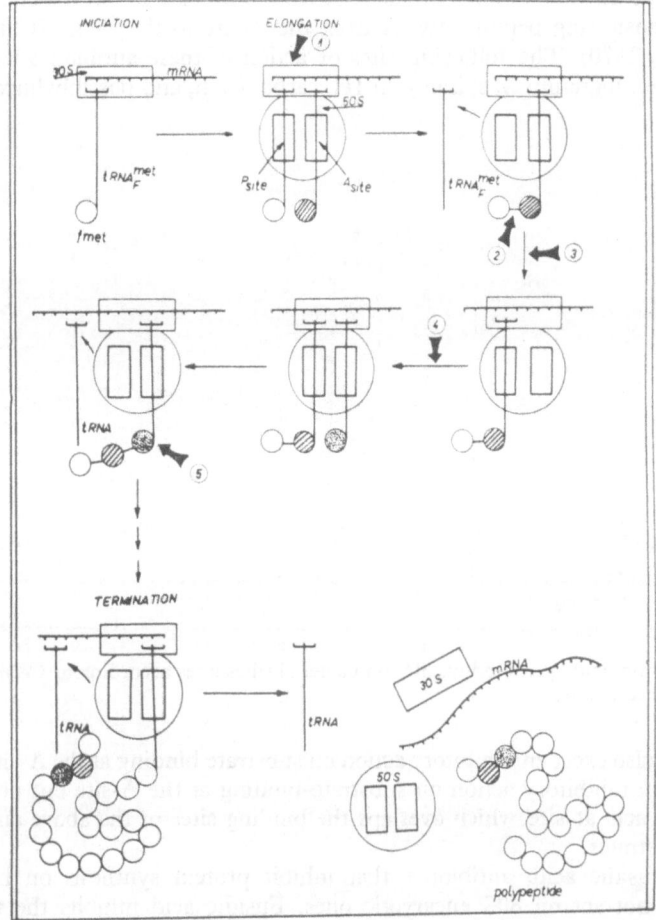

Figure 3 Interferences of antibiotics with protein synthesis. Thick arrows indicate effects of: (1) streptomycin, (2) chloramphenicol, (3) fusidic acid, (4) erythromycin, and (5) puromycin. See text for explanations.

(3) Fusidic acid blocks the activity of the G factor which is responsible for hydrolysis of GTP (TANAKA, KINOSHITA and MASUKAWA, 1968) and which is involved in moving ribosomes along mRNA (NISHIZUKA and LIPMANN, 1966) — the translocation step.

(4) Erythromycin and some other antibiotics combine with 50S subunits which will be discussed in more details later.

(5) Puromycin is structurally related to the amino-acyl end of the complex aminoacyl-tRNA. As a structural analogue of aminoacyl-tRNA, puromycin accepts growing polypeptide chains intended to transfer to the next aminoacyl-tRNA, thus terminating

further extension of the polypeptide. The demonstration that puromycin becomes linked to the carboxyl group of peptide chains by means of a peptide bond suggested that this reaction might serve as a model for specifically studying peptide bond formation in protein synthesis and is widely used indeed (NATHANS, 1967).

Erythromycin and other macrolide antibiotics together with chloramphenicol and lincomycin bind to 50S subunits of bacterial ribosomes and act on the enzyme peptidyl transferase transferring peptidyl-tRNA from the A-site to the P-site (CELMA, MONRO and VAZQUEZ, 1970). The following sites of action of these antibiotics were proposed (Figure 4). Streptogramin A, spiramycin III, carbomycin, and possibly lincomycin block

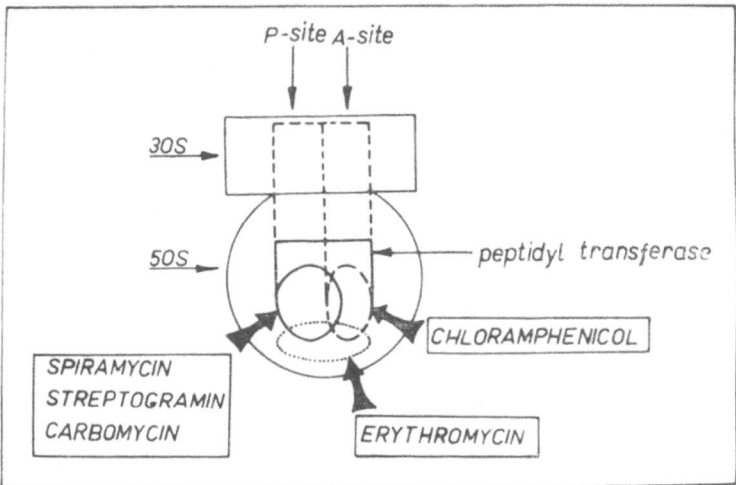

Figure 4 Antibiotics and their binding sites on bacterial ribosomes according to *Celma* et al (1970). See text for explanations.

the P-site and also exert an inhibitory action on substrate binding at the A-site. Chloramphenicol has an inhibitory action on substrate-binding at the A-site but not the P-site. Erythromycin acts at site which overlaps the binding sites of the above antibiotics but not of the substrates.

Except of fusidic acid, antibiotics that inhibit protein synthesis on bacterial 70S ribosomes do not act on 80S eucaryotic ones. Fusidic acid inhibits the translocation reaction both in bacterial and animal cells (TANAKA et al., 1968) and both in procaryotic and eucaryotic cell-free systems (BODLEY and LIN, 1970). Cycloheximide (actidione) is an antibiotic which inhibits protein biosynthesis in cells and systems that utilize ribosomes of the 80S type (for references see OBRIG, CULP, McKEEHAN and HARDESTY, 1971). It was demonstrated by OBRIG et al. (1971) that cycloheximide and related glutarimide antibiotics inhibit peptide synthesis on reticulocyte ribosomes at two different stages: initiation and elongation, the former being inhibited at lower concentrations of these antibiotics. At the elongation stage, the above antibiotics inhibit the translocation of aminoacyl-tRNA or peptidyl-tRNA from the A-site to the P-site at the 60S subunit. One might expect that cycloheximide inhibits the translocation step by a mechanism which is different to that of fusidic acid.

However, in eucaryotic cells there exist two types of ribosomes. Ribosomes working in the cytoplasm are of the 80S type and their function is sensitive to cycloheximide. On the other hand, in mitochondria and in chloroplasts there are ribosomes of the 70S (pro-caryotic) type and they can be specifically affected by inhibitors of bacterial protein synthesis. It is therefore possible to differentiate with antibiotics *in vivo* cytoplasmic and mitochondrial (or chloroplast) protein synthesis in eucaryotic cells (CLARK-WALKER and

Table 1

DIFFERENTIATION OF PROTEIN SYNTHESIS BY ANTIBIOTICS

Antibiotics	Inhibition of protein synthesis in			
	Procaryotic cells	Eucaryotic cells		
		Cytoplasm	Mitochondria	Chloroplasts
Chloramphenicol	+	−	+	+
Erythromycin	+	−	+	+
Fusidic acid	+	+	+	+
Cycloheximide	−	+	−	−

LINNANE, 1966; HOFFMANN and WALTER, 1970). Based on data collected from the literature, Table 1 presents possibilities of differential inhibition of protein synthesis by some antibiotics.

Inhibitors of intermediary metabolism

Antibiotics may act as antimetabolites and by doing so they can inhibit various reactions of intermediary metabolism. Examples of such antibiotics, inhibiting *de novo* purine synthesis, are given in Table 2. Their inhibitory effects can be overcome by addition of proper metabolites in the growth media.

Table 2

ANTIBIOTICS WITH ANTIMETABOLIC PROPERTIES

Antibiotics	Antimetabolites of	References
Azaserine	Glutamine	Pittillo and Hunt, 1967
Cordycepin	Adenosine, Guanosine	Guarino, 1967
Hadacidin	L-Aspartic acid	Shiguera, 1967
Psicofuranine	Guanine	Hanka, 1967

Melinacidin and albocycline are known as inhibitors of nicotinic acid synthesis and addition of nicotinic acid or nicotin-amide to *B. subtilis* cultures effectively reverses the inhibitory activity of these antibiotics (REUSSER, 1968, 1969).

Sideromycins, iron containing antibiotics, are competitive inhibitors of sideramines which are believed to play a role in iron metabolism (ZÄHNER, 1965).

Effects of antibiotics on cell wall synthesis

Several antibiotics are known to interfere with bacterial cell wall synthesis. Bacterial cell walls are synthesized in three distinct stages which occur at three different sites in the bacterial cell (for details and references see STROMINGER, 1967). Antibiotics are known which specifically inhibit the activity of enzymes at each of these sites (Figure 5).

In the first stage which proceeds in the cytoplasm two uridine nucleotide precursors of the bacterial cell wall, UDP-acetylglucosamine (UDP-GlcNAc) and UDP-acetyl-muramyl-pentapeptide (UDP-MurNAc-pentapeptide), are synthesized. The antibiotic, D-cycloserine, inhibits the biosynthesis of the latter by inhibiting two sequential reactions catalyzed by alanineracemase and D-alanyl-D-alanine synthetase which are essential for synthesis of this nucleotide.

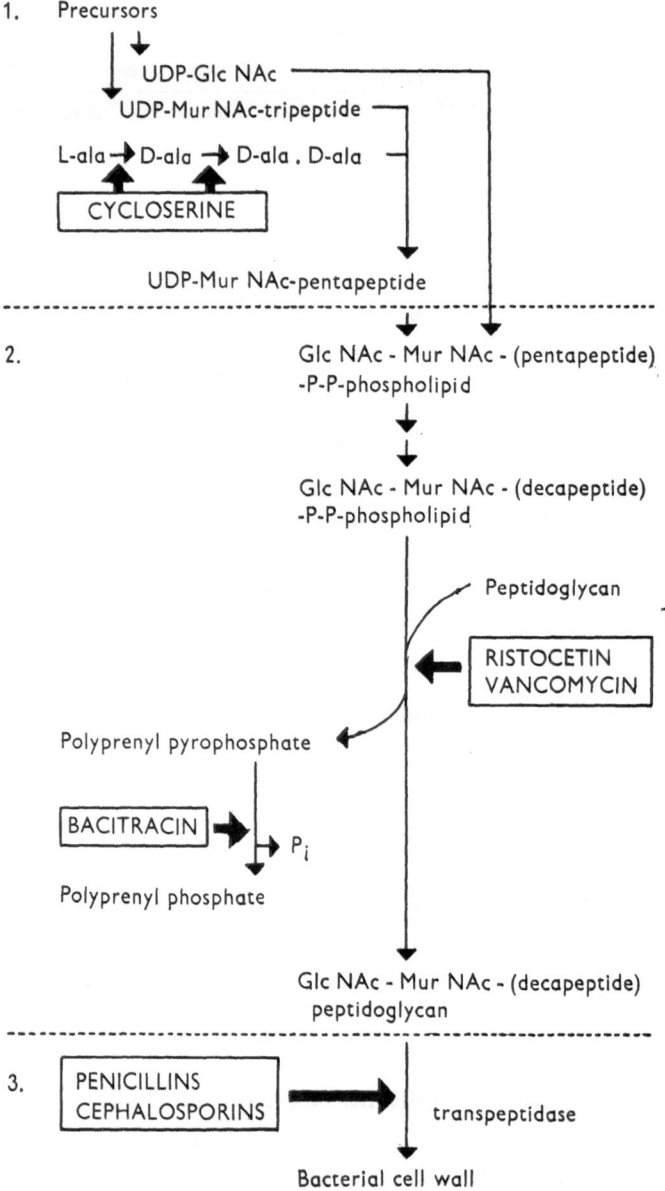

Figure 5 Antibiotics as inhibitors of bacterial cell wall synthesis (schematically). Three sequential stages of the synthesis are indicated by numbers 1, 2 and 3. For details see text.

The second stage of cell wall synthesis is the utilization of these two uridine nucleotide precursors and other substrates for the introduction of new disaccharide-pentapeptide units into a growing peptidoglycan in the bacterial cell wall. Ristocetin and vancomycin are specific inhibitors of the utilization of the lipid intermediates for peptidoglycan synthesis. Bacitracin is another specific inhibitor of the dephosphorylation of polyprenyl pyrophosphate which is liberated during attachement of the disaccharide units to peptidoglycan (ANONYMOUS, 1970).

The third stage in cell wall synthesis is the cross-linking of the linear peptidoglycan strands in a transpeptidation reaction. The latter is inhibited by penicillins and cephalosporins which results in protoplast or sphaeroplast formation from growing bacteria with damaged cell walls. The above processes were elucidated due to the use of antibiotics as specific tools interfering with these reactions.

Effects of two antibiotics, polyoxin A and polyoxin D on cell wall synthesis in fungi have been described recently. Both inhibitors block chitin synthetase playing an essential role in synthesis of chitin which is a major component of fungal cell wall (KELLER and CABIB, 1971).

Studies of cell wall synthesis in yeast protoplasts under appropriate conditions revealed that both wall components, i. e. fibrillar network consisting of glucan and amorphous matrix containing proteins, are synthesized synchronously and complete cell wall regenerate (NEČAS, 1971). It has been found that cycloheximide does not interfere with the synthesis of neither mannans in a cell-free system (FARKAŠ, SVOBODA and BAUER, 1970) nor the fibrillar network of regenerated cell wall of *Saccharomyces cerevisiae* but it inhibits completely the formation of the matrix (NEČAS, SVOBODA and KOPECKÁ, 1968). This is in good agreement with the effect of the antibiotic on the synthesis of wall components in normal cells. SENTANDREU and NORTHOCTE (1969) found that cycloheximide inhibits the incorporation of labelled threonine into the wall but only partially inhibits the incorporation of labelled glucose. From these experiments it was concluded that only synthesis of cell wall proteins (i. e. components of the amorphous matrix) is inhibited by cycloheximide while the synthesis of glucan, which forms the fibrillar network, is relatively independent of protein synthesis (NEČAS, 1971).

Changes of cell membranes and energy metabolism by antibiotisc

Many antibiotics may interfere with cell membranes and cause damage of their functions. Polyene antibiotics, e. g. nystatin, amphotericin B etc., damage cytoplasmic membranes in eucaryotic cells. Their interactions with fungal and animal cell membranes were described by many authors (for references see LAMPEN, 1966 and KINSKY, 1967). Permeability alterations caused by some polyene antibiotics in plant cells have been observed in our laboratory (NEMEC and BETINA, 1968; BETINA, BARÁTHOVÁ, BARÁTH and NEMEC, 1969). Such permeability alterations induced by polyene antibiotics are ascribed mainly to binding of these substances to sterols in eucaryotic cell membranes. Bacterial cytoplasmic membrane, because of absence of sterols in its structure, is insensitive to polyene antibiotics (LAMPEN, 1966).

Antibacterial antibiotics are known to affect procaryotic cell membrane and to alter its permeability and transport functions. They include polypeptide and macrotetrolide antibiotics such as valinomycin, gramicidin, polymyxin, the actins and nigericidin. It was proposed that a common feature of the mode of action of these membrane-active antibacterial compounds is their initial adsorption on the sensitive membrane. Although it seems certain that, once adsorbed, the action of tyrocidine and polymyxin is in fact to destroy non-specifically the membrane's permeability barrier to low-molecular-weight substances, other antibiotics mentioned above demonstrate a considerable degree of specifity in their action on the bacterial plasma membrane. Some of them have been found to act as uncouplers of oxidative phosphorylation in both bacterial and mitochondrial systems. The most striking results of recent studies has been the finding that these antibiotics can render the mitochondrial, bacterial and even lipid bilayer membranes specifically permeable to various monovalent cations (HAMILTON, 1970).

The above antibiotics and certain others became useful tools in studies of energy metabolism. Antimycin A and oligomycins are perhaps their best known representatives. Others may be found listed and well documented in a recent book dealing with mechanisms of action of antibiotics (GOTTLIEB and SHAW, 1967).

Effects of antibiotics on cell organelles

Extensive studies on the effects of various antibiotics on the formation of mitochondrial proteins have made contributions toward elucidating the genetic control mechanisms of mitochondrial biogenesis. Amino acid incorporation into protein by isolated ribosomal systems from eucaryotic cells has been established as not being affected by chlorapmhenicol but the antibiotic inhibited protein synthesis in mitochondria which were isolated from protozoa (MAGER, 1960), yeast (WINTERSBERGER, 1965) and rat liver (WHEELDON and LEHNINGER, 1966). It has been shown that chloramphenicol inhibits the formation of cytochrome a, a_3, b and c_1 and the inner membrane of mitochondria in yeast and HeLa cells, but not that of cytochrome c and the outer membrane of the particles (CLARK-WALKER and LINNANE, 1966; HUANG, BIGGS and LINNANE, 1966; CLARK-WALKER and LINNANE, 1967; FIRKIN and LINNANE, 1968; LINNANE, BIGGS, HUANG and CLARK-WALKER, 1967). On the other hand, cycloheximide suppressed protein synthesis in yeast ribosomes but not that of mitochondria (CLARK-WALKER and LINNANE, 1966).

Interresting results have been obtained in studies on biogenesis of mitochondria during aging of sliced sweet potato root tissue (ASAHI and MAJIMA, 1969). The results with chloramphenicol and cycloheximide suggest a possible differentiation of ribosomal and mitochondrial protein synthesis in sweet potato root tissue: peroxidase synthesis in cytoplasmic ribosomes (inhibited by cycloheximide) and cytochrome oxidase synthesis in mitochondria (inhibited by chloramphenicol). The reproduction of mitochondria may be controlled by protein synthesis in mitochondria but is not controlled by protein synthesis in cytoplasmic ribosomes. Mitomycin C inhibited mitochondrial reproduction but did not protein synthesis. Thus it has been inferred that the biogenesis of mitochondria during aging of sliced sweet potato root tissue is controlled by mitochondrial genes.

Strong evidence has been provided to support the hypothesis that reversible bone marrow suppression from large doses of chloramphenicol results from inhibition by the drug of mitochondrial protein synthesis (MARTELO, MANYAN, SMITH and YUNIS, 1969). Electron-microscopic examination of bone marrow mitochondria derived from patients before and after chloramphenicol therapy have also shown that the antibiotic induces an ultrastructural modification resulting in an increase in the density of the mitochondrial matrix. These changes have been interpreted in terms of mitochondrial protein synthesis (SMITH, SMITH and YUNIS, 1970).

Important results have been obtained in studies on effects of antibiotics on chloroplasts. Inhibitors of DNA replication or of protein synthesis of the procaryotic type have been shown to specifically interfere with chlorophyl synthesis and reproduction of chloroplasts. Streptomycin, erythromycin and other antibiotics induced changes leading to mutants of *Euglena gracilis* which have lost the inherent ability to reproduce chloroplasts

(EBRINGER, 1971; EBRINGER, NEMEC, SANTOVÁ and FOLTÍNOVÁ, 1970). Thus, photoautotrophic organisms have been changed into heterotrophic ones.

Cytotoxic and cancerostatic antibiotics have strong effects on the mitotic cycle. Mitomycin C and actinomycin D have been studied in this respect (TRUHAUT and DEYSSON 1960; MERTZ, 1961; BAL and GROSS, 1963). Finding in this field obtained in our laboratory might also be mentioned here. In the presence of the antibiotic cyanein (BETINA, NEMEC, DOBIAS and BARÁTH, 1962) mitosis in root meristem in *Vicia faba* ceases after about 4 hours. Cyanein causes a considerable decrease of colchicine-metaphases after 2 hours and prevents the second mitotic cycle acting as a pre-prophase inhibitor (BETINA and MURIN, 1964).

Cytochalasin B is known to cause several types of animal cells to become multinucleate. Many other biological processes are sensitive to the drug which can be interpreted that contractile microfilament machinery is reversibly inhibited by cytochalasin B (see a review of WESSELLS, SPOONER, ASH, BRADLEY, LUDUENA, TAYLOR, WRENN and YAMADA, 1971). Cytochalasin B is now widely used in studies of morphogenesis and differentiation of animal cells and tissues.

Antibiotics in studies of morphogenesis of slime molds and fungi

The cellular slime mold, *Dictyostellium discoideum*, is a widely used model for studying morphogenesis. Its life cycle is characterized by at least two phases of development: vegetative reproduction and morphogenesis. During the morphogenetic phase, the myxamoebae stop growing and form multicellular agregates which differentiate into complete fruiting bodies with spore masses and supporting tissue ensheathed in cellulose (BONNER, 1959). Actinomycin D inhibits both development of amoebae and RNA formation in the early stage of morphogenesis. Cycloheximide prevents both overall morphogenesis and protein synthesis. These results suggest that RNA and protein syntheses are responsible for morphogenesis in the slime mold. Experimental data are available that during development from interphase to the migration stage formation of mRNA greatly predominates over those of tRNA and ribosomal RNA. Thus mRNA synthesis in the early stage of morphogenesis may well be inhibited considerably or completely by actinomycin D. Protein synthesis in the early stage was not prevented by actinomycin treatment. A possible explanation for this is that protein synthesis in the early stage of morphogenesis may be controlled by mRNA synthesized in the previous not the same stage (MIZUKAMI and IWABUCHI, 1970).

Morphology and morphogenesis of true fungi can also be affected by antibiotics. BRIAN, CURTIS and HEMMING (1946) observed curling of *Botrytis cinerea* hyphae after contact with griseofulvin. Scopamycins induced branching of hyphae of the same fungus (HÜTTER, KELLER-SCHIERLEIN, NÜSCH and ZÄHNER, 1965). With Drs. Segretain and Drouhet at the Pasteur Institute we found that cyanein induces yeast-like growth *in vitro* of the dimorphic fungus *Paecilomyces viridis* (BETINA, DROUHET and SEGRETAIN, 1965). This phenomenon was studied in more detalis by BETINA, BETINOVÁ and KUTKOVÁ (1966). When *P. viridis* growing in the presence of cyanein was transferred onto agar plates without the antibiotic, filamentous growth was again obtained. The observed transformations of *P. viridis* were characterized as follows:

Filamentous		Yeast-like		Filamentous
form	$\xrightarrow[\text{added}]{\text{cyanein}}$	form	$\xrightarrow[\text{removed}]{\text{cyanein}}$	form
(saprophytic)		(parasitic)		(saprophytic)

Cyanein and some other antibiotics induced various morphological changes of pathogenic fungi, e. g. strong ramification of hyphae of *B. cinerea*.

When studying morphological effects of about 30 antibiotics on *B. cinerea* we found that 18 of them induced changes which have been classified as branching, curling, narrowing, broadening and bulging (BARÁTHOVÁ, BETINA and NEMEC, 1969). Besides of cyanein, other antibiotics belonging to the same group of aglycosidic macrolide antibiotics (monorden, cytochalasin A, zygosporin A) induce branching of *B. cinerea* hyphae (BETINA and MIČEKOVÁ, 1971). Ramihyphins, a complex of antibiotics with antifungal properties are characterized by branching effects on filamentous fungi (BARÁTH, BARÁTHOVÁ, BETINA and NEMEC, in preparation). Ramihyphin A causes a rapid hyphal branching in *Neurospora sitophila* which is accompanied by changes in the ratio of aminohexoses to neutral hexoses in mycelial cell walls (HUDEC, BARÁTH and BETINA, in preparation).

Morphology of *P. viridis* can be deeply influenced by several antibiotics (BARÁTHOVÁ et al., 1969). When composition of cell walls of the filamentous and cyanein-induced yeast-like forms *P. viridis* was analyzed significant differences in the ratio of aminohexoses to neutral hexoses were found and cell walls of the latter form were much thicker than those of the former (BARÁTH, BARÁTHOVÁ, KOMAN and BETINA, in preparation). Further work is in progress on this problem as we feel that antibiotics may be helpful agents in studying morphogenesis of fungi.

REFERENCES

ANONYMOUS (1970): —. New Scientist, **48**, 113.

ASAHI, T. and MAJIMA, R. (1969): Effect of antibiotics on biogenesis of mitochondria during aging of sliced sweet potato root tissue. Plant and Cell Physiology, **10**, 317.

BAL, A. K. and GROSS, P. R. (1963): Mitosis and differentiation in roots treated with actinomycin. Science, **139**, 584.

BARÁTHOVÁ, H., BETINA, V. and NEMEC, P. (1969): Morphological changes induced in fungi by antibiotics. Folia microbiologica, **14**, 475.

BETINA, V. and MIČEKOVÁ, D. (1971): Morphological changes in Botrytis cinerea induced by macrolide antibiotics from molds. Folia microbiologica, **16**.

BETINA, V. and MURÍN, A. (1964): Inhibition of mitotic activity in root tips of Vicia faba by the antibiotic cyanein. Cytologia, **29**, 370.

BETINA, V., BETINOVÁ, M. and KUTKOVÁ, M. (1966:) Effects of cyanein on growth and morphology of pathogenic fungi. Archiv für Mikrobiologie, **55**, 1.

BETINA, V., DROUHET, E. and SEGRETAIN, G. (1965): Action de la cyanéine in vitro sur des champignons pathogènes. Annales de l'Institut Pasteur, **109**, 933.

BETINA, V., BARÁTHOVÁ, H., BARÁTH, Z. and NEMEC, P. (1969): Effects of polyene antibiotics on plant, fungal and animal cell membranes. Biológia (Bratislava), **24**, 450.

BETINA, V., NEMEC, P., DOBIAS, J. and BARÁTH, Z. (1962): Cyanein, a new antibiotic from Penicillium cyaneum. Folia microbiologica, **7**, 353.

BODLEY, J. W. and LIN, L. (1970): Studies on translocation. V.: Fusidic acid stabilization of a eukaryotic ribosome-translocation factor-GDP complex. FEBS Letters, **11**, 153.

BONNER, J. T. (1959): *The cellular slime mold.* Princeton University Press, Princeton, N. J.

BRIAN, P. W., CURTIS, P. J. and HEMMING, H. G. (1946): A substance causing abnormal development of fungal hyphae produced by Penicillium janczewskii. Transactions of the British Mycological Society, **29**, 173.

CELMA, M. L., MONRO, R. E. and VAZQUEZ, D. (1970): Substrate and antibiotic binding sites at the peptidyltransferase centre of E. coli ribosomes. FEBS Letters, **6**, 273.

CHAMBERLIN, M., McGRATH, J. and WASKELL, L. (1970): New RNA polymerase from Escherichia coli infected with bacteriophage T7. Nature, **228**, 227.

CHANDRA, P., ZIMMER, Ch. and THRUM, H. (1970): Effect of distamycin A on the structure and template activity of DNA in RNA-polymerase system. FEBS Letters, **7**, 90.

CLARK-WALKER, G. D. and LINNANE, A. W. (1966): In vivo differentiation of yeast cytoplasmic and mitochondrial protein synthesis with antibiotics. Biochemical and Biophysical Research Communications, 25, 8.

CLARK-WALKER, G. D. and LINNANE, A. W. (1967): The biogenesis of mitochondria in Saccharomyces cerevisiae. A comparison between cytoplasmic respiratory-deficient mutant yeast and chloramphenicol-inhibited wild type cells. Journal of Cell Biology, 34, 1.

CRICK, F. (1970): Central dogma of molecular biology. Nature, 227, 561.

DEZELÉE, S., SENTENAC, A. and FROMAGEOT, P. (1970): Study on yeast RNA polymerase. Effect of α-amanitin and rifampicin. FEBS Letters, 7, 220.

EBRINGER, L. (1971): The action of inhibitors of nucleic acid synthesis on Euglena. Experientia, 27, 586.

EBRINGER, L., NEMEC, P., SANTOVÁ, H. and FOLTÍNOVÁ, P. (1970): Changes of the plastid system of Euglena gracilis induced with streptomycin and dihydrostreptomycin. Archiv für Mikrobiologie, 73, 268.

ELLEM, K. A. O. and RHODE, S. L. (1970): Selective inhibition of ribosomal RNA synthesis in HeLa cells by nogalamycin, a dA: dT binding antibiotic. Biochimica et Biophysica Acta, 209, 415.

FARKAŠ, V., SVOBODA, A. and BAUER, Š. (1970): Secretion of cell wall glycoproteins by yeast protoplasts. The effect of 2-deoxy-D-glucose and cycloheximide. Biochemical Journal, 118, 755.

FIRKIN, F. C. and LINNANE, A. W. (1968): Differential effects of chloramphenicol on the growth and respiration of mammalian cells. Biochemical and Biophysical Research Communications, 32, 398.

GADALETA, M. N., GRECO, M. and SACCONE, C. (1970): The effect of rifampicin on mitochondrial RNA polymerase from rat liver. FEBS Letters, 10, 54.

GOTTLIEB, D. and SHAW, P. D. (Editors) (1967): Antibiotics, Vol. I, Mechanism of Action, pp. 764 to 765. Springer-Verlag, Berlin.

GUARINO, A. J. (1967): Cordycepin. In: Antibiotics, Vol. I, Mechanism of Action, pp. 468—480. Editors: D. Gottlieb and P. D. Shaw. Springer-Verlag, Berlin.

GURGO, C., APIRION, D. and SCHLESSINGER, D. (1969): Polyribosome metabolism in Escherichia coli treated with chloramphenicol, neomycin, spectinomycin, or tetracycline. Journal of Molecular Biology, 45, 205.

HAMILTON, W. A. (1970): Membrane-active antibacterial compounds. Biochemical Journal, 118, 46P.

HANKA, L. J. (1967): Psicofuranine. In: Antibiotics, Vol. I, Mechanism of Action, pp. 457—463. Editors: D. Gottlieb and P. D. Shaw. Springer-Verlag, Berlin.

HOFFMANN, P. and WALTER, G. (1970): Der Einfluss von Chloramphenicol und Streptomycin auf die Entwicklung des photosynthetischen Apparates bei Weizenkeimpflanzen. Biologisches Zentralblatt, 89, 163.

HUANG, M., BIGGS, D. R., CLARK-WALKER, G. D. and LINNANE, A. W. (1966): Chloramphenicol inhibition of the formation of particulate mitochondrial enzymes of Saccharomyces cerevisiae. Biochimica et Biophysica Acta, 114, 434.

HÜTTER, R., KELLER-SCHIERLEIN, W., NÜSCH, J. and ZÄHNER, H. (1965): Stoffwechselprodukte von Mikroorganismen. 48. Mitteilung. Scopamycine. Archiv für Mikrobiologie, 51, 1.

KELLER, F. A. and CABIB, E. (1971): Chitin and yeast budding. The Journal of Biological Chemistry, 246, 160.

KERSTEN, H. and FEY, G. (1972): On the mechanism of tetracycline action and resistance: Association of tetracyclines with ribosomes and ribosomal subunits studied by a fluorometric method. These Proceedings.

KINSKY, S. (1967): Polyene antibiotics. In: Antibiotics, Vol. I, Mechanism of Action, pp. 122—141. Editors: D. Gottlieb and P. D. Shaw. Springer-Verlag, Berlin.

LAMPEN, J. O. (1966): Interference by polyenic antifungal antibiotics (especially nystatin and filipin) with specific membrane functions. In: Biochemical Studies of Antimicrobial Drugs, pp. 111—130. Editor: E. F. Gale. Cambridge University Press, Cambridge.

LASKIN, A. I. (1967): Tetracyclines. In: Antibiotics, Vol. I, Mechanism of Action, pp. 752—754. Editors: D. Gottlieb and P. D. Shaw. Springer-Verlag, Berlin.

LINNANE, A. W., BIGGS, D. R., HUANG, M. and CLARK-WALKER, G. D. (1967): The effect of chloramphenicol on the differentiation of the mitochondrial organelle. In: Aspects of Yeast Metabolism, pp. 217—242. Editor: A. K. Mills. Blackwell Scientific Publications, Oxford.

LOSICK, R., SHORENSTEIN, R. G. and SONENSHEIM, A. L. (1970): Alteration of RNA polymerase during sporulation. Nature, 227, 910.

MAGER, J. (1960): Chloramphenicol and chlortetracycline inhibition of amino acid incorporation into proteins in a cell-free system from Tetrahymena pyriformis. Biochimica et Biophysica Acta, 38, 150.

MARINO, P., BALDI, M. I. and TOCCHINI-VALENTINI, G. P. (1968): Effect of rifampicin on DNA-dependent RNA polymerase and on RNA phage growth. Cold Spring Harbor Symposia on Quantitative Biology, **33**, 125.

MARTELO, O. J., MANYAN, D. R., SMITH, U. and YUNIS, A. A. (1969): Chloramphenicol and bone marrow mitochondria. Journal of Laboratory and Clinical Medicine, **74**, 927.

MCCARTHY, B. J. and HOLLAND, J. J. (1965): Denaturated DNA as a direct template for in vitro protein synthesis. Proceedings of the National Academy of Sciences U.S.A., **49**, 551.

MCDONNELL, J. P., GARAPIN, A. C., LEVINSON, W. E., QUINTRELL, N., FANSHIER, L. and BISHOP, J. M. (1970): DNA polymerases of Rous sarcoma virus: delineation of two reactions with actinomycin. Nature, **228**, 433.

MERTZ, T. (1961): Effect of mitomycin C on lateral root tip chromosomes of Vicia faba. Science, **133**, 329.

MIZUKAMI, Y. and IWABUCHI, M. (1970): Effects of actinomycin D and cycloheximide on morphogenesis and syntheses of RNA and protein in the cellular slime mold, Dictyostelium discoideum. Experimental Cell Research, **63**, 317.

MIZUNO, N. S. and GILBOE, D. P. (1970): Binding of streptonigrin to DNA. Biochemica et Biophysica Acta, **224**, 319.

MODRIGUEZ-LÓPEZ, M. and MUNOZ, M. L. (1970): The effects of the rifamycin antibiotics on algae. FEBS Letters, **9**, 171.

NASS, G. and HASENBANK, R. (1970): Effect of borrelidin on the threonyl-tRNA-synthetase activity and the regulation of threonine-biosynthetic enzymes in Saccharomyces cerevisiae. Molecular and General Genetics, **108**, 28.

NASS, G., PORALLA, K. and ZÄHNER, H. (1969): Effect of the antibiotic borrelidin on the regulation of threonine biosynthetic enzymes in E. coli. Biochemical and Biophysical Research Communications, **34**, 84.

NATHANS, D. (1967): Puromycin. In: *Antibiotics, Vol. I., Mechanism of Action*, pp. 259—277. Editors: D. Gottlieb and P. D. Shaw. Springer-Verlag, Berlin.

NEČAS, O. (1971): Cell wall synthesis in yeast protoplasts. Bacteriological Reviews, **35**, 149.

NEČAS, O., SVOBODA, A. and KOPECKÁ, M. (1968): The effect of cycloheximide (actidione) on cell wall synthesis in yeast protoplasts. Experimental Cell Research, **53**, 291.

NEMEC, P. and BETINA, V. (1953): Permeability alterations in beet root Beta vulgaris var. rubra caused by amphotericin B. The Journal of Antibiotics, **21**, 626.

NISHIZUKA, Y. and LIPMANN, F. (1966): The interactioning between guanosine triphosphate and amino acid incorporation. Archives of Biochemistry and Biophysics, **116**, 344.

OBRIG, T. G., CULP, W. J., MCKEEHAN, W. L. and HARDESTY, B. (1971): The mechanism by which cycloheximide and related glutarimide antibiotics inhibit peptide synthesis on reticulocyte ribosomes. The Journal of Biological Chemistry, **246**, 174.

OCHOA, S. (1968): Translation of the genetic message. Naturwissenschaften, **55**, 505.

PITTILLO, R. F. and HUNT, D. E. (1967): Azaserine and 6-Diazo-5-Oxo-L-Norleucine (DON). In: *Antibiotics, Vol. I, Mechanism of Action*, pp. 481—493. Editors: D. Gottlieb and P. D. Shaw. Springer-Verlag, Berlin.

PUSCHENDORF, B. and GRUNICKE, H. (1969): Effect of distamycin A on template activity of DNA in a DNA polymerase system. FEBS Letters, **4**, 355.

PUSCHENDORF, B., PETERSEN, E., WOLF, H., WERCHAU, H. and GRUNICKE, H. (1971): Studies on the effect of distamycin A on the DNA dependent RNA polymerase system. Biochemical and Biophysical Research Communications, **43**, 617.

REICH, E., CERAMI, A. and WARD, D. C. (1967): Actinomycin. In: *Antibiotics, Vol. I, Mechanism of Action*, pp. 714—725. Editors: D. Gottlieb and P. D. Shaw. Springer-Verlag, Berlin.

REUSSER, F. (1969): Mode of action of melinacidin, an inhibitor of nicotinic acid biosynthesis. Journal of Bacteriology, **98**, 1285.

REUSSER, F. (1969): Mode of action of albocycline, an inhibitor of nicotinate biosynthesis. Journal of Bacteriology, **100**, 11.

REUSSER, F. (1970): Tirandamycin: inhibition of ribonucleic acid polymerase. Infection and Immunity, **2**, 77.

SAKAI, F. and TAKEBE, I. (1970): RNA and protein synthesis in protoplasts isolated from tobacco leaves. Biochimica et Biophysica Acta, **224**, 531.

SCHLESSINGER, D. (1969): Ribosomes: development of some current ideas. Bacteriological Reviews, **33**, 445.

SENTANDREU, R. and NORTHCOTE, D. H. (1969): Yeast cell wall synthesis. The Biochemical Journal, **115**, 231.

SHIGUERA, H. T. (1967): Hadacidin. In: *Antibiotics, Vol. I, Mechanism of Action*, pp. 451—456. Editors: D. Gottlieb and P. D. Shaw. Springer-Verlag, Berlin.

170

SMITH, U., SMITH, D. S. and YUNIS, A. A. (1970): Chloramphenicol-related changes in mito-chondrial ultrastructure. Journal of Cell Science, **7**, 501.

SONENSHEIM, A. L. and LOSICK, R. (1970): RNA polymerace mutants blocked in sporulation. Nature, **227**, 906.

STROMINGER, J. L. (1967): Enzymatic reactions in bacterial cell wall synthesis sensitive to penicillins, cephalosporins, and other antibacterial agents. In: *Antibiotics, Vol. I, Mechanism of Action*, pp. 705–713. Editors: D. Gottlieb and P. D. Shaw. Springer-Verlag, Berlin.

SZYBALSKI, W. and IYER, V. N. (1967): The mitomycins and porfiromycins. In: *Antibiotics, Vol. I., Mechanism of Action*, pp. 211–245. Editors: D. Gottlieb and P. D. Shaw. Springer-Verlag, Berlin.

TANAKA, N., KINOSHITA, T. and MASUKAWA, H. (1968): Mechanism of protein synthesis inhibition by fusidic acid and related antibiotics. Biochemical and Biophysical Research Communications, **30**, 278.

TRUHAUT, R. and DEYSSON, G. (1960): Etude de propriétés antimitotiques de la mitomycine C sur les cellules méristématiques d',,Allium sativum" L. Comptes Rendus de la Société de Biologie (Paris), **154**, 718.

WESSELLS, N. K., SPOONER, B. S., ASH, J. F., BRADLEY, M. O., LUDUENA, M. A., TAYLOR, E. L., WREEN, J. T. and YAMADA, K. M. (1971): Microfilaments in cellular and developmental processes. Contractile microfilament machinery of many cell types is reversibly inhibited by cytochalasin B. Science, **171**, 135.

WHEELDON, L. W. and LEHNINGER, A. L. (1966): Energy-linked synthesis and decay of membrane protein in isolated rat liver mitochondria. Biochemistry, **5**, 3533.

WINTERSBERGER, E. (1965): Protein synthesis in isolated yeast mitochondria. Biochemisches Zeitschrift, **341**, 409.

WINTERSBERGER, E. and WINTERSBERGER, U. (1970): Rifamycin insensitivity of RNA synthesis in yeast. FEBS Letters, **6**, 58.

ZÄHNER, H. (1965): *Biologie der Antibiotika*, pp. 80–84. Springer-Verlag, Berlin.

A GENETIC ANALYSIS OF CONJUGATIONAL TRANSFER
AND ITS CONTROL

N. S. WILLETTS and D. J. FINNEGAN*

MRC Molecular Genetics Unit, Department of Molecular Biology, University of
Edinburgh, Great Britain

ABSTRACT

A model is proposed for the inhibition of *Flac* transfer by R100. A product of R100
(called I) first interacts with a product of *Flac* (called P_F) to form the F transfer inhibitor.
This then prevents the synthesis or function of the F*traJ* gene product. *traJ* is probably
a control gene whose product is necessary for the synthesis or function of several of the
ten or more other transfer genes whose products are required for conjugational DNA
transfer. Thus both the transfer inhibitor and *traJ* mutations affect plasmid-specific
transfer products, F-pilus formation, and surface exclusion. The model predicts three
types of inhibitor-insensitive *Flac* mutants, all of which have been isolated.

INTRODUCTION

The many sex factors now known, including the *E. coli K12* sex factor F and numerous
colicinogenic and resistance transfer factors, share two major properties. One is the ability
to replicate autonomously in the host cell, and the other is the ability to transfer from one
cell to another by the process known as conjugation.

The mechanism of *Flac* transfer has been subjected to genetic analysis by isolation of
transfer-deficient (Tra⁻) mutants, determination of their phenotype, arrangement into
complementation groups, and mapping on the *Flac* linkage group. Although this analysis
was fundamentally equivalent to genetic analysis of any other process involving a sequence
of enzymic steps, the properties of F such as surface exclusion and incompatibility, as well
as the transfer-deficient phenotype of the mutants studied, necessitated modification of
the techniques normally used. For example, because of incompatibility, stable F/F
heterozygotes carrying two Tra⁻ *Flac* mutants could not be isolated for the complementation analysis: instead, the transfer ability of F/F heterozygotes in transient populations
was measured. Also, mutants had to be transferred from one cell to another either by P1
transduction or by using *amber*-suppressible Tra⁻ mutants in a Su⁺ host.

The analysis is described in full by ACHTMAN, WILLETTS and CLARK (1971 and manuscript in preparation) and WILLETTS and ACHTMAN (manuscript in preparation). Eleven
cistrons necessary for transfer were identified. Eight are required for formation of the
F-pilus, since mutants in these cistrons were resistant to male-specific phage. Mutants in
traD and *traI* still formed the F-pilus and were sensitive to male-specific phage (except
that certain RNA phages could adsorb to, but not infect, cells carrying *traD* mutants);
they may be defective in conjugational DNA metabolism. Some mutants in *traG* were

* Supported by a George Murray Scholarship from the University of Adelaide, Australia.

sensitive to male-specific phage while others were resistant, and the product of this gene may be bifunctional, required both for F-pilus formation and DNA metabolism. These eleven cistrons were mapped by complementation between the point mutants and a series of Hfr deletions extending different distances into F. The order was: *traJ traA traE traK traB traC traF traH traG traD traI* (IPPEN, ACHTMAN, WILLETTS, and FOMITCHEV, manuscript in preparation).

Although F was chosen as a representative sex factor, it lacks one property frequently found in others: the ability to inhibit its own transfer and that of related sex factors. Transfer inhibition was therefore studied using R100, which inhibits both its own transfer and that of F (EGAWA and HIROTA, 1962). A mutant of this R factor called R100-1, which has lost the ability to produce the transfer inhibitor (*op. cit*) was used in studies comparing the transfer systems of F*lac* and R100 (WILLETTS, 1971).

RESULTS

The properties of traJ mutants. Mutations in *traJ* are of particular interest in the study of F transfer and its control, since they are pleiotropic. Not only are such mutants transfer-deficient and unable to form the F-pilus, but they have lost surface exclusion (Table 1, lines 1 and 5). The latter property, leading to poor recipient ability in matings, is probably due to the product of a different gene (WILLETTS and ACHTMAN, unpublished experiments). In addition, R100-1 is unable to provide the *traJ* function either for transfer or for formation of the F-type of pilus (Table 1, line 6). This would be expected if the *traJ* product were necessary both for *traI* function (the only other gene whose transfer function

Table 1

THE PHENOTYPES OF STRAINS CARRYING R AND *Flac* ELEMENTS

Plasmids carried [a] Flac	R100	Flac transfer [b]	R100 transfer [b]	Malespecific phage sensitivity [c]	Surface Exclusion index [d]
1. Flac	—	145	0	S	300
2. —	R100	0	0.3	R	3
3. —	R100−1	0	100	R/S	4
4. Flac	R100−1	130	140	S	50
5. Flac traJ	—	10^{-4}	0	R	2
6. Flac traJ	R100−1	1	130	R/S	11
7. Flac	R100	1	1	R	6
8. Flac traP	R100	160	1	S	250
9. Flac traO	R100	130	1	S	550
10. (ColB4)	R100−1	—	1	R	—

a) These are derivatives of JC3272 (His⁻ Trp⁻ Lys⁻ Lac⁻ Str[r] Spc[s]) except for (ColB4 R100−1) which is a derivative of JC5455 (His⁻ Trp⁻ Lac⁻ Str[s] Spc[r]).

b) These were measured in 30 min 1:10 donor: recipient matings at 37°, using ED24 (prototrophic, Lac⁻ Spc[r]) as recipient, selecting Lac⁺ (His⁺ Trp⁺ Lys⁺ Spc[r]) and Tet[r] (His⁺ Trp⁺ Lys⁺) progeny. The results are expressed per 100 donor cells. For the (ColB4, R100−1) cross, JC3051 (His⁻ Trp⁻ Str[r]) was used as recipient, selecting Tet[r] (Str[r]) progeny.

c) Measured by the efficiency of plaque formation with the RNA phages M12, f2, and Q3 on LC agar. R/S indicates the lower efficiency (~5 %) shown by R100−1, as compared with *Flac* (Willetts, 1971).

d) Measured in 60 min. exponential phase 1 : 1 crosses with KL98 as the Hfr donor, selecting His⁺(Str[r]) progeny. The surface exclusion index is the number of such progeny obtained with the F⁻ strain, JC3272, divided by the number obtained with the strain in question (Achtman, Willetts, and Clark, 1971).

cannot be provided by R100-1) and *traA* function (the only other gene whose F-pilus forming ability cannot be provided by R100-1) (WILLETTS, 1971).

The simplest explanation for these results is that *traℑ* is a control gene whose product is necessary for the synthesis or function of the products of the two plasmid-specific transfer genes, *traI* and *traA*, as wel as of the surface exclusion gene. It might also control other transfer genes.

The properties of R100/Flac strains. In these strains, transfer of F*lac* is inhibited, as is formation of the F-pilus and surface exclusion (Table 1, line 7; WILLETTS and FINNEGAN, 1970). Such strains therefore have a phenotype similar to that of F*lac traℑ* mutants.

This similarity was further emphasized by the properties of inhibitor-insensitive mutants of F*lac* (FINNEGAN and WILLETTS, 1971). As expected, these showed F*lac* transfer, F-pilus production, and surface exclusion even in the presence of R100 (Table 1, lines 8 and 9). However, despite the presence of a fully-operational F*lac* transfer system, transfer of R100 itself was still inhibited. This showed that the transfer-inhibitor was acting upon a plasmid-specific transfer component of the type described above.

This similarity in phenotype of F*lac traℑ* mutants and R100/F*lac* strains is most simply explained by assuming that the transfer inhibitor prevents synthesis or function of *traℑ* the absence of which in turn prevents synthesis or function of several other transfer genes and the surface exclusion gene.

Dominant and recessive inhibitor-insensitive mutants. Although strains carrying an inhibitor-insensitive F*lac* mutant and R100 all showed the same phenotype, two classses of such mutants could be distinguished in dominance tests carried out in cells containing the mutant F*lac*, a wild-type F*his*, and R100. Mutants in one class were dominant, and in

Table 2

PLASMID RETRANSFER ABILITY

	Incoming plasmid	Resident plasmids	Retransfer of incoming plasmid
1.	Flac	−	20
2.	Flac	Fhis + R100	1
3.	Flac traP	−	20
4.	Flac traP	Fhis + R100	1
5.	Flac traO	−	20
6.	Flac traO	Fhis + R100	15
7.	Flac	R100	55
8.	R100−1	−	20
9.	R100−1	ColB4	20

Exponential cultures of the incoming plasmid derivative of JC6255 (Trp⁻ Lac⁻ T6ˢ Strˢ Spcˢ) were mated with stationary-phase recipient cultures of the resident plasmid derivatives of JC5455 (His⁻ Trp⁻ Lac⁻ T6ʳ Strʳ Spcʳ), for 45 min (0.6 ml: 1.4 ml). This mating was interrupted with T6, and the retransfer ability of the incoming plasmid immediately determined by mixing 0.2 ml of the T6-treated mating mixture with 1.8 ml of an exponential culture of JC3051 (His⁻ Trp⁻ Lac⁻ T6ʳ Strʳ). After 30 min, dilutions were plated to select the appropriate Strʳ progeny of JC3051. Retransfer is expressed as a percentage of the number of JC5455 cells which had received the incoming plasmid. This was measured by selecting the appropriate Spcʳ progeny of JC5455, or, in the case of F*lac* and F*his*, counting sectored colonies on lactose tetrazolium plates. (FINNEGAN and WILLETTS, 1971).

the other, recessive (Table 2, lines 1−6). Recessive mutations are in a gene designated *traP*, whose product (called P_F) may be necessary, together with an R100 product (called I), for inhibition of F transfer. Dominant mutations, in a gene designated *traO*, are presumed to be mutant at the site of action of the transfer inhibitor (see Discussion and FINNEGAN and WILLETTS, 1971).

Although the above results show that inhibition of F transfer requires P_F, they do not indicate whether R100 transfer is inhibited by I alone, or needs an analogous R100 product (called P_R). This question was resolved in a further series of experiments depending upon the slow production of P (or its slow interaction with I to give the transfer inhibitor) after transfer of a sex factor to a cell not previously carrying it. Thus F*lac* re-transfers from an intermediate cell carrying R100 at the same frequency as from an F$^-$ intermediate: if the intermediate carries both R100 and F*his*, however, retransfer is inhibited (Table 2, lines 1, 2 and 7). In similar experiments the retransfer of R100-1 from intermediate cells carrying ColB4 was measured. ColB4 inhibits R100-1 transfer when both are present in the same cell (Table 1, line 10). Retransfer, however, was as efficient from an intermediate cell carrying ColB4 as from an F$^-$ intermediate (Table 2, lines 8 and 9). This indicated that a slowly-produced (or interacting) R100-1 product, presumably

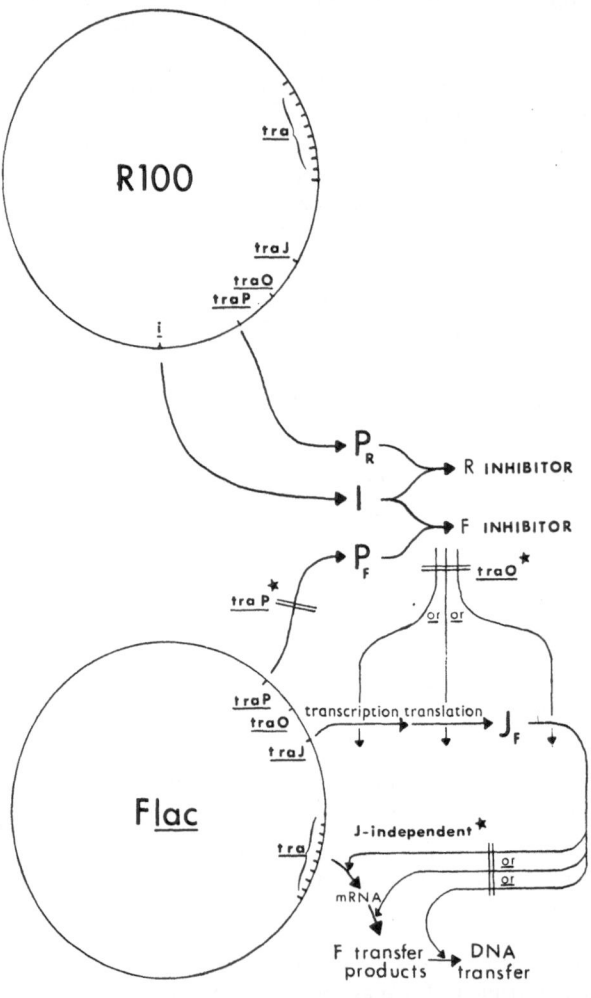

Fig. 1. A model for the control of F transfer

176

P_R, was required together with the I product made by ColB4 for inhibition of R100-1 transfer.

The slow synthesis of a plasmid-specific P product, or its slow interaction with I to give the transfer inhibitor, may be a general phenomenon. It provides an alternative explanation for the formation of HFT preparations, previously supposed to be due to slow I production.

DISCUSSION

From the above experimental results, we propose the model shown in Fig. 1 for the control of F transfer. The I product of R100 first interacts with the P_F product of F*lac* to form the F transfer inhibitor. (An analogous scheme for inhibition of R100 transfer is not shown). This prevents the synthesis or function of the F *traJ* product which in turn prevents the synthesis or function of several F transfer gene products needed for conjugational DNA transfer.

The model explains the existence of three types of inhibitor-insensitive mutants of F*lac* (* in Fig. 1). Two of these, in *traO* and *traP*, have been described above, and a third type are mutants not requiring the *traJ* product for synthesis or function of the F transfer gene products which *traJ* normally controls. Such mutants, called J-independent mutants, have recently been isolated by M. Achtman (personal communication).

As indicated in the model, the level of action of the F transfer inhibitor (or of the *traJ* product) is not known. It could prevent transcription or translation of *traJ*, or inactivate the *traJ* product or its site of action. *traO* mutants would be expected whichever explanation were correct, and only biochemical studies will resolve this point.

Acknowledgement

The model for the mechanism of action of *traJ* was developed in conjunction with Dr. M. ACHTMAN.

REFERENCES

ACHTMAN, M. A., WILLETS, N. S. and CLARK, A. J. (1971): Beginning a genetic analysis of conjugational transfer determined by the F factor in *E. coli* by isolation and characterisation of transfer-deficient mutants. Journal of Bacteriology, **106**, 529.

EGAWA, R. and HIROTA, Y. (1962): Inhibition of fertility by multiple drug-resistance factor in *E. coli* K12. Japanese Journal of Genetics, **37**, 66.

FINNEGAN, D. J. and WILLETTS, N. S. (1971): Two classes of F*lac* mutants insensitive to transfer inhibition by an F-like R factor. Molecular and General Genetics, **111**, 256.

WILLETTS, N. S. (1971): The plasmid-specificity of two proteins required for conjugation in *E. coli* K12. Nature New Biology, **230**, 183.

WILLETTS, N. S. and FINNEGAN, D. J. (1970): Characterisation of *E. coli* K12 strains carrying both an F-prime and en R factor. Genetical Research, **16**, 113.

DRUG RESISTANCE FACTORS: THE ROLE OF HOST-SPECIFIC RESTRICTION AND MODIFICATION OF DNA

S. W. GLOVER

MRC Molecular Genetics Unit, Department of Molecular Biology, University of Edinburgh, Mayfield Road, Edinburgh EH9 3JR, Great Britain.

When asked by the organising committee to speak about the mechanism of host-specific restriction and modification of DNA at a Symposium of Infectious Antibiotic Resistance, I was faced with a problem. R-factors with which this Symposium is concerned may, because they are composed of DNA, become substrates for restriction and modification enzymes when they are transmitted to new host bacteria. On the other hand they may themselves code for restriction and modification enzymes. In other words they may be both the victims and the villains. To explain how this comes about I have to divide my contribution into two parts. In the first part I will summarize the restrictions which R-factors can exercise over invading foreign DNA molecules mainly confining my remarks to bacteriophage DNA, and where appropriate discuss the modification of DNA which some R-factors direct. In the second part I will deal with the mechanism of restriction and modification of DNA and its genetic control.

Abortive infection of bacteriophages in R+ hosts

Restriction of the growth of bacteriophages in bacteria carrying R-factors has been widely reported (YOSHIKAWA and AKIBA, 1962₃ WATANABE, NISHIDA, ARAI, SATO and OGATA, 1964; MOLINA, 1964; ANDERSON and LEWIS, 1965; WATANABE, TAKANO, ARAI, NISHIDA and SATO, 1966; SICCARDI, 1966; ANDERSON, 1966; GUINÈE and WILLEMS, 1967; BANNISTER and GLOVER, 1968). It is certain that these observations cloak a large number of widely different mechanisms which may operate at quite different stages during the growth of a bacteriophage to stop its normal development. We know very little about some of these mechanisms while others are well understood, and have been investigated in some detail. In this section some of these diverse mechanisms of restriction will be described using examples from our own work with R-factors.

Some years ago we undertook a survey of a large number of R+ strains of *Escherichia coli* for their ability to limit the growth of eight different bacteriophages. It turned out that just under one half of them reduced the efficiency of plating of one or more of these phages, and on the basis of the pattern of phage plating on these strains, it proved possible to divide them into ten groups (BANNISTER and GLOVER, 1968). It became apparent subsequently that this was an over-simplication because many of the R+ strains carried two or more plasmids; frequently *fi+* and *fi-* R-factors were present in the same strain and the presence of two *fi-* R factors was detected in some strains (BANNISTER, 1970a, 1970b; ROMERO and MEYNELL, 1969). Therefore it is necessary to exercise some caution in ascribing the pattern of phage plating to particular classes of R-factor, and rather than concentrate on this rather tenuous classification, a few examples of abortive infection will be examined to determine what is known about the underlying mechanism.

R⁻ strains in the original classification of BANNISTER and GLOVER (1968), assigned to group III, reduce the efficiency of plating of phage λ (Table 1). On these strains phage λ

Table 1

RESTRICTION OF BACTERIOPHAGES BY R⁺ STRAINS OF *Escherichia coli*

R-factor Group	T3	W31	∅I	BF23	λ	∅80	P2	P1
I	—	—	—	—	+	+	+	+
II	—	—	—	—	+	+	+	+
III	—	—	—	—	+	+	—	—
IV	—	—	—	—	+	—	—	—
V	+	+	+	+	+	—	—	—
VI	+	+	+	+	+	—	—	—
VIII	+	+	+	+	+	—	—	—
IX	+	+	+	+	+	—	—	—

+ indicates that the phage plates less efficiently on the R⁺ strain than on the same host bacteria without the R-factor.

− indicates that the phage plates with equal efficiency on the R⁺ strain and on the same host bacteria without the R-factor.

For details of efficiencies of plating see *Bannister* and *Glover* (1968).

produces very small plaques at a low efficiency. The phage adsorbs well to these strains, but only a small fraction of the infected bacteria lyse, and they produce small bursts of progeny λ particles which, like the parental phage, is unable to initiate successful lytic infection of the R⁺ strain. It proved easy to isolate phage λ mutants at a frequency of about 10^{-6} which grew normally on group III R⁺ hosts. Phage λ mutants isolated on any one of the four R⁺ strains in this group are able to plaque efficiently on all of them, so it is likely that all group III R⁺ strains block the same specific step in λ development. This block, whatever it is, is clearly different from the block imposed on λ development by R⁺ strains from several other groups which are also characterised, at least in part, by their ability to block phage λ development since mutants isolated for their ability to plaque efficiently on group III R⁺ strains, are not improved in their ability to plaque on other restricting host strains.

There are several well-known examples in which phage λ growth is blocked in certain host bacteria to which the phage can adsorb. *Escherichia coli* strain W contains a prophage, W∅, which does not permit the growth of phage λ. In this case the DNA of the infecting phage is rapidly degraded after infection and, as in the case of abortive infection by group III R-factor strains, it is possible to isolate mutants which grow normally and which are not recessive to wild-type in mixed infection (KERZSMAN, GLOVER and ARONOVITCH, 1967). Strains of bacteria lysogenic for prophage P2 which is related to W∅, also fail to permit λ growth, but the mechanism is clearly different. In this case λ DNA is not degraded, but DNA replication is blocked (LINDAHL, SIRONI, BIALY and CALENDAR, 1970). Mutants of λ can be isolated which plaque efficiently on P2 lysogenic hosts, but these mutants are unable to grow on bacteria lysogenic for W∅, and unlike the λ mutants which can grow in W∅ lysogens these mutants behave as recessives in mixed infection with wild type λ. Which, if either, of these two mechanisms blocks the development of λ in group III R⁺ strains remains to be elucidated.

Another group of R⁺ strain, group IV (Table 1) also block phage λ development although λ adsorbs normally to such strains. Mutants of λ isolated for their ability to plaque on group III R+ strains, are unable to plaque on group IV R+ strains so that these two groups appear to exercise quite different mechanisms of restriction. This group which contains only a single *fi*+ R factor has not been further investigated.

Two other groups of R+ strains may be taken together, groups VI and IX (Table 1). One feature which characterizes these groups is the abortive infection of phage BF 23. This phage adsorbs well, but only a small fraction of the infected bacteria produce progeny phage. Of the 12 strains in these two groups, ten are colicinogenic and carry *colIb* determinants. Of the remaining two, one is *colIb* resistant though not demonstrably colicinogenic, and the other is *colIb* sensitive. This associatin of colicinogeny with certain R-factor has been observed previously by Siccardi (1966), who also observed that R+ strains which were resistant to *colIb* were also subject to abortive infection by phages BF 23 and W 31.

The growth of phage BF 23 *colI*+ strains has been investigated by STROBEL and NOMURA (1966) and by NISIOKA and OZEKI (1968). These authors showed that *colIb*+ strains lyse prematurely following infection with BF 23, and that a phage function is required for premature lysis. The phage injects normally and the injected DNA is not degraded, but no new DNA synthesis takes place and host-cell DNA is degraded. Group VI and group IX R+ strains infected with BF 23 also lyse prematurely about 12 minutes after adsorption, and it seems likely that it is the association of the R-factors in these strains with *colIb*+ which is responsible for the abortive infection by BF 23. All group VI and group IX strains appear to block phage BF 23 development by the same mechanism, since all the mutants of BF 23 isolated for their ability to plaque efficiently on one or other of these strains plaque efficiently on all of them. NISIOKA and OZEKI (1968) isolated what is probably a similar BF 23 mutant which can grow normally on *ColIb*+ strains, and showed that it was recessive to wild type in respect to premature lysis.

R+ strains belonging to groups V and VIII may be taken together (Table 1). R+ strains in these two groups are characterised, among other things, by their ability to cause a marked reduction in the efficiency of plating of several female-specific phages, $\emptyset$I (DETTORI, MACCACARO and PICCININ, (1961); W31 (WATANABE and OKADA, 1964); and T3 (SCHELL, GLOVER, STACEY, BRODA and SYMONDS, 1963). These phages form large plaques with well-defined halos on F− bacteria with an efficiency which is defined as 1:0. On male strains of *E. coli* they form very small plaques without clearly defined halos at a very much reduced efficiency. The plaques formed by these phages on group V and group VIII R+ strains resemble closely the plaques produced on male hosts, and the efficiency is similarly reduced. Cultures of these strains infected with page T3 are not killed, the infected bacteria are not lysed, and they recover from the infection and appear to continue to grow normally. Although one of these strains contains an *fi*+ R-factor which could mask the presence of an *fi*− R-factor, the others do not and contain only *fi*− R-factors. Nevertheless it is tempting to suppose that the F-mediated abortive infection with female-specific phages may provide a model for the restriction of these same phages by R− factors belonging to these two groups. Recently, MORRISON and MALAMY (1971) have produced evidence that the female-specific phage T7 is blocked in its development in F-*lac*+ hosts by sex-factor coded products, which act to prevent the translation of certain classes of T7 protein from T7 messenger RNA which is synthesised normally. Like group V and group VIII, R+ strains normal F+ strains are not lysed following infection with female-specific phages, but F-factor mutants can be isolated for their ability to permit lysis by T7. They are also lysed by another female-specific phage $\emptyset$II and progeny phage are produced.

R-factors may thus block the development of bacteriophages at quite different levels. They may be able to degrade phage DNA as happens when λ infects strains lysogenic for phase Wø; they may prevent the replication of phage DNA as happens following infection of P2 lysogenic hosts; they may block normal development by triggering premature lysis as happens when BF 23 infects *collb*+ strains, or strains containing R-factors associated with *Collb*+; they may interfere with normal translational control mechanisms as happens when female-specific phages infect F+ hosts.

Whether these diverse mechanisms have developed in specific response to phage infection as protective defence mechanisms, or whether they reflect the effects on phage development of R factor gene products whose normal function is concerned in some as yet undiscovered normal activity cannot be decided. However, the group specificity of these mechanisms, that is, the ability of a group of R factors to block the development of several quite different phages, and the ability of several groups of R-factors to restrict the same phage by what are clearly different mechanisms, make it unlikely to my mind that R-factors have evolved these complex restriction mechanisms solely as devices to ward off infection by bacteriophages, but rather that these abortive infections are the result of the effects, incidental if you like, of R factor gene products on phage development. Since R factors show such diversity of properties in this respect, at one extreme, some having little or no effect on the growth of any phages tested, it means that many of the gene products which affect phage development are non-essential, and that R-factors show considerable heterogeneity in the distribution of the genes that code for them.

The mechanisms by which the R factors , in those groups of strains considered so far in this section, prevent the growth of bacteriophages, still require further elucidation. For two groups of R+ strains, groups I and II the mechanism is much better understood. These two groups of R-factors exercise host-specific restrictions and modifications of DNA (Table 2), like those exercised by certain prophages and by certain strains of *E. coli*

Table 2

RESTRICTION AND MODIFICATION OF PHAGE λ BY R+ STRAINS OF *E. coli* K
CARRYING GROUP I AND GROUP II R FACTORS

Phage*	None	R factor Group I	R factor Group II
λ.K	1.0**	4×10^{-4}	2×10^{-2}
λ.KRI	1.0	1.0	1×10^{-2}
λ.KRII	1.0	2×10^{-4}	1.0

* The nomenclature of *Arber* and *Linn* (1969) is used to indicate the host specificity of the strain on which the phage was last grown.
** The results are expressed as efficiencies of plating.

(BERTANI and WEIGLE, 1953; LEDERBERG, 1957; DUSSOIX and ARBER, 1962; ARBER and DUSSOIX, 1962; GLOVER, SCHELL, SYMONDS and STACEY, 1963; WOOD, 1966). Group I contains a single R-factor R 124 which restricts the growth of phages λ, ø80, P1, P2 and T1 (BANNISTER and GLOVER, 1968). Phage which is grown on hosts containing this R-factor is host-modified so that it is able to grow successfully in a second infection of the same R+ strain. This modification does not affect its ability to grow in any of the other restricting hosts, and is thus specific to group I R-factors. The group I R-factor, R124, is *fi*+ and is the only *fi*+ R factor known to carry genetic determinants for the host-specific restriction and modification of DNA.

Group II contains eleven R-factors which are also able to restrict the growth of phages λ, ø80, P1, P2 and T1. These R-factors confer a host modification upon phages grown in group II R+ hosts so that they are able to initiate successful infection of any group II R+

bacteria. This modification is group-specific and group II modified phage is not able to grow in other restricting hosts. Initially, several of the group II R factors were believed to be fi^+, but subsequent analysis of the R-factors carried by these strains has shown that they contain both fi^+ and fi^- R factors, and the host-specificity determinants designated *hspII* are associated in each case with the fi^- R-factor. Thus R 124 fi^+ remains the only exception to the observation made originally by WATANABE, NISHIDA, OGATA, ARAI and SATO (1964), that only fi^- R factors were associated with the restriction of bacteriophages.

The mechanisms of restriction and modification of DNA

The molecular mechanisms of the restriction and modification of DNA by bacteria, have been analysed in some detail in recent years largely as a result of the isolation and characterization of two enzymes, a restriction endonuclease and a modification methylase. The first demonstration of *in vitro* restriction was carried out using crude extracts from an R-factor containing host. These extracts displayed a specific ability to inactivate infectious molecules of phage λ DNA (TAKANO, WATANABE, and FUKASAWA, 1966). Subsequently, MESELSON and YUAN, (1968), LINN and ARBER (1968) and ROULLAND-DUSSOIX and BOYER (1969) have investigated the mechanism of restriction using purified enzymes.

MESELSON and YUAN (1968) purified the restriction endonuclease III.K from *E. coli* K 12 and showed that the enzyme has the required specificity; it attacks λ . C DNA and not λ . K DNA. The enzyme has important specific co-factor requirements for Mg^{++}, ATP and S-adenosylmethionine (SAM) and from analysis of the partial and limit products, these authors were able to show that the enzyme first causes single-strand breaks at a limited number of sites on λ . C DNA, and then rapidly breaks the second strand at a point more or less directly opposite the first break thus cleaving the duplex. The requirements for Mg^{++} and ATP are not unique among nucleases, but the requirement for SAM is unique and will be reffered to again later.

Independently, LINN and ARBER (1968) and ROULLAND-DUSSOIX and BOYER (1969) have studied the *in vitro* activity of a similar restriction endonuclease isolated from *E. coli* B. It appears that this enzyme acts in a similar manner to the restriction endonuclease III. K and has identical co-factor requirements.

LARK and ARBER (1970) have divided strains with restriction endonucleases into two classes. One class contains the specificity types 15 (from *E. coli* strain 15), N3 (an R-factor of *hsp* II specificity) and P1 (the specificity determined by phage P1). Strains with this class of host-specific restriction all show DNA breakdown when grown in the presence of ethionine. The second class contains the *E. coli* specificity types K, B and A. There is no detectable breakdown of DNA when these strains are grown in the presence of ethionine. These authors suggest that this difference may be a reflection of the activity of the restriction endonucleases possessed by these two classes of strains. They suggest that the first class possessed restriction endonucleases which are independent of SAM for activity, and thus can breakdown DNA under conditions of methionine starvation induced by growth in ethionine. On the other hand the second class of strains possess restriction endonucleases which are dependent upon SAM for activity, and are thus inactive under conditions of growth in ethionine. However, this correlation is not complete since there is both indirect and direct evidence that the P1 restriction endonuclease is SAM-dependent (HIRSCH-KAUFFMAN and SAUERBIER, 1968; MESELSON and YUAN, (1968). In this respect it would be of interest to know the SAM-dependence of the *hspI* and *hspII* restriction endonucleases. Preliminary experiments (BANNISTER, unpublished results) indicate that methionine starvation leads to a partial loss of host-specific restriction and modification, but this indirect evidence has not been confirmed by *in vitro* characterization of the enzymes. Similarly it would be of interest to know the SAM-dependence of the *hspLT* and *hspS* restriction endonucleases of *Salmonella typhimurium* (COLSON, COLSON and VAN PEL, 1970; COLSON, 1971). Several lines of evidence point clearly to a correlation between enzymatic methylation of DNA, and host-specific modification. Methionine starvation can lead to loss of ability to host-modify phage λ DNA (ARBER, 1965) and infection with phage T3 which produces an enzyme, SAMase, able to cleave S-adenosyl methionine, leads to loss of ability to restrict as well as to host-modify phages λ and T1 (KLEIN and SAUERBIER, 1965; HIRSCH-KAUFMANN and SAUERBIER, 1968). Direct evidence that host-specific modification is the result of methylation of DNA was obtained by ARBER and SMITH (1966), and ARBER and KÜHNLEIN (1967). They showed that the chemical basis of B-specific modification was the methylation of a few adenine residues in the DNA of phage *fd*. KÜHNLEIN, LINN and ARBER (1969) have purified an extract of *E. coli* B which has the enzymatic activity of a B-specific host modification methylase *in vitro*. As expected this host-specific methylase requires SAM as a co-factor.

The restriction endonucleases and modification methylases act on specific nucleotide sequences on DNA. These sequences are short, perhaps only six to eight nucleotide pairs in length, and are distributed at mapable locations along the chromosome of phage λ (FRANKLIN and DOVE, 1969). There are apparently two such sequences on the DNA of phage *fd* recognised by the B-specific enzymes, and apparently no sequence recognised by the K-specific enzymes (ARBER and LINN, 1969). The distribution of these sites is different in different phages, for example, the K-specific sites in phages $\varnothing$80 and λ can be exchanged by recombination (FRANKLIN and DOVE, 1969). Specificity sites can be altered as might be expected by mutations which presumably alter the base sequence (FRANKLIN and DOVE, 1969, ARBER and LINN, 1969). Normally $\varnothing$X174 DNA does not contain a B-specific site, but SCHNEGG and HOFFSCHNEIDER (1969) have succeeded in inducing such a site following proflavin mutagenesis of the phage.

Recently, a rather different restriction endonuclease has been isolated and characterised from *Haemophilus influenzae* (SMITH and WILCOX, 1970; KELLY and SMITH, 1970). This enzyme does not require ATP and SAM as co-factors for activity. It produces about 40 double strand 5′ phosphoryl, 3′ hydroxyl cleavages in the DNA of the *E. coli* phage T7 and cleaves the nucleotide sequence:

$$5'\ \overset{*}{\text{G}}\ \text{T Py Pu A C}\ 3'$$

$$3'\ \underset{*}{\text{C}}\ \text{A Pu Py T G}\ 5'$$

at a point between the unspecified purine-pyrimidine base pairs. The most interesting feature of this sequence is its symmetry, the implications of which have been discussed in general by ARBER and LINN, (1969), and in particular by KELLY and SMITH (1970). The *Haemophilus* enzyme is active not only on T7 DNA, but also on the DNA of the *Salmonella* phage P22, *Bacillus subtilis* DNA and salmon sperm DNA, but not on the DNA of *Haemophilus influenzae* itself (SMITH and WILCOX, 1970). It is apparently active on the DNA of the virus SV40 (ADLER and NATHANS, 1970). The fact that *Haemophilus influenzae* DNA is not attacked may mean that this organism like many others protects its DNA from restriction by a specific modification. Recently we have been able to show that many serotypes of *H. influenzae* possess host-specific restriction and modification systems active on *H. influenzae* phages (PIEKAROWICZ and GLOVER, unpublished results).

The genetic control of restriction and modification

There is now convincing evidence that at least three genes designated *hss*, *hsr* and *hsm* are concerned in the control of host-specific restriction and modification. This evidence derives from the isolation and characterisation of mutants deficient in restriction and/or modification in *E. coli* (GLOVER et al., 1963; WOOD, 1966, COLSON, GLOVER, SYMONDS and STACEY, 1965; GLOVER and COLSON, 1969) and in *Salmonella typhimurium* (COLSON, COLSON and VAN PEL, 1970). Similar mutants have been isolated for the two R-factor specified restriction and modification types *hspI* and *hspII* (Bannister and Glover, 1970) and Table 3 illustrates the properties of these mutants.

Table 3

PHENOTYPES OF R+ STRAINS OF *E. coli* CARRYING RESTRICTION-DEFICIENT MUTANTS OF R FACTOR HOST SPECIFICITY TYPES *hspRI* AND *hspRII*

R factor	Host specificity type	Host specificity phenotype of *E. coli* R+ strains*	
R124	*hspRI*	r_I^+	m_I^+
R124−1	*hspRI*	r_I^-	m_I^+
R124−2	*hspRI*	r_I^-	m_I^-
R313	*hspRII*	r_{II}^+	m_{II}^+
R313−1	*hspRII*	r_{II}^-	m_{II}^+
R132−2	*hspRII*	r_{II}^-	m_{II}^-

* r^+ indicates restriction, m^+ indicates modification and the appropriate specifity is indicated by a subscript.

Additional evidence comes from examination of the restriction and modification phenotypes of recombinants obtained between these mutants (GLOVER and COLSON, 1969). These three genes map close together on the *E. coli* chromosome (COLSON, GLOVER, SYMONDS and STACEY, 1965; WOOD, 1966), but nevertheless it has proved possible to obtain recombination between them. It was shown that the specificity of both restriction and modification expressed by recombinants obtained from P1-mediated transduction between *E. coli* K and *E. coli* B was invariably that of the parent which contributed the *hss* gene to the recombinant. Therefore it is this gene which confers the strain specificity to the restriction and modification enzymes presumably by the role it plays in recognising the appropriate sequences on DNA (GLOVER and COLSON, 1969).

This conclusion has been reinforced by the results of complementation analysis of mutants of *E. coli* K and *E. coli* B (GLOVER, 1968; BOYER and ROULLAND-DUSSOIX, 1969; GLOVER, 1970, and ARBER and LINN, 1969). These results, taken together with an analysis of the behaviour of temperature-sensitive host-specificity mutants in complementation experiments (HUBACEK and GLOVER, 1970) enable us to conclude that the *hsp* gene cluster comprises three interacting genes, *hss*, *hsr* and *hsm*. For restriction the activity of all three genes is required, while for modification only *hss* and *hsm* are necessary. We envisage that the restriction endonuclease is an oligomeric enzyme composed of three different types of sub-unit specified by the genes *hss*, *hsr* and *hsm*, while the modification methylase is a simpler oligomer containing only two types of sub-unit specified by the genes *hss* and *hsm*. This conclusion is in keeping with the observation made by many investigators that both restriction and modification may be SAM-dependent indicating that methylation may be an important step in restriction as well as in modification, and reflecting the presence of the *hsm* directed polypeptide in both enzymes. It is to be expected that both enzymes are large and this appears to be the case (MESELSON and YUAN, 1968; ROULLAND-DUSSOIX and BOYER, 1969; ARBER and LINN, 1969). Furthermore from their similar structures, in terms of common subunits it is not surprising that they co-purify to some degree (MESELSON and YUAN, 1968; ROULLAND-DUSSOIX and BOYER, 1969; LINN and ARBER, 1968; ARBER and LINN, 1969).

Of considerable interest is the extent to which these host-specificity types are functionally related to one another. Complementation tests of the type referred to above, allow one to test whether mutants of one host specificity type can be complemented by another. It is clear from these experiments that the *hsr* and *hsm* genes from *E. coli* K and B can complement one another more or less fully, and that the P1 host-specificity determinants are not functionally related to those of *E. coli* K or B since no complementation can be detected between P1 and *E. coli* K or B. Strain 15 of *E. coli* has been shown to possess two host specificity types, one *hspA*, is determined by chromosomal genes which are allelic with *hspK* and *hspB* and another, *hsp15*, is determined by a P1-like defective plasmid. These two host-specificity types do not interact with one another, their effects are additive in host cells that carry both, they do not appear to complement one another, nor at the genetic level is there any exchange between *hsp15* and *hspA* genes (ARBER and WAUTERS-WILLEMS, 1970). There is however, a close relationship between type 15 host specificity and P1 host-specificity, genetic recombination can take place between *hsp15* and *hsp1* genes, and a close functional relationship is revealed in complementation experiments (ARBER, to be published). A similar close relationship is to be expected between *hspK* and *hspB*.

Salmonella typhimurium also possess two host specificity types, one designated S is determined by chromosomal genes allelic to *hspK* and *hspB*, and another designated LT also determined by chromosomal genes which map close to *proC*. These two types do not appear to be closely related, they do not complement one another and are additive in host bacteria that possess both, in the same manner as K and P1 host-specificity types

Table 4

EFFICIENCIES OF PLATING OF PHAGE λ ON *E. coli* STRAINS K, B, 15 AND C CARRYING GROUP I AND GROUP II R FACTORS

Host strain	$\lambda . K$	$\lambda . B$	$\lambda . 15$	$\lambda . CRI$	$\lambda . CRII$	$\lambda . K(P1)$
K	1.0	5×10^{-4}	$\star -$	1×10^{-4}	1×10^{-4}	1.0
KRI	4×10^{-4}	7×10^{-5}	—	6×10^{-5}	2×10^{-5}	3×10^{-4}
KRII	2×10^{-2}	7×10^{-5}	—	1×10^{-4}	1×10^{-3}	5×10^{-2}
B	2×10^{-4}	1.0	—	5×10^{-4}	2×10^{-4}	—
BRI	2×10^{-4}	7×10^{-5}	—	2×10^{-4}	1×10^{-4}	—
BRII	7×10^{-4}	2×10^{-3}	—	7×10^{-4}	7×10^{-2}	—
15	—	—	1.0	5×10^{-2}	1×10^{-2}	—
15RI	—	—	1×10^{-2}	1×10^{-2}	1×10^{-4}	—
15RII	—	—	1×10^{-2}	1×10^{-2}	1×10^{-2}	—
C	1.0	1.0	1.0	1.0	1.0	1.0
CRI	5×10^{-6}	7×10^{-6}	1×10^{-3}	1.0	1×10^{-4}	—
CRII	4×10^{-3}	1×10^{-4}	1×10^{-2}	1×10^{-2}	1.0	—
K(P1)	1×10^{-4}	—	—	—	—	1.0

$\star$ — = not tested.

are additive in *E. coli* K (P1) (COLSON, COLSON and VAN PEL, 1970; COLSON, 1971). Preliminary evidence indicates that the *Salmonella* S system may be functionally related to the *E. coli* K and B host specificity types (VAN PEL, pers. comm.), and it would be interesting to know the functional relationship if any, between the LT system and the P1 and 15 host specificity types. A simple classification may turn out to be possible. On the one hand the chromosomal host specificity types genetically mapped near *thr* on the chromosome which include the *E. coli* K, B and A types, and the *S. typhimurium* S type, and on the other hand the P1, 15 and LT types of which P1 and 15 are certainly related. It is relevant in this context to consider where the R-factor host-specificity types *hspI* and *hspII* fit. Genetic analysis by mutant isolation and characterization has shown that in their genetic control they resemble other host specificity systems. They can be expressed in the presence of the K, B, 15 and P1 systems, but they are only weakly additive in their quantitative effects to the K, B, 15 and P1 restrictions, and they do not show any functional relationship to the K, B or P1 host-specificity types in complementation tests (Tables 4

Table 5

PHENOTYPES OF STRAINS OF *E. eoli* CARRYING GROUP I AND GROUP II
R FACTORS AND MUTANT R FACTORS

* Strain and host specificity phenotype

R factor	Host specificity phenotype	K r_K^+ m_K^+			7K r_K^- m_K^+			K RII r_K^+ m_K^+ r_{II}^+ m_{II}^+						
R124	r_I^+ m_I^+	r_K^+ m_K^+ r_I^+			m_I^+ r_K^- m_K^+ r_I^+			m_I^+ r_K^+ m_K^+ r_{II}^+ m_{II}^+ r_I^+ m_I^+						
R124—1	r_I^- m_I^+	r_K^+ m_K^+ r_I^-			m_I^+ r_K^- m_K^+ r_I^-			m_I^+ r_K^+ m_K^+ r_{II}^+ m_{II}^+ r_I^- m_I^+						
R124—2	r_I^+ m_I^-	r_K^+ m_K^+ r_I^+			m_I^- r_K^- m_K^+ r_I^+			m_I^- r_K^+ m_K^+ r_{II}^+ m_{II}^+ r_I^+ m_I^-						
R313	r_{II}^+ m_{II}^+	r_K^+ m_K^+ r_{II}^+			m_{II}^+ r_K^- m_K^+ r_{II}^+			m_{II}^+	n. t.					
R313—1	r_{II}^- m_{II}^+	r_K^+ m_K^+ r_{II}^-			m_{II}^+ r_K^- m_K^+ r_{II}^+			m_{II}^+	n. t.					
R132—2	r_{II}^- m_{II}^-	r_K^+ m_K^+ r_{II}^-			m_{II}^- r_K^- m_K^+ r_{II}^+			m_{II}^-	n. t.					

* Similar experiments using *E. coli* strains 4K r_K^- m_K^-; B r_B^+ m_B^+; B6 r_B^- m_B^+; B8 r_B^- m_B^- and K (P1) r_K^+ m_K^+ r_{P1}^+ m_{P1}^+ each containing the R factors listed in the table gave phenotypes which were qualitatively additive (see *Bannister* and *Glover*, 1970).
n. t. = not tested.

and 5). However, the R-factor *hspII* type shares two properties with the P1 system, both lead to breakdown of host DNA following a period of growth in ethionine and both are able to restrict phage T1. On the other hand *hspI* and *hspII* like *E. coli* K and B permit the growth of phage T3 while P1 does not.

.When together in the same host strain the two R-factor host-specificity types are additive, no recombinants have been detected between them, and they show no functional relationship to one another (Table 5), in that mutants of one system are not complemented by the other (BANNISTER and GLOVER, 1970).

The situation then is that the two R-factor host-specificity types *hspRI* and *hspRII* are clearly different from one another, and not closely related to any of the other host-specificity types tested. The origin of these R-factor host specificity genes, like the origin of many other R-factor genes, remains obscure. It is clear that they did not acquire them from any of the commonly used laboratory strains of *E. coli*, and this is hardly surprising since the R-factors themselves were only transferred to *E. coli* K12 just prior this study.

Most likely they were acquired from previous hosts which carried these R factors and we would therefore anticipate that it should prove possible to isolate from nature strains of bacteria which possess DNA host-specificities identical to or very closely related to the R-factor specificities *hspRI* and *hspRII*.

REFERENCES

ADLER, S. P. and NATHANS, D. (1970): Cleavage of simian virus 40 DNA by bacterial restricting enzymes. Federation Proceedings, **29**: 2708.

ANDERSON, E. S. (1966): Influence of the Δ transfer factor on the phage sensitivity of Salmonellae. Nature, **212**, 795−799.

ANDERSON, E. S. and LEWIS, M. J. (1965): Characterisation of a transfer factor associated with drug resistance in *Salmonella typhimurium*. Nature, **208**: 843−849.

ARBER, W. (1965): Host specificity of DNA produced by *Escherichia coli*. V. The role of methionine in the production of host specificity. Journal of Molecular Biology, **11**: 247−256.

ARBER, W. and DUSSOIX, D. (1962): Host specificity of DNA produced by *Escherichia coli*. I. Host controlled modification of bacteriophage λ. Journal of Molecular Biology, **5**: 18−36.

ARBER, W. and KÜHNLEIN, U. (1967): Mutationeller Verlust B-spezifischer Restriktion des Bacteriophagen *fd*. Path. microbiol. **30**: 946−952.

ARBER, W. and LINN, S. (1969): DNA modification and restriction. Annual Review of Biochemistry, **38**: 467−500.

ARBER, W. and SMITH, J. D. (1966): Host controlled modification of phage and its correlation with specific methylation of deoxyribonucleotides. *IXth* International Congress of Microbiology, p. 5.

ARBER, W. and WAUTERS-WILLEMS, D. (1970): Host specificity of DNA produced by *Escherichia coli*. XII. The two restriction and modification systems of strain 15T. Molecular and General Genetics, **108**: 203−217.

BANNISTER, D. (1970a): Analysis of an R⁺ strain carrying two *fi⁻* sex factors. Journal of General Microbiology, **61**: 273−281.

BANNISTER, D. (1970b): Explanation of the apparent association of host specificity determinants with *fi⁺* R factors. Journal of General Microbiology, **61**: 283−287.

BANNISTER, D. and GLOVER, S. W. (1968): Restriction and modification of bacteriophages by R⁺ strains of *Escherichia coli* K12. Biochemical and Biophysical Research Communications, **30**, 735−738.

BANNISTER, D. and GLOVER, S. W. (1970): The isolation and properties of non-restricting mutants of two different host specificities associated with drug resistance factors. Journal of General Microbiology, **61**, 63−71.

BERTANI, G. and WEIGLE, J. J. (1953): Host-controlled variation in bacterial viruses. Journal of Bacteriology, **65**: 113−121.

BOYER, H. W. and ROULLAND-DUSSOIX, D. (1969): A complementation analysis of the restriction and modification of DNA in *Escherichia coli*. Journal of Molecular Biology, **41**: 459−472.

COLSON-CORBISIER, A. M. (1971): Restriction et Modification de l'ADN chez *Salmonella typhimurium*. Thesis University od Louvain.

COLSON, C., COLSON, A. M. and van PEL, A. (1970): Chromosomal location of host specificity in *Salmonella typhimurium*. Journal of General Microbiology, **60**: 265−271.

COLSON, C., GLOVER, S. W., SYMONDS, N. and STACEY. K. A. (1965): The location of the genes for host controlled modification and restriction in *Escherichia coli* K-12. Genetics, **52**: 1043−1050.

DETTORI, R., MACCACARO, G. A., and PICCININ, G. L. (1961): Sexspecific bacteriophages of *Escherichia coli* K12. Giornale di Microbiologia, **9**: 141−150.

DUSSOIX, D. and ARBER, W. (1962): Host specificity of DNA produced by *Escherichia coli*. I. Control over acceptance of DNA from infecting phage λ. Journal of Molecular Biology, **5**: 37−49.

FRANKLIN, N. C. and DOVE, W. F. (1969): Genetic evidence for restriction targets in the DNA of phages λ and ⌀80. Genetical Research, **14**: 151−157.

GLOVER, S. W. (1968): Host specificity in F'heterogenotes of *Escherichia coli*. Journal of General Microbiology, **53**, 1−11.

GLOVER, S. W. (1970): Functional analysis of host-specificity mutants in *Escherichia coli*. Genetical Research, **15**, 237−250.

GLOVER, S. W. and COLSON, C. (1969): Genetics of host controlled restriction and modification in *Escherichia coli*. Genetical Research, **13**, 227−240.

GLOVER, S. W., SCHELL, J., SYMONDS, N., and STACEY, K. A. (1963): The control of host induced modification by phage P1. Genetical Research, 4, 480−482.

GUINÉE, P. A. M. and WILLEMS, H. M. C. C. (1967): Restriction and modification of phage 47 and lambda by R factors. Antonie van Leeuwenhoek, 33: 397−406.

HIRSCH-KAUFFMAN, M. and SAUERBIER, W. (1968): Inhibition of modification and restriction for phages λ and T1 by co-infecting T3. Molecular and General Genetics, 102: 89−94.

HUBACEK, J. and GLOVER, S. W. (1970): Complementation analysis of temperature-sensitive host specificity mutations in Escherichia coli. Journal of Molecular Biology, 50: 111−127.

KELLY, T. J. and SMITH, H. O. (1970): A restriction enzyme from Haemophilus influenzae II. Base sequence of the recognition site. Journal of Molecular Biology, 51: 393−409.

KERSZMAN, G., GLOVER, S. W., and ARONOVITCH, J. (1967): The restriction of bacteriophage λ in Escherichia coli strain W. Journal of General Virology, 1: 333−347.

KLEIN, A. and SAUERBIER, W. (1965): Role of methylation in host controlled modification of phage T1. Biochemical and Biophysical Research Communications, 18: 440−445.

KÜHNLEIN, V., LINN, S. and ARBER, W. (1969): Host specificity of DNA produced by Escherichia coli. XI. In vitro modification of phage fd replicative form. Proceedings of the National Academy of Sciences, U.S.A. 63, 556−562.

LARK, C. and ARBER, W. (1970): Host specificity of DNA produced by Escherichia coli. XIII. Breakdown of cellular DNA upon growth in ethionine of strains with r_{15}^+, r_{P1}^+ or r_{N13}^+ restriction phenotypes. Journal of Molecular Biology, 52: 337−348.

LEDERBERG, S. (1957): Suppression of the multiplication of heterologous bacteriophages in lysogenic bacteria. Virology, 3: 493−513.

LINDAHL, G., SIRONI, G., BIALY, H. and CALENDAR, R. (1970): Bacteriophage lambda: Abortive infection of bacteria lysogenic for phage P2. Proceedings of the National Academy of Sciences, U.S.A. 66: 587−594.

LINN, S. and ARBER, W. (1968): Host specificity of DNA produced by Escherichia coli. X. In vitro restriction of phage fd replicative form. Proceedings of the National Academy of Sciences, U.S.A. 59: 1300−1306.

MESELSON, M. and YUAN, R. (1968): DNA restriction enzyme from E. coli. Nature, 217: 1110 to 1114.

MOLINA, A. M. (1964): Genetic elements with cytoplasmic location controlling drug and phage T1 resistance in Enterobacteriaceae. Transfer of resistance factors by conjugation. Giornale di microbiologia, 12: 107−120.

MORRISON, T. G. and MALAMY, M. H. (1971): T7 translational control mechanisms and their inhibition by F factors. Nature New Biology, 231: 37−41.

NISIOKA, T. and OZEKI, H. (1968): Early abortive lysis by phage BF 23 in Escherichia coli K12 carrying the colIb factor. Journal of Virology, 21: 1249−1254.

ROMERO, E. and MEYNELL, E. (1969): Covert fi− R factors in fi+ R+ strains of bacteria. Journal of Bacteriology, 97: 780−786.

ROULLAND-DUSSOIX, D., and BOYER, H. W. (1969): The Escherichia coli B restriction endonuclease. Biochemica et Biophysica Acta 195: 219−229.

SCHELL, J., GLOVER, S. W., STACEY, K. A., BRODA, P. M. A., and SYMONDS, N. (1963): The restriction of phage T3 by certain strains of Escherichia coli. Genetical Research 4: 483−484.

SCHNEGG, B. and HOFSCHNEIDER, P. H. (1969): Mutant of ⌀X174 accessible to host controlled modification. Journal of Virology, 3, 541−542.

SICCARDI, A. G. (1966): Colicin resistance associated with resistance factors in Escherichia coli. Genetical Research, 8: 219−228.

SMITH, H. O., and WILCOX, K. W. (1970): A restriction enzyme from Haemophilus influenzae. I. Purification and general properties. Journal of Molecular Biology, 51: 379−391.

STROBEL, M. and NOMURA, M. (1966): Restriction of the growth of bacteriphage BF 23 by a colicin I (Col I−P9) factor. Virology, 28: 763−764.

TAKANO, T., WATANABE, W., and FUKASAWA, T. (1966): Specific inactivation of infectious λDNA by sonicates of restrictive bacteria with R factors. Biochemical and Biophysical Research Communications, 25: 192−198.

WATANABE, T., NISHIDA, H., OGATA, C., ARAI, T., and SATO, S. (1964): Episome-mediated transfer of drug resistance in Enterobacteriaceae VII. Two types of naturally occuring R factors. Journal of Bacteriology, 88: 716−726.

WATANABE, T., NISHIDA, H., ARAI, T., SAITO, S. and OGATA, C. (1964): Restriction and host-induced modification of phages λ and T1 by certain types of R factors in Escherichia coli. Struktur und Funktion des genetischen Materials. Ed. H. Stubbe.

WATANABE, T., and OKADA, M. (1964): New type of sex-factor specific bacteriophage of Escherichia coli. Journal of Bacteriology, 87, 727−736.

189

WATANABE, T., TAKANO, T., ARAI, T., NISHIDA, H., and SATO, S. (1966): Episome-mediated transfer of drug resistance in *Enterobacteriaceae*. *X*. Restriction and modification of phages by fi⁻ R factors. Journal of Bacteriology, **92**: 477—486.

WOOD, W. B. (1966): Host specificity of DNA produced by *Escherichia coli*. Bacterial mutations affecting the restriction and modification of DNA. Journal of Molecular Biology, **16**, 118—133.

YOSHIKAWA, M. and AKIBA, T. (1962): Studies on transferable drug resistance in bacteria. *IV*. Suppression of plaque formation of phages by the resistance factor. Japanese Journal of Microbiology, **6**: 121—132.

HIGH-FREQUENCY TRANSDUCTION OF TETRACYCLINE RESISTANCE MARKER OF R FACTOR BY BACTERIOPHAGE P22 IN SALMONELLA TYPHIMURIUM

TSUTOMU WATANABE and YASUKO OGATA

Department of Microbiology, Keio University School of Medicine, Tokyo, Japan

ABSTRACT

Transduction of R factor 222 with the markers of resistance to sulfanilamide (*sul*) streptomycin (*str*), chloramphenicol (*cam*) and tetracycline (*tet*) in *Salmonella typhimurium* LT-2 by phage P22 results in the segregation of these drug-resistance markers into *tet* and the other three. The *tet* marker was found to be integrated at the proline region of the recipient chromosome in confirmation of the previous result of Dubnau and Stocker with a different R factor carrying similar drug-resistance markers. The *sul*, *str* and *cam* markers were found to be integrated together near the galactose region in the transductants. Some of the *tet* transductants produced HFT lysates for *tet* transduction upon ultraviolet induction but none of the *sul . str . cam* transductants gave rise to HFT lysates for these markers. The HFT lysates for *tet* contained about 100 times more *tet*-transducing particles than normal P22. The *tet*-transducing phage was defective (P22 *dtet*) in that it could not replicate without the helper action of normal P22. Single infection with P22 *dtet* seems to result in abortive transduction in a majority of recipient cells, and the cells destined to become abortive by infection with P22 *dtet* seem to be converted to complete ransductants by the helper action of normal P22.

INTRODUCTION

R factors (WATANABE, 1963) can be transduced by phage P1 in *Escherichia coli* and by phage P22 in *Salmonella typhimurium* (WATANABE, FUKASAWA, 1961; WATANABE et all., 1968). The patterns of transduction of R factors in these two systems are considerably different from each other; generally speaking, the whole structures of R factors can be transduced *en bloc* by phage P1, whereas only portions of structures of R factors are transduced by phage P22. The difference in the patterns of transduction of R factors is dependent on the transducing phage rather than on the bacterial species employed (OKADA, WATANABE, 1968). In the transduction of R factor 222, which we have been using as one of our standard R factors, by phage P22 in *S. typhimurium*, the drug-resistance markers of 222, which are the markers of resistance to sulfanilamide (*sul*), streptomycin (*str*), chloramphenicol (*cam*) and tetracycline (*tet*), are invariably segregated into *tet* and the other three markers (WATANABE, FUKASAWA, 1961ab). A remarkable property of the drug-resistant transductants obtained by transduction of 222 is that a majority of them are unable to transfer their drug-resistance markers by causing conjugation (WATANABE, FUKASAWA, 1961b). The P22-transduced *tet* marker was found to be integrated into the chromosome of recipient bacteria by Dubnau and Stocker (DUBNAU,

STOCKER, 1964), using a different R factor with drug-resistance markers similar to those of 222, and this finding has later been confirmed by us with 222. However, the precise location, even whether cytoplasmic or chromosomal, of the other drug-resistance markers transduced by phage P22 has not been known. We have attempted to disclose the location of these P22-transduced markers in the present study and have found that they are integrated together into the chromosome of recipient bacteria close to the galactose (*gal*) region.

R factors can be transduced also by phage epsilon in *Salmonella anatum* and *Salmonella newington* and the patterns of transduction of the drug-resistance markers of a four-drug-resistance R factor are very similar to those of the transduction system of *S. typhimurium* and phage P22 (HARADA et al., 1963). In other words, the *sul*, *str*, *cam* and *tet* markers are invariably segregated into *tet* and the other three, and none of the drug-resistant transductants obtained were able to transfer their drug-resistance markers by causing conjugation. Furthermore, their drug-resistance markers could not be eliminated by treatment with acriflavine unlike ordinary R factors (HARADA et al. 1963). It was further found that ultraviolet (UV)-induced lysates of a *tet* transductant obtained by phage epsiolon caused high-frequency transduction (HFT (KAMEDA et al., 1965), although the nature of the transducing phage was not studied in detail. We have undertaken to study if similar HFT may be possible with the system of transduction of R factor 222 by phage P22 and have succeeded in demonstrating HFT of the *tet* marker, the detail of which will be reported here. HFT lysates could not be obtained, however, with drug-resistance markers other than *tet*.

MATERIALS AND METHODS

Media and antibiotics. These were the same as those described in a previous paper (12). In addition, tryptone broth (pH 6.9) containing 1% of Bacto-tryptone (Difco) and 0.5% of sodium chloride was used.

Strains of bacteria, phages and R factors. S. *typhimurium* LT-2 wild type, DB47, a recombination-deficient (*rec⁻*) mutant of LT-2, *proA36* (*pro⁻* F⁻), TR92 (*trpA*, *purE*, *hisA*, *mtl⁻*, *str^r*, F⁻) and DB46 (*his⁻*, *gal⁻*, Hfr B2) were used. A simplified chromosome map with the origin and direction of chromosome transfer of Hfr B2 is shown in Figure 1. Phage P22 wild type and an integration-deficient (*int⁻*) mutant of P22 were used for transduction. R factors used were 222 and S-a. S-a has recently been found to have kanamycin-resistance marker (*kan*) in addition to *sul*, *str* and *cam* which were already reported (WATANABE et all. 1968).

Procedure for conjugal transfer of R factors. The procedure for conjugal transfer of R factors was described previously (WATANABE, FUKASAWA, 1961a).

Procedure for transduction of R factors. The procedure for transduction of R factors in *S. typhimurium* LT-2 by phage P22 was described in a previous paper (WATANABE, FUKASAWA, 1961b).

Procedure of UV induction of phage P22 in lysogenic bacteria. Drug-resistant transductants and other lysogenic bacterial strains of *S. typhimurium* LT-2 were grown in tryptone broth to about 1×10^8 cells per ml with gentle shaking at 37° C, and 6 ml of each culture was irradiated in a petri dish with a germicidal lamp (National, 60 watts) in the dark for 20 seconds from a distance of 30 cm. The UV-irradiated cultures were aerated at 37° C in the dark for 2.5 hours. The partially lysed cultures were centrifuged at 8,000 rpm for 3 min and the supernatants were treated with chloroform and used as lysates.

Other general phage techniques. Other general phage techniques followed were those described by Adams (ADAMS, 1959).

192

Procedure for mating. Drug-resistant transductants of *S. typhimurium pro A36* and TR92 were mated with DB46 (Hfr) following the procedure of Sanderson and Demerec (SANDERSON, DEMEREC, 1965).

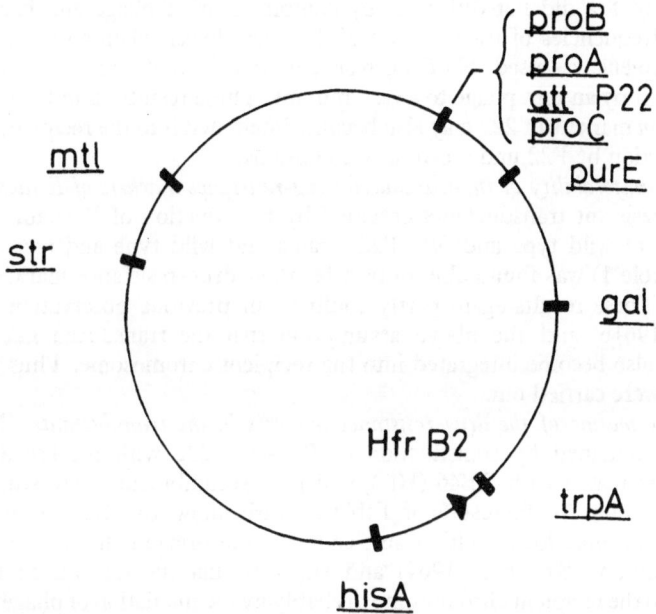

Fig. 1. *A simplified chromosome map of Salmonella typhimurium with the origin and direction of chromosome transfer of Hfr B2*
Modified from *Sanderson* (6). *pro:* proline; *att:* attachement site; *pur:* purine; *gal:* galactose; *trp:* tryptophan; *his:* histidine; *str:* streptomycin; *mtl:* mannitol.

RESULTS

Frequencies of transduction of R factors 222 and S-a by wild type and an int⁻ mutant of phage P22 in wild type and a rec⁻ mutant of S. typhimurium LT-2. As the results are shown in Table 1, the frequencies of transduction of R factor S-a were much higher than those

Table 1.

FREQUENCIES OF TRANSDUCTION OF R FACTORS 222 (sul, str, cam, tet) AND S-a (sul, str, cam, kan) BY WILD TYPE (int⁺) AND AN int⁻ MUTANT OF PHAGE P22 IN *Salmonella typhimurium* LT-2 WILD TYPE (rec⁺) AND rec⁻ MUTANT.

Donor / Recipient	P22 *int⁺* gronw on LT-2 *rec⁺* (222)		P22 *int⁻* grown on LT-2 *rec⁺* (222)		P22 *int⁺* grown on LT-2 *rec⁺* (S-a)	P22 *int⁻* grown on LT-2 *rec⁺* (S-a)
	Selected by Cm*	Selected by Tc*	Selected by Cm	Selected by Tc	Selected by Cm	Selected by Cm
LT-2 *rec⁺*	1.2×10^{-7}	4.3×10^{-9}	2.7×10^{-9}	7.1×10^{-10}	3.2×10^{-6}	2.9×10^{-6}
LT-2 *rec⁻*	2.1×10^{-0}	1.9×10^{-10}	$<1.7 \times 10^{-10}$	$<1.7 \times 10^{-10}$	4.4×10^{-6}	3.5×10^{-6}

* Cm: chloramphenicol. Tc: tetracycline.
Frequencies of transduction are expressed per plaque-forming unit.

of R factor 222 in any combinations of phage and bacterial strains. These results in part are in accordance with our previous findings (WATANABE et al., 1968). Another remarkable difference noted between the transduction data of 222 and S-a is that the frequencies of transduction of S-a did not differ in any combinations of phage and bacterial strains, whereas the frequencies of transduction of 222 were lower when an *int*⁻ mutant phage or a *rec*⁻ recipient was used. No drug-resistant transductant could be found when 222 was transduced by an *int*⁻ phage to a *rec*⁻ mutant. These results seem to suggest that the *sul, str* and *cam* markers of 222 may also become integrated into the recipient chromosome after transduction by P22 under ordinary conditions.

Conjugal transferability of the transduced drug-resistance markers of R factor 222. None of the drug-resistant transductants obtained by transduction of R factor 222 with any combinations of wild type and *int*⁻ P22 strains and wild type and *rec*⁻ LT-2 strains (shown in Table 1) was found able to transfer their drug-resistance markers by causing conjugation. These results again partly confirm our previous observation (WATANABE, FUKASAWY, 1961b) and the above assumption that the transduced *sul, str* and *cam* markers may also become integrated into the recipient chromosome. Thus the following experiments were carried out.

Mapping by mating of the drug-resistance markers in the transductants. Drug-resistant transductants obtained by transduction of R factor 222 with *proA36* and TR92 as recipients were mated with DB46 (Hfr), and *pro*⁺ recombinants were studied for their genetic constitution. As the results of Table 2 clearly show, the transduced *tet* marker is closely linked to *proA* locus. This result confirms the previous finding of Dubnau and STOCKER (DUBNAU, STOCKER, 1964) and suggests that the transduced *tet* marker is integrated into the recipient chromosome probably by the mediation of phage P22 genome,

Table 2.

MATING BETWEEN *Salmonella typhimurium* DB46 (Hfr) AND *tet* TRANSDUCTANTS OBTAINED BY PHAGE P22 IN *S. typhimurium* PRO A36.

Strain of *tet* transductant	Markers of *pro*⁺ recombinants*			
	tet P22⁺	*tet* P22⁻	*tet*⁻ P22⁺	*tet*⁻ P22⁻
TC-1	0	0	0	88
TC-2	0	1	0	97

* P22⁺ and P22⁻ indicate the presence and absence of prophage P22, respectively, which was checked by the ability and inability to liberate infectious P22 particles upon UV irradiation.

Table 3.

MATING BETWEEN *Salmonella typhinuriun* DB46 AND *sul . str . cam* TRANSDUCTANTS OBTAINED BY PHAGE P22 IN *S. typhinuriun* PRO A36

Strain of *sul. str. cam* transductant	Markers of *pro*⁺ recombinants*			
	sul. str. cam P22⁺	*sul. str. cam* P22⁻	*sul.*⁻*.str*⁻*.cam*⁻ P22⁺	*sul*⁻*.str*⁻*.cam*⁻ P22⁻
CM-1	48	33	0	1
CM-2	88	0	0	0
CM-3	58	0	30	0

* P22⁺ and P22⁻ indicate the presence and absence of prophage P22, respectively, which was checked by the ability to liberate infectious P22 particles upon UV irradiation.

because the *pro* region is known to be the attachement site of prophage P22 (SMITH, 1968; SMITH, STOCKER, 1962). The results of recombination between Hfr and *sul . str . cam* transductants are in contrast to those with *tet* transductants and indicate that the *sul, str* and *cam* markers are not closely linked to *proA* locus (Table 3). These results also suggest that prophage P22 in the *sul . str . cam* transductants may be located at some site other than the ordinary prophage site.

Table 4.

GENETIC CONSTITUTION OF PUR⁺ RECOMBINANTS OBTAINED IN THE
MATING BETWEEN *Salmonella typhimurium* DB46 AND sul . str . cam
TRANSDUCTANT No. 5 OF *S. typhimurium* TR92

Genetic marker							No. of recombinants
pur	gal	trp	str	mtl	cam		
1	0	0	0	0	0		57 (64.8%)
1	1	0	0	0	0		28 (31.8%)
1	1	0	0	0	1		2 (2.3%)
1	0	1	0	0	0		1 (1.1%)
						Total	88

Genetic markers of donor and recipient strains.
   DB46: *pur⁺ gal⁻ trp⁺ str^s mtl⁺ sul⁻ . str⁻ . cam⁻* Hfr.
   TR92: *pur⁻ gal⁺ trp⁻ str^r mtl⁻ sul . str . cam* F⁻.
Donor markers are expressed as 1 and recipient markers as 0.
The frequency of *pur⁺* recombinants was 3.0×10^{-3} per introduced Hfr cell in this experiment.

Then the following experiments were performed: R factor 222 was first transduced to strain TR92 and the *sul . str . cam* transductants obtained were mated with DB46 (Hfr). The results with one such transductant (KONDO, MITSUHASHI, 1964) are shown in Tables 4, 5 and 6. These results suggest that the *sul . str . cam* markers are integrated into

Table 5.

GENETIC CONSTITUTION OF TRP⁺ RECOMBINANTS OBTAINED IN THE MATING
BETWEEN *Salmonella typhimurium* DB46 AND sul . str . cam TRANSDUCTANT
No. 5 OF *S. typhimurium* TR92

Genetic marker							No. of recombinanst
pur	gal	trp	str	mtl	cam		
0	0	1	0	0	0		31
0	0	1	0	0	1		23
1	1	1	0	0	1		21
1	1	1	0	0	0		10
1	0	1	0	0	1		6
0	1	1	0	0	1		3
1	0	1	0	0	0		3
0	1	1	0	0	0		3
						Total	100

Genetic markers of donor and recipient strains.
   DB46: *pur⁺ gal⁻ trp⁺ str^s mtl⁺ sul⁻ . str⁻ . cam⁻* Hfr.
   TR92: *pur⁻ gal⁺ trp⁻ str^r mtl⁻ sul . str . cam* F⁻.
Donor markers are expressed as 1 and recipient markers as 0.
The frequency of *trp⁺* recombinants was 1.5×10^{-4} per introduced Hfr cell in this experiment.

Table 6.

GENETIC CONSTITUTION OF pur⁺ trp⁺ RECOMBINANTS OBTAINED IN THE
MATING BETWEEN *Salmonella typhimurium* DB46 AND sul . str . cam
TRANSDUCTANT No. 5 OF *S. typhimurium* TR92

Genetic marker						No. of recombinants
pur	*gal*	*trp*	*str*	*mtl*	*cam*	
1	1	1	0	0	1	61
1	0	1	0	0	1	15
1	1	1	0	0	0	15
1	0	1	0	0	0	9
					Total	100

Genetic markers of donor and recipient strains.
  DB46: *pur⁺ gal⁻ trp⁺ str*ˢ *mtl⁺ sul⁻ . str⁻ . cam⁻* Hfr.
  TR92: *pur⁻ gal⁺ trp⁻ str*ʳ *mtl⁻ sul . str . cam* F⁻.
Donor markers are expressed as 1 and recipient markers as 0.
  The frequency of *pur⁺ trp⁺* recombinants was 5.0×10^{-5} per introduced Hfr cell in this experiment.

the recipient chromosome between *gal* and *trpA* (see Fig. 1). The data of a similar cross of another *sul . str . cam* transductant (No. 47) of TR92 with DB46 are shown in Tables 7, 8 and 9. These results suggest that the *sul . str . cam* markers of this transductant are integrated between *purE* and *gal* rather than between *gal* and *trpA*.

Table 7.

GENETIC CONSTITUTION OF pur⁺ RECOMBINANTS OBTAINED IN THE MATING
BETWEEN *Salmonella typhimurium* DB46 AND sul . str . cam TRANSDUCTANT
No. 47 OF *S. typhimurium* TR92

Genetic marker						No. of recombinants
pur	*gal*	*trp*	*str*	*mtl*	*cam*	
1	0	0	0	0	0	39
1	0	0	0	0	1	28
1	1	0	0	0	0	20
1	1	0	0	0	1	13
					Total	100

Genetic markers of donor and recipient strains.
  DB46: *pur⁺ gal⁻ trp⁺ str*ˢ *mtl⁺ sul⁻ . str⁻ . cam⁻* Hfr.
  TR92: *pur⁻ gal⁺ trp⁻ str*ʳ *mtl⁻ sul . str . cam* F⁻.
Donor markers are expressed as 1 and recipinet markers as O.
  The frequency of *pur⁺* recombinants was 5.6×10^{-4} per introduced Hfr cell in this experiment.

Failure to obtain HFT lysates from sul . str . cam transductants. We have attempted to obtain HFT lysates for *sul . str . cam* markers using 27 independently isolated *sul . str . cam* transductants but without success, although all of these transductants except one liberated infectious phage particles upon UV irradiation.

Success to obtain HFT lysates from tet transductants. Three out of 26 independently isolated *tet* transductants gave rise to HFT lysates upon UV irradiation. The titers of plaque-forming units (PFU) contained in these lysates were much lower as compared with those contained in the lysates obtained by UV-induction of normal P22-lysogens

Table 8.

GENETIC CONSTITUTION OF trp⁺ RECOMBINANTS OBTAINED IN THE MATING BETWEEN *Salmonella typhimurium* DB46 AND sul . str . cam TRANSDUCTANT No. 47 OF *S. typhimurium* TR92

Genetic marker							No. of recombinants
pur	*gal*	*trp*	*str*	*mtl*	*cam*		
0	0	1	0	0	0		29
1	1	1	0	0	1		21
1	1	1	0	0	0		18
1	0	1	0	0	0		15
1	0	1	0	0	1		7
0	0	1	0	0	1		7
0	1	1	0	0	0		2
0	1	1	0	0	1		1
						Total	100

Genetic markers of donor and recipient strains.

DB46: *pur⁺ gal⁻ trp⁺ str⁸ mtl⁺ sul⁻ . str⁻ . cam⁻* Hfr.

TR92: *pur⁻ gal⁺ trp⁻ strʳ mtl⁻ sul . str . cam* F⁻.

Donor markers are expressed as 1 and recipient markers as 0.

The frequency of *trp⁺* recombinants was 4.0×10^{-5} per introduce Hfr cell in this experiment.

and *sul . str . cam* transductants; they were between 10^4 and 10^5 PFU per ml and the frequencies of *tet* transduction per PFU were about 10^0. The *tet* transductants obtained by HFT lysates were then irradiated with UV to see if HFT lysates could be obtained

Table 9.

GENETIC CONSTITUTION OF pur⁺ trp⁺ RECOMBINANTS OBTAINED IN THE MATING BETWEEN *Salmonella typhimurium* DB46 AND sul . str . cam TRANSDUCTANT No. 47 OF *S. typhimurium* TR92

Genetic marker							No. of recombinants
pur	*gal*	*trp*	*str*	*mtl*	*cam*		
1	1	1	0	0	1		32 (32.7%)
1	1	1	0	0	0		30 (30.6%)
1	0	1	0	0	0		21 (21.4%)
1	0	1	0	0	1		15 (15.3%)
						Total	98

Genetic markers of donor and recipient strains.

DB46: *pur⁺ gal⁻ trp⁺ str⁸ mtl⁺ sul⁻ . str⁻ . cam⁻* Hfr.

TR92: *pur⁻ gal⁺ trp⁻ strʳ mtl⁻ sul . str . cam* F⁻.

Donor markers are expressed as 1 and recipient markers as 0.

The frequency of *pur⁺ trp⁺* recombinants was 1.1×10^{-5} per introduced Hfr cell in this experiment.

successively. As shown in Table 10, many of the *tet* transductants obtained by an HFT lysate for *tet* again gave rise to HFT lysates upon UV induction, but some *tet* transductants did not produce either *tet*-transducing particles or PFU. This kind of data were obtained successively by using the obtained *tet* transductants as the sources of transducing phage.

Prophage immunity of tet transductants obtained by HFT lysates. Phage P22 was spotted on each *tet* transductant culture seeded in soft tryptone agar (containing 0.6% agar) and the plate was incubated at 37° C overnight. P22-lysogenic and non-lysogenic cultures of

Table 10.

FREQUENCIES OF tet TRANSDUCTION WITH LYSATES OBTAINED BY ULTRAVIOLET INDUCTION OF tet HFT TRANSDUCTANTS

Strain of tet transductant*	Titer of PFU** (per ml)	Frequency of tet transductants (per PFU)	Immunity to phage
TC-10-11	0	0	—
TC-10-12	1.2×10^4	1.5×10^0	±
TC-10-13	9.7×10^3	1.1×10^0	±
TC-10-14	1.8×10^4	1.0×10^0	±
TC-10-15	2.7×10^4	1.2×10^0	±
TC-10-A	2.4×10^4	1.2×10^0	±
TC-10-B	9.3×10^4	$5 4 \times 10^{-1}$	±
TC-10-C	3.0×10^4	9.0×10^{-1}	±
TC-10-D	1.5×10^4	8.8×10^{-1}	±
TC-10-E	9.2×10^4	8.5×10^{-1}	±

* The first five transductants were obtained in one experiment and the following five transductants in the other experiment.
** PFU: plaque-forming unit.

LT-2 wild type were used as controls in this test. All of the *tet* transductants, which were obtained by HFT lysates and which no longer gave HFT lysates upon UV irradiation, were found sensitive to P22 like non-lysogenic LT-2 wild type. In contrast, all of the *tet* transductants, which were obtained by HFT lysates and which again gave HFT lysates upon UV induction, were found partially sensitive to P22 unlike P22-lysogenic LT-2 wild type which was completely immune to P22 in the spot test. The *tet* transductants

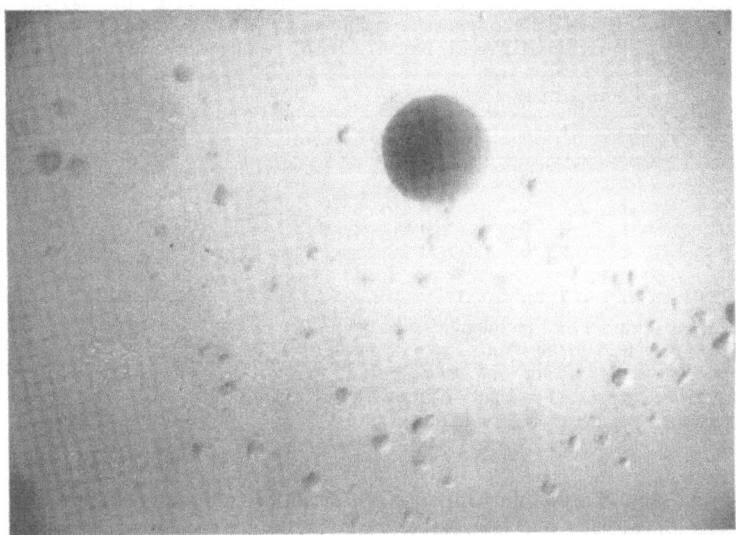

Fig. 2 Colonies of complete and abortive tet transductants produced by an HFT lysate of P22 in Salmonella typhimurium LT-2.
These colonies developed on nutrient agar containing 25 µg/ml of tetracycline hydrochloride. A large colony is thought to be a complete transductant and the other minute colonies are assumed to be abortive transductants.

partially sensitive to P22 were found, upon plating on nutrient agar, to spontaneously and frequently segregate clones completely sensitive to P22. These P22-sensitive clones no longer produced HFT lysates upon UV irradiation. The frequencies of segregation of such P22-sensitive clones were not accurately determined.

Superinfection with normal P22 of P22-sensitive tet transductants. The above-described P22-sensitive *tet* transductants, which did not produce HFT lysates upon UV irradiation, were lysogenized with wild type P22 by growing them in tryptone broth containing high titers of wild type P22. The P22-lysogenic *tet* clones thus obtained were then induced with UV and the phage lysates obtained were tested for the frequencies of *tet* transdugtion and PFU. It was found that high titers of PFU ($10^8 - 10^9$ per ml) and relatively low titers of *tet*-transducing particles (about 10^{-4} per PFU) are contained in these lysates. These frequencies of *tet* transduction are still higher than the ordinary low frequencies of transduction (LFT) of *tet* by ordinary, lytically grown phage (see Table 1) or phage lysates obtained by UV induction of lysogens for normal P22.

Table 11.

HELPER EFFECT OF NORMAL PHAGE P22 ON THE COMPLETE TRANSDUCTION
OF tet BY AN HFT LYSATE OF P22 IN *Salmonella typhimurium* LT-2

PFU* in transduction donor (per ml)		Frequency of complete *tet* transductants per PFU contained in HFT lysate
HFT lysate	Normal P22 added as helper	
5.0×10^0	0	8.0×10^0
5.0×10^0	1.1×10^{10}	7.3×10^2
5.0×10^0	1.1×10^9	4.0×10^2
5.0×10^0	1.1×10^8	2.3×10^2
5.0×10^0	1.1×10^7	3.0×10^1
5.0×10^0	1.1×10^6	8.0×10^0
5.0×10^0	1.1×10^5	1.4×10^0
2.6×10^{-1}	0	$<3.8 \times 10^1$
2.6×10^{-1}	1.6×10^{10}	1.5×10^4
2.6×10^{-1}	1.6×10^9	6.5×10^3
2.6×10^{-1}	1.6×10^8	6.1×10^2
2.6×10^{-1}	1.6×10^7	1.2×10^2
2.6×10^{-1}	1.6×10^6	$<3.8 \times 10^1$
2.6×10^{-1}	1.6×10^5	$<3.8 \times 10^1$
3.3×10^{-2}	0	$<3.0 \times 10^2$
3.3×10^{-2}	1.7×10^{10}	1.7×10^4
3.3×10^{-2}	1.7×10^9	7.3×10^3
3.3×10^{-2}	1.7×10^8	3.0×10^2
3.3×10^{-2}	1.7×10^7	$<3.0 \times 10^2$
3.3×10^{-2}	1.7×10^6	$<3.0 \times 10^2$
3.3×10^{-2}	1.7×10^5	$<3.0 \times 10^2$

Minute tet transductants observed on tetracycline-containing nutrient agar seeded with S. typhimurium LT-2 infected with HFT lysates for tet. LT-2 cells infected with HFT lysates for *tet* gave rise to minute colonies on nutrient agar containing 25 μg per ml of tetracycline hydrochloride in addition to colonies of the ordinary size (Figure 2). These minute colonies were about 100 times more frequent than the large colonies. The minute colonies were suspected to be abortive transductants, because no such colonies developed in the plating of non-infected cells on tetracycline-containing medium.

Increase in number of large tet colonies by the addition of normal P22 to HFT lysates. Normal P22 grown on LT-2 wild type was added to HFT lysates for *tet* at varying ratios, and transduction of *tet* was performed to LT-2 wild type with these mixtures. As the results are shown in Table 11 and Figure 3, the frequencies of large *tet* transductants were markedly increased by the addition of high titers of normal P22 to the HFT lysates.

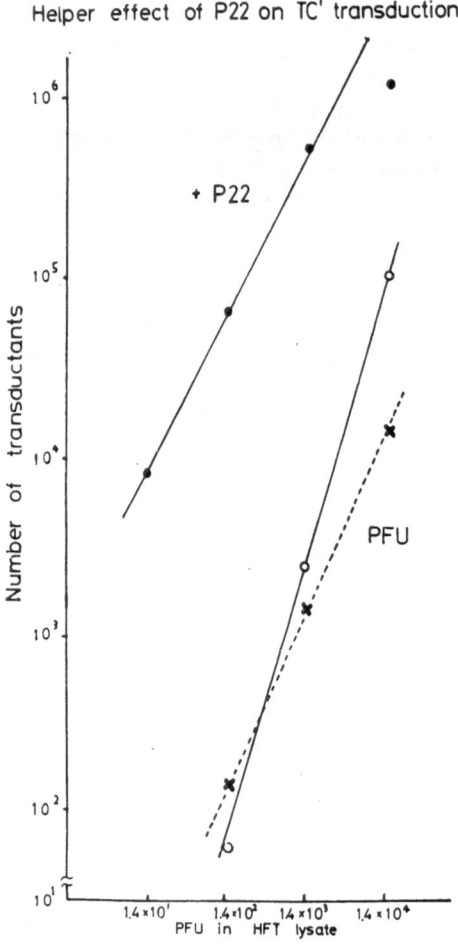

Helper effect of P22 on TC^r transduction

Fig. 3 Helper effect of normal phage P22 on the complete transduction of tet by an HFT lysate of P22 in Salmonella typhimurium LT-2.

PFU: plaque-forming unit.

○ : number of tet transductants obtained with a certain dilution of an HFT lysate.

● : number of *tet* transductants obtained with a certain dilution of an HFT lysate mixed with 3.3×10^9/ml of normal P22.

The maximal increase in number of the large *tet* transductants was nearly 100 times of the original transduction frequency. This result together with the frequency of minute *tet* colonies suggests that the original HFT lysates contain about 100 times more *tet*-transducing particles than PFU.

DISCUSSION

As we have reported here as well as previously (WATANABE, FUKASAWA, 1961b; WATANABE et al., 1968), transduction of R factor 222 by phage P22 in *S. typhimurium* results in the segregation of the drug-resistance markers and their integration into the chromosome of the recipient bacteria and the loss of their conjugal transferability. These unusual patterns of transduction of 222 by P22 as compared with transduction of the same R factor by phage P1 can be ascribed to the small size of P22. P22, unlike P1, cannot incorporate both drug-resistance markers and RTF (resistance transfer factor) (WATANABE, 1963) together into single transducing particles. The *sul, str* and *cam* markers are closely linked to each other and they are usually transduced together. The *tet* marker, however, is not located close enough to other drug-resistance markers on the structure of R factor to be picked up together by P22. The drug-resistance markers should become abortive unless they are integrated into the recipient chromosome (WATANABE, OGATA, 1970). In contrast, R factor S-a is small enough to be incorporated *en bloc* into a transducing particle of P22 as reported previously (WATANABE et al., 1968) and the present data of transduction of this R factor by an *int⁻* mutant of P22 to a *rec⁻* mutant of LT-2 seem to confirm our previous conclusion.

We have shown here that not only the *tet* marker but also *sul . str . cam* markers together become integrated into the recipient chromosome. The integration of the *tet* marker at the *pro* region is most likely due to the mediation of P22 genome but the mechanism of integration of the other three markers near the *gal* region is not yet known. This region may contain homologies with either these drug-resistance genes of R factor 222 or with P22 genome attached to the drug-resistance genes.

HFT lysates for *tet* were obtained by UV induction of three out of 26 independently isolated *tet* transductants, but none of the 27 independently obtained *sul . str . cam* transductants studied produced HFT lysates for these drug-resistance markers upon UV induction, although most of them liberated infectious phage particles. The *tet* transductants which produced HFT lysates were partially immune to P22 and produced both *tet*-transducing, defective particles (P22 *dtet*) and non-transducing, infectious particles. To the contrary, the *tet* transductants which did not give rise to HFT lysates upon UV irradiation produced neither *tet*-transducing particles nor non-transducing, infectious particles. The HFT lysates obtained from the first type *tet* transductants again produced two types of *tet* transductants; one of them was similar to the first type and the others were similar to the second type. Thus it can be assumed that the *tet* transductants which give rise to HFT lysates may be doubly lysogenic for normal P22 and P22 *dtet*, which requires the helper action of normal P22 for its growth, and that the *tet* transductants which do not produce HFT lysates for *tet* may be single lysogens for P22 *dtet*. The absence of prophage immunity in these probable single lysogens may be due to the absence of the immunity region in the defective prophage. The partial prophage immunity observed in the supposedly doubly lysogenic *tet* transductants seems to be due to rather frequent, spontaneous loss of normal prophage from the double lysogens. Superinfection with normal P22 of the singly lysogenic *tet* transductants is in fact easy, although the frequencies of lysogenization with normal P22 has not been studied quantitatively. The double lysogens thus obtained produce high titers of normal P22 upon UV induction but the ratios of *tet*-transducing particles contained in these lysates are much lower than those contained in the ordinary HFT lysates. The reason for this curious finding will be discussed in a following paper.

HFT lysates for *tet* seem to contain about 100 times more P22 *dtet* particles than normal P22 particles assuming from the frequencies of "abortive" plus complete *tet* transductants and the titers of PFU, and also from the finding that the cells destined to become abortive in single infection can be converted to complete *tet* transductants by simultaneous infection with normal phage. This result may indicate that P22 *dtet* is so defective that it has a low probability of integration, and that its integration may be promoted by the helper action of normal phage. The mechanism of liberation of more P22 *dtet* particles than normal P22 by HFT lysate-producing *tet* transductants is under current investigation and will be reported in a following paper.

The origin of P22 *dtet* is assumed to be a result of genetic recombination between phage P22 genome and R factor 222 probably when both of them are in autonomous states, because the *tet* transducing particles are already contained in lytically prepared HFT lysates. Thus P22 *dtet* is thought analogous to P1*CM* in that both of them are assumed to have developed as a result of vegetative recombination between phage genome and R factor (KONDO, MITSUHASHI, 1964), but the genetic defect of P22 *dtet* is apparently more severe than P1*CM* that can replicate for itself without the help of normal P1. The reason of the failure to obtain HFT lysates for *sul . str . cam* markers remains to be disclosed.

This investigation was supported by U. S. Public Health Service research grant AI-08078 form National Institute of Allergy and Infectious Diseases.

REFERENCES

ADAMS, M. H. (1959): *Bacteriophages*. Interscience Publishers, Inc., New York.

DUBNAU, E. and STOCKER, B. A. D (1964): Genetics of plasmids in *Salmonella typhimurium*. Nature **204**: 1112—1113.

HARADA, K, M, KAMEDA, M, SUZUKI, and MITSUHASHI, S. (1963): Drug resistance of enteric bacteria. II. Transduction of transmissible drug-resistance (R) factors with phage epsilon. J. Bacteriol. **86**: 1332—1338.

KAMEDA, M. K. HARADA, M. SUZUKI, and S. MITSUHASHI (1965): Drug resistance of enteric bacteria. V. High frequency of transduction of R factor with bacteriophage epsilon. J. Bacteriol. **90**: 1174—1181.

KONDO, E., and S. MITSUHASHI (1964): Drug resistance of enteric bacteria. IV. Active transducing bacteriophage P1CM produced by the combination of R factor with bacteriophage P1. J. Bacteriol. **88**: 1266—1276.

SANDERSON, K. E. (1970): Current linkage map of *Salmonella typhimurium*. Bacteriol. Rev. **34**: 176—193.

SANDERSON, K. E., and M. DEMEREC (1965): The linkage of map *Salmonella typhimurium*. Genetics **51**: 897—913.

OKADA, M., and T. WATANABE (1968): Transduction with phage P1 in *Salmonella typhimurium*. Nature **218**: 185—187.

SMITH, H. O. (1968): Defective phage formation by lysogens of integration-deficient phage P22 mutants. Virology **34**: 203—223.

SMITH, S. M., and B. A. D. STOCKER (1962): Colicinogeny and recombination. Brit. Med. Bull. **18**: 46—51.

WATANABE, T. (1963): Infective heredity of multiple drug resistance in bacteria. Bacteriol. Rev. **27**: 87—113.

WATANABE, T., and T. FUKASAWA (1961a): Episome-mediated transfer of drug resistance in *Enterobacteriabeae*. I. Transfer of resistance factors by conjugation. J. Bacteriol. **81**: 669—678.

WATANABE, T., and T. FUKASAVA (1961b): Episome-mediated transfer of drug resistance in *Enterobacteriaceae*. III. Transduction of resistance factors. J. Bacteriol. **82**: 202—209.

WATANABE, T., C. FURUSE, and S. SAKAIZUMI (1968): Transduction of various R factors by phage P1 in *Escherichia coli* and by phage P22 in *Salmonella typhimurium*. J. Bacteriol. **96**: 1791 to 1795.

WATANABE, T., and Y. OGATA (1970): Abortive transduction of resistance factor by bacteriophage P22 in *Salmonella typhimurium*. J. Bacteriol. **102**: 596—597.

GENETICS OF COLICINOGENIC FACTORS AND THEIR RECOMBINATION WITH R FACTORS

P. FREDERICQ and E. DELHALLE

University of Liège, Belgium.

GENETICS OF COLICINOGENIC FACTORS

The property to produce a colicine is a highly stable hereditary characteristic of some strains of Enterobacteriaceae and must therefore be governed by genetic determinants which have been called colicinogenic factors (Col factors). Several of these colicinogenic factors can be transferred from one strain to another, in mixed cultures, by conjugation and also by phage mediated transduction. The recipient strain always produces a colicine identical to that of the donor strain and can in turn transfer the Col factor to other recipients. Several different Col factors can be transmitted to the same strain which will then produce several distinct colicines. They can be transferred by conjugation to *Escherichia* strains but also to *Shigella, Klebsiella, Salmonella, Providencia, Proteus* and *Serratia* strains. (FREDERICQ (1954), FREDERICQ (1958), FREDERICQ (1959).

In such crosses Col factors are transferred, sometimes at a high rate, but without linkage to any chromosomal genes. They appear therefore as autonomous units, independent from the chromosome and belong to the class of genetic determinants known as plasmids. Integration into the chromosome has been demonstrated on rare occasions, showing that some Col factors are indeed true episomes (FREDERICQ (1965), KAHN (1968)).

When a donor produced several distinct colicines, these properties were generally tranferred independently by conjugation but, in some cases, they were always transferred together as if carried by a single genetic unit. In such cases, transduction could split some of these complex Col factors but not others (for example a Col VBM factor could be split into VM, BM, V, B and M but a ColVI could not be split (FREDERICQ (1969)).

Col factors have been isolated by gradient centrifugation. They were characterized as double-stranded, covalently linked, circular DNA molecules with contour lengths ranging from $2.3\,\mu$ for $ColE_1$ to $32.0\,\mu$ for ColIB, and even more for more complex factors (CLEWEL and HELINSKI (1970), ROTH and HELINSKI (1967)).

From the size of even the smallest Col factors, it is evident that they can code for much more than a single protein. Besides the structural gene(s) for the synthesis of one or several colicines they probably carry some other information. As Col factors are potentially lethal agents they must be normally repressed by regulatory genes in order to permit survival of their host. Very little is known about the mechanism involved, except that colicine synthesis is inducible by U. V. irradiation and other mutagenic agents and probably results from unregulated Col factor DNA replication (AMATI (1964)).

Another property found by all Col factors is a more or less pronounced immunity, specific of the particular colicine whose synthesis they govern. The mechanism is still very poorly understood but quite different from those involved in resistant or tolerant mutations (FREDERICQ (1963), NOMURA (1967)). Immune cells keep functional receptors and differ from tolerant mutants by level and specificity of their partial resistance. Furthermore, immunity is a dominant character while resistance or tolerance were shown to be recessive. Immunity is clearly due to the presence of the Col factor, for it always parallels loss or acquisition of that agent, but it is independent from colicine production itself. Indeed 2 types of mutants from a ColV factor have been found, one which had lost immunity but was still producing colicine while the other was still immune but did not produce colicine anymore. Strains harboring the former type grew very poorly on ordinary media, because they were poisoned by the colicine that they produce, but normal growth could be restored by adding trypsin to destroy the colicine. When 2 mutants of the second type, obtained independently, were put in the same cell, there was no complementation but fully colicinogenic clones appeared in the progeny, probably by intragenic recombination (FREDERICQ (1971), FREDERICQ and DELHALLE: to be published).

Some but not all Col factors may also govern still other properties. Several of them were found to carry a fertility determinant promoting their self-transfer by conjugation. These experiments were done in the absence of the E. coli K12 F factor and clearly showed that 2 different kinds of Col factor were occuring: one which is infectious like F (capable of self-transfer) and the other which is not, but can be transferred as an independent plasmid with the help of the former or of any other transfer agent (CLOWES (1961), FREDERICQ (1969), FREDERICQ et BETZ-BAREAU (1953), OZEKI and HOWARTH (1961).

The fertility determinant of Col factors seems to act like the F agent of E. coli K12 by inducing synthesis of sex pili. Indeed, 2 classes of fertile Col factors have been found: a) Governing sex pili very similar to those produced by F (F-like pili) and thus inducing susceptibility to the so-called sex-specific phages; b) governing another type of pili (I-like pili because first met by a ColI factor) morphologically different and unable to adsorb these phages. A new type of sex-specific phage has however been found which is adsorbed by these I-like but not by the F-like pili (LAWN, MEYNELL E., MEYNELL G. G. and DATTA (1967).

Fertility is regulated by a repressor, also carried by the Col factor. Derepressed cultures could be obtained, giving rise to HFC systems, that are transferring their Col factors at a very high frequency. By way of that repressor, Col factors may interfere with the high fertility of the F factor when they are of the F like type. They are called fi+ (fertility inhibiting) while their derepressed mutants or the I-like type are fi- (EDWARDS and MEYNELL (1968), FREDERICQ et BETZ-BAREAU (1956)).

Other properties which were found to be carried by some Col factors include restriction of certain phages and increased resistance to U. V. irradiation (HOWARTH (1965), STROBEL and NOMURA (1966)).

Col factors are thus more or less complex genetical units in which structural genes governing the synthesis of one or several different proteins (colicines) are associated to regulatory genes and eventually to genes governing other properties. All properties carried by a Col factor are generally transferred together by conjugation but may be separated by transduction and get lost independently by mutation. Col factors may also recombine, thus associating on a single unit properties originally carried by 2 independent units (FREDERICQ 1969).

It is therefore evident that Col factors are very similar to R factors and clearly built on the same model. That they belong to the same class of agents was further strengthened by complex interactions. Incompatibilities between Col and R factors have often been reported as well as their more or less frequent associated transfer in conjugation. Indeed non-self-transferable Col factors can be mobilized by fertile R-factors just as non-self-transferable R-factors can be mobilized by fertille Col factors (FREDERICQ, KRCMÉRY and KETTNER (1971), IIJIMA (1962)).

Still more stable associations have been observed, in which permanent recombination appears to have occured between Col and R factors, thus associating on a single genetic structure colicine and resistance genes which were originally carried by 2 independent plasmids (FREDERICQ et al., (to be published)). Such recombination phenomena will be considered in the next section.

RECOMBINATION OF COL FACTORS WITH R FACTORS

A particularly complex Col factor originating from the wild *E. coli* strain K260 has been used to study recombination with R factors. This Col factor did carry the structural genes for colicines V, B and M, linked to a fertility determinant and was generally transferred independently from the chromosomes by conjugation. On a rare occasion, a recipient marked by a *trp* deletion received a complex structure associating the Col factor markers to a segment of the donor chromosome, including the complete *trp* operon as well as the *cysB* and *tonB* genes which lie either side of it. This complex structure remained stable and could be transferred *en bloc*, at a high rate (10^{-1} to 10^{-2}) in crosses with K12F-derivatives, which, in turn, could transfer it at the same rate. It was therefore very similar to F′ episomes, except that the concomitant transfer of the chromosome was very low and was not oriented, probably due to lack of homology of the chromosomal genes of the episome, originating from strain K260, with the corresponding region of K12 (FREDERICQ (1965), FREDERICQ (1969)).

This complex episome was well suited for recombination experiments because it carried many different markers, was highly fertile and transfer of Trp$^+$ could be easily selected, even in transduction experiments. As the colicine B and M genes were highly linked, even in transduction, and difficult to score separately, only B has been considered in the following experiments. A segregant having lost the ColV gene was also used and we shall call these episomes ColVBTry or ColBTry accordingly.

In conjugation experiments colicinogeny was always transferred in very close association with the tryptophan genes and with fertility but, in transduction experiments, cotransfer of colicinogeny was highly dependent on the presence of other episomes in the recipient. Rates were 2% for V and 0.1% for B if no episome was present, and only exceptional transductants receiving both V and B were fertile. Cotransfer of V was not much affected, but cotransfer of B increased to 40% and more when the recipient already carried Fd, F′lac or a fertile ColV factor. In many such transductants, the transduced episome could be further transferred, by conjugation, independently of the preexisting one. But in others, the transduced episome appeared to recombine with the preexisting one, as these transductants could transfer, at a high rate and in very close association, markers originating from both parental episomes, such as Trp and Lac or ColV. If other Col factors (E_1, E_2 or Ib) were present in the recipient, there was no effect on cotransfer of ColB with *trp* genes, but one rare transductant was found to recombine ColIb with the transduced *trp* genes, thus forming a ColIbTry episome.

If R factors were present in the recipient, there was no effect, either, on cotransfer of ColB but, as with ColIb, one rare transductant was found to recombine the preexisting resistance to tetracycline with the transduced *trp* genes and could transfer both markers in very close association.

In order to increase the chances of recombining R with Col, a ColBTry episome was then transduced to a recipient carrying both an R factor, R(STCK) and a ColV factor, known to increase considerably the cotransfer of ColB. Results are presented in table 1.

Table 1

ANALYSIS OF Trp+ TRANSDUCTANTS OBTAINED BY TRANSDUCING A ColBTry EPISOME TO A RECIPIENT CARRYING ColV AND R (STCK)

Markers present							Fertility Type[1]	Frequency (percentage)
ColV	ColB	Trp	R(S)	R(T)	R(C)	R(K)		
+	+	+	+	+	+	+		66
+	−	+	+	+	+	+	I	27
+	+	+	+	−	+	+		1
+	+	+	−	+	−	−	II	1
+	−	+	−	+	−	−		1
+	+	+	−	−	−	−	III	3
+	−	+	−	−	−	−		1

(1) see text

All transductants kept the preexisting ColV episome and 70% received ColB in addition to Trp+. They can be divided into 3 classes according to resistance and fertility type:

a) In class I (94%), the original R factor is still present (the one without R(T) was probably a spontaneous segregant). By conjugation they transfer Trp+ (and colicinogeny) at a much higher frequency than the resistances, indicating that both episomes are still independent.

b) In class II (2%) the original R factor has segregated into R(T) only. They transfer by conjugation Trp+ (and colicinogeny) and R(T) in very close association, showing that the transduced segment has probably recombined not only with ColV but also with the tetracycline resistance part of the R factor.

c) In class III (4%) the original R factor has been completely eliminated. By conjugation, they transfer Trp+ (together with colicinogeny) only.

Table 2

MARKERS PRESENT IN A VARIETY OF RECOMBINANT EPISOMES

R(S)	R(T)	R(C)	ColB	ColV	Trp	Lac
+	+	+	+	+	+	
+	+	+	+	+	−	
+	+	+	+	−	−	
+	+	+	−	+	−	
+	−	+	+	−	+	
+	−	+	+	−	−	
+	−	+	−	+	−	
−	+	−	+	+	+	
−	+	−	+	−	+	
−	+	−	+	+	−	
−	+	−	+	+	−	
−	+	−	−	+	−	
−	+	−	+	+	+	+
−	+	−	+	−	−	+

Very similar results have been obtained by transducing the same ColBTry episome to a recipient carrying another R factor, R(STC), together with ColV. Again 4% of the Trp$^+$ transductants have also recombined ColBTry with the R(T) part of the R factor. This time however, transductants of class I (88%) did transfer, by conjugation, their resistances at a higher rate than Trp$^+$. Furthermore among recombinants from such crosses, which received the complete set of resistances together with Trp$^+$ and colicinogeny, some were found to have apparently recombined ColVBTry with the complete R factor. They were now able to transfer all their markers at the same rate and in close association, as did transductants of class II. When such hybrid episomes were further transduced to a recipient carrying F'Lac, recombination with *lac* genes could also be observed occasionally. A large variety of hybrid episomes carrying, on a single genetic structure and in many different combinations, markers originating from Col and R factors as well as from the chromosome have thus been obtained. (Table 2).

Linkage of markers originating from Col and R factors as well as from the chromosome on a single genetic structure was confirmed by the following observations:

1. All markers from the presumably hybrid episomes were transferred en bloc by conjugation. Segregation was extremely rare and did never involve preferential elimination of one of the constituent plasmid. As an example, results obtained by transferring an hybrid episome carrying R(STC), ColVB, Try, Cys to an antibiotic-susceptible Trp-, Cys- strain are given in table 3.

Table 3

TRANSFER BY CONJUGATION OF AN R(STC)COLVBTryCys HYBRID EPISOME TO AN ANTIBIOTIC-SUSCEPTIBLE, TRP-, CYS- STRAIN

Selection	Rate of transfer	Markers transferred							Frequency (in %)
		R(S)	R(T)	R(C)	ColB	ColV	Trp	Cys	
R(S)	10^{-4}	+	+	+	+	+	+·	+	100
R(T)	10^{-4}	+	+	+	+	+	+	+	86
		−	+	−	+	+	+	+	14
R(C)	10^{-4}	+	+	+	+	+	+	+	98
		+	+	+	+	+	−	−	1
		+	+	+	−	+	−	−	1
Trp+	10^{-4}	+	+	+	+	+	+	+	98
		−	+	−	+	+	+	+	2
Cys+	10^{-4}	+	+	+	+	+	+	+	100

Similar results were also obtained with several other hybrid episomes. An R(T) ColBTryLac, for example, could be transferred not only to *E. coli* but also to *Sh. sonnei* and *S. panama*. In the latter case, rates of transfer were much decreased but all recombinants receiving R(T) also received the associated *lac*, *trp* and ColB genes.

2. Colicine and resistance genes carried by such hybrid episomes could be cotransduced by phage P1, after selecting either Trp$^+$ or R(T) transfer. Results of one experiment are given in table 4. It can be seen that transductants receiving ColB, Trp and R(T) together were obtained by both types of selection and that some R(T) transductants also received ColV, alone or in addition to ColB. All transduced markers were linearly linked in groups which overlapped to form a circular map. Analysis by transduction of 2 other hybrid episomes carrying R(T), ColB, Trp, Lac or R(SCT), ColVB, Trp genes gave similar results.

207

3. Association of colicine and resistance genes on a single genetic structure was also confirmed by segregation. The hybrid episomes studied were quite stable. Spontaneous segregants were very rare but could be selected for loss of *tonB*, by resistance to phage T1.

Table 4

NUMBER OF TRANSDUCTANTS (in %) RECEIVING MARKERS FROM AN R(T), COLVB, TRP EPISOME WHEN TRANSFER OF EITHER TRP+ OR R(T) HAS BEEN SELECTED

Markers received				Selection	
ColB	Trp	ColV	R(T)	Trp+	R(T)
−	+	−	−	68	−
−	+	+	−	3	−
+	+	−	−	10	−
+	+	−	+	19	56
+	−	+	+	−	2
+	−	−	+	−	18
−	−	+	+	−	1
−	−	−	+	−	23

Results of an experiment are given in Table 5. Loss of *tonB*, a marker from one of the parental episome incorporated into the hybrid, often involved complete elimination of all markers (93%), thus indicating a close association. In less frequent classes loss was not complete, but resistance genes remained associated to ColV, ColB or both in all cases.

Table 5

MARKERS PRESENT IN SPONTANEOUS SEGREGANTS FROM AN R(STC), COLVB, TRP HYBRID EPISOME, SELECTED FOR LOSS OF *tonB* BY RESISTANCE TO PHAGE T1

Markers present							Frequency
tonB	Trp	ColB	ColV	R(S)	R(T)	R(C)	(in %)
−	+	+	+	+	+	+	4,5
−	−	+	+	+	+	+	0,5
−	+	−	+	+	+	+	1,5
−	−	−	+	+	+	+	0,5
−	−	−	−	−	−	−	93,0

In nature many R factors bearing strains are colicinogenic. In most cases the two properties appear to be carried by independent units, though associated transfer by conjugation may occur more or less frequently. In other cases however both properties are always transferred together by conjugation, indicating close linkage of colicine and resistance genes on a single genetic structure. Linkage of R factors with ColIb has been demonstrated by Siccardi (1966) and Romero and Meynell (1969). Linkage with ColIa, ColBM, ColVM, and ColM was also found in more recent experiments (FREDERICQ, KRCMÉRY, KNOTHE and WIEDEMANN to be published).

Such R factors in which resistance genes are associated to colicinogeny, appear to carry colicine resistance since the Col factor part of them is governing immunity to the particular colicine produced. Some naturally occurring R factors, which are non colicinogenic, also seem to carry colicine resistance (FREDERICQ (1971), SICCARDI (1966)).

These R factors could originate by a mutation affecting colicine production but not immunity of an associated Col factor, as independent loss of colicinogeny and of immunity governed by Col factors has been experimentally demonstrated.

CONCLUSIONS

Colicinogenic factors are independent genetic units of varying complexity in which the structural genes for the synthesis of one or several different colicines are associated with genes governing other properties such as repression, immunity, fertility, inhibition of fertility, restriction of phages and resistance to U. V. irradiation. They are clearly build on the same model as R factors and belong to the same class of agents. Association of genes governing colicine synthesis and resistance to antibiotics on a single genetic structure is sometimes found in nature and has been experimentally reproduced by recombination of Col and R factors. Colicinogenic factors appear therefore to have played an important role in the emergence and dissemination of R factors, not only in providing a natural source of transfer agents for the mobilization and spread of resistance determinants but also by endowing colicinogenic strains, and particularly R factors which include colicine genes, with a selective advantage, which is operating even in the absence of antibiotic drugs.

Acknowledgment

The experimental work reported in this paper was aided by a grant from the "Fonds de la Recherche fondamentale collective" from Belgium.

REFERENCES

AMATI, P. (1964): Vegetative multiplication of colicinogenic factors after induction in Escherichia coli. Journal of Molecular Biology, 8, 239.

ANDERSON, E. S. and LEWIS, M. J. (1965): Characterization of a transfer factor associated with drug resistance in Salmonella typhimurium. Nature, 208, 843.

CLEWELL, D. B. and HELINSKI, D. R. (1970): Existence of the colicinogenic factor-sex factor ColIB- P9 as a supercoiled circular DNA-protein relaxation complex. Biochemical and Biophysical Research Communications, 41, 150 .

CLOWES, R. C. (1961): Colicine factors as fertility factors in Bacteria. Escherichia coli K12. Nature, 190, 988.

DUBNAU, E. and STOCKER, B. A. D. (1964): Genetics of plasmids in Salmonella typhimurium. Nature, 204, 1112.

EDWARDS, S. and MEYNELL, G. G. (1968): General method for isolating de-repressed bacterial sex factors. Nature, 219, 869.

FREDERICQ, P. (1954): Transduction génétique des propriétés colicinogènes chez Escherichia coli et Shigella sonnei. Comptes rendus des séances de la Société de biologie, 148, 399.

FREDERICQ, P. (1958): Colicins and colicinogenic factors. Symposia of the Society for Experimental Biology, 12, 104.

FREDERICQ, P. (1959): Transduction par bactériophage des propriétés colicinogènes chez Salmonella typhimurium. Comptes rendus des séances de la Société de biologie, 153, 357 .

FREDERICQ, P. (1963): Colicines et autres bactériocines. Ergebnisse der Mikrobiologie, Immunitäts- forschung und experimentellen Therapie, 37, 114.

FREDERICQ, P. (1965): Genetics of colicinogenic factors. Zentralblatt für Bakteriologie, Parasitenkunde, Infektionskrankheiten und Hygiene, I Original, 196, 142.

FREDERICQ, P. (1969): The recombination of colicinogenic factors with other episomes and plasmids. In Ciba Foundation Symposium on Bacterial Episomes and Plasmids, pp. 163–174. Editors: G. E. W. Wolstenholme and M. O'Connor. Churchill Ltd, London.

FREDERICQ, P. (1971): Colicine resistance associated with R factors. VII International Congress of Chemotherapy, Praha. Abstracts of Communications.

FREDERICQ, P. et BETZ-BAREAU, M. (1953): Transfert génétique de la propriété colicinogène en rapport avec la polarité F des parents. Comptes rendus des séances de la Société de biologie, **147**, 2043.

FREDERICQ, P. et BETZ-BAREAU, M. (1956): Influence de diverses propriétés colicinogènes sur la fertilité d'Escherichia coli. Comptes rendus des séances de la Société de biologie, 150, 615.

FREDERICQ, P., KRČMÉRY, V. and KETTNER, M. (1971): Transferable colicinogenic factors as mobilizing agents for extrachromosomal streptomycin resistance. Zeitschrift für Allgemeine Mikrobiologie, **11**, 11.

HOWARTH, S. (1965): Résistance to the bactericidal effect of ultraviolet radiation conferred on Enterobacteria by the colicine factor colI. Journal of General Microbiology, **40**, 43.

IIJIMA, T. (1962): Transfer of a colicinogenic factor with multiple resistance factor in Escherichia coli K12. Japanese Journal of Genetics, **37**, 187.

KAHN, P. L. (1968): Isolation of high-frequency recombining strains from Escherichia coli containing the V colicinogenic factor. Journal of Bacteriology, **96**, 205.

LAWN, A. M., MEYNELL, E., MEYNELL, G. G. and DATTA N. (1967): Sex pili and the classification of sex factors in the Enterobacteriaceae. Nature, **216**, 343.

NOMURA, M. (1967): Colicins and related bacteriocins. Annual Review of Microbiology, **21**, 257.

OZEKI, H. and HOWATH, S. (1961): Colicin factors as fertility factors in Bacteria. Salmonella typhimurium strain LT2. Nature, **190**, 986.

ROMERO, E. and MEYNELL, E. (1969): Covert fi- R factors in fi+R+strains of bacteria. Journal of Bacteriology, **97**, 780.

ROTH, T. F. and HELINSKI, D. R. (1967): Evidence for circular DNA forms of a bacterial plasmid. Proceedings of the National Academy of Sciences, USA, **58**, 650.

SICCARDI, A. G. (1966): Colicin resistance associated with resistance factors in Escherichia coli. Genetical Research, **8**, 219.

STROBEL, M. and NOMURA, M. (1966): Restriction of the growth of bacteriophage BF23 by a colicine I (colI-P9) factor. Virology, **28**, 763.

THE REGULATION OF REPLICATION OF EPISOMAL DNA

D. NOACK and S. KLAUS

Institute of Microbiology, Academy of Science, Jena, G. D. R.

The replication system of lambda phage DNA is regarded as a model for the replication systems of episomal and bacterial DNA. For the following statements the lysogenic cells can be characterized by two facts:

1. The genome of the lambda phage is linearely inserted into the bacterial genome as so called prophage the genetic information of which is repressed by repressor molecules.

2. The replication of the prophage DNA is controlled by these repressor molecules. When these repressors are inactivated the replication of prophage DNA is initiated.

After all treatments resulting in a stop of host DNA synthesis for example after UV irradiation, thymine starvation, mitomycine C application etc., the phage repressors are inactivated. In alysogenic cells these agents lead to a reinitiation of host DNA replication after the lift of replication inhibition (WORCEL, 1970). From this it is assumed that the replication of phage DNA and host DNA are controlled by the same principle. Results of GOLDTHWAIT and JACOB (1964) and KIRBY, JACOB and GOLDTHWAIT (1967) led to the conclusion, that these repressor inactivating substances accumulated after a stop of DNA synthesis are one or some precursors of DNA synthesis. The induction rate of the mutant strain E. coli C600 T44 lysogenized with several UV-sensitive lambda phages can be influenced by precursors of DNA metabolism after addition to the culture medium.

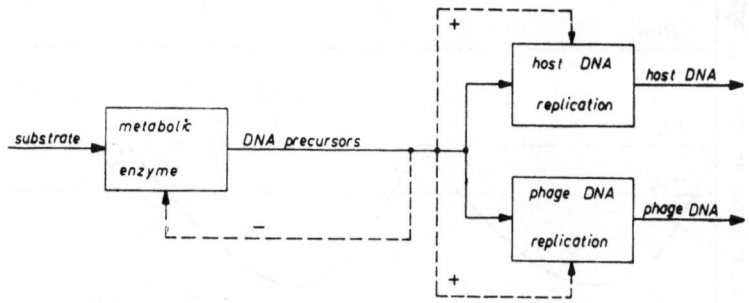

Fig. 1 A regulatory model for the control of DNA replication in lambda lysogenic cells.

On the base of these findings a regulatory model is proposed. Fig. 1 shows the influx of substrate molecules into a metabolic enzyme system, which produces DNA precursors. The concentration of these precursors acts as regulatory signal via a feedback loop upon the production rate of DNA precursors resulting in an end product inhibition. The DNA precursors are used by the replication systems of both the host DNA and the phage DNA respectively. According to the findings, the concentration of DNA precursors must act as initiating signal for the replication of both the host DNA and phage DNA. The information fluxes are indicated with dotted arrows and the substance fluxes with solid arrows. A mathematical model of this regulatory scheme yields a differential equation for the amount M of DNA precursors present in a cell:

$$\frac{dM}{dt} = \frac{aV}{b+m} - R$$

where V is the volume of the cell, m is the concentration of DNA precursors within the cell and R is the rate of DNA synthesis. The volume V in the first terme of the equation regards the fact that the capacity of precursor synthesis is proportional to the cell volume. The precursor concentration in the denominator stands for the feedback inhibition. With the relation

$$M = m \cdot V$$

and the assumption

$$\frac{dV}{dt} = \mu V$$

for the exponential growth of the cell, an equation for the precursor concentration is obtained

$$\frac{dm}{dt} = \frac{a}{b+m} - \mu m - \frac{R}{V} \, .$$

It is proposed that a new replication cycle of host DNA is initiated when the precursor concentration m reaches a critical value m_i. Herewith the solution of the differential equation for the precursor concentration m in dependence on time shows a periodical shape as it is demonstrated in Fig. 2. The periode of this solution is a regulatory function

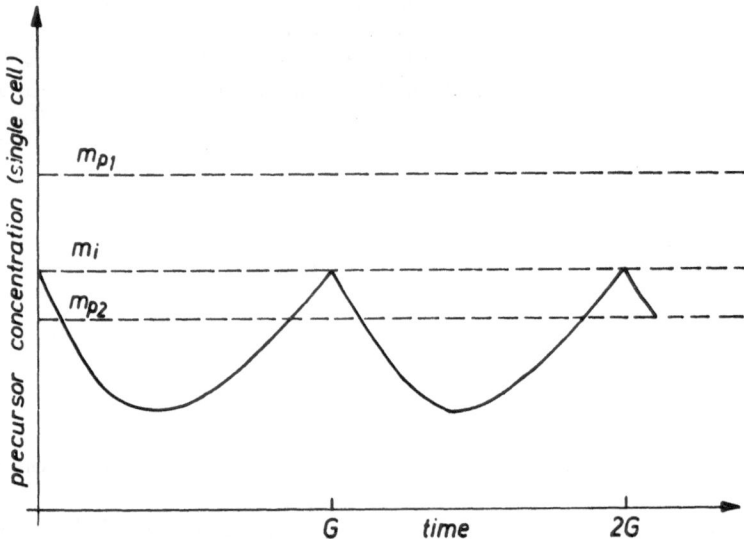

Fig. 2 DNA precursor concentration in a single cell in dependence on time. m_i is the turn on concentration for host DNA replication. m_{p1} and m_{p2} are the effective DNA precursor concentrations for the initiation of episomal DNA replication.

and equals the doubling time G of cell volume. So the timing of DNA replication is related to the growth rate μ of cell volume V.

When an other autonomous replicon is present in a cell and its replication is initiated by the same DNA precursors as it is for the host DNA, the number of these additional autonomous replicons per cell will depend on the critical value of precursor concentration at which the replication is initiated. For example when this critical concentration m_{p1} is greater than m_{l_j}, the autonomous replicons will be diluted out because no replication takes place. On the other hand when this critical value m_{p2} is smaller than m_{l_j}, the number of replicons per cell will depend on the time during which the precursor concentration is greater than m_{p2}. Within this time interval the initiation of replicon replication is allowed to take place.

This concept is investigated on lysogenic cells, which bear the genome of the temperate phage lambda as prophage. This prophage is induced when the DNA synthesis is inhibited. This effect is measured on a population of lysogenic cells after treatment with an agent resulting in a stop of DNA synthesis. In order to obtain a quantitative picture of related processes, only it is necessary to calculate a mean value for the precursor concentration in a statistical population. With other words the solution function of the differential equation must be averaged over the distribution of replication timing resulting in the value m_h in Fig. 3. In the exponential growth phase of the population m_h is constant with time.

After the disturbance of the regulatory circuit in Fig. 1 the precursors concentration show a reaction which is characteristic for the nature of the disturbing agent. There are three possibilities. At first for example when the feedback loop representing the end product inhibition is inactivated at time indicated by the arrow, the precursor con-

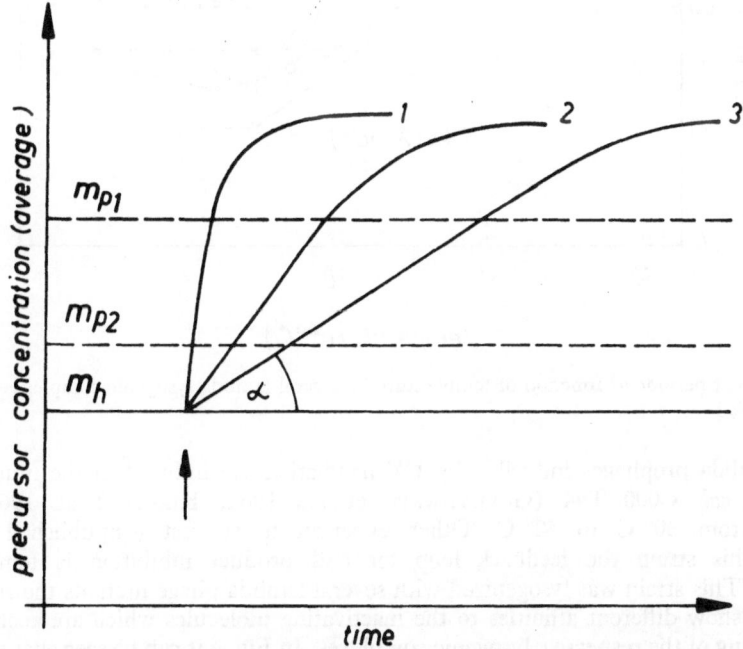

Fig. 3 DNA precursor concentration in a statistical population after 1. inactivation of end product inhibition, 2. absolute stop of DNA synthesis, 3. slowering of the rate of DNA synthesis.

centration will increase very rapidly until a upper value is reached depending on the maximal production rate. This behaviour is demonstrated by the curve 1 in Fig. 3. When in the second case the DNA synthesis is inhibited absolutely, the precursor concentration will increase slower according to curve 2. And in the third case when the DNA synthesis is only slowed for example after UV irradiation, the precursor concentration must show a accumulation rate α which depends on the irradiation dose (curve 3).

According to our model, the critical value of the precursor concentration for allowing the autonomous replication of prophage to be initiated shall be m_{p1}. From Fig. 3 it can be seen that the delaying time between disturbance of the regulatory circuit indicated by the arrow and the time of initiation of replication of prophage must depend on the nature of the disturbing agent. Furthermore this delaying time should be changed when a prophage mutant is included the repressor of which exhibits an altered affinity to the DNA precursors. When for example the critical value of the prophage mutant is m_{p2}, the delaying times must be shortened. These proposals resulting from the model are proved with the following bacterial strains lysogenic with different lambda phage mutants.

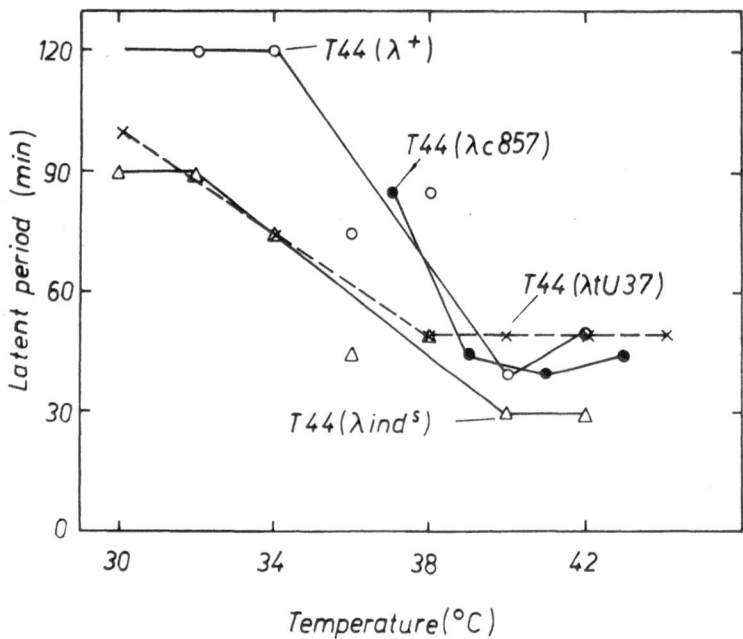

Fig. 4 Latent periode as function of temperature in several lambda lysogenic complexes of E. coli C 600 T44.

All lambda prophages inducible by UV irradiation are induced in the mutant host strain *E. coli* C600 T44 (GOLDTHWAIT et al., 1964, KIRBY et al. 1967) after heating from 30° C to 42° C. Other experiments suggest (unpublished results) that in this strain the feedback loop for end product inhibition is temperature sensitive. This strain was lysogenized with several lambda phage mutants the repressors of whose show different affinities to the inactivating molecules which are accumulated after heating of the respective lysogenic complexes. In Fig. 4 it can be seen that the latent period, this is the time interval between inducing treatment and lysis of cells, reaches at 42° C the shortest value which can be obtained at lambda lysogenic cells. The complex

E. coli C600 T44 (λ ind^s) shows the shortest latend periode due to the highest affinity of the repressors to the inactivating molecules.

The dependence of latent period of these lysogenic complexes on the UV dose is shown in Fig. 5. The UV sensitive complexes exhibit shorter latent periods than the wild

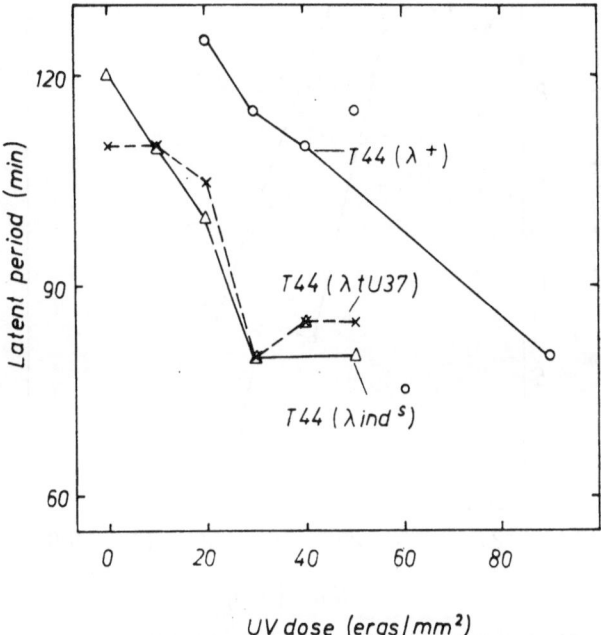

Fig. 5 Latent period as function of UV dose in several lambda lysogenic complexes of E. coli C 600 T 44.

typ lysogene. All latent periodes decrease with UV dose according to the proposals of the model.

The effect of an absolute inhibition of host DNA replication was studied on a temperature sensible replication mutant E. coli K12 Hfr H 165 (LANKA and SCHUSTER, 1970). Here the colony forming ability is tested as measure for the repressor inactivating event after heating of the lysogenic complexes from 30° C to 42° C as it is designated with the arrow in Fig. 6. The alysogenic strain (solid circles) shows the arrest of cell division due to the stop of DNA synthesis. The complex lysogenic with wild type lambda phage (asterisced curve) shows a delaying time of 20–25 min between heating and inactivation of phage repressors. The complex lysogenic with the UV sensitive phage λ ind^s is induced at most 5 min after heating (empty circles). These results are also in an agreement with the proposals of the model.

Summarizing it can be postulated that the repressor inactivating substance which is accumulated after a stop of DNA synthesis or after a disturbance of DNA metabolism shows a kinetical behaviour which must be demanded from the DNA precursors according to the regulatory model. Therefore it can be suggested that the replications of host DNA and episomal DNA are controlled by the same principle.

Acknowledgements: The autors are much indebted to Mrs. A. Schulze and Mrs. B. Ziegler for their excellent technical assistance.

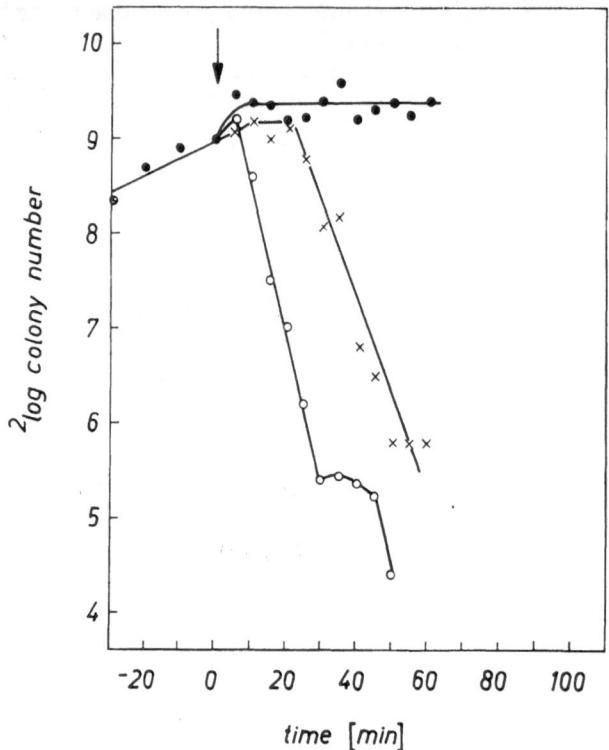

Fig. 6 Inactivation kinetics of several lambda repressors in the temperature sensitive replication mutant E. coli K12 Hfr H 165 after heating indicated by the arrow.

●——● alysogenic strains   x——x lysogenic complex with wild type λ^+ ○——○ lysogenic complex with the phage mutant λind[s].

REFERENCES

GOLDTHWAIT, D. and JACOB, F. (1964): Sur le mécanisme de l'induction du développment du prophage chez les bactéries lysogénes. Comptes rendus hedbomandaires des séances de l'academie des sciences, Paris, **259**, 661.

KIRBY, E. P., JACOB, F. and GOLDTHWAIT, D. (1967): Prophage induction and filament formation in a mutant strain of E. coli. Proceedings of the National Academy of Sciences U.S.A. **58**, 1903.

LANKA, E. and SCHUSTER, H. (1970): Replication of bacteriophages in Escherichia coli mutants thermosensitive in DNA synthesis. Molecular and General Genetics, **106**, 274.

Worcel, A. (1970): Induction of chromosome reinitiations in a thermosensitive DNA mutant of E. coli. Journal of Molecular Biology, **52**, 371.

RECOMBINATIONS BETWEEN DIFFERENT R(f) AND R(i) PLASMIDS AND BETWEEN R-PLASMIDS AND THE CHROMOSOME IN E. COLI AND P. p MIRABILIS

H. TSCHÄPE and H. BÖHME

Institut für experimentelle Epidemiologie, Wernigerode, and Zentralinstitut für Genetik und Kulturpflanzenforschung der DAW, Gatersleben, DDR

INTRODUCTION

Plasmids with different genetic properties are common and widespread among bacteria (Novick 1969). These extrachromosomal DNA elements are characterized by their autonomous replication, their ability to maintain their extrachromosomal state, and their determination of non-essential cell functions. One of these functions is the resistance against various drugs; plasmids with drug resistance determinants are called R-plasmids. As far as known R-plasmids are of a composite nature (heterogeneity of R-DNA). Their somatic functions have been suggested to be arisen from various bacterial species, the exact origin of either the resistance genes or the R-plasmids itself, however, are unknown. Several predictions or models exist to explain R-plasmid evolution (Watanabe 1969, Novick 1969, Anderson 1969).

In order to learn more about R-plasmid origin and nature, studies on plasmid-host-interactions would be suitable. Recombination experiments may reveale a considerable information on plasmid-chromosome relationships.

In this paper presented recombination studies between different R-plasmids and between R-plasmids and the chromosome were summarized (Tschäpe and Böhme, to be published).

Whereas recombinations between the chromosome and R-plasmids (measured as activity of chromosome mobilization in E. coli and integrative-excisive recombination with a tet-region in Proteus mirabilis) depend on a fully functioning REC-system, additive as well as reciprocal recombinations between R-plasmids of the R(f) and R(i) types after compatible and incompatible crosses were independent of the bacterial REC-function.

Recombinations between various R(f) and R(i) plasmids

In order to evaluate the influence of the REC-system of the bacterial host on recombinations between various R-plasmids of the R(f) as well as of R(i) type the experiments were carried out in rec⁺ and rec⁻ (recA) strains of E. coli. The formation of both additive and reciprocal recombinant R-plasmids after compatible and incompatible crosses occured with the same frequency in rec⁻ (recA) and rec⁺ strains (Table 1). These results confirm and amplify experiments accomplished by Takano (1966) that recombinations between different R-plasmids are independent of the REC-function of the bacterial host.

In addition, the results summarized in table 1 have revealed that all genes proved behaved as single determinants in all crosses. It has been possible therefore to construct plasmids which were never found among wild type strains such as fer(i)sul tet from R(i)E-1 X R(i)2 or fer(f) chl str sul mer tet collb from R(f)187 X R(i) D4 crosses.

Table 1

SUPERINFECTION AND RECOMBINATION FREQUENCIES OF R(f) AND R(i) PLASMIDS CARRYING VARIOUS DRUG RESISTANCE GENES

No R-plasmid crosses	parental properties	super infection frequency in %	recom- bination frequency in %	recombined properties
1 R(i)1 × R(i)218/45(rec⁺)	str sul tet ✕	8.5×10^{-5}	0.5	chl str sul tet
2 R(i)1 × R(i)218/46(rec⁻)	chl str-s sul-s tet	8.8×10^{-5}	0.2	chl str sul tet
3 R(i)2 × R(f)187/45(rec⁺)	tet ✕	6.2×10^{-2}	10.0	chl tet
			3.6	chl str sul mer tet
4 R(i)2 × R(f)187/46(rec⁻)	chl str sul mer	3.1×10^{-2}	4.5	chl str sul mer tet
5 R(i)2 × R(i)E−1/45(rec⁺)	tet	36.0	4.0	sul tet
6 R(i)2 × R(i)E−1/46(rec⁻)	× sul	30.0	7.0	sul tet
7 R(i)2 × R(f)225/45(rec⁺)	tet ✕	39.0	8.5	str sul tet
8 R(i)2 × R(f)225/46(rec⁻)	str sul	35.0	3.5	str sul tet
9 R(f)4 × R(f)187/45(rec⁺)	chl-s str-s sul-s mer-s tet ✕	0.1	0.3	chl str sul mer tet
10 R(f)4 × R(f)187/46(rec⁻)	chl str sul mer	0.1	0.5	chl str sul mer tet
			0.2	str sul tet
11 R(f)4 × R(f)225/45(rec⁺)	chl-s str-s sul-s mer-s tet	1.5×10^{-3}	10.0	str sul tet chl mer
12 R(f)4 × R(f)225/46(rec⁻)	× str sul	2.7×10^{-3}	8.0	chl str sul mer tet
13 R(f)4 × R(i)E−1/45(rec⁺)	chl-s str-s sul-s mer-s tet ✕	1.5	1.0	sul tet
			0.3	chl sul tet
			0.9	chl str sul mer tet
14 R(f)4 × R(i)E−1/46(rec⁻)	sul	0.9	0.1	chl str sul mer tet
			0.4	sul tet
15 R(i)218 × R(f)225/45(rec⁺)	chl str-s sul-s tet ✕	12.0	4.1	chl str sul tet
			2.0	chl sul str
16 R(i)218 × R(f)225/46(rec⁻)	str sul	16.0	3.5	chl str sul tet
			3.0	chl str sul
17 R(i)D4 × R(f)187/45(rec⁺)	tet collb ✕	0.7	5.5	chl tet
			5.0	chl tet collb
			0.3	chl str sul mer tet collB
18 R(i)D4 × R(f)187/46(rec⁻)	chl str sul mer	0.1	2.3	chl tet

Additive as well as reciprocal recombinations between R-plasmids have been demonstrated by several authors (WATANABE and LYANG 1962, HASHIMOTO and MITSUHASHI 1966, HASHIMOTO and HIROTA 1966, WATANABE 1969, and WATANABE, FUROSE and SAKAIZUMI 1968) could not found recombinant formation in crosses between R(f) X R(i) type plasmids unless using transduction.

Physical studies of R-DNA have shown the heterogenous nature of the multiple drug resistance plasmids. (FALKOW, HAAPALA and SILVER 1969, NISIOKA, MITANI and CLOWES 1969, 1970, COHEN and MILLER 1970 b). It is reasonable to assume therefore that multiple R-plasmids arose by recombination between different monomer or oligomer resistance plasmids of R(f) as well as of R(i) types (NOVICK 1969, NISIOKA, MITANI and CLOWES 1970).

For explanation of the origin of extrachromosomal resistance genes, however, the hypothesis of gene pick up of chromosomal genes has been developed by WATANABE (1969). If this hypothesis is correct integration of R-plasmids into the chromosome or at least any molecular homologies between corresponding sites on plasmid and chromosome should be demonstrable.

Mobilization of E. coli host chromosome by recombinational integration of R-plasmids

It has been supposed and proved experimentally that integration of different plasmids is necessary as a first step for chromosomal mobilization (SCAIFE and GROSS 1963, CLOWES and MOODY 1966, BÖHME, ADLER and STÄBER 1967, SCAIFE 1967, CURTISS 1969, FALKOW, JOHNSON and BARON 1967, WILLETTS and BRODA 1969, WILKINS 1969, KAHN 1969, CURTISS and RENSHAW 1969). For ColI induced chromosome mobilization, however, occuring with very low frequency, CLOWES and MOODY (1966), MEYNELL and EDWARDS (1969) and EDWARDS and MEYNELL (1969) did not found integration of the ColI plasmid.

On the other site the mechanism (whether or not integration) of R(f) and R(i) plasmid induced chromosome mobilization is not yet fully understood (MEYNELL, MEYNELL and DATTA 1968, PEARCE and MEYNELL 1968, COOKE and MEYNELL 1969, MEYNELL and DATTA 1969).

Table 2

THE INFLUENCE OF THE BACTERIAL REC-FUNCTION ON THE CHROMOSOMAL
MOBILIZATION BY DIFFERENT R(f) AND R(i) PLASMIDS IN E. COLI

donors	Pa209		CSH-2	
	trp	thr	pro	str
R(f)6 chl str sul mer tet/45(rec⁺)	350	270	210	—
R(f)6 chl str sul mer tet/46(rec⁻)	3	0.5	5	—
R(f)187 chl str sul mer/45(rec⁺)	22	9	11	—
R(f)187 chl str sul mer/46(rec⁻)	1.5	0.1	2	—
R(i)D4 colIb tet/45(rec⁺)	440	180	290	195
R(i)D4 colIB tet/46(rec⁻)	2	7	3	7
R(i)2 tet/45(rec⁺)	580	210	35	240
R(i)2 tet/46(rec⁻)	6	1	3	3
F—lac/45(rec⁺)	21000	22000	24000	18000
F—lac/46(rec⁻)	8	7	11	2
R⁻/45(rec⁺)	3	1	0.5	5
R⁻/46(rec⁻)	1.5	2	3	4

(all R-plasmids have been used in the repressed state; the numbers correspond to recombinant per 10^8 R-plasmid infected recipient cells)

Results presented in table 2 show that frequencies of chromosomal mobilization by different R(f) as well as R(i) plasmids were reduced by a factor of 10^2 to the level of background in rec⁻ (recA) E. coli as compared with the isogenic rec⁺ strain. The activities of chromosomal mobilization of R-plasmids used in these experiments seem to depend on the fully functioning REC-system of the bacterial host. These results speak for an occurence of an integration event before chromosomal transfer to F⁻ strains.

PEARCE and MEYNELL (1963) supposed a high degree of homology between the transfer region rather than any of the resistance genes of the R1drd plasmid and the chromosome as an evidence for integration of this plasmid into the chromosome.

By using different R-plasmid deletions within the R-genote of R(f)6 and R(i)D4 we demonstrated (table 3) a reduced R-mating activity if the tet-region of the plasmid is

Table 3

MOBILIZATION OF THE E. COLI CHROMOSOME BY DIFFERENT R-PLASMIDS WITH AND WITHOUT TET-REGION

donors	Pa209			G45	
R+CSH-2	trp	his	leu	leu	arg
R(f)6 chl str sul mer tet	400	260	20	30	520
R(f)6d12 tet	390	320	35		
R(f)6d8 chl str sul mer	12	8	2	5	1.2
R(i)D4 collb tet	440	320	80		
C(i)D4 collb	3	2	− 1		
R(f)187 chl str sul mer	7	5	1.5	1.5	3
R(f)187 chl str sul mer tet−193	240	140	8	130	410
R(f)187 chl str sul mer tet−2	610	220	4		
R(f)187 chl str sul mer tet−D4	280	190	10		
F−lac(1485b)	21000	19000	220000	23000	16000
R−	2.3	1	0.1	0.6	3.3

(all R-plasmids have been used in the repressed state; the numbers correspond to recombinants per 10^8 R-plasmid infected recipient cells)

absent but an increase of chromosomal mobilization of a tet-delation R-plasmids (R(f)187 after recombinational introduction of the tet-region into the plasmid (R187Tc-193, R187Tc-2, R187Tc-D4). These results point to a possible homology of the tet-region with the chromosomal integration site.

R-plasmid recombination with a chromosomal tet-gene in Proteus mirabilis

The mapping of integration site of R-plasmids should be possible by "spread-off" experiments rather than by interupted matings. In such experiments, however, neither addition nor substitution of neighbouring regions could be demonstrated with 14 genetically different R-plasmids and several chromosomal genes locating around the supposed integration site (unpublished results). GINOZA and PAINTER (1964), however, have described a possible recombination between an R-plasmid and a chromosomal tet gene in E. coli. Additionally, HARADA, KAMEDA and MITSUHASHI (1967) and HARADA, KAMEDA, SHIGENARA, NAKAJIMA and MITSUHASHI (1970) showed recombinations of transferable plasmids with nontransferable chromosomal integrated Rtet plasmid in *Salmonella*. Both physical homology between the tet and the fer regions (FALKOW, CITARELLA, WOHLHIETER and WATANABE (1966), the results presented by GINOZA and PAINTER (1964), HARADA et al. (1967, 1970) and the reduced chromosomal mobilization frequencies of different R-plasmids with tet-deletions seem to make attempts possible to look for recombinations between different R-plasmids and a chromosomal tet-gene.

In the course of investigations of R-mating activity with the tet-deletion plasmid R187 in E. coli CSH-2/Tc-2 carrying a resistance mutation in the chromosomal tet locus plasmids were isolated with the constitution str sul tet fer(f) in very low frequencies.

228

These recombinants had lost the chl-determinant, but transmission of all other genes linked was observed.

On the other hand HOFEMEISTER and BÖHME (to be published) have demonstrated a very similar resistance mechanism for R-plasmid determined TET-resistance and the naturally occurring TET-resistance in *Proteus mirabilis* which is presumably a species specific property of the *Proteus* genus, and COHEN and MILLER (1970a) described a recombination between pen-gene of *Proteus mirabilis* and an unloaded transfer factor. It was therefore interesting to look for chromosomal tet-recombination in different *Proteus mirabilis* strains with different tet-deletion plasmids.

The results presented in table 4 indicate that the described tet recombination is possible with two tet deletions plasmids of the fer(f) type but it proved impossible with two fer(i) plasmids. One R(f) plasmid, R225, exhibits a so high tendency to segregate in the *Proteus* strains used that backtransfer to E. coli was difficult to demonstrate.

Table 4

RECOMBINATION BETWEEN DIFFERENT R(f) AND R(i) PLASMIDS AND THE CHROMOSOMAL TET GENE IN *Proteus mirabilis* REC+ AND REC- STRAINS

plasmids	recombinant types	193rec+	273rec+	672rec-
R187(f) chl str sul mer	chl str sul mer tet fer	0.55	0.60	0.00
	chl str sul mer fer	0.20	0.15	0.63
	chl str sul mer tet[1])	0.25	0.25	0.37
R6d8(f) chl str sul mer	chl str sul mer tet fer	0.58	0.52	0.00
	chl str sul mer fer	0.30	0.30	0.70
	chl str sul mer tet[1])	0.12	0.12	0.30
R15(i) str sul mer	str sul mer tet fer	0.00	0.00	0.00
	str sul mer fer	0.85	0.90	0.88
	str sul mer tet[1])	0.15	0.10	0.12
RE−1(i) sul	sul tet fer	0.00	0.00	0.00
	sul fer	0.50	0.45	0.45
	sul tet[1])	0.50	0.55	0.55
R225(f) str sul	str sul tet fer	0.00	0.00	0.00
	str sul fer	0.15	0.12	0.20
	str sul tet[1])	0.85	0.88	0.80

notes: [1]) we do not know the real genetic structure only that transmissibility was lost.

In contrast, as shown in table 4 in a rec- strain of *P. mirabilis* (BÖHME 1968) recombinations with the tet-deletion plasmids R187(f) and R6d8(f) could not be found.

All R-plasmid clones that acquired the tet-determinant from *Proteus* hosts behave as stable plasmids transfering resistance genes linked.

We suppose that the R(f) plasmids R187 and R6d8 integrate into the host chromosome and according to Campbell's model wrong pairing leads during excision to tet-substitution in E. coli CSH-2/Tc-2 and tet-addition in *P. mirabilis*.

These results of recombination between the host chromosome and plasmids represent a further indication of R-plasmids' integration into the chromosome and support on the other side the gene pick up theory developed by WATANABE (1969).

SUMMARY

Additive as well as reciprocal recombinations between different R(f) and R(i) plasmids have been shown to be independent of the bacterial REC-function in E. coli.

In contrast, integrative recombination (measured as chromosomal mobilization) of

221

R-plasmids both of the R(f) and R(i) types is reduced to the background in rec⁻ (recA) strains of E. coli. The same dependence on a fully REC-function of the bacterial host could also be demonstrated in recombination experiments between R-plasmids and the chromosome of *Proteus mirabilis*. In rec⁺ strains of *P. mirabilis* recombinations between the chromosomal tet-region and the tet-deletion plasmids R(f) 187 and R(f)6d8 were shown but not in a rec⁻ strain. The same recombinations were proved impossible with two fer(i) plasmids (R15, RE-1).

REFERENCES

ANDERSON, E. S. (1969): Ecology and Epidemiology of transferable drug resistance. In: Bacterial plasmids and episomes. A Ciba Foundation Symposium, pp. 102—115, Editors: G. E. W. Wolstenholme and M. O'Connor. Churchill LTD, London.

BÖHME, H. (1968): Absence of repair of photodynamically induced damage in two mutants of Proteus mirabilis with increased sensitivity to monofunctional alkylating agents. Mutation Research **6**, 166.

BÖHME, H., ADLER, B., STÄBER, H. (1967): Resistenz-Übertragungsfaktoren als extrachromosomale Informationsträger bei Bakterien. Biologisches Zentralblatt (Supplement) **86**, 25.

CAMPBELL, A. M. (1969): Episomes. Harper and Row, New York.

CLOWES, R. C. and MOODY, E. E. M. (1966): Chromosomal transfer from recombination deficient strain of E. coli K-12. Genetics **53**, 717.

COHEN, S. N. and MILLER, Ch. A. (1970a): Characterization of autonomous R-factor segregants lacking drug resistance markers. X. International Congress of Microbiology, Mexico, *VIII*, 58.

COHEN, S. N. and MILLER Ch. A. (1970b): Non-chromosomal antibiotics resistance in bacteria. II. Molecular nature of R-factors isolated from Proteus mirabilis and E. coli. Journal of molecular Biology **50**, 671.

COOKE, M. and MEYNELL, E. (1969): Chromosome transfer by drd R-factors in F⁻ E. coli K-12. Genetical Research **14**, 79.

CURTISS, R. (1969): Bacterial conjugation. Annual Review of Microbiology **23**, 68

CURTISS, R. and RENSHAW, J. (1969): Kinetics of F⁺ transfer and recombination production in F⁺ × F⁻ matings in E. coli K-12. Genetics **63**, 39.

EDWARDS, S. and MEYNELL, G. G. (1969): I sex factors and chromosomal recombination in S. typhimurium. Genetical Research **13**, 321.

FALKOW, S., CITARELLA, R. V., WOHLHIETER, J. A., and WATANABE, T. (1966): The molecular nature of R-factor. Journal of molecular Biology **17**, 102.

FALKOW, S., JOHNSON, E. M., and BARON, L. S. (1967): Bacterial conjugation and extrachromosomal elements. Annual Review of Genetics **1**, 87.

FALKOW, S., HAAPALA, D. K., and SILVER R. P. (1969): Relationships between extrachromosomal elements. In: Bacterial episomes and plasmids, pp. 136—158. Ciba Foundation Symposium. Editors: G. E. W. Wohlstenholme and M. O'Connor. Churchill LTD, London.

GINOZA, H. S. and PAINTER, R. B. (1964): Genetic recombination between resistance transfer factors and the chromosome. Journal of Bacteriology **87**, 1339.

HARADA, K., KAMEDA, M., and MITSUHASHI, S. (1967): Drug resistance of enteric bacteria. X. Recombination of defective R(Tc) factor with other episomes. Japanese Journal of Microbiology **11**, 143.

HARADA, K., KAMEDA, M., SHIGELLARA, S., NAKAJIMA, T. and MITSUHASHI, S. (1970): Genetic structure of F-lac-tet factor. Japanese Journal of microbiology **14**, 423.

HASHIMOTO, H. and HIROTA, Y. (1966): Gene recombination and segregation of resistance factor in E. coli. Journal of Bacteriology **91**, 51.

HASHIMOTO, H. and MITSUHASHI, S. (1966): Drug resistance of enteric bacteria. VII. Recombination of R-factors with tetracycline-sensitive mutants. Journal of Bacteriology **92**, 1351.

KAHN, P. L. (1968): Isolation of high frequency recombining strains from E. coli containing the V colicinogenic factor. Journal of Bacteriology **96**, 205.

MEYNELL, E. and DATTA, N. (1969): Sex factor activity of drug resistance factors. In: Bacterial episomes and plasmids. Ciba Foundation Symposion. p. 120—133. Editors: G. E. W. Wolstenholme and M. O'Connor. Churchill LTD, London.

MEYNELL, E., MEYNELL, G. G., and DATTA, N. (1968): Phylogenetic relationship of drug resistance factors and other transmissible bacterial plasmids. Bacteriological Reviews **32**, 55.

MEYNELL, G. G. and EDWARDS, S. (1969): Failure of ColI factor to integrate in the bacterial chromosome. Proceedings of the Society of general Microbiology.

Nisioka, T., Mitani, M., and Clowes, R. C. (1969): Composite circular forms of R-factor DNA molecules. Journal of Bacteriology **97**, 376.

Nisioka, T., Mitani, M. and Clowes, R. C. (1970): Molecular recombination between R-factor DNA molecules in E. coli host cells. Journal of Bacteriology **103**, 166.

Novick, R. P. (1969): Extrachromosomal inheritance in bacteria. Bacteriological Reviews **33**, 210.

Pearce, L. E. and Meynell, E. (1968): Specific chromosomal affinity of a resistance factor. Journal of general Microbiology **50**, 159.

Scaife, J. (1967): Episomes. Annual Review of Microbiology **21**, 601.

Scaife, J. and Gross, J. D. (1963): The mechanism of chromosome mobilization by an F-prime factor in E. coli K-12. Genetical Research **4**, 328.

Takano, T. (1966): Behaviour of some episomal elements in a recombination deficient mutant of E. coli. Japanese Journal of Microbiology **10**, 201.

Watanabe, T. (1969): Transferable drug resistance in bacteria: the nature of the problem. In: Bacterial episomes and plasmids. A Ciba Foundation Symposion. pp. 81—97. Editors: G. E. W. Wolstenholme and M. O'Connor. Churchill LTD, London.

Watanabe, T. and Lyang, K. W. (1962): Episome mediated transfer of drug resistance in Enterobacteriaceae. V. Spontaneous segregation and recombination of resistance factors in Salmonella typhimurium. Journal of Bacteriology **84**, 422.

Watanabe, T., Furose C., and Sakaizumi, S. (1968): Superinfection with R-factors by transduction in E. coli and S. typhimurium. Journal of Bacteriology **96**, 1791.

Wilkins, S. M. (1969): Chromosome transfer from F-lac+ strains of E. coli K-12 mutant at recA, recB, or recC. Journal of Bacteriology **98**, 509.

Willetts, N. and Broda, P. (1969): The E. coli sex factor. In: Bacterial episomes and plasmids. A Ciba Foundation Symposion. pp. 32—48. Editors: G. E. W. Wolstenholme and M. O'Connor. Churchill LTD, London.

TRANSFER OF STREPTOMYCIN RESISTANCE BY THE PLASMID R222

C. HURWITZ, V. KRCMERY, C. B. BRAUN, and E. AGUIRREGOITIA

Research Service, Veterans Administration Hospital, Albany, N. Y., and the Research Institute of Hygiene, Bratislava, Czechoslovakia.

That R factors behave differently in different host cells has been known for some time (1). We have become interested in this phenomenon and will present data from some of our preliminary studies on this subject.

We have obtained from Dr. H. ROSENKRANZ a strain of *E. coli* CSH-2 containing R factor 222 which differs from Dr. WATANABE'S original culture in its resistance to streptomycin. Whereas WATANABE'S original strain is inhibited by concentrations above 20 μg/ml., ROSENKRANZ'S strain grows at 100 μg/ml.

We had observed that when transferred to either of two K-12 recipient strains (*E. coli* 711 or *E. coli* 185), the R factor from Dr. ROSENKRANZ'S strain appeared to infer a low-level resistance to the antibiotic. Of several possible explanations, we have so far examined the following three: (1) Dr. Rosenkranz's strain might contain more than one R factor per cell, some inferring higher levels of resistance than others, and the recipient strains might restrict entry of the R factors inferring the higher levels; (2) strains in which the R factor infers higher levels of resistance may contain more than one R factor per cell, resulting in higher levels of enzyme production by the host cell; and (3) different host cells may interact differently with the same R factor and may thereby modify the expression of the plasmid genes.

We attempted to decide among these possibilities by the following stratagems.

1. Dr. ROSENKRANZ'S strain, which we will refer to as *E. coli* CSH-2 (222R) or as 222R for short, is resistant to streptomycin (S) at 100 μg/ml; to chloramphenicol (C) at 75 μg/ml; and to tetracycline (T) at 20 μg/ml. It is also resistant to sulfonamides, but we did not include this inhibitor in our studies. The strain is an auxotroph, requiring proline, tryptophane, methionine and niacin for growth in minimal medium, and it is lac⁺.

2. Dr. WATANABE'S strain, which we obtained directly from him and which we will refer to as 222W, is identical except that only rare colonies will appear on plates containing 50 or 100 μg S per ml.

3. *E. coli* CSH-2 (R⁻), also obtained from Dr. WATANABE, is the original recipient into which R factor 222 was transferred to produce 222 W. It is, of course, sensitive, lac⁺ and has the same growth requirements as the other *E. coli* CSH-2 strains.

4. *E. coli* 711 and *E. coli* 711 Nx are recipient K-12 strains obtained from Dr. William SMITH. *E. coli* 711 Nx is a naldixic acid resistant (Nx) mutant obtained from *E. coli* 711. *E. coli* 711 is also an auxotroph, requiring proline, histidine and tryptophane. Unlike the other strains, it is lac⁻.

The strategy was to transfer the R factor from 222R (Dr. ROSENKRANZ'S strain) to *E. coli* 711 Nx and then back into *E. coli* CSH-2 (R⁻), taking advantage of the different growth requirements for the latter transfer. If the R factor which infers high-level resistance in the original CSH-2 host, infers low-level resistance in *E. coli* 711 Nx and again infers high-level resistance when transferred back into *E. coli* CSH-2, one could conclude that host cell modification of the infecting gene may account for the differing levels of resistance to S. Transfer of R factor from *E. coli* CSH-2 to *E. coli* 711 Nx was made by using as the selective medium phenol red lactose agar containing Nx (20 μg/ml), S (20, 50 or 100 μg/ml as indicated), C (75 μg/ml), and T (15 μg/ml). Further transfer of R factor from *E. coli* 711 Nx to *E. coli* CSH-2 was made by using as a selective medium, minimal medium containing S, C, and T as indicated above, and supplemented with the

Table 1

RESISTANCE PROFILES OF R FACTOR INFECTED *E. coli* CSH-2

| R factor | Nutrient agar | Number of Macrocolonies | | |
		$S_{20}CT$	$S_{50}CT$	$S_{100}CT$
222R	1.2×10^9	4.7×10^8 (39%)	4.7×10^8 (39%)	5.0×10^8 (42%)
222W	1.9×10^9	1.2×10^9 (63%)	0	0
$222W_h$	1.8×10^9	1.9×10^9 (100%)	1.5×10^9 (83%)	8.6×10^8 (48%)

Cultures incubated overnight in nutrient broth were diluted and plated on nutrient agar and on phenol red lactose agar containing 75 μg/ml of chloramphenicol, 15 μg/ml of tetracycline, and either 20, 50 or 100 μg/ml of streptomycin as indicated.

growth requirements for *E. coli* CSH-2 (proline, methionine, tryptophane and niacin at 10 μg/ml). *E. coli* 711 Nx does not grow in the absence of histidine.

Table I shows the resistance profiles of R factor infected *E. coli* CSH-2 strains. 222 W_h is a strain derived from 222W by plating large numbers in the presence of $S_{100}CT$.

Table 2

R FACTOR TRANSFER FROM *E. coli* CSH-2 TO *E. COLI* 711 Nx

| R factor | Number of Macrocolonies | | |
	$S_{20}CT$	$S_{50}CT$	$S_{100}CT$
222R	1.0×10^7	2.1×10^5	1.1×10^5
222W	5.3×10^5	0	0
$222W_h$	3.7×10^5	1.6×10^5	0

Donor and recipient cells were grown out in nutrient broth to 10^8 cells per ml. Equal volumes were mixed and incubated overnight in the same medium to allow for transfer of R factors; and the cells were diluted and plated on phenol red lactose nutrient agar containing nalidixic acid (20 μg/ml) and other antibiotics as indicated.

Table 2 illustrates the pattern of transfer of resistance to streptomycin from these *E. coli* CSH-2 strains to *E. coli* 711 Nx. Donor and recipient cells, growing at 10^8/ml in nutrient broth were mixed, incubated overnight, and the suspensions were then plated on selective media. The table shows the cell count per ml. of *E. coli* 711 Nx recipients which grew out to form macrocolonies. Only about 1% of the *E. coli* 711 Nx infected with

226

222R are resistant to 100 µg/ml of streptomycin. Strain 222W transfers at a much lower frequency, no colonies appearing on S_{50} or S_{100} plates, while $222W_h$ transferred intermediate resistance levels.

Table 3 shows the resistance profiles of three different clones selected from outgrowth of infected *E. coli* 711 Nx cells on $S_{20}CT$ medium. Similar results are obtained with

Table 3

RESISTANCE PROFILE OF *E. coli* 711 Nx INFECTED WITH R FACTOR 222R

	Inc. Time (hours)	Nutrient agar	Number of Macrocolonies		
			$S_{20}CT$	$S_{50}CT$	$S_{100}CT$
≠1 large colony	48	1.4×10^9	2.1×10^8	4.4×10^6	6×10^3
	72	$-\star$	$-$	9.1×10^7	3.8×10^5
	96	$-$	$-$	$-$	3.8×10^7
≠2 medium size colony	48	1.3×10^9	4.7×10^8	2.6×10^6	1.1×10^5
	72	$-$	$-$	3.5×10^8	3.7×10^6
	96	$-$	$-$	$-$	1.1×10^8
≠3 small colony	48	1.5×10^9	3.7×10^8	7.4×10^6	2×10^4
	72	$-$	$-$	$-$	4.3×10^6
	96	$-$	$-$	$-$	$-$

$\star$ — indicates no change
Conditions as described in legend for Table 1.

E. coli 711 Nx cells infected with R factors from 222W. Three interesting facts can be observed. Firstly, there was a marked variation in colony size of the outgrowth of infected *E. coli* 711 Nx cells on SCT media. Secondly, 2 of the clones ultimately show high-level resistance patterns, while one shows a low-level pattern. And thirdly, there appears to be a pronounced effect on onset of growth at the higher levels of S, a surprising finding in view of the bactericidal nature of S. On the other hand, the resistance profiles of *E. coli* 711 Nx clones selected from the $S_{100}CT$ plates are uniformly high level with no evidence of delayed growth; i. e. all cells grow out within 48 hours at all levels of S.

Table 4

R FACTOR TRANSFER TO *E. coli* CSH-2

Clone Number	Hours Incubation	Number of Macrocolonies		
		$S_{20}CT$	$S_{50}CT$	$S_{100}CT$
≠1	48	4.2×10^3	5.8×10^3	4.9×10^3
≠2	48	5.3×10^4	3.3×10^4	4.4×10^4
≠3	48	$1.4 + 10^5$	1.5×10^5	8.5×10^4

There was no change on further incubation.
Donor and recipient cells were grown out in nutrient broth to 10^8 cells per ml. Equal volumes were mixed and incubated overnight in the same medium to allow for transfer of R factors; and the cells were then diluted and plated on phenol red lactose minimal medium supplemented with proline, methionine, tryptophane, niacin, and antibiotics as indicated.
Clone number refers to the 3 colonies of Table III.

Table 4 illustrates the next step, transfer of the R factor back into *E. coli* CSH-2 (R⁻). All three infected *E. coli* 711 Nx strains transferred only high-level resistance, at lower frequency, back to *E. coli* CSH-2. Transfer of R factor from *E. coli* 711 Nx, selected on S_{100}CT plates, to *E. coli* CSH-2 yielded the same results. One further note. All the newly infected *E. coli* CSH-2 strains tested have intermediate-level resistant profiles after outgrowth on nutrient agar and nutrient broth

S_{20}CT	S_{50}CT	S_{100}CT
3.8×10^8	7.8×10^7	2.3×10^4

and when they in turn serve as donors to *E. coli* 711 Nx, only uniformly high-level resistant infected *E. coli* 711 Nx cells are obtained.

S_{20}CT	S_{50}CT	S_{100}CT
6.8×10^5	6.4×10^5	1.8×10^5

Like all other high-level resistant strains, they show no delay in appearance as macro-colonies.

The possibility that the variation in S resistance might result from variation in the number of R factors per cell was investigated as follows: Since Dr. WATANABE's R factor

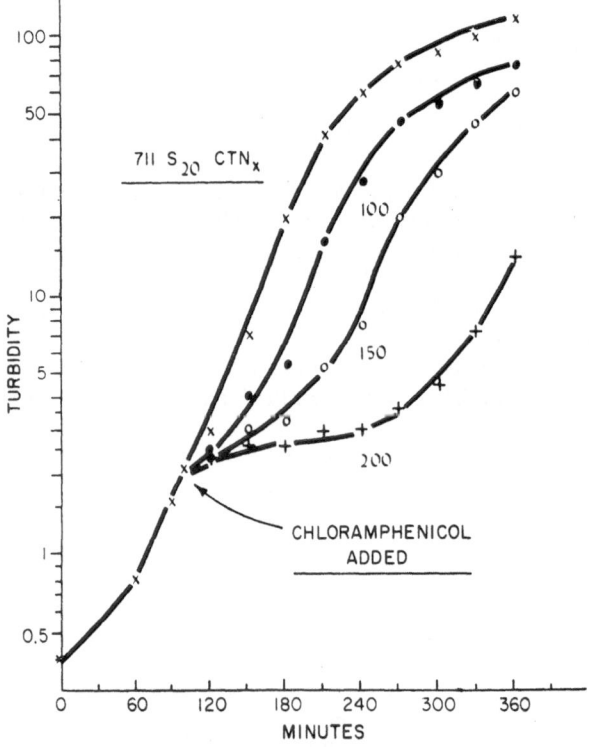

Fig. 1 Growth of *E. coli* 711 Nx (S$_{20}$CT) in the presence of chloramphenicol. This strain received its plasmid from *E. coli* CSH-2 (222R). It grows at 20 μg/ml of streptomycin, but not at 50 μg/ml.

222 transfers its resistance determinants as a unit, a double dose of S inactivating genes would be accompanied by a double dose of C inactivating genes. We therefore compared the ability of *E. coli* 711 Nx S$_{20}$CT to inactivate C to that of *E. coli* 711 Nx S$_{100}$CT. Each

cell population was grown out to log phase (2×10^7/ml) and separated into four portions, to one of which was added 100 µg/ml CM, to another 150 and to a third, 200 µg/ml. The rationale was that growth could not begin again until the excess C was inactivated. If *E. coli* 711 $S_{100}CT$ contained more C inactivating enzyme than 711 $S_{20}CT$, growth should regain its former rate more quickly in the former. Figures 1 and 2 indicate that the level of C inactivating enzyme appears to be the same in both cell types.

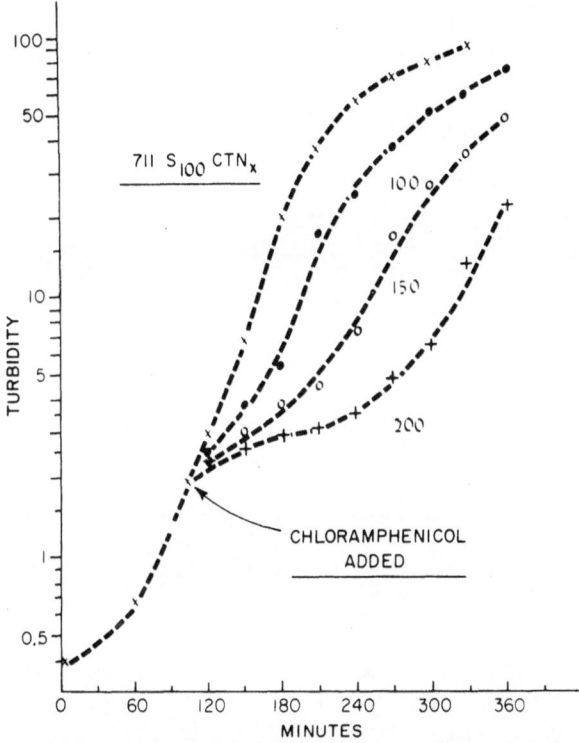

Fig. 2 Growth of *E. coli* 711 Nx ($S_{100}CT$) in the presence of chloramphenicol. This strain also received its plasmid from *E. coli* CSH-2 (222R), but grows at 100 µg/ml of streptomycin.

Of the 3 possibilities examined, the first, that the 222R population contains a mixture of R factors, some inferring higher levels of resistance to S than others, and that *E. coli* 711 Nx is preferentially infected by R factors inferring low-level resistance to S, appears to be contraindicated since further transfer of the R factor to *E. coli* CSH-2 (R⁻) did not result in a population resistant to the low levels of S. The possibility that the different levels of resistance to S result from differences in the number of homologous R factors per cell is also contraindicated by the failure to discover concomitant differences in ability to inactive C. Our results indicate that host modification appears to play a role in the expression of R factor genes, since the R factor, 222R, infers high-level resistance to S in *E. coli* CSH-2 and predominantly low-level resistance in *E. coli* 711 Nx. That the story is probably more complex than this, however, is inferred by the low resistance of 222W in the original *E. coli* CSH-2 and its high-level resistance when transferred to newly infected *E. coli* CSH-2 via *E. coli* 711 Nx. It should also be noted that we were unable to reconstitute either 222R or 222W after passage of their respective R factors through *E. coli* 711.

REFERENCE

WATANABE, T. and T. FUKASAWA (1961): Episome-mediated transfer of drug resistance in *Enterobacteriaceae*. I. Transfer of resistance factors by conjugation. J. Bacteriol. **81**: 669—678.

PHENOTYPIC EXPRESSION OF β-LACTAMASE ACTIVITY IN DIFFERENT STRAINS CARRYING THE TEM R-FACTOR

A. ROSSELET, F. KNÜSEL, and W. ZIMMERMANN

Biological Research Laboratories, Pharmaceuticals Division CIBA-GEIGY, Basle
Switzerland

SUMMARY

The investigation included four strains of *E. coli* and one *Salmonella typhimurium*. The amount of β-lactamase synthesized by each of the strains carrying the TEM R-factor differs widely. Two groups of β-lactamase producers can be distinguished, the first showing a high specific activity ($\sim$ 100 units/mg dry wt.), the second one exhibiting only a low activity ($\sim$ 15 units/mg dry wt.). In the high activity group, an elevated increase in resistance to cephaloridine was found, whereas the corresponding value remained small in the low activity group. An increase in streptomycin-resistance, which is also coded for by the TEM R-factor, was only found in the group of high β-lactamase-activity. These results are discussed in terms of a possible relaxed or stringent R-factor replication in the two activity groups.

By means of cloxacillin-inhibition of the TEM β-lactamase in intact and sonicated cells, the decreased accessibility of the enzyme to penicillins in intact cells was shown to be due to a substantial barrier.

Osmotic shock experiments confirmed that the enzyme is located outside the cell membrane. Based on a theoretical model, enzyme kinetic measurements performed on intact and disrupted cells are interpreted in terms of unaltered kinetic properties of the cell-bound enzyme. As a consequence, in the high activity group, the substrate concentration at the site of enzyme location is expected to be much lower than in the surrounding medium. The determination of cephaloridine concentrations allowing half-maximal growth of R+-strains confirms this assumption. Diffusion is therefore a limiting factor of substrate supply in the high activity group. The importance of a functionally optimal distribution of the β-lactamase is discussed.

INTRODUCTION

Considerable effort has been put into the study of R-factor mediated β-lactamases RICHMOND et al. (1971), SAWAI and MITSUHASHI (1971), class III-β-lactamase being the most common (RICHMOND et al. 1971). Its most thoroughly investigated vector is the TEM-R-factor (DATTA and KONTOMICHALOU 1965), DATTA and RICHMOND (1966), KONTOMICHALOU (1967), SMITH (1969), JACK and RICHMOND (1970), KONTOMICHALOU et al. (1970). A wide range of β-lactamase activity has been found upon introducing this R-factor into several host strains (RICHMOND et al. 1971), DATTA and KONTOMICHALOU (1965, 1967), SMITH (1969). It seemed difficult to detect a linear relationship between the increase in resistance and the β-lactamase activity established by an R-factor in different hosts (RICHMOND et al. 1971), KONTOMICHALOU (1967). However a clear correlation was found as an average of eight different cephalosporins (ROSSELET 1971). This uncertainty suggests that the host cell environment greatly influences the working conditions of the enzyme molecule. At least the R_{TEM}-mediated β-lactamase seems to be located outside the cell membrane (DATTA and KONTOMICHALOU 1965), DATTA and RICHMOND (1966) and it may be reasonably assumed to be adsorbed to some supporting structure. Thereby, the kinetic properties of the enzyme may alter. Diffusion phenomena are likely to be involved in the phenotypic expression of β-lactamases. The existence of a decreased accessibility to β-lactamase for penicillins in *Enterobacteriacea* has been described by several workers (DATTA and KONTOMICHALOU 1965), SMITH (1963), HAMILTON-MILLER et al. (1965). This permeability barrier seems to be influenced by ethylene-diamine-tetra-acetate and sub-inhibitory concentrations of penicillins (HAMILTON-MILLER 1965, 1966).

The purpose of the present work was to establish, which of the described possibilities is most likely to influence the phenotypic expression of β-lactamase activity.

MATERIALS AND METHODS

Antibiotics

Penicillin G, ampicillin, cloxacillin, cephaloridine and streptomycin were obtained from commercial sources. Rifampicin (Rimactan[B]) is a product of Ciba-Geigy Ltd.

Organisms

E. coli TEM harboring the TEM-R-factor DATTA and ¦KONTOMICHALOU (1965), recently termed R6K KONTUMICHALOU et al. (1970), its plasmidless variant *E. coli* TEM R−, and *E. coli* K_{12} W 3110, phosphatase derepressed LEE and RICHMOND (1969), were kindly provided by Prof. Richmond (Bristol).

E. coli 2018, *E. coli* 205 and *Salmonella typhimurium* 277 are Ciba-Geigy screening strains.

In this paper, the strains will be referred to by their numbers. R_{TEM} carries markers coding for a defined β-lactamase (DATTA and RICHMOND 1966) and resistance to streptomycin (DATTA and KONTOMICHALOU 1965). The R− strains are sensitive to β-lactam antibiotics and to streptomycin and do not produce a detectable β-lactamase.

Media and culture conditions

Liquid and solid (1.5% agar) CY-medium (DATTA and RICHMOND 1966) were used throughout this work. Liquid cultures were incubated at 37° C on a rapid rotary shaker. The biomass of the cultures was determined photometrically at 675 nm using a calibrated curve.

R-factor transfers

E. coli TEM R+ was the donor in all transfer experiments. The recipients were rifampicin-resistant mutants of 205, 2018, 277 and 3110.

Donor and recipients were grown in CY-medium to a cell density of 10^8/ml and mixed in the ratio 1:10 respectively. After overnight stationary growth at 37° C, culture samples were plated on CY-agar containing ampicillin and rifampicin each at a concentration of

232

100 μg/ml. Single colonies were purified by streaking once on selective plates. A clone of each recipient harboring R_{TEM} was investigated further. Their identity with the R^- recipient was controlled by the following criteria:

3110: staining for phosphatase (14)

2018, 205: sensitivity to chloramphenicol

277: lac⁻, no indole formation

The R^+ strains were kept on agar containing ampicillin (100 μg/ml).

Ultrasonic disruption

Cells were ultrasonically treated by a Branson B12 sonifier at 20 kcyc/sec. for 3 min. under refrigeration. Preliminary experiments showed that after 2 min. sonication, all the β-lactamase activity remained in the supernatant after 15 hours centrifugation at 100,000 g. It was possible to extend sonication to 6 min. without any loss of activity.

Osmotic shock

Osmotic shock was performed according to NEU and CHOU (1967). Stationary-phase cells were washed twice with 0.85% NaCl at 20° C and taken up in 0.5 M sucrose — 0.03 M Tris-HCl (pH 7.3) —10^{-3} M EDTA. After 10 min. mixing at 20° C, the cells were spun down at 0° C. The pellet was resuspended in ice-cold distilled water and mixed for 10 min. A sample was then removed for ultrasonic disruption. The remaining suspension was centrifuged and the supernatant assayed for β-lactamase activity.

ß-lactamase assay

For the determination of β-lactamase activity, the cells were centrifuged and resuspended in 0.1 M phosphate buffer pH 7.0. Whole cells and sonicated samples were assayed iodometrically according to PERRET (1954). Enzyme kinetics were measured on substrate concentrations ranging from 10^{-2} to 10^{-3} M in 0.1 M phosphate buffer pH 7.0. Care was taken not to hydrolyse more than 1/4 of the substrate, since it was found that reaction velocity remained almost constant over this concentration range. The reaction time was kept minimal to avoid enzyme inactivation. To increase the accuracy of the iodometric titrations for low substrate concentrations, low thiosulphate-concentrations were used. Activity calculations based on the finding that each mole of penicilloic acid reacts with eight equivalents of iodine, whereas each mole of hydrolysed cephaloridine was assumed to react with four equivalents of iodine ALICINO (1961). The activity unit is defined as the amount of enzyme hydrolysing 1 μm of substrate per hour. Km- and Vmax-values were extrapolated from Lineweaver-Burk plots.

Cloxacillin inhibition

Penicillin G and cephaloridine ($8 . 10^{-3}$ M) were subjected to β-lactamase hydrolysis alone or in presence of $0.5 . 10^{-3}$ M cloxacillin. The hydrolysis of cloxacillin at $8 . 10^{-3}$ M was negligible.

Electrophoresis of crude cell extracts

A β-lactamase containing cell extract was prepared from each R^+ strain according to DATTA and RICHMOND (1966). The steps included concentration of the cells ten times in 0.1 M phosphate buffer pH 7.0, ultrasonic disintegration, centrifugation at 100'000 g and overnight dialysis against 0.1 M phosphate buffer pH 7.0. The extracts were applied (2 μl) to cellulose acetate membranes soaked with 0.03 M borate buffer (pH 8.5). The electrode vessels of a Shandon electrophoresis apparatus Kohn U 77 were filled with 0.3 M borate buffer (pH 8.5). The membranes were then subjected to a potential difference of 50 V/cm for 10 min. After the run they were briefly dipped in a 2% starch solution and in a solution of 0.008 M J_2 + 0.06 M KJ + 0.6 % penicillin G in 0.1 M phosphate buffer pH 7.0. The position of β-lactamase activity developed to sharp white bands.

Measurement of the changes in resistance in R⁺ strains

Twofold serial dilutions of the antibiotics in CY-medium were inoculated to give a cell density of 10^7/ml. After 3 hrs. incubation at 37° C in a water-bath, growth was stopped with 4% formaldehyde. The turbidity was measured at 580 nm. The initial inoculum (10^7/ml) corresponds to an OD of 0.05. The OD's attained at the different concentrations were represented graphically. The concentrations giving an OD of 0.5 were read from the graphs and were defined as concentrations allowing half-maximal growth, since a culture without antibiotic reached on OD of about 1 under these conditions.

RESULTS

The strains investigated showed considerable differences in their β-lactamase activity (table 1). The stationary-phase cultures may be divided into a high activity group (TEM,

Table 1

β-LACTAMASE ACTIVITIES OF DIFFERENT R⁺ TEM STRAINS

	Penicillin G Log units/mg		Penicillin G Stationary² units/mg		Ampicillin Log		Ampicillin Stationary		Cephaloridine Log		Cephaloridine Stationary	
Strain	A		A		A		A		A		A	
INTACT CELLS												
TEM	17		0.8		16		0.5		54		61	
205	24		1.4		16		1.8		144		101	
3110	9.4		4.6		8.5		3.6		32		22	
2018	13		2.4		5.9		2.6		24		22	
277	2.6		1.3		2.3		3.9		6.9		12	
	A	B	A	B	A	B	A	B	A	B	A	B
SONICATED CELLS												
TEM	46	2.7	60	75	54	3.4	55	110	55	1.0	85	1.4
205	179	7.5	77	55	184	11.5	80	44	236	1.6	136	1.3
mean		5.1³)		65		7.5		77		1.3		1.4
3110	27	2.9	15	3.3	40	4.7	12.5	3.5	34	1.1	20	0.9
2018	25	1.9	13	5.4	23	3.9	21	8.1	32	1.3	22	1.0
277	5.7	2.2	9.2	7.1	6.9	3.0	11.3	2.9	7.2	1.0	12.5	1.0
mean		2.3		5.3		3.9		4.8		1.1		1.0

β-lactamase activity (units/mg dry wt.)
B: activity increase after sonication
[1]) Log phase: cell density of 5 . 10^8 cells/ml
[2]) Stationary phase: 16 hr. culture (∼3−4 . 10^9 cells/ml)
[3]) mean activity increase
  The cells were centrifuged and resuspended on 0.1 m phosphate buffer pH 7.0.
Substrate concentration: 5 . 10^{-3} M
  The results concerning log- and stationary-phase cells are derived from the same culture.

205) and a low activity group (3110, 2018, 277). From log-to stationary-phase, the activity varied maximally by a factor of two.

Upon cell disruption, the β-lactamase activity measured with the penicillins increased with all strains. In the case of TEM and 205 this activity increase enhanced on an average 10 times from log-to stationary-phase. This enhancement was not clear-cut in the low activity group. With cephaloridine, there was no activity increase upon sonication. These results suggest the presence of an accessibility barrier for penicillins, whereas cephaloridine has free access to the β-lactamase.

With TEM, the dependence of this barrier on the culture age was investigated further. Fig. 1 shows that there was a steady decrease of penicillin accessibility with increasing

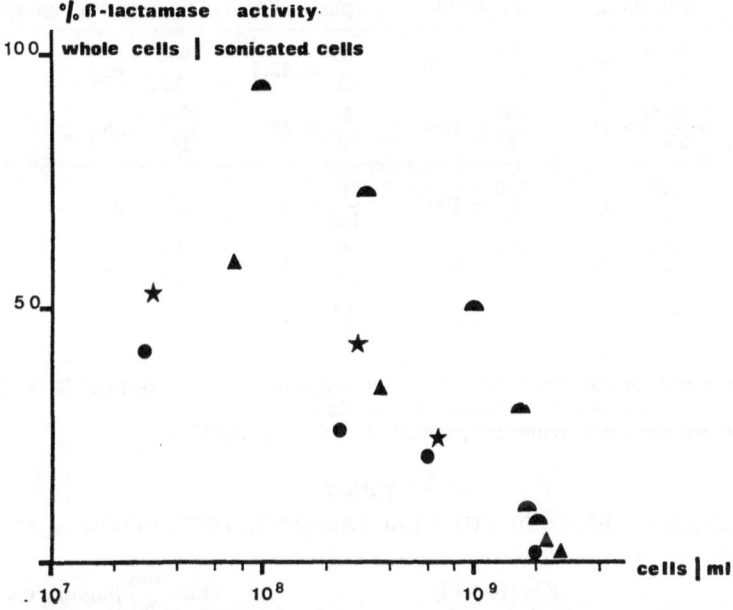

Fig. 1 Dependence of the accessibility to penicillins on the cell density of *E. coli* TEM R+. Four overnight cultures were diluted 100 fold into prewarmed CY-medium and shaken at 37° C. The first samples were withdrawn after 1 hr. incubation, the others at 1 hr. intervals. The cells were taken up in 0.1 M phosphate buffer pH 7.0. Intact and disrupted cells were assayed with $5 \cdot 10^{-3}$ M penicillin G. The β-lactamase activity of whole cells is expressed in percentage of the activity of sonicated cells.

cell density. This diminution began in full log-phase. All cultures reached minimal accessibility at a cell density of 2.10^9/ml. The highest value of accessibility varied greatly amongst different cultures.

As concerns electrophoretic mobility, the β-lactamase produced by the 5 strains was indistinguishable. In the system described, the mobility attained 3 mm/min. towards the anode.

The β-lactamase activity in the supernatant of log-phase cultures remained below 4 % of the total activity. The TEM-β-lactamase seems not to be excreted actively. All strains released 90—100% of their β-lactamase when subjected to osmotic shock, pointing thus at this periplasmic location.

Table 2 shows the R_{TEM}-induced increases in resistance to several antibiotics. With cephaloridine, they were closely connected to the specific β-lactamase activities, whereas with the penicillins a strict correlation was missing. Only TEM and 205 exhibited a resistance increase to streptomycin. The resistance levels in R^+ and R^- strains were also determined as minimal inhibitory concentrations (MIC) after overnight incubation. All MIC-values of penicillin G and ampicillin measured with R^+ strains exceeded 1000 μg/ml.

Table 2

R_{TEM} INDUCED CHANGES IN RESISTANCE

$$\frac{[R^+]}{[R^-]}$$

Strain	Penicillin G	Ampicillin	Cephaloridine	Streptomycin	units/mg dry wt.[1]
TEM	$\frac{>4000}{20} > 200$	$\frac{380}{2.5} = 152$	$\frac{85}{2} = 42.5$	$\frac{900}{20} = 45$	90
205	$\frac{>4000}{25} > 160$	$\frac{160}{1} = 160$	$\frac{46}{2} = 23$	$\frac{1200}{14} = 86$	113
3110	$\frac{300}{20} = 15$	$\frac{200}{2} = 100$	$\frac{6}{1.5} = 4$	$\frac{4}{7} = 0.6$	19
2018	$\frac{320}{8} = 40$	$\frac{150}{1} = 150$	$\frac{6}{1.5} = 4$	$\frac{14}{24} = 0.6$	16
277	$\frac{1250}{14} = 89$	$\frac{32}{5} = 6.4$	$\frac{12}{6} = 2$	$\frac{3}{5} = 0.6$	7.4

(R^+), (R^-): antibiotic concentrations (μg/ml) allowing half maximal growth of R^+ and R^- strains respectively. For experimental conditions see methods.
[1] units/mg dry wt: Vmax-values for penicillin G, taken from table 3.

Table 3

ENZYME KINETICS OF THE β-LACTAMASE IN DIFFERENT R_{TEM} STRAINS

Strain	S	n	Km (10^{-4} M)		Vmax $\frac{dm}{60}$ /mg dry wt. (10^{-6} M)	
			intact	sonicated	intact	sonicated
TEM	P	5	18.7 ± 4.2[1]	3.5 ± 1.5	5.2 ± 1.7	90 ± 4.7
	C		197 ± 38	14.3 ± 1.8	380 ± 65	153 ± 16
205	P	4	20 ± 6.3	2.3 ± 0.9	2.9 ± 0.7	113 ± 21
	C		150 ± 27	16.4 ± 2.8	362 ± 73	197 ± 27
3110	P	4	8.8 ± 1.7	3.4 ± 0.8	3.1 ± 0.2	19.1 ± 2.7
	C		15.3 ± 0.4	11 ± 1.1	35 ± 7	35 ± 11
2018	P	1	10	3.5	1.6	16
	C	2	25 ± 10.3	13 ± 1.6	33 ± 0.9	29 ± 8
277	P	2	177 ± 29	2.7 ± 1.8	2.5 ± 0.8	7.4 ± 0.2
	C		14.5 ± 0.5	7.8 ± 1.1	10.9 ± 5.7	11.7 ± 3.4
Mean	P	16		3.0 ± 0.5		
	C	17		13.1 ± 1.0		

[1] standard error
S: substrate
P: penicillin G

C: cephaloridine
n: number of different cultures examined

236

The $\dfrac{\text{MIC R}^+}{\text{MIC R}^-}$ ratios determined with cephaloridine confirmed the correlation of resistance increase to enzyme activity.

R$^-$ segregants occured in all strains with a frequency less than 1%, as determined by replica-plating on ampicillin (100 μg/ml).

The results of enzyme kinetic measurements carried out on intact and sonicated cells (stationary phase) are shown in table 3. The Km-values determined with disrupted cells are very similar in all strains and their mean value corresponds closely to the Km measured with a sonic extract of TEM, free of particles and low molecular weight compounds (Km penicillin G 4.2 . 10^{-4} M, Km cephaloridine 17.4 . 10^{-4} M). The Vmax-values are expressed in μm substrate hydrolysed per hr. per mg dry wt.; when determined with broken cells, they allow a clear-cut division into a high (TEM, 205) and a low activity group (3110, 2018, 277).

Table 4

COMPARISON OF β-LACTAMASE KINETICS IN INTACT AND SONICATED CELLS

Strain	Penicillin G		Cephaloridine	
	$\dfrac{\text{Km int.}}{\text{Km son.}}$	$\dfrac{\text{Vmax int.}}{\text{Vmax son.}}$	$\dfrac{\text{Km int.}}{\text{Km son.}}$	$\dfrac{\text{Vmax int.}}{\text{Vmax son.}}$
TEM	5.3	0.058	13.1	2.48
205	8.7	0.026	9.1	1.84
3110	2.6	0.16	1.4	1.0
2018	2.9	0.10	1.9	1.14
277	65.6	0.34	1.9	0.93

int.: intact cells
son.: sonicated cells

The ratios $\dfrac{\text{Km intact}}{\text{Km sonicated}}$ and $\dfrac{\text{Vmax intact}}{\text{Vmax sonicated}}$ (table 4) show the resemblance of TEM to 205 on the one hand, and of 3110 to 2018 on the other hand. These properties coincide with the capacity of enzyme production. The cell-bound β-lactamase of 3110, 2018 and 277 exhibited almost similar kinetics of cephaloridine hydrolysis as the free enzyme. The maximal velocity of penicillin G hydrolysis measured with the cell-bound enzymes was in all strains smaller than when determined with sonicated cultures. A striking feature

Table 5

COMPARISON OF SINGLE Vmax-VALUES MEASURED ON INTACT AND SONICATED CELLS WITH CEPHALORIDINE

Strain	$\dfrac{\text{Vmax int.}}{\text{Vmax son.}}$					mean ± SE
TEM	1.92	1.95	2.51	2.80	3.01	2.15 ± 0.17
205	1.38	1.81	1.98	2.01		
3110	0.85	0.93	1.19	1.32		
2018	0.95	1.44				1.06 ± 0.08
277	0.71	1.08				

is the enhanced Vmax of cephaloridine break-down in intact cells of TEM and 205. This apparent activity increase is only about twofold, but nevertheless significant on comparing the single $\dfrac{\text{Vmax intact}}{\text{Vmax sonicated}}$ ratios (table 5) of the high activity group with those of the low activity group. It will be shown in the discussion that the Km and Vmax-values of cell-bound enzyme are apparent, if they differ markedly from those of free enzyme.

They are indicative of an elevated substrate concentration gradient between the surrounding medium and the site of enzyme location.

The inhibition of β-lactamase activity by cloxacillin both in intact and sonicated cells is represented in fig. 2. Cloxacillin ($0.5 \cdot 10^{-3}$ M) inhibited the splitting of penicillin

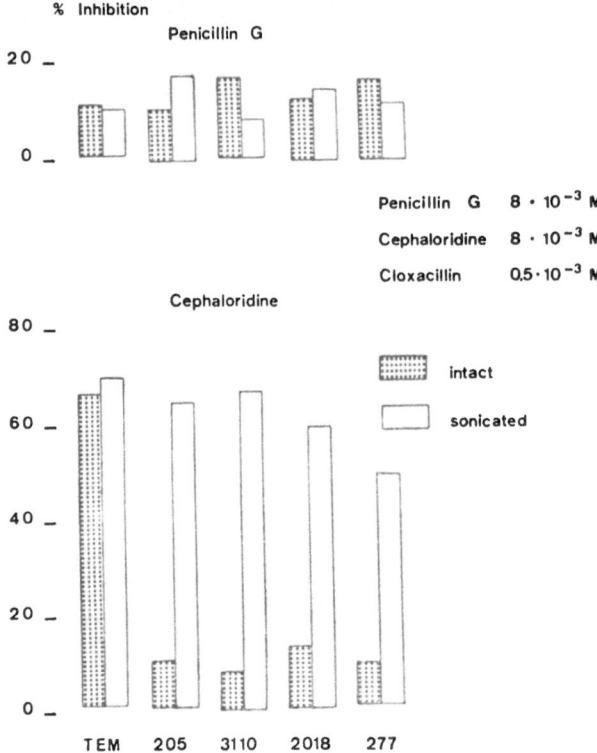

Fig. 2 Levels of cloxacillin-inhibition of the β-lactamase activity in intact and sonicated cells.

G ($8 \cdot 10^{-3}$ M) only to a small extent very similar on average, whether measured on whole or broken cells. With all strains, except TEM, cloxacillin inhibition of cephaloridine hydrolysis was low ($\sim 10\%$) in intact and high in disrupted cells ($\sim 60\%$). With TEM however, inhibition of cephaloridine break-down attains the same high level both with intact and sonicated cultures.

DISCUSSION

The amount of β-lactamase synthesized by different R_{TEM} strains may reflect the number of R-factor copies per cell or the rate of transcription of the β-lactamase gene. E. coli $K_{12}RC$ 85 produces about 13 R_{TEM}-copies per cell in the logarithmic phase and 38 in the stationary phase (KONTOMICHALOU 1970). Thus in one strain of E. coli, R_{TEM} replicates under relaxed control, a feature which seemed specific to Proteus sp. (KASAMATSU and ROWND 1970). E. coli K_{12} RC 85 R_{TEM} exhibits a β-lactamase activity of 120 units/mg dry wt. (ampicillin) (KONTOMICHALOU 1970), which corresponds to the activity of TEM and 205. This might indicate a relaxed R_{TEM}-replication in these two strains, whereas the R-factor presumably replicates under stringent control in the low activity group. The disappearance of streptomycin-resistance in the low activity group is not in contradiction to this assumption, although the possibility of a loss of the str-marker during the transfer cannot be excluded. A mechanism of β-lactamase repression within the low activity group seems improbable, since the R_{TEM}-mediated increase in resistance to cephaloridine depends on the amount of β-lactamase synthesized without inducer. Whatever the correct interpretation may be, it is clear that the quantity of TEM-β-lactamase synthesized is determined by the host strain. Cloxacillin-inhibition is one of the characteristic features of TEM-β-lactamase (RICHMOND et al. 1971). This peculiarity enables us to prove that the reduced accessibility of penicillins to the cell-bound β-lactamase is based on a substantial barrier. The results obtained with 3110 and 2018 can be interpreted quantitatively. The mean $\dfrac{\text{Vmax intact}}{\text{Vmax sonicated}}$ ratio of these two strains determined with penicillin G (table 4) indicates that 13% of the total β-lactamase is accessible to this antibiotic. Since the cloxacillin-inhibition of penicillin G hydrolysis is approximately equal in whole and disrupted cells (fig. 2), we may admit that both cloxacillin and penicillin G are similarly accessible to β-lactamase. About 65% of the β-lactamase-mediated splitting of cephaloridine is inhibited in disrupted cultures (fig. 2). The same fraction of the cloxacillin-accessible enzyme (8.5%) should therefore be inhibited in intact cells. The average value of 10% inhibition measured on intact cells of 3110 and 2018 (fig. 2) shows this assumption to be true.

Strains 205 and 277 show a similar inhibition figure, but quite unexpectedly, cephaloridine hydrolysis in whole cells of TEM is inhibited to the same extent as in a broken cell preparation. The TEM cell-envelope could possibly be rendered permeable to penicillins by cephaloridine. This peculiarity points to a different organisation of the TEM cell-envelope in comparison with the other strains. At least for TEM, the accessibility barrier for penicillins is much more pronounced in stationary phase cultures than in log phase cultures with small cell densities. Since a decrease of penicillin accessibility can be measured throughout log phase, this barrier is possibly induced by a fermentation product accumulating in the batch culture with increasing culture age.

For the determination of enzyme kinetic data we used the Perret method and not the microiodometric assay of NOVICK (1962), since the TEM-β-lactamase is known to be very sensitive to iodine-potassium-iodide solution (DATTA and RICHMOND 1966). The average Km-value obtained for cephaloridine with broken cells by the Perret method (13.1 . . 10^{-4} M) is in close accordance with the value determined by a UV-method (ROSSELET et al. 1971). The Km-values of penicillin G determined with sonicated cells are probably too high. The slopes of the Lineweaver-Burk plots are very small for this compound, thus excluding an accurate measurement, since the Perret method can hardly be used for substrate concentrations lower than $5 . 10^{-4}$ M. Nevertheless, the Vmax determinations for penicillin G are accurate and it is possible to detect differences in Km-values determined on intact and sonicated cells. Several characteristics must be considered when measuring enzyme kinetics on intact cells. First of all, the very high local concentration of the cell-bound enzyme. Whole cells were assayed at a density of approximately 10^9 cells/ml corresponding to a total cell volume of about 1 mm³/ml. The β-lactamase is localized outside the plasma membrane in the complex cell-envelope, which is roughly

239

estimated to represent 10% of the cell volume at the most. The β-lactamase escaping its compartment upon sonication is therefore diluted at least 10'000 fold. Developing the Michaelis-Menten equation one gets:

$$\frac{[E]_T}{[ES]} = \frac{Km}{[S[} + 1 \qquad v = -\frac{d[S]}{dt} = \frac{d[P]}{dt}$$

$$v \propto [ES]$$

$[E]_T$ intact cells $= 10^4 [E]_T$ disrupted cells. Assuming that the Km-values are identical for free and cell-bound enzyme and that [S] at the active site is equal in both enzyme-states.

$$[ES]_{intact} = 10^4 [ES]_{disrupted}$$

$$v_{intact} = 10^4 v_{disrupted}$$

The reaction product formed by the cell-bound enzyme is diluted 10'000 fold when released into the medium, which means that the velocities measured with intact and sonicated cells are identical.

Since diffusion is likely to be the sole transport mechanism outside the cell membrane, we may postulate it to be the vector supplying the cell-bound β-lactamase with new substrate. The substrate concentration $[S]_i$ at the active site of the β-lactamase in whole cells is lower than $[S]_o$ in the surrounding medium. $[S]_i$ is the result of a steady-state equilibrium between the velocity of substrate hydrolysis and the diffusion rate at which the enzyme is provided with new substrate.

$$\left(\frac{dS}{dt}\right)_{diffusion} = \left(\frac{dS}{dt}\right)_{enzyme} \tag{1}$$

$$\left(\frac{dS}{dt}\right)_{diffusion} = A \cdot D \frac{[S]_o - [S]_i}{L} = C([S]_o - [S]_i) \tag{2}$$

$$C = \frac{A \cdot D}{L}$$

A = diffusion area
D = diffusion constant
L = diffusion length

$$\left(\frac{ds}{dt}\right)_{enzyme} = \frac{[S]_i}{Km + [S]_i} Vmax \tag{3}$$

$$C([S]_o - [S]_i) = \frac{[S]_i}{Km + [S]_i} Vmax \tag{4}$$

Equation (DATTA and RICHMOND 1966) has been used by Koch and Coffman for a rational approach to the activity of β-galactosidase in intact E. coli cells (KOCH and COFFMAN 1970). However, they eliminated the quantity $[S]_i$, which is difficult to measure.

Fig. 3 shows a graphical representation of equation (DATTA and RICHMOND 1966). The Lineweaver-Burk transforamtion of this hypothetical model is shown in fig. 4.

The enzyme kinetics, determined with penicillin G on whole cells are complicated by the accessibility barrier. However, 277 excepted, the $\frac{Km \text{ intact}}{Km \text{ sonicated}}$-ratios accord with the theoretical model (tables 3 and 4). The enzyme kinetic results obtained with cephaloridine on intact cells correspond exactly with the theoretical model (tables 3, 4 and 5). The $\dfrac{\text{Km intact}}{\text{Km sonicated}}$ - and $\dfrac{\text{Vmax intact}}{\text{Vmax sonicated}}$ - ratios give high values in strains of high β-lactamase activity and tend towards unity in the low activity group. There is therefore strong evidence that the kinetic properties of free TEM-β-lactamase remain unaltered if the enzyme functions in the cell-bound state. Although the β-lactamase is

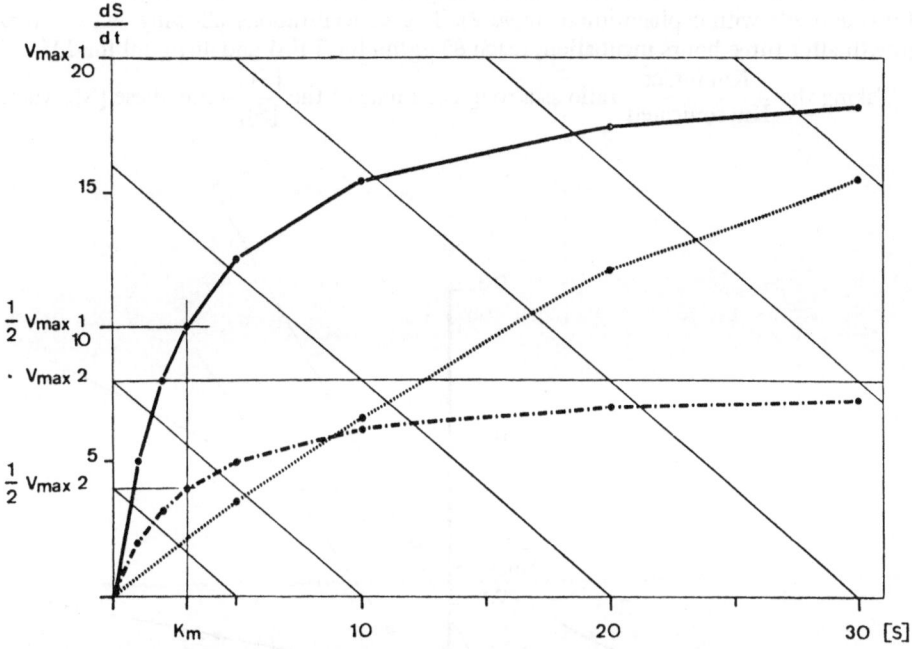

Fig. 3 Graphical representation of the velocity of substrate-diffusion, $\left(\dfrac{dS}{dt}\right)$ diff., and enzyme-catalysed substrate hydrolysis, $\left(\dfrac{dS}{dt}\right)$ enz., versus substrate concentration (S). Arbitrary units are used $\left(\dfrac{dS}{dt}\right)$ diff. $= C[(S)_o - (S)_i]$ is represented by thin diagonal straight lines for different $(S)_o$ values. For C, an arbitrary value of $\dfrac{4}{5}$ was assumed.

$(S)_i$: substrate concentration at the active site for the β-lactamase in intact cells.

$(S)_o$: substrate concentration in the surrounding medium. The intersection of $\left(\dfrac{dS}{dt}\right)$ diff. with the abscissa corresponds to $(S)_o$. $\left(\dfrac{dS}{dt}\right)$ enz. $= \dfrac{(S)_i}{Km + (S)_i}$ Vmax is represented for 2 different Vmax-values, analogous to 2 strains producing different amount of enzyme. Km is arbitrarily set at 3 for the 2 plots.

$\bullet$ ———————— $\bullet$ Vmax 1 = 20
$\bullet$ — $\cdot$ — $\cdot$ — $\cdot$ — $\bullet$ Vmax 2 = 8

These plots correspond to measurements with free enzyme. The intersection of $\left(\dfrac{dS}{dt}\right)$ enz.-plots with $\left(\dfrac{dS}{dt}\right)$ diff.-plots give the $(S)_i$values resulting from a steady-state equilibrium between substrate supply and substrate hydrolysis.

Upon plotting $\left(\dfrac{dS}{dt}\right)$ enz. versus $(S)_i$, a curve, represented by the dotted line, is obtained $\bullet$ $\cdots\cdots\cdots$ $\bullet$ for Vmax$_1$ = 20), which corresponds to a measurement on intact cells. This plot does not fit into Michaelis-Menten kinetics, although ultimately the same Vmax-value is reached.

241

located outside the cell membrane, diffusion is a limiting factor in substrate supply in the high activity group. This means that the higher the local enzyme concentration is, the lower is the antibiotic concentration at this site. If the TEM-β-lactamase was located in the same compartment as the target of β-lactam antibiotics (STROMINGER 1970), the cells would grow in a medium containing concentrations much higher than the minimal inhibitory concentrations of the corresponding R$^-$ strain. This seems to be the case for TEM and 205 with cephaloridine (table 2). The concentrations allowing half-maximal growth after three hours incubation, reach 85 μg/ml for TEM and 46 μg/ml for 205.

Taking the $\dfrac{\text{Km intact}}{\text{Km sonicated}}$-ratio as a rough estimate of the $\dfrac{[S]_o}{[S]_i}$-ratio, these $[S]_o$-values

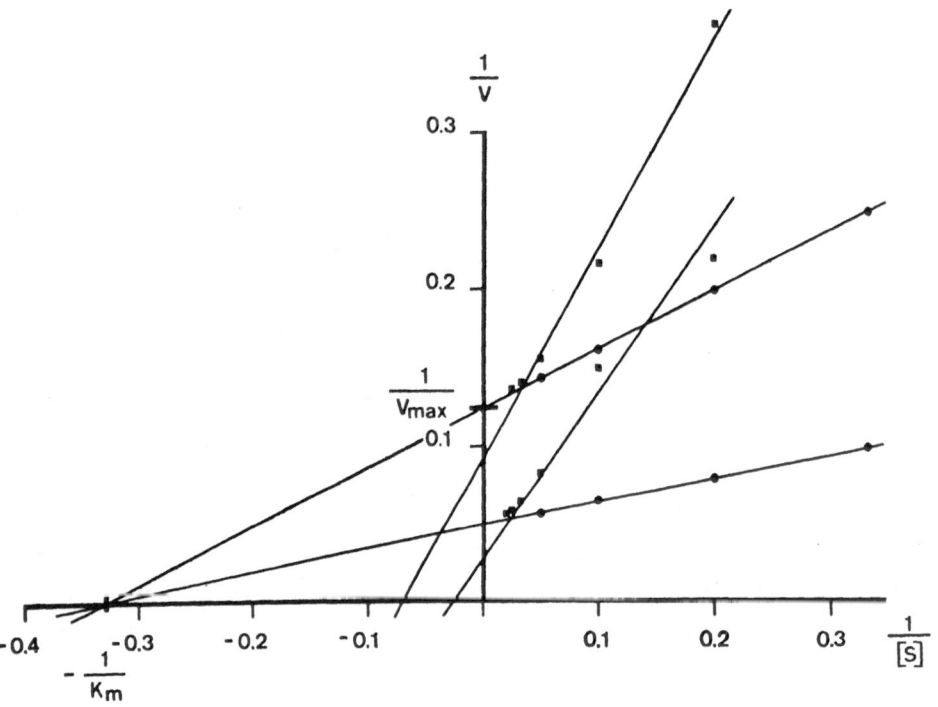

Fig. 4 Lineweaver-Burk transformation of the $\left(\dfrac{dS}{dt}\right)$ enzyme versus (S) plots represented in fig. 3.

Each pair of values corresponding to Michaelis-Menten kinetics, measured with free enzyme, are represented by ●, those measured on intact cells by ■.
The arbitrary units are the same as for fig. 3.
It is possible to fit a straight line to the value-pairs measured on intact cells, resulting in apparent Vmax- and Km-values.
Km (free):   obtained with free enzyme (sonicated culture),
Km (intact):   obtained with intact cells.
The following features emerge from the graph:
Km (intact) > Km (free). With decreasing Vmax (free),
Km (intact) tends towards Km (free).
Vmax (intact) > Vmax (free). With decreasing Vmax (free),
Vmax (intact) tends towards Vmax (free).

The ratio $\dfrac{\text{Km (intact)}}{\text{Km (free)}}$ is a rough estimate of the $\dfrac{(S)_o}{(S)_i}$ ratio for $(S)_i <$ Km (free) (see fig. 3).

242

result in inner concentrations $[S]_i$ of 5.7 µg/ml for TEM and 4.0 µg/ml for 205. These figures correspond approximately to the MIC's, which strongly emphasizes the importance of a functionally optimal distribution of β-lactamases. Two main possibilities of β-lactamase utilization seem to have evolved in bacteria. Either a large production of inducible enzyme, which is excreted in high amounts, typical for *Staphylococci* and *Bacilli*, or a constitutive synthesis of relatively small amounts of optimally located enzyme as found in *Enterobacteriaceae* (CITRI and POLLOCK 1966).

REFERENCES

ALICINO, J. F. (1961): Jodometric assay of natural and synthetic penicillins, 6-aminopenicillanic acid and cephalosporin C. Anal. Chem. **33**: 648−649.

CITRI, N., and M. R. POLLOCK. (1966): The biochemistry and function of β-lactamase (penicillinase). Advanc. Enzymol. **28**: 237−323.

DATTA, N., and P. KONTOMICHALOU. (1965): Penicillinase synthesis controlled by infectious R factors in Enterobacteriaceae. Nature **208**: 239−241.

DATTA, N., and M. H. RICHMOND. (1966): The purification and properties of a penicillinase whose synthesis is mediated by an R-factor in Escherichia coli. Biochem. J. **98**: 204−249.

HAMILTON-MILLER, J. M. T., J. T. SMITH, and R. KNOX. (1965): Interaction of cephalorodine with penicillinase-producing Gram-negative bacteria. Nature **208**: 235−237.

HAMILTON-MILLER, J. M. T. (1965): Effect of EDTA upon bacterial permeability to benzyl-penicillin Biochem. Biophys. Res. Commun. **20**: 688−691.

HAMILTON-MILLER, J. M. T. (1966): Damaging effects of ethylenediaminetetra-acetate and penicillins on permeability barriers in Gram-negative bacteria. Biochem. J. **100**: 675−682.

JACK, G. W., and M. H. RICHMOND. (1970): A comparative study of eight distinct β-lactamases synthesized by Gram-negative bacteria. J. gen. Microbiol. **61**: 43−61.

KASAMATSU, H., and R. ROWND. (1970): Replication of R-factors in Proteus mirabilis: Replication under relaxed control. J. Mol. Biol. **51**: 473−489.

KOCH, A. L., and R. COFFMAN. (1970): Diffusion, permeation, or enzyme limitation: A probe for the kinetics of enzyme induction. Biotechnology and Bioengineering **12**: 651−677.

KONTOMICHALOU, P. (1967): Transmissible extrachromosomal resistance to the penicillins in E. coli K_{12} and Falkow's Proteus host. 5th International Congress of Chemotherapy, Vol. 4: 251−255.

KONTOMICHALOU, P., M. MITANI, and R. C. CLOWES. (1970): Circular R-factor molecules controlling penicillinase synthesis, replicating in Escherichia coli under either relaxed or stringent control. J. Bacteriol. **104**: 34−44.

LEE, P. A., and M. H. RICHMOND. (1969): Method for assessing the frequency of transfer of an R-factor on solid media and for isolating cells of the donor type from a predominantly repressed culture. J. Bacteriol. **100**: 1131−1132.

NEU, H. C., and J. CHOU. (1967): Release of surface enzymes in Enterobacteriaceae by osmotic shock. J. Bacteriol. **94**: 1934−1945.

NOVICK, R. P. (1962): Micro-iodometric assay for penicillinase. Biochem. J. **83**: 236−240.

PERRET, C. J. (1954): Jodometric assay of penicillinase. Nature **174**: 1012−1013.

RICHMOND, M. H., G. W. JACK, and R. B. SYKES. (1971: The β-lactamases of Gram-negative bacteria including Pseudomonads. Ann. N. Y. Acad. Sci. **182**: 243−257.

ROSSELET, A., F. KNÜSEL, and W. ZIMMERMANN. (1971): The susceptibility of 6 derivatives of 7-cyanacetamido cephalosporanic acid to hydrolysis by the β-lactamase of E. coli R_{TEM} 7_{th} International Congress of Chemotherapy, in press.

SAWAI, T., and S. MITSUHASHI. (1971): Mechanism of ampicillin resistance, p. 136−142. In S. Mitsuhashi (ed.). Transferable drug resistance factor R. University Park Press, Baltimore.

SMITH, J. T. (1969): R-factor gene expression in Gram-negative bacteria. J. gen. Microbiol. **55**: 109−120.

SMITH, J. T. (1963): Penicillinase and ampicillin resistance in a strain of Escherichia coli. J. gen. Microbiol. **30**: 299−306.

STROMINGER, J. L. (1970): Penicillin-sensitive enzymatic reactions in bacterial cell wall synthesis. The Harvey Lectures, Series 64, p. 179−213. Academic Press, New York.

R FACTORS CARRYING GENES
GOVERNING RESISTANCE TO β-LACTAM DRUGS, STUDIED
IN DIFFERENT BACTERIAL HOSTS

P. KONTOMICHALOU, A. EFSTRATIADIS and G. LEVIS

School of Medicine, Department of Clinical Therapeutics, "Alexandra" Hospital, Athens, Greece.

INTRODUCTION

Besides the variations of the epidemiology of infective diseases, the policy on the use of antibiotics in everyday clinical practice animal husbandry, and veterinary medicine varies in different countries. Hence, the selective pressure by drugs, which influences the emergence of drug-resistant and R^+ bacteria, diversifies in the environment of the bacterial populations in different parts of the world.

In our previous publications on infective drug-resistance (KONTOMICHALOU, 1967 a, b), from material composed exclusively from R factors found in this laboratory in Greece, we have shown that wild *Enterobacteriaceae*, isolated from clinical practice since 1963, possessed a high proposition of R factors, which carried a variety of combinations of resistance-determinants, including the genes governing resistance to the penicillins. Since 1965, when it was shown by DATTA and KONTOMICHALOU that the genetic information for penicillinase synthesis can be carried on R factors, penicillinase plasmids became a very convenient system for studies on episomal enzymes (DATTA and KONTOMICHALOU 1965). Episomal penicillinases have been purified and elegantly studied by different investigators (DATTA and RICHMOND (1966); YAMAGISHI, O'HARA, SAWAI and MITSUHASHI (1969); SAWAI TAKAHASHI, YAMAGISHI and MITSUHASHI (1970); LINDQUIST and NORDSTRÖM (1970)). It has often been claimed that the episomal penicillinases in *Enterobacteriaceae* are, as a rule, constitutive enzymes (DATTA et al. (1965)); BURMAN, NORDSTRÖM and BOMAN (1968); SAWAI, MITSUHASHI and YAMAGISHI (1968); LINDQUIST et al. (1970)).

We first reported in 1967 the host-dependence of the expression of episomal resistance to the penicillins, as well as the difference in this aspect between K12 and PM 1 hosts, carrying four of our R factors (KONTOMICHALOU (1967)c).

On the basis of his molecular studies on the nature of R factors, ROWND reported in 1966 the existence of two possible states of the intracellular R factors: a multicopy state, found by him in *Proteus* and another state, characterised by a small number of R copies per cell, found in K12R$^+$ and *Serratia* R$^+$ strains. He suggested that these states, representing cases of "relaxed" and "stringent" control of replication of the R factors respectively, were characteristic for the R$^+$ state of each of the above hosts (ROWND, NAKAYA and NAKAMURA (1966); ROWND (1969)).

In 1970 we showed that a multicopy state of R factors, i. e. a "relaxed" control of R factor replication, can also be found in K12 host (KONTOMICHALOU, MITANI and CLOWES (1970)).

Since the levels of drug-resistance of bacteria have direct implications on clinical chemotherapy, investigations on the differences among bacterial hosts in the expression of episomal drug resistance are of extreme significance for clinical bacteriologists, in addition to their purely biological interest.

In this communication we report results based on the study of 10 R factors, investigated in different bacterial hosts. We show the peculiarity of individual R factors, carrying genes governing resistance to the β-lactam drugs and the host-dependence of the expression of some of their functions. Results on the incorporation of ³H-thymidine into episomal and chromosomal DNA are also presented.

Material, characters and genetic study of the R factors

Ten R factors of this study have been taken at random from our collection of drug-resistant plasmids, carrying the gene A (resistance to the penicillins) (KONTOMICHALOU (1971)). The designation, origin and characters of these R factors are given in Table 1.

Table 1

DESIGNATION, ORIGIN AND CHARACTERS OF THE R FACTORS: CLASS OF TRANSFER FACTOR AND COMPOSITION FOR RESISTANCE DETERMINANTS

Designation of R factors	Original hosts of the R factors	Year of isol- ation	Resistance patterns		fi character	Association with other plasmids	R+ clones tested for fi class
			of clinical strains	of R factors			
R4K	Escher. coli	1963	ASSu	ASSu	fi⁻	col Ia	A
*R6K	Escher. coli	1963	AS	AS	fi⁻		AS
R7K	Proteus rettgeri	1964	ASSu	ASSu	fi⁻		A
R8K	Proteus rettgeri	1964	ASTCSu	ASTCSu	fi⁻		A
R9K	Escher. coli	1963	ASCT	ASC	fi⁻		AS
R22K	Proteus mirabilis	1963	ASCT	AS	fi⁻		S
R28K	Citrobacter	1965	ASK	ASK	fi⁻		A
R59K	Escher. coli	1968	ASCKTSu	ASKCSu	fi⁺		ACSSu
R62K	Citrobacter	1968	ASCTSu	ASSu	fi⁻		ASSu
R102K	Klebsiella	1969	ASCTNaSu	ACSSu	fi⁺		ACSSu

* : previously designated R TEM		C : resistance to Chloramphenicol
A : resistance to Ampicillin		T : resistance to Tetracycline
S : resistance to Streptomycin		K : resistance to Kanamycin
Su: resistance to the Sulfonamides		Na: resistance to Nalidixic acid

The fi character of the plasmids was tested by the inhibition of plating of the male specific phage MS2 on F⁺R⁺ and HfrR⁺ strains. It is shown that, in this material, the fi⁻ R factors predominated, and that only two R factors (R59K and R102K), carrying the gene C in close linkage with the gene A, belonged to the fi⁺ class. The R⁺ clones tested for fi character possessed always the marker A, and in some cases the resistance-markers counter-selected with A. Only in one case (factor R22K) did the fi character reported concern the S-resistant R⁺ clones, because the A gene of this plasmid, after entering the F⁻ K12 strain, became non-transmissible and could not be introduced to F⁺ or Hfr strains. In R factors found in *Escherichia coli* strains isolated from other countries the fi⁺ class R factors predominated (ROMERO and MEYNELL (1969)). Our R factors were selected for carrying the gene A; it is probable that this gene may be more often associated with fi⁻ than with fi⁺ transfer factors. The ASTΔ R factors, isolated by Anderson from *Salm. typhimurium* strains, belonged also to the fi⁻ class (ANDERSON (1969)).

Tests for purity of the R factors, i. e. for association with other plasmids, showed that a colicinogenic factor, which was identified as ColIa, was transferred en bloc with factor

R4K. Using HFCT system, we were able to get independent transfer of the col factor, deprived of the resistance plasmid; we have not, however, succeeded in separating the R factor from the col factor of this associated plasmid, even by use of treatment with curing agents.

All ten R factors of this study possessed, in addition to the A gene, the marker for streptomycin resistance, in most cases together with additional resistance-determinants. During the experiments of conjugal transfers, we selected the R+ clones of the newly infected recipients by A and S separately, and the phenotype of resistance of 100 of each of the A and S selected clones was tested in each experiment. Each of the 10 R factors was transferred to three, until more than six host strains, i. e. to F− K12, to Proteus PM1, to Hfr and F+ K12 (for the MS2 inhibition test) and half of them to Salm. typhi as well. Table 2 shows a rough summary from results of these transfer experiments, performed with conventional methods. It is seen that, under our experimental conditions with established cultures, our factors varied in the extension of the repression of their transfer activity; they could be distinguished to those which, in some crosses, reached almost derepression (transfer frequencies 10^{-1} or 10^{-2} per recipient population) and those which were in all crosses considerably repressed (transfer frequencies not exceeding 10^{-4}). Nevertheless, it is worth mentioning that, in both groups, a negative outcome of the transfer of all or some of their resistance-determinants was repeatedly found. The crosses which gave highest or lowest transfer frequencies varied also with the individual R factor. Though highest frequencies were found in most cases in crosses with K12R+ × K12R− derivatives and in crosses of K12 derivatives with Salm. typhi, in some cases they also occurred with PM1 cultures, PM1R+ cells, behaving as highly-efficient donors.

The data of Table 2 provide also some indications on the probable structure of these R factors, concerning the linkage of the A and S genes to each other, to their genes with sex factor activity, and to their remaining resistance determinants. It is seen that, in the above aspect, the 10R factors varied considerably. The only stable R factor, with definite linkage in all hosts of its two A and S resistance determinants, was factor R6K. Another R factor, R59K, was stable as far as the linkage of the A and S markers is concerned but not its remaining resistance genes. In the case of factor R8K the marker A was carried in an independent plasmid (fi− class) whereas the S marker, in close linkage with its remaining resistance genes, composed another plasmid of fi+ class. Factor R22K was exceptional in that it entered K12F− and Salmonella typhi with close association of the A and S markers and, then, in both hosts dissociated spontaneously to a nontransmissible replicon, carrying the gene A, and a transmissible plasmid carrying the marker S. The results obtained from the remaining R factors are consistent with Anderson's model, suggesting that the transfer factor and the resistance determinants may not be originally associated in one molecule, but might exist as independent replicons, potentially linked. Nevertheless, frequencies and patterns of dissociation of the resistance determinants of the above R factors exhibited during their conjugal transfer a dual, R factor and host-dependence. It is therefore suggested that, besides the differences in structure which influence the actual transfer, post-transfer conditions and events, determining the establishment of the entering plasmids to their new hosts, played also a fundamental role. This is shown in the following results: Two R factors, R4K and R28K, had their A gene closely linked to their transfer factor, whereas the transfer and establishment in their new host of their S marker, together with their accessory resistance determinants, depended on the sex factor of their A plasmid. With two other R factors (R59K, R102K), the host-dependence of the resistance patterns, found during their conjugal transfer, predominated. In general, K12 derivates and Salmonella typhi behaved similarly — whereas PM1 cells behaved differently — as hosts of the entering plasmids: for 5 out of the 10 R factors

Table 2

CONJUGAL TRANSFER FREQUENCIES OF THE R FACTORS, IN CROSSES OF DIFFERENT HOSTS, AND RESISTANCE PATTERNS OF NEWLY INFECTED R+ CLONES, SELECTED BY AMPICILLIN (A) AND STREPTOMYCIN (S)

R factors	Range of conjugal transfer frequencies	Crosses with — higher transfer	Crosses with — lower frequencies	Selection by	Resistance patterns of clones selected by A, in different hosts	Resistance patterns of clones selected by S
R4K	10^{-1} – n.d.	Salm. × K12F–; K12F– × K12Hfr	PM1 × K12F+ K12Hfr	A>S	A, 77–100% — K12, Salm., PM1	ASSu, 100%; SSu, 100% — K12, Salm., PM1
R6K	10^{-4} – 10^{-6}	Salm. × K12F–; PM1 × K12F+ K12Hfr	K12F– × K12F–; PM1	A=S	AS, 100% all hosts	AS, 100% all hosts
R7K	10^{-4} – n.d.	Pr. ret. × K12F–	K12F– × Prot. PM1	A<S	A, 90% K12F–	SSu. 100% — K12F–, PM1
R8K	10^{-3} – n.d.	K12F– × K12F+ K12Hfr	PM1 × K12F+ K12Hfr	A=S	A, 100% — K12F–, Salm.	CSSu, 85%; TCSSu, 15% — K12F–
R9K	10^{-3} – 10^{-7}	Wild E. coli × Salm.	PM1 × K12Hfr	A>S; A=S	ASC, 90%; A, 90% PM1 — K12F–, Salm.	AS, 100% or n.t. — K12
R22K	10^{-2} – n.d.	K12F– × Salm.; K12F– × PM1 (S)	Pr. mir. × Salm.; K12F– × K12F– K12Hfr PM1 (A)	A=S; A<S	AS, 100% — K12F–, Salm.	AS, 100%; S, 100% — Salm., K12F–, PM1, K12F+, K12Hfr
R28K	10^{-1} – 10^{-8}	PM1 × K12F– K12F+ K12Hfr	Citr. × Salm. (ASK); PM1 × K12Hfr (S)	A=S; A>S	A, 90% all hosts	AS, 65–100% all hosts
R59K	10^{-2} – 10^{-6}	PM1 × K12Hfr	Wild E. coli × PM1	A=S	AS, 100%; ASSu, 50–100% all hosts	n.t.
R62K	10^{-2} – n.d.	PM1 × K12Hfr	Klebs. × PM1	n.t.	A, 80% PM1; ASSu 50% K12; AS	n.t.
R102K	10^{-4} – n.d.	Citr. × PM1 K12F–	K12F– × K12Hfr	A>S; A<S	ACS, 60% K12F–; ACSSu, 100% K12Hfr	CS, 60% PM1

n.d.: not detectable   n.t.: not tested

248

(R4K, R7K, R9K, R59K and R102K) the segregants encountered in newly infected PM1R+ cultures were either not found or very rare in the other tested hosts. For 3 out of 10 R factors, it was imposible to introduce the A marker in PM1 host, whereas the remaining of their resistance-determinants were successfully transferred to this host. The mechanism involved in this failure may not be the same in all cases; we assume, however, that it is mostly due to a post-transfer event, leading to the exclusion of the A marker. Molecular studies have demonstrated recently that episomal molecules, which are found in K12 host with physical integrity, tend to dissociate in PM1 host (NISIOKA, MITANI and CLOWES (1969); (1970); HAAPALA and FALKOW (1971)). Breakages, separating in PM1 host the resistance determinants A from the genes coding for their replication and establishment, could account for the above exclusion.

Besides the above three cases, stability tests for the A marker performed in all PM1 R+ and K12R+ cultures, showed that in all R factors the plasmids carrying the A marker, once established in PM1 host, were permanently found in it; the same was observed with the A resistance-determinant of all R factors in K12 hosts.

Resistance to the β-lactam drugs conferred to the three hosts by the individual R factors.

The resistance of the R− and R+ cultures, towards 12 β-lactam drugs, was tested in solid media and with two inocula (2×10^3 and 2×10^5 bacteria per ml). The MICs from the light inoculum of the R− host strains are given in Table 3. All 6 F−, F+ and Hfr

Table 3

MINIMAL INHIBITORY CONCENTRATIONS OF THE b-LACTAM DRUGS FOR THE R− HOST CULTURES, TESTED WITH LIGHT INOCULA (10^3 BACTERIA PER ml)

b-lactam drugs	E. coli K12*	R− host strains Proteus PM1	Salmonella typhi
Benzylpenicillin	16	2	2
Ampicillin	1	0.25	0.12
Carbenicillin	2	0.5	0.5
6 – APA	16	16	8
Phenoxymethylpenicillin	62	62	62
Phenoxyethylpenicillin	125	125	8
Phenoxypropylpenicillin	125	125	8
Methicillin	125	30	62
Cloxacillin	125	500	125
Cephaloridine	1	1	0.5
Cephalothin	0.5	0.5	0.25
Cephalexin	4	4	4

* K12 derivatives = F− : 58161, RC85, RC711. F+ : W1655. Hfr C, Hfr H.

K12 derivatives, used in these experiments, had the same sensitivity to all β-lactam drugs and exhibited also the same changes in their R+ state. They will, therefore, be mentioned from now on as one host. It is observable that *Salm. typhi* in the R− state was more sensitive than the two other hosts to most b-lactam drugs, and that smaller differences were found in the MICs of R− K12 and R− PM1 cultures.

Table 4 shows the increase in resistance conferred to the above hosts by the acquisition of our R factors, expressed in ratios of the MICs of the R+:R− state for each culture. It is shown that each R factor determines the presence of a specific resistance pattern to the β-lactam drugs tested. This pattern — the same for all 9 out of the 10 R factors tested,

Table 4

Resistance patterns to the β- lactam drugs specified by the individual R factors, and R factors and host dependence of the magnitude of the changes introduced by each R factor.

R factors	R8K	R4K	R6K	R7K	R9K	R28K	R59K	R62K	R102K	R22K
				In E. coli K12 F⁻, F⁺, Hfr hosts						
		Class I				Class II				
Benzylpenicillin	250	125	125	16	16	32	32	62	32	8
Ampicillin	4000	1000	1000	125	250	250	250	500	125	32
Carbenicillin	8000	8000	8000	500	2000	2000	1000	2000	1000	4
6- APA	62	32	32	32	32	32	16	16	16	2
Phenoxymethylpenicillin	125	64	64	8	16	8	8	8	8	4
Phenoxyethylpenicillin	64	125	64	32	16	32	16	16	8	4
Phenoxypropylpenicillin	125	62	125	16	16	32	8	16	16	4
Methicillin	64	32	16	4	16	8	8	8	8	4
Cloxacillin	4	4	4	2	4	4	2	2	2	2
Cephaloridine	16	8	8	4	4	2	4	4	4	8
Cephalothin	16	8	8	8	4	4	4	4	4	250
Cephalexin	1	1	1	1	1	1	1	1	1	8

In Proteus PM1 host

	Class I		Class II					
Benzylpenicillin	500	8	8	4	4	4	8	
Ampicillin	4000	125	125	32	32	64	64	
Carbenicillin	1000	125	125	250	32	64	32	
6- APA	32	4	4	8	8	2	2	
Phenoxymethylpenicillin	32	2	2	2	2	2	2	
Phenoxyethylpenicillin	62	8	8	4	4	4	8	
Phenoxypropylpenicillin	62	8	4	4	4	4	8	
Methicillin	32	4	4	4	2	8	8	
Cloxacillin	2	2	2	2	1	1	1	
Cephaloridine	32	2	2	2	1	2	1	
Cephalothin	16	2	4	4	2	2	4	
Cephalexin	2	2	2	1	2	2	1	

In Salmonella typhi host

	Class I		Class II					
Benzylpenicillin	250	500	62	125				
Ampicillin	4000	8000	1000	1000				
Carbenicillin	16000	8000	4000	4000				
6- APA	62	62	32	62				
Phenoxymethylpenicillin	32	64	8	8				
Phenoxyethylpenicillin	1000	1000	250	125				
Phenoxypropylpenicillin	1000	2000	250	125				
Methicillin	32	64	32	16				
Cloxacillin	2	4	2	2				
Cephalorodine	4	16	8	4				
Cephalothin	8	16	8	4				
Cephalexin	1	1	1	1				

Resistance patterns to the β- lactam drugs specified by the individual R factors, and R factor and host dependence of the magnitude of the changes introduced by each R factor.

The figures in the Table are ratios of the M I C s of the R⁺ : R⁻ state for each culture.

and unusual for only one factor (R22K) — is not influenced by the host carrying the R factors, to a large extent. This common resistance pattern is characterized by degrees of resistance, decreasing in the following order: highest against carbenicillin, followed by ampicillin and benzylpenicillin, the other penicillins, 6APA and the cephalosporins were intermediate and with least changes, concerning resistance to cloxacillin and cephalexin. The difference in this pattern for the three hosts is: a) that in PM1 host resistance towards carbenicillin it was not considerably higher, or, in some cases, it was lower than the increase in resistance towards ampicillin; b) there was not any change detected towards cephalexin, as to the increase in resistance for all K12 and *Salm. typhi* R+ cultures, whereas the PM1R+ cultures had, in most cases, double MICs than in their R− state.

Factor R22K was unique in its pattern of resistance: it had the highest increase in resistance towards cephalothin and a considerable increase in resistance towards cephalexin.

The magnitude of the changes introduced by the acquisition of the R factors by the three hosts had apparently a dual R factor and host-dependence. Thus, in K12R+ cultures, three R factors (R8K, R4K, R6K, characterized as class I) conferred very high resistance levels and 6 R factors (R7K, R9K, R28K, R59K, R62K, and R102K, characterized as class II) conferred considerably lower resistance levels, although all 9R factors had the same resistance patterns. Factor R22K conferred also to K12R+ cultures rather low levels of resistance.

In PM1 host only one factor (R8K) was expressed as class I, conferring almost equally high resistance levels as in the K12R8K+ cultures. All other 6, out of 7, R factors, i. e. two of those expressed in K12R+ cultures as class I and 4 out of those expressed in K12 as class II, conferred to PM1 host considerably lower levels of resistance than in the K12R+ cultures, harboring the same R factors.

Salmonella typhi behaved as host similarly to K12 derivatives, the levels of resistance to the b-lactam drugs in K12R+ and *Salmonella typhi* R+ cultures — harboring the same R factors — being the same. Since *Salmonella typhi* was in the R− state more sensitive than the K12R− cultures, the increase in resistance found in *Salm. typhi* R+ was higher than in K12R+ cultures.

An existing difference in inoculum size of 10^2 bacteria per ml did not cause any inoculum size effect in all the K12R+ and *Salm. typhi* R+ cultures, for all the β-lactam drugs tested (MICs ratio for $10^5 : 10^3$ inocula = 1—2). In the PM1 R+ cultures and with the same differences in the inocula used there was a higher figure ($\geqslant 4$) for inoculum size effect, for 6APA and most of the penicillins tested.

Substrate profile and activity levels of the R factors β-lactamases

The results pertaining to enzymic activities of the R− and R+ cultures refer to assays performed with ultrasonically disrupted, late log phase (5 hour shaking) cultures, growing in CY 1% medium, tested with the iodometric method of Perret at 30° C and pH 7, expressed in Units per hour per mg dry weight of bacteria.

There was not any detectable hydrolytic activity in the R− *Salmonella typhi* culture; the K12R− and PM1R− strains had a slightly detectable activity ($\leqslant 0.3$ units) towards certain of the substrates tested, only.

The substrate profiles of the b-lactamases found in the R+ cultures are given in Table 5. The substrate specificity of the b-lactamases was always the same in the three hosts (K12, PM1, S. *typhi*), infected with the same R factor. It was also the same in the R+ cultures of these hosts harboring seven out of the nine R factors, exhibiting the same pattern of resistance to the β-lactam drugs. The β-lactamase of these seven R factors was active against penicillins and cephalosporins, hydrolysing ampicillin and cephaloridine at higher rates than benzylpenicillin and the remaining β-lactam substrates at lower rates, as shown in column (a) of Table 5. This substrate specificity has been reported in 1965 by DATTA and KONTOMICHALOU as characteristic of the episomal β-lactamases of two out of three R factors studied by them. One of these two R factors — R6K, previously

Table 5

β- lactam substrates	Relative rates of hydrolysis (%)					
	Common type β-lactamase	Specific β- lactamases of				
		Factor R9K	Factor R28K	Factor R22K	Wild donor of R7K I	Wild donor of R7K II
	a	b	c	d	e	f
Benzylpenicillin	100	100	100	100	100	100
Cephaloridine	115−160	77−88	130−146	280	348	1.1
Ampicillin	102−160	68−89	130−140	6.5	80	129
6- APA	70−110	65−82	82−89	3.4	34.8	5.1
Phenoxymethylpenicillin	39−75	49−60	48−52	39	62.5	101
Phenoxyethylpenicillin	22−32	21−28	38−48	7.4	6.7	50.5
Cephalothin	6−22	15−19	32−42	560	118	0.8
Phenoxypropylpenicillin	6−13.5	7−10	16−20	6	2.3	50.7
Carbenicillin	5−12	6−9.5	21−23	1	12	43.5
Cephalexin	2−11	1.2−2.2	5−10	34	n. t.	0.7
Cloxacillin	0.6−3.5	0.6−1.2	3−5.2	−	1.2	1.8
Methicillin	0.2−1.4	0.2−0.6	0.6−1.4	−	0.4	1.8

Substrate profiles of the β- lactamases of the R+ cultures tested.

a: found in all hosts infected with factors: R6K, R8K, R59K, R62K, R102K and in K12R7K+ culture.
b: found in all hosts infected with factors: R9K
c: found in all hosts infected with factors: R28K
d: found in K12R22K+ culture
e: found in the culture of donor Proteus 7KR+ in 1968
f: found in the culture of donor Proteus 7KR+ in 1971
n.t.: not tested

designated RTEM — is also included to the material of this communication. It was subsequently shown by other authors that β-lactamases of this substrate profile prevailed among the episomal penicillinases of R factors found in other countries, namely Japan and Britain (SAWAI et al. (1968); JACK and RICHMOND (1970)) and that they were also common as chromosomal penicillinases of a variety of Enterobacteriaceae (JACK et al. (1970)). Our results with R factors encountered in another country confirm the finding that episomal penicillinases are predominantly of the above type.

In further work, with purified, or crude enzyme preparations, where more characters were searched for, it has been shown that episomal β-lactamases of this common profile, which has been designated as type I, might differ in other characters and therefore they must not be considered always as the same enzyme (SAWAI et al. (1968); (1970); JACK et al. (1970)).

The substrate profiles of the remaining two β-lactamases of our R factors, with a common pattern of resistance to the b-lactam drugs was different, but not considerably, from the common type β-lactamase, as shown in Table 5. The 9 R factors of the same or similar b-lactamase substrate specificity have been found in nature in *E. coli* (4), *Citrobacter*

(2), *Klebsiella* (1), and *Proteus rettgeri* (2), from a wide range of sources, which is not the same as to the origin of episomal β-lactamases of the same type with that described by other authors (SAWAI et al. (1968); JACK et al. (1970)).

The last of our R factors (R22K), having the exceptional resistance pattern, also had a unique substrate profile: it was a cephalosporinase with the highest hydrolytic activity against cephalotin (cephalothinase). This R factor, with a substrate specificity which has not been reported for other episomal β-lactamases, had a *Proteus mirabilis* strain for

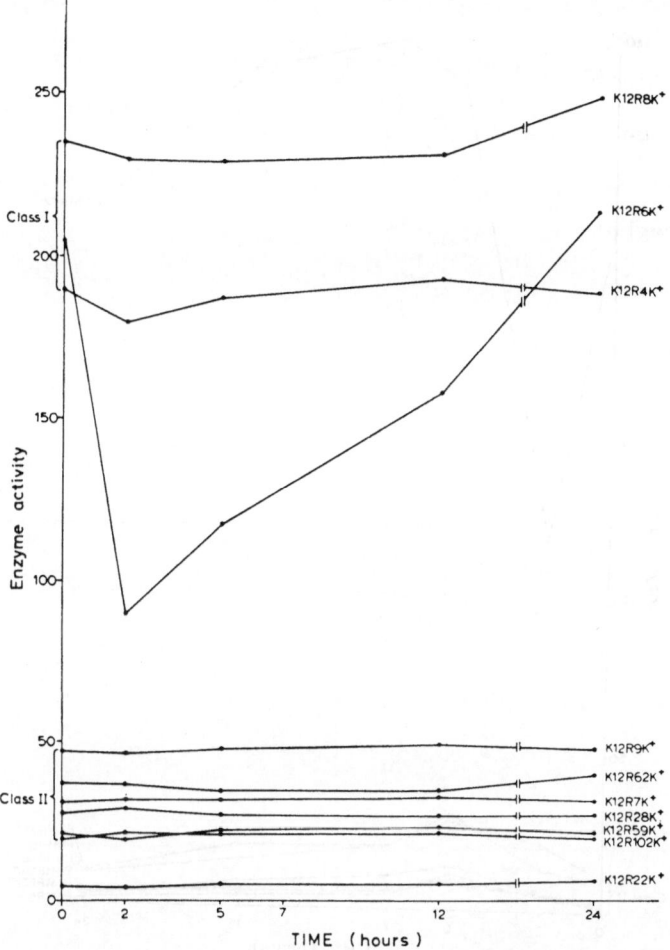

Fig. 1 Activity of β- lactamases from K12R+ cultures, at different stages of growth. Enzyme activity was assayed, with benzylpenicillin as substrate, as described in the text and expressed in units per mg dry weight of bacteria.

original host. Studies on the species-specific chromosomal penicillinases in *Enterobacteriaceae* have shown the existence of cephalosporinases as chromosomal enzymes of a variety of *Enterobacteriaceae*, but not of *Proteus mirabilis* (SAWAI et. al. (1968); JACK et al. (1970); OOKA, HASHIMOTO and MITSUHASHI (1970)). This is an indication that the R22K β-lactamase plasmid was foreign to its original host.

The specific activity of our R+ cultures in enzyme units per mg dry weight of organisms, when determined with benzylpenicillin as substrate, was found quite parallel to the increase in resistance introduced to all hosts by these R factors. Thus, the 6 R+ cultures of class I, i. e. 3 out of the 10 K12R+; 1 out of the 7 PM1R+; and 2 out of the 4 *Salm. typhi* R+ cultures had a specific hydrolytic activity of 100—300 units; the 6 K12R+ and 2 *Salm. typhi* R+ cultures of class II had an activity of 20—50 units; on the other hand, the activity of the remaining 6 PM1R+ cultures and that of the K12R22K+ strain ranged between 5—30 units (see later, Figures 1 and 2). Such a direct correlation between drug

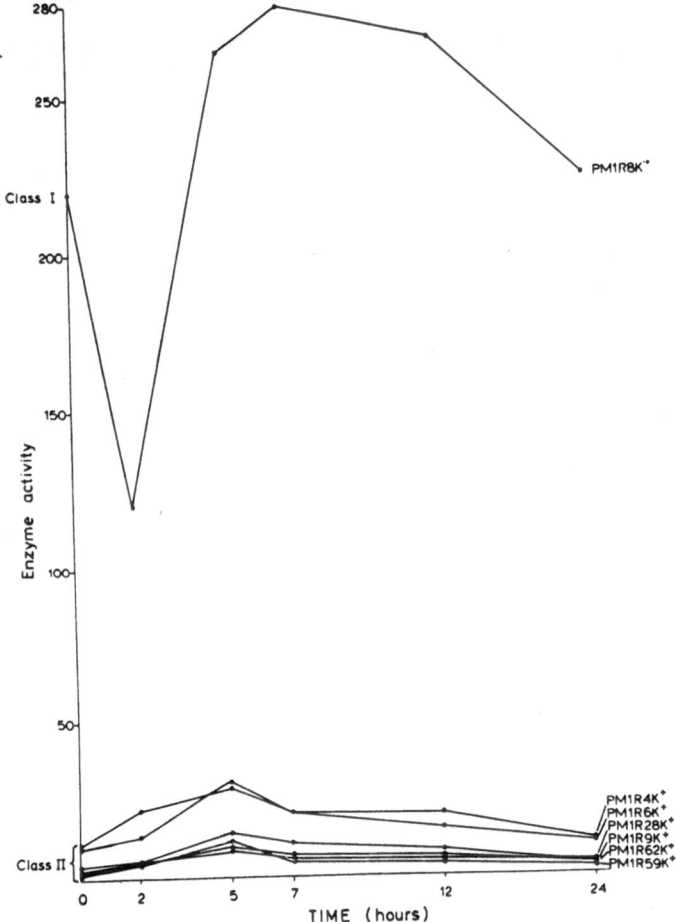

Fig. 2 Activity of β- lactamases from PM1R+ cultures at different stages of growth. Substrate benzylpenicillin.

destruction and levels of resistance conferred was not found for most of the other β-lactam drugs tested, and as far as the 9 factors of common pattern of resistance to the β-lactam drugs are concerned. Specifically, carbenicillin, towards which the highest degree of resistance was conferred by these 9 R factors, was hydrolysed by the R factors penicillinases at a very low rate, slightly higher from that of cephalexin, towards which no increase in resistance was conferred. In the case of factor R22K, with cephalosporinase specificity, the highest degree of resistance conferred as well as the highest hydrolytic activity, were towards the same drug cephalothin.

Tests for crypticity of the β-lactamases, performed by parallel estimation of the activity of undisrupted and disrupted R⁺ cultures, showed that the three cephalosporins and 6-APA were accessible to the ezymes in all hosts and with all R factors, whereas the penetration of the penicillins in the R⁺ cells was impaired. (Carbenicillin was not tested in this aspect.)

Resistance and β-lactamases of the wild strains, donors of the R factors, compared with the K12R⁺ cultures.

The wild E. coli donor strain 6KR⁺ and the K12R⁺ cultures harboring factor R6K were the same, as far as all four characters are concerned: the resistance pattern to the b-lactam drugs, the resistance levels, the substrate specificity and the absolute activity of β-lactamase. In all other cases, the wild strains —E. coli, Klebsiella, Citrobacter and Proteus — were more resistant and, in most cases, exhibited a different resistance-pattern from the K12R⁺ cultures harboring the same R factors. The substrate specificity of the β-lactamases of the donor strains in all other cases, except one, was the same with that of the enzymes of K12R⁺ — and all other hosts — carrying their R factors. Only in one case (factor R7K) the substrate specificity of the enzymes of the donor, Proteus rettgeri and the K12R7K⁺ culture, were different. As shown in Table 5, the donor culture hydrolysed the cephalosporins at a rate 3 to 5 times higher than the K12R7K⁺ culture, e. t. c. The presence of a second, non-transmissible enzyme, with a cephalosporinase specificity in the donor culture, masking the presence of the common-type episomal β-lactamase in this strain, could account for the above difference. The donor culture was repeatedly tested, always with negative results, for transferability of its cephalosporinase marker, while it was kept in stock culture, for years. Recently we came across a complete inversion in the substrate profile of the enzyme of this donor culture, which lost completely its cephalosporinase activity and acquired an unusual profile — shown in Table 5 — and an almost 20 times higher activity, as compared to that previously found in this culture.

Mutational changes of the substrate specificities of β-lactamases have been reported first by POLLOCK (1967) for strains of Bacillus licheniformis submitted to mutagen treatment and by SAWAI et al. (1968) for a strain of Escherichia freundii.

The absolute activity of the β-lactamases of the wild strains in most cases was the same with that of the K12R⁺ cultures, despite their differences in levels and patterns of resistance of these cultures. — For the sake of brevity we omit Tables referring to the wild strains (see KONTOMICHALOU (1971)).

Molecular properties of some of our R factors and correlation of these results to the resistance and the enzyme activity.

Two of the R factors of this material, namely factors R6K and R28K, expressed in K12 host as class I and II respectively, have been choosen for a molecular study of their properties. This work was done in the Division of Biology of the University of Texas at Dallas, and published by KONTOMICHALOU, MITANI and CLOWES (1970). It has been shown that the two R factors differed in the overall base composition of their DNA (R6K: G + C = 45%, R28K G + C = 50%), the contour length of their molecules (R6K = 12,8 µm, R28K = 21,6 µm) and the mode of their replication in K12 host. Factor R6K was found in a number of 13 copies in log phase, increasing in stationary phase to 38 copies per chromosome, whereas factor R28 was represented in the K12R⁺ cells by a small number of R copies, 2—3 per chromosome, stable in all phases of growth.

Thus these two R factors represent the two models of episomal replication, i. e. under relaxed and stringent control respectively in K12 cells. Factor R6K was the first R factor reported to have that type of replication in K12 host and an overall base composition distinct for R factor.

We have also shown that the specific activities of the β-lactamases, coded by these two R factors, measured either per mg dry weight of bacteria, or per mg of total protein, exhibited changes parallel to the number of copies of the R factors at different stages of growth of their K12R+ cultures. Thus the amounts of enzymes produced per gene were constant in all stages of growth of the above cultures and their difference in levels of enzyme and resistance was a direct consequence of the difference in number of R copies in the K12R+ cells.

Since it was found that changes of the presumably constitutive episomal enzymes paralleled the changes of episomal DNA, b-lactamase assays were used as an indirect approach for the investigation of possible changes of episomal DNA in K12 and PM1 hosts during growth.

The measurement of the specific β-lactamase activity in different stages of growth of all the K12R+ and PM1R+ cultures, tested with benzylpenicillin as substrate, are given in Figures 1 and 2 for the two hosts, respectively. It is seen that, among the K12R+ strains, the only culture with sharp decrease of its activity in log phase, followed by progressive increase towards the end of stationary phase, was strain K12R6K+. All other K12R+ cultures of high (class I), low (class II) or very low (K12R22K+) activity had, in all times of sampling, a stable specific activity measured either per mg dry weight or per mg of total protein and towards all the β-lactam substrates.

In PM1 hosts the β-lactamase of factor R8K (class I) exhibited a pattern of fluctuation in specific activity similar to that of K12R6K+ culture, characterised by the sharp decrease of its activity in log phase cultures. The difference in the fluctuation pattern of K12R6K+ and PM1R8K+ cultures was that a fall in its activity was found in the stationary phase of the latter. The remaining six PM1R+ cultures had their own pattern of fluctuation of their penicillinases, which was different from that of the K12R+ cultures, and in which the same fall of activity in stationary phase cultures with that in PM1R8K+ strain occurred. Tests for the appearance of R− clones or of extracellular enzyme activity in this phase of growth were negative and, thus, it seems that an apparent fall in the production of enzymes takes place in PM1R+ cells at the stationary phase.

The results of the above experiments show a dual, R factor and host dependence of the fluctuation on β-lactamase specific activity during growth.

These findings, when interpreted on the basis of variations of enzyme biosynthesis during growth, besides other biological implications suggest that experimental attempts, to correlate episomal DNA with enzyme activity and levels of resistance should preferably take place not with late stationary phase cultures.

In this respect, the direct dye buoyant density centrifugation technique was used to separate episomal from chromosomal DNA. This technique was applied as described by NISIOKA, MITANI and CLOWES (1970) with a modification only in the radioisotope counting procedure. Middle stationary phase cultures, of K12 F− (RC85) and PM1 carrying factors R8K, R6K, R4K (col Ia) and R28K, were labeled for several generations with ³H-thymidine and then subjected to the above procedure. Cultures K12R6K+ and K12R28K+, which had been also used before with the above method and a PM1R− culture were included as controls for this technique. A good resolution between a main DNA band (host chromosomal DNA) and a heavier satellite band, (episomal DNA), separated due to their differential bindings to ethidium bromide, has been achieved in 18 out of 22 experiments performed (82%). The distance between the chromosomal and the heavier, satellite band (table 6) was in the cultures tested for the first time, identical to that found in the control R+ cultures, for which it was previously proved that the satellite band consisted of episomal molecules. This finding provides a good evidence that with

Table 6

RELATIVE POSITIONS AND RADIOACTIVITY PERCENTAGE OF DNA BANDS, SEPARATED BY CsCl EQUILIBRIUM DENSITY GRADIENT CENTRIFUGATION IN THE PRESENCE OF ETHIDIUM BROMIDE, FROM CRUDE, ^{3}H-THYMIDINE LABELED LYSATES, OF E. COLI RC85 AND PM1 STRAINS, CARRYING DIFFERENT R FACTORS

Cultures	Experiment	Franction number		Peak fraction of		Distance of peaks in fractions	Radioactivity of satellite to chromosomal band %	Class*
		Satellite band	Chromosomal band	Satellite band	Chromosomal band			
K12R28K+	1	7—13	14—21	9	15	6	2.32	II
K12R8K+	1	7—12	13—23	10	16	6	1.40	I
K12R8K+	2	13—19	20—32	16	23	7	6.92	I
K12R8K+	3	10—16	19—26	11	20	9	10.90	I
K12R6K+	1	5—10	14—21	7	15	8	16.21	I
K12R4K+col Ia+	1	5—13	14—23	9	16	7	14.00	I
K12R4K+col Ia+	2	1—8	9—27	7	12	5	4.80	I
PM1R8K+	1	9—13	14—24	12	18	6	0.67	I
PM1R8K+	2	11—17	22—31	15	24	9	1.26	I
PM1R8K+	3	3—10	11—21	8	13	5	2.52	I
PM1R6K+	1	11—16	20—28	13	21	8	5.40	II
PM1R4K+col Ia+	1	4—11	12—27	9	15	6	0.59	II
PM1R28K+	1	14—18	19—27	16	21	5	0.81	II

* Phenotype of β- lactamase activity and resistance to the penicillins.

the use of the above technique, episomal DNA in the form of covalently closed circular molecules has been separated from the chromosomal DNA of all the above K12R+ and PM1R+ cultures. Our first impression was that a difference in unsuccessful experiments between PM1R+ and K12R+ cultures was significantly greater for PM1 host, however by increasing the number of our experiments, this aspect was ruled out. The unsuccessful experiments consisted in either a fragmentation of the single heavy satellite band to several heavy peaks, or in a doubtful resolution between the two bands, or in disappearence of the satellite band. The latter case was accompanied by a heavily labeled, usually fragmented shoulder or tail of the main band.

The radioactivity curves obtained with certain cultures of K12R+ and PM1R+ strains are presented in Fig. 3 and 4 respectively. Table 6 shows the percent H³ labeling of satellite to chromosomal bands for each culture as well as the distances between the two radioactive peaks.

It is obvious that no satellite band was detected in PM1R⁻ culture. The percent labeling of satellite bands in the K12R+ cultures, used as controls, was for K12R28K+ the same as previously found (2,3%) and for K12R6K+ at a lower limit of that expected with this strain (16,21%), less than half of what we previously found with it in stationary phase cultures.

In the strains examined for the first time, K12 host posessing the associated plasmid R4KcolIa (resistance and enzyme of K12R4K+ = class I) gave a percent satellite labeling in one experiment of the same order with that found in K12R6K+ cultures

(14%), but in another experiment it gave a much lower proportion (4,8%). Factor R8K, which conferred to both K12 and PM1 hosts high levels of enzyme and resistance (class I), was manifested in both hosts with a low proportion of episomal to chromosomal labeling, ranging in K12R8K+ cultures from 1,40 to 10,90% and in PM1R8K+ cultures from 0,67

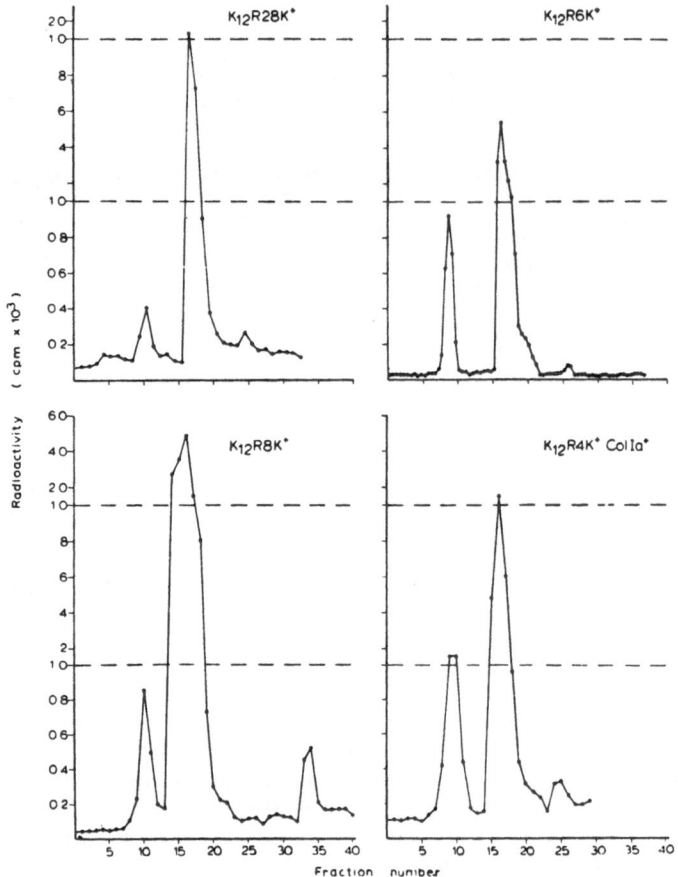

Fig. 3 Fractionation of DNA from K12(RC85)R+ strains. The cultures were incubated for several generations with H³-thymidine and the sarkosyl lysate from the washed cells was subjected to buoyant density cesium chloride centrifugation in the presence of ethidium bromide, in a Beckman preparative ultracentrifuge, Model L, and a fixed angle rotor, type 50. After centrifugation at 40 000 rpm for 60 hours fractions of 8 drops were collected from the bottom of the tube and diluted with TES buffer (0.4 ml). 0.1 ml was used for radioactivity counting in 10 ml mixture of equal volumes of INSTA-GEL (Packard Cat. No 6002173) and of distilled water in a Packard Liquid Scintilation Counter.

to 2,52%. Thus, in general, there was a wide range in the episomal to chromosomal labeling in different experiments of each culture. The three PM1R+ cultures of class II examined, PM1R6K+, PM1R4K colIa+ and PM1R28K+ had proportions of episomal labeling 5,4% 0,59% and 0,81% respectively.

If it is assumed that the episomal and chromosomal DNAs in each host have the same specific radioactivity, then radioactivity ratios could be directly interpreted to DNA ratios for each R+ culture. With this assumption the above results would indicate a) that the amount of episomal DNA in R+ cells varies considerably from experiment to experiment for each culture; b) that of all cultures studied, K12R6K+ culture possesses the higher load of episomal DNA and c) that the amount of episomal DNA in PM1R+ cells is for all plasmids studied less than that of the K12R+ cells, harboring the same R factors.

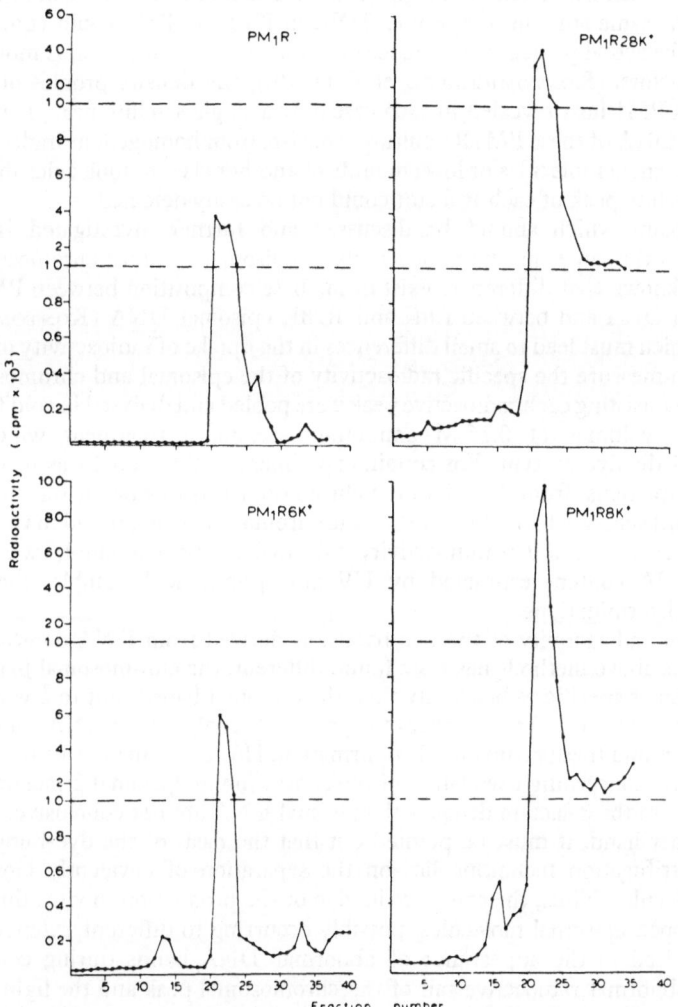

Fig. 4 Fractionation of DNA from PM1R- and PM1R+ cultures. Other experimental conditions are the same as described in Fig. 3.

The difference found on episomal labeling between K12R+ and PM1R+ cultures harboring factors R6K, R28K and the composite plasmid R4KcolIa are broadly parallel to the differences in β-lactamase specific activity between these two cultures. This would mean that the amount of the β-lactamase enzymes produced per R factor copy (gene dose) is broadly the same for K12 and PM1 hosts, harboring each R factor. Therefore these R factors, with a lower proportion of episomal DNA in PM1 than in K12 cells, behave in this aspect in the opposite way as compared to what other authors have

259

found with other R factors (ROWND et al. (1966) ROWND (1969), FALKOW et al. (1969)).

However, recent molecular studies, pointing out to the dissociating tendency of R factors in PM1, have shown that the dissociated small replicons are met in PM1R+ cells in different ratios of copies per chromosome (FALKOW, HAAPALA and SILVER (1969). COHEN (1969). HAAPALA and FALKOW (1971)). Therefore, if our factors dissociate in PM1 host, the same amount of episomal DNA in K12 and PM1 could contain different numbers of the actual penicillin-resistance determinants. In our previous molecular study of these R factors, (KONTOMICHALOU et al. (1970)), the density profiles of factor R6K and R28K in PM1 host revealed in each case only a single satellite peak, hence probably the episomal DNA of these PM1R+ cultures consists from homogenous molecular species. Nevertheless, small molecules or low amounts of another class of molecules masked under the single satellite peak of each R factor could not be easily detected.

Another point which should be discussed and further investigated is the initial assumption on the same specific radioactivity of episomal and host chromosomal DNAs. It is already known that differences exist in the base composition between PM1 and K12 chromosomal DNA and between R6K and R28K episomal DNA (KONTOMICHALOU et al. (1970)) which must lead to small differences in the uptake of radioactivity of thymidine.

In order to measure the specific radioactivity of the episomal and chromosomal bands the fractions consisting each radioactive peak were pooled and dialysed in cold for 48 hours, against large volumes of 0.15 M ammonium acetate, a treatment which removed 80—100% of the dye present. For certain experiments a third pool was made also from a number of fractions, from the tail of the chromosomal band when it was highly labeled or, from a third separate band, lighter than the chromosomal one, found in the sedimentation profiles in some cases. The radioactivity of the dialysed pooled samples was remeasured and their DNA content estimated by UV absorption, acid soluble phosphate and deoxyribose determinations.

The specific radioactivity of the two bands, as derived from DNA determinations by all three of the above methods has been found different, the chromosomal bands showing as a rule a higher specific radioactivity than the episomal bands, but to a variable extent for the different cultures. The number of experiments analysed for DNA content is small at the moment, and these results need confirmation. However, due to this fact, the results presented here, concerning correlation of the expression of episomal β-lactamase activity and resistance to the β-lactam drugs with episomal DNA are not conclusive.

On the other hand, it must be pointed out that the basis of the dye-buoyant density gradient centrifugation technique lies on the separation of covalently closed circular episomal molecules. Thus, the existence in vivo or the production in vitro during lysis or shearing of open episomal molecules, possibly occurring to different extents in the two hosts, could lead to the appearance of abnormal DNA bands during centrifugation. Indeed the abnormal radioactive tail of the chromosomal peak and the light radioactive peaks, observed in certain experiments were found to consist of considerable amount of DNA, but of unknown as yet identity. This fact should be taken into consideration in the evaluation of the differences found in the episomal labeling of the present study.

Our results are not adequate yet to explain the function of factor R8K, conferring to both K12 and PM1 hosts the same high levels of β-lactamase specific activity, while it had a rather low proportion of episomal H^3 labeling in K12 host and still lower in PM1 cultures. We are reluctant to come up with any conclusion on the decrease in enzyme activity in log phase cultures found in the pattern of the β-lactamase during growth of the PM1R8K+ culture. This R factor, upon further investigation will probably show that codes for an enzyme of high specific activity, similar to that already found by SAWAI et al. (1970), designated by them as type Ib.

A point connected with our study also requiring further investigation, is the question whether the episomal resistance to the penicillins is only of enzymatic origin. We have shown that our cultures of type I, conferred huge levels of resistance to carbenicillin, although this substrate was hydrolysed by their enzymes at a very low rate. Single colonies of the R^+ cultures tolerated also very high levels of most of the β-lactam drugs tested, a fact which seems to be irrelevant to enzymatic resistance. These findings provide an indication that the R factors inside their host cells, in addition to their function in the hydrolysis of the β-lactam drugs, may confer resistance through an other mechanism. If R factor products become involved into the mucopeptide forming system, substituting penicillin-sensitive cell-wall synthetising systems, they could confer to the R^+ cells a considerable degree of "intrinsic" in addition to their enzymic resistance. If the non-enzymatic resistance is expressed to a different degree in the different host bacteria, this could account for the inability of $PM1R^+$ cells to become as highly resistant to carbenicillin, as $K12R^+$ and *Salmonella typhi* R^+ cells.

In conclusion, the similarity between K12 derivatives and *Salmonella typhi* and their difference to PM1 as hosts of the R factors of the above study must be attributed to evolutionary relations of these species.

SUMMARY

The R factors conferring resistance to the β-lactam drugs, have been investigated each one in two to four different bacterial hosts. Genetic study of the R factors, levels of resistance and hydrolytic activity, resistance patterns and substrate specificities to the β-lactam drugs, pointed out to the peculiarities of the individual R factors and the host dependence of the expression of some of the above functions. As a rule, K12 derivatives and *S. typhi* behaved as R factors' hosts similarly, and *Proteus* PM1 differently. Wild donor bacteria also behaved as a rule each one differently in the expression of the episomal resistance to the β-lactam drugs.

Type I β-lactamases predominated in the above material, but one transmissible cephalosporinase has been also found. The β-lactamase of one donor strain mutated during our experiments from a predominately cephalosporinase to complete loss of activity towards cephalosporins.

The resistance pattern to the β-lactam drugs, specified by the β-lactamases type I, was characterised by high degree of increase in resistance towards carbenicillin, associated with low rate of hydrolysis of this substrate.

Levels of enzyme and resistance to the penicillins were R-factor and host dependent and as a rule in PM1 host were lower than in the other hosts harboring the same R factors. Low level episomal β-lactamases predominated in our material.

The specific activity of β-lactamases expressed by the ten R factors was measured during growth in two hosts. It was found that the fluctuation of activity, as a function of the age of the culture, was both, R factor and host dependent.

The ethidium bromide — density gradient centrifugation technique was used to separate episomal from chromosomal DNA, labeled with ^{3}H-thymidine. This technique was applied to $K12R^+$ and $PM1R^+$ strains carrying four out of the ten R factors and to $PM1R^-$ culture. Attempts have been made to correlate the results of the above technique with episomal β-lactamase and penicillin resistance findings.

Acknowledgments

This work was suppored by grants from: a) the World Health Organisation, grant No R/00022, and b) the Wellcome Foundation.

REFERENCES

ANDERSON E. S. (1969): Ecology and epidemiology of transferable drug resistance. Symposium on: Bacterial Episomes and Plasmids. Ciba Foundation, ed. by Wolstenholme G. and O'Connor, M. Churchill, London: 102—115.

BURMAN, L. G., NORDSTRÖM, K. and BOMAN, N. G. (1968): Resistance of Escherichia coli to penicillins. V. Physiological comparison of two isogenic strains, one with chromosomally and one with episomally mediated ampicillin resistance. Journal of Bacteriology 96: 438—446.

COHEN, S. (1969): Isolation and characterization of R factor DNA. Bacteriological Proceedings, 49.

DATTA, N. and KONTOMICHALOU, P. (1965): Penicillinase synthesis controlled by infectious R factors in Enterobacteriaceae. Nature. 208: 239—242.

DATTA, N. and RICHMOND, M. H. (1966): The purification and properties of a penicillinase whose synthesis is mediated by an R factor in Escherichia coli. Biochemical Journal. 98: 204—209.

FALKOW, S., HAAPALA, D. K. and SILVER, R. P. (1969): Relationships between extrachromosomal elements. Symposium on: Bacterial Episomes and Plasmids. Ciba foundation. ed. by Wolstenholme G. and O'Connor M., Churchill, London, 136—158.

HAAPALA, D. and FALKOW, S. (1971): Physical studies on the Drug Resistance Transfer Factor in Proteus. Journal of Bacteriology, 106: 294—295.

JACK, G. W. and RICHMOND, M. H. (1970): A comparative study of eight distinct b-lactamases synthesized by gram-negative bacteria. Journal of Bacteriology, 61: 43—61.

KONTOMICHALOU, P. (1967a): Studies on resistance transfer factors. Pathologia et Microbiologia. 30: 71—93.

KONTOMICHALOU, P. (1967b): Studies on resistance transfer factors. II. Transmissible resistance to eight antibacterial drugs in a strain of Escherichia coli. Pathologia et Microbiologia. 30: 185—200.

KONTOMICHALOU, P. (1967c): Transmissible extrachromosomal resistance to the penicillins in E. coli K12 and Falkow's Proteus host. 5th International Congress of Chemotherapy. C2/5: 251—255.

KONTOMICHALOU, P. (1971): R factors controlling resistance to the penicillins. Habilitation Thesis. Athens.

KONTOMICHALOU, P., MITANI, M. and CLOWES, R. C. (1970): Circular R factor molecules controlling penicillinases synthesis, replicating in Escherichia coli under either relaxed or stringent control. Journal of Bacteriology, 104: 34—44.

LINDQVIST, C. and NORDSTRÖM, K. (1970): Resistance of Escherichia coli to penicillins. VII. Purification and characterization of a penicillinase mediated by the R Factor R1. Journal of Bacteriology. 101: 232—239.

NISIOKA, T., MITANI, M. and CLOWES, R. C. (1969): Composite circular forms of R factors deoxyribonucleic acid molecules. Journal of Bacteriology. 97: 376—385.

NISIOKA, T., MITANI, M., and CLOWES, R. C. (1970): Molecular recombination between R factors deoxyribonucleic acid molecules in Escherichia coli host cells. Journal of Bacteriology. 103: 166—177.

OOKA, T., HASHIMOTO, H., and MITSUHASHI, S. (1970): Comparison of penicillinases produced by R factors isolated from ampicillin-resistant gram negative bacteria. Japanese Journal of Microbiology. 14: 123—128.

POLLOCK, M. R. (1967): Origin and function of penicillinase: a problem in biochemical evolution. British Medical Journal 4: 71—77.

ROMERO, E. and MEYNELL., E. (1969): Covert fi⁻ factors in fi+ R+ strains of bacteria. Journal of Bacteriology. 97: 780—786.

ROWND, R. (1969): Replication of a bacterial episome under relaxed control. Journal of Molecular Biology. 44: 387—402.

ROWND, E., NAKAYA, R. and NAKAMURA, A. (1966): Molecular nature of the drug resistance factors of the Enterobacteriaceae. Journal of Molecular Biology. 17: 376—393.

SAWAI, T., MITSUHASHI, S. and YAMAGISHI, S. (1968): Drug resistance of enteric bacteria. XVI. Comparison of b-lactamases in gram negative rod bacteria resistant to aminobenzyl penicillin. Japanese Journal of Microbiology, 12: 423—434.

SAWAI, T., TAKAHASHI, K., YAMAGISHI, S. and MITSUHASHI, S. (1970): Variant of penicillinase mediated by an R factor in Escherichia coli. Journal of Bacteriology. 104: 620—629.

YAMAGISHI, S., O'HARA K., SAWAI, T. and MITSUHASHI, S. (1969): The purification and properties of penicillin b-lactamases mediated by transmissible R factors in Escherichia coli. The Journal of Biochemistry. 66: 11—20.

BETA-LACTAMASE GENE EXPRESSION IN ENTERIC BACTERIA INFECTED WITH R-FACTORS

M. M. BOBROWSKI, D. DZIERZANOWSKA, M. LACHMAJER and
J. BOROWSKI

University Medical School, Białystok and University Medical School, Gdańsk, Poland.

Resistance to ampicillin and to other β-lactam antibiotics has been reported in many R-factor harbouring enteric bacteria including strains of *Salmonella* (ANDERSON and DATTA, 1965; DATTA and KONTOMICHALOU, 1965; LACHMAJER, 1970), Shigella (TANAKA, NAGAI, SAWAI, HASHIMOTO and MITSUHASHI, 1966; quoted by SAWAI, MITSUHASHI and YAMAGISHI, 1968; DAVIES, FARRANT and TOMLINSON, 1968), E. coli (DATTA and KONTOMICHALOU, 1965; EGAWA, SAWAI and MITSUHASHI, 1967; SAWAI et al., 1968; EVANS, GALINDO, OLARTE and FALKOW, 1968) and Pseudomonas (LOWBURY, KIDSON, LILLY, AYLIFFE and JONES, 1969; SYKES and RICHMOND, 1970; FULLBROOK, ELSON and SLOCOMBE, 1970).

The studies of DATTA and KONTOMICHALOU (1965) have shown that the resistance is due to β-lactamase formation and the ability to produce the enzyme may be transferred from the donor to the recipient strains by conjugation. Further investigations of DATTA and RICHMOND (1966) and by other authors (YAMAGISHI, O'HARA, SAWAI and MITSUHASHI, 1969; LINDQVIST and NORDSTRÖM, 1970; SAWAI, TAKAHASHI, YAMAGISHI and MITSUHASHI, 1970; NEU and WINSHELL, 1970; DALE and SMITH, 1971; DALE, 1971) resulted in purification and determination of properties of several distinct types of β-lactamases, the synthesis of which was episomally-mediated by R-factors.

It has been demonstrated that the activity of β-lactamase mediated by particular R-factor is similar, though not absolutely identical, for a number of host species as E. coli, Salmonella, Klebsiella, Serratia, Alkalescens and Shigella (DATTA and KONTO-MICHALOU, 1965; KONTOMICHALOU, 1967; SMITH, 1969; MEDEIROS and O'BRIEN, 1968, NEU and WINSHELL, 1970). Some of the β-lactamases specified by the same R-factors when harboured by different host gave been consequently purified by NEU and WINDSHELL (1970) and as well as by DALE (1971). The results obtained by the authors revealed that practically all the physico-chemical characteristics including specific activities, molecular weights, kinetic constants, substrate profiles and electrophoretic mobilities, were very same for different preparations of the same R-factor mediated β-lactamase.

In contrast, great differences have been found when the levels of β-lactamase activity controlled by the same R-factor gene were compared in E. coli and Proteus mirabilis hosts (KONTOMICHALOU, 1967; SMITH, 1969; NEU and WINSHELL, 1970). Namely, the specific activities of the enzyme synthesized in P. mirabilis cells were from 20 to 100 times lower than those produced in E. coli cells.

In order to clarify the reason for the extremely low activity in P. mirabilis DALE and

SMITH (1971) have obtained highly purified preparations of the β-lactamase and compared the properties of this preparations derived from *E. coli* and that from *P. mirabilis* cultures. The data presented by the authors lead to conclusion that the same enzyme is synthesized in both hosts but the amount of the active enzyme produced per cell is much more higher in *E. coli* than in *P. mirabilis*. Furthermore, the presence of relatively high amounts of proteins which were hardly separated from the β-lactamase in preparations obtained from *P. mirabilis* culture, strongly suggests that some errors in transcription of the R-factor DNA by *Proteus* RNA polymerase are involved.

Recent studies of KONTOMICHALOU, MITANI and CLOWES (1970) have shown that the regulation of the R-factor replication is different in both hosts being more relaxed in *P. mirabilis* and less relaxed or more stringent in *E. coli*. Thus, the impaired regulatory system in *P. mirabilis* is probably unable to control the β-lactamase synthesis. In our previous studies (LACHMAJER and BOBROWSKI, 1969; BOBROWSKI and LACHMAJER, 1970) it has been found that β-lactamases activities in E. coli K12 populations carrying R-factor transferred from a given Salmonella donor strains varied widely from clone to clone being at the same time different from those activities of original isolates.

The present work was undertaken to investigate the levels of expression of the R-factor mediated β-lactamase genes when they are transferred into the hosts which either do not produce any considerable amounts of the enzyme or synthesized already other β-lactamase.

Table 1

BACTERIAL STRAINS CARRYING R-FACTORS

R-factor	Species in which isolated	Resistance pattern transferred	Reference
R 11	S. typhimurium	AST	Lachmajer
R 14	S. typhimurium	AST	(1970)
R 17	S. enteritidis	ASCTN/K	
R 19	S typhimurium	AST	
R 21	S. enteritidis	ASCTN/K	
R 31	S. sonnei	ACT	Borowski
R 35	S. sonnei	ACT	et. al.
R 38	S. sonnei	ACT	(1971)

A — ampicillin S — streptomycin C — chloramphenicol T — tetracycline N — neomycin
K — kanamycin

The R-factor donors used are listed in Table 1. In addition, the resistance patterns of the strains are presented.

The transfer of the R-factors into E. coli K12 recipients was performed as previously described (LACHMAJER, 1970). For the introduction of the R-factors into the Pseudomonas aeruginosa strains a selective medium containing acetamide, 2%, to prevent the growth of the donor cells, and carbenicillin, 200 μg/ml, to inhibit the growth of the unconverted recipient cells, were employed.

Since our preliminary experiments have indicated that with some organisms the enzyme activity was increased until the culture reached the stationary phase of growth, the bacterial cells obtained from a 12-hr culture were used with the aim of preparing cell-free β-lactamase samples. The activities of β-lactamases in the samples using benzylpenicillin, ampicillin and cephaloridine as substrates were measured by the modified hydroxylamine method (BOBROWSKI and LACHMAJER, 1970) and were expressed in the terms of the international enzyme units per mg of protein. One unit is equivalent to 1 μmole of substrate hydrolysed per 1 minute at 30 C and pH 7.0 and corresponds to 60 cnits expressed according to POLLOCK and TORRIANI (1953). Every determination was repeated five times at least using different batches of culture and the results presented as their average values. Substrate profiles were calculated and expressed in the manner described by JACK and RICHMOND (1970).

Table 2

ACTIVITIES AND SUBSTRATE PROFILES OF R FACTOR-MEDIATED
β-LACTAMASES IN THE ORIGINAL CULTURES AND IN E. COLI K 12 CULTURES

R-factor	Original host			E. coli K12 host		
	Specific enzyme activity (units per mg protein)	Relative rates of hydrolysis P A C		Specific enzyme activity (units per mg protein)	Relative rates of hydrolysis P A C	
R 11	1.90 ± 0.16	100 115 78		0.54 ± 0.10	100 104 73	
R 14	2.52 ± 0.23	100 110 89		0.96 ± 0.13	100 108 98	
R 19	2.21 ± 0.22	100 110 78		2.12 ± 0.21	100 110 80	
R 17	3.15 ± 1.07	100 104 74		6.12 ± 0.69	100 109 80	
R 21	4.09 ± 1.50	100 116 86		6.22 ± 0.83	100 116 89	
R 31	0.66 ± 0.07	100 135 66		0.65 ± 0.02	100 138 62	
R 35	0.685± 0.07	100 106 77		0.595± 0.03	100 100 75	
R 38	0.555± 0.03	100 126 88		0.45 ± 0.01	100 114 84	

Table 2 compares the specific activities of the R-factor β-lactamases in the original cultures and in *E. coli K12* cultures. The levels of the enzyme activity in the E. coli K12 cultures which acquired the R-19, R-31, R-35 and R-38 R-factors were the same as in the original isolates. After introduction of the R-17 and R-21 R-factors frcm parent *S. enteritidis* strains into the *E. coli* K12 recipient, however, the β-lactamase activity apparently increased being about 1.5 times or twice as high as in the respective donors. This finding may suggest that the number of R-factor copies should be different in the hosts and that the replication of these R-factors is more relaxed in *E. coli* than in *S. enteritidis*. On the other hand, the activity of the enzymes specified by the R-11 and R-14 factors in the E. coli K12 host represented only 28.5 and 38 per cent, respectively, of the activity exhibited by the original *S. typhimurium* donors. In this case, the release of a repressor the action of which was more pronounced in E. coli than in *S. typhimurium* hosts is offered to explain the decrease in the rate of the β-lactamase synthesis.

It should be noted that apart from the variations in the levels of β-lactamase activity no differences in the substrate profiles of the enzyme mediated by the same R-factor were observed.

Significant differences in the β-lactamase activity have been found when the R-factors were transferred into the three *P. aeruginosa* strains (Table 3). For example, the expression of the activity of the β-lactamase mediated by the R-factor R-31 was ten times higher in the *P. aeruginosa* P77 than in the *P. aeruginosa* P72 recipients. In contrast, the activity of the enzyme specified by the R-21 R-factor was much lower in this former host than in that latter.

A considerable shift in substrate profile has been observed when the relative rates of hydrolysis of ampicillin or of cephaloridine were compared in the original host and in the *P. aeruginosa* strains which acquired an R-factor. For instance, the β-lactamase mediated by the R-31 R-factor has a substrate profile of 100:135:66 when it is synthesized in the parent *Sh. sonnei* host, while the over-all substrate profile of 100:92:85 in one

P. aeruginosa host or of 100:112:101 in the other was demonstrated. Thus, the relative rates of hydrolysis of ampicillin lowered in P. aeruginosa hosts, the same time as the rates of cephaloridine hydrolysis enhanced.

Table 3

ACTIVITIES AND SUBSTRATE PROFILES OF R FACTOR-MEDIATED
β-LACTAMASES IN THREE P. AERUGINOSA STRAINS

R-factor	Enzyme activity in host culture (units/mg protein)			Relative rates of hydrolysis (benzylpenicillin: ampicillin: cephaloridine)		
	P 72	P 77	P 96	P 72	P 77	P 96
R 21	5.65	1.87	3.09	100:118:88	100:104:103	100: 99:98
R 19	0.72	2.00	—	100:105:80	100:110:105	—
R 31	0.64	5.75	—	100: 94:92	100:111: 71	—
R 35	0.40	1.47	—	100: 92:85	100:112:101	—
R 38	0.715	—	1.20	100:111:93	—	100:117:96

The P. aeruginosa recipients used produced themselves undetectable amounts of β-lactamase until they were induced. After induction with benzylpenicillin at the concentration of 1 mg/ml the enzyme activity of the strains was of the order of 0.4 units/mg of protein. The enzymes were predominantly active against cephalosporins and the relative rates of hydrolysis were as follows: benzylpenicillin — 100, ampicillin — from 6 to 30, and cephaloridine — about 400.

All these facts mentioned above lead to conclusion that in *P. aeruginosa* strains infected with R-factors there are two different components; one with broad-spectrum β-lactamase or penicillinase activity which is characteristic of R-factor mediated enzymes, and second with preferential cephalosporinase activity which is chromosomally mediated and species-specific. Moreover, considering that practically no enzyme is produced in uninduced *P. aeruginosa* cultures, it may be predicted that introduction of an R-factor into *P. aeruginosa* cells results in stimulation of species-specific β-lactamases.

The β-lactamase activities were also determined in R-factor harbouring bacteria superinfected with another R-factor. Such organisms carrying two R-factors were obtained due to the fact that the R-11 and R-14 R-factors lacked the chloramphenicol and neomycin/kanamycin resistance markers which were carried by the R-17 and R-21 R-factors.

The results achieved are summarized in Table 4.

Table 4

β-LACTAMASE ACTIVITIES IN E. COLI K 12 STRAINS CARRYING R-FACTORS
BEFORE AND AFTER ACQUISITION OF ANOTHER R-FACTOR

R-factor in E. coli K 12 host	Enzyme activity before acquisition of another R-factor*)	Enzyme activity after acquisition of another R-factor*)	
		R 17	R 21
R⁻ (control)	0.01	6.12 + 0.69	6.22 + 0.83
R 11	0.54 + 0.10	3.64 + 1.06	4.40 + 0.86
R 14	0.96 + 0.13	2.63 + 0.78	4.39 + 0.84

*) μmoles of benzylpenicillin hydrolysed at 30 °C and pH 7.0 per min. per mg protein

The levels of the β-lactamase activity in the cultures of the *E. coli* K12 carrying two R-factors were obviously higher than the activity of enzymes mediated by the R-11 and R-14 R-factors in the same host. This indicates that the superinfection was effective. On the other hand, the activities in the *E. coli* K12 strains infected with two R-factors were lower than in the same host carrying the superinfecting R-17 or R-21 R-factors. Two possible explanations therefore arised. First — the repressor associated with the R-11 and R-14 R-factors still reduces the rates of the β-lactamases synthesis mediated by the R-17 and R-21 R-factors. Second — it may be speculated that in S. enteritidis R-17 and R-21 there are two distinct R-factors controlling β-lactamase production and only one of them is compatible with the R-11 or R-14 R-factors. No evidence for that latter hypothesis has been so far produced.

In conclusion, the results of the present studies indicate that many efforts will be needed to elucidate all the problems reported here.

Acknowlegments

The authors are grateful for the technical assistance of Mrs. Nina Chamienia, and Mrs. Elzbieta Markiewicz.

REFERENCES

ANDERSON E. S. and DATTA N. (1965): Resistance to penicillins and its transfer in Enterobacteriaceae. Lancet, **1**, 407.

BOBROWSKI M. and LACHMAJER M. (1970): The transfer of intrinsic resistance to penicillins mediated by an R-factor. Archivum Immunologiae et Therapiae Experimentalis, **18**, 225.

DALE, J. W. (1971): Characterization of the β-lactamase specified by the resistance factor R-1818 in E. coli K12 and other gram-negative bacteria. Biochemical Journal (in the press).

DALE J. W. and SMITH J. T. (1971): The purification and properties of the β-lactamase specified by the resistance factor R-1818 in Escherichia coli and Proteus mirabilis. Biochemical Journal (in the press).

DATTA N. and KONTOMICHALOU P. (1965): Penicillinase synthesis controlled by infectious R factors in Enterobacteriaceae. Nature, **208**, 239.

DATTA N. and RICHMOND M. H. (1966): The purification and properties of a penicillinase whose synthesis is mediated by an R-factor in Escherichia coli. Biochemical Journal, **98**, 204.

DAVIES J. R., FARRANT W. N. and TOMLINSON A. J. (1968): Further studies on antibiotic resistance of Shigella sonnei. Journal of Hygiene, **66**, 479.

EGAWA R., SAWAI T. and MITSUHASHI S. (1967): Drug resistance of enteric bacteria. XII. Unique substrate specificity of penicillinase produced by R factor. Japonese Journal of Microbiology, **11**, 173.

EVANS J., GALINDO E., OLARTE J. and FALKOW S. (1968): β-Lactamase of R factors. Journal of Bacteriology, **96**, 1441.

FULLBROOK P. D., ELSON S. W. and SLOCOMBE B. (1970): R-factor mediated β-lactamase in Pseudomonas aeruginosa. Nature, **26**, 1054.

JACK G. W. and RICHMOND M. H. (1970): A comparative study of eight distinct β-lactamases synthesized by gram-negative bacteria. Journal of General Microbiology, **61**, 43.

KONTOMICHALOU P. (1967): Transmissible extrachromosomal resistance to the penicillins in E. coli K12 and Falkow's Proteus host. Proceedings of the V-th International Congress of Chemotherapy (Viena), **4**, 251.

KONTOMICHALOU P., MITANI M. and CLOWES R. C. (1970): Circular R-factor molecules controlling penicillinase synthesis, replicating in Escherichia coli under either relaxed or stringent control. Journal of Bacteriology, **104**, 34.

LACHMAJER M. (1970): Infectious resistance to antibiotics in Salmonella strains isolated in Poland. Medycyna Doświadczalna i Mikrobiologia, **22**, 10.

LACHMAJER M. and BOBROWSKI M. (1969): The nature of resistance to penicillins mediated by R-factor. Archivum Immunologiae et Therapiae Experimentalis, **17**, 633.

LINDQVIST R. C. and NORDSTRÖM K. (1970): Resistance of Echerichia coli to penicillins. VII.

Purification and characterization of a penicillinase mediated by the R-factor RI. Journal of Bacteriology, **101**, 232.

LOWBURY E. J. L., KIDSON A., LILLY G. A. J., AYLIFFE G. A. J. and JONES R. J. (1969): Sensitivity of Pseudomonas aeruginosa to antibiotics: emergence of strains highly resistant to carbenicillin. Lancet, **2**, 448.

MEDEIROS A. A. and O'BRIEN T. F. (1968): R factor-mediated increments in levels of resistance to and enzymatic degradation of penicillins and cephalosporins. Antimicrobial Agents and Chemotherapy, **7**, 271.

NEU H. C. and WINSHELL E. B. (1970): Characterization of penicillinases of various Enterobacteriaceae in which synthesis is episomally mediated. Archives of Biochemistry and Biophysics, **139**, 278.

SAWAI T., MITSUHASHI S. and YAMAGISHI S. (1968): Drug resistance of enteric bacteria. XIV. Comparison of β-lactamases in gram-negative rod bacteria resistant to α-aminobenzylpenicillin. Japanese Journal of Microbiology, **12**, 423.

SAWAI T., TAKAHASHI K., YAMAGISHI S. and MITSUHASHI S. (1970): Variant of penicillinase mediated by an R factor in Escherichia coli. Journal of Bacteriology, **104**, 620.

SMITH J. T. (1969): R-factor gene expression in gram-negative bacteria. Journal of General Microbiology, **55**, 109.

SYKES R. B. and RICHMOND M. H. (1970): Intergeneric transfer of a β-lactamase gene between Ps. aeruginosa and E. coli. Nature, **226**, 952.

TANAKA T., NAGAI Y., SAWAI T., HASHIMOTA H., and MITSUHASHI S. (1966): Transferable resistance to aminobenzylpenicillin derived from Shigella strains isolated in Japon. Japanese Journal of Bacteriology, **21**, 591.

YAMAGISHI S., O'HARA K., SAWAI T. and MITSUHASHI S. (1969): The purification and properties of penicillin β-lactamases mediated by transmissible R factors in Escherichia coli. Journal of Biochemistry (Tokyo), **66**, II.

INVESTIGATIONS OF THE MOLECULAR STRUCTURE
OF R-FACTORS

S. N. COHEN

Department of Medicine Stanford University School of Medicine, Stanford, California

P. A. SHARP and N. DAVIDSON

Gates-Crellin-Church Laboratories of Chemistry California Institute of Technology,
Pasadena, California U.S.A.

INTRODUCTION

During the twelve years that have elapsed since appearance of the first Japanese reports of transfer of drug resistance among different species of Enterobacteriaceae by cell-to-cell contact (OCHIAI, YAMANAKA, KIMURA and SAWADA (1959); AKIBA, KOYAMA, ISHIKI, KIMURA and FUKUSHIMA (1960); WATANABE and FUKASAWA, (1960)), the biological and medical importance of R-factors has become increasingly evident. Extensive genetic studies carried out in a number of laboratories throughout the world have established that transfer of multiple resistance to a variety of antibiotics is mediated by autonomously replicating units of inheritance which are functionally and physically distinct from the bacterial chromosome. The genetic properties of R-factors and their biological interactions with host bacteria and with other extrachromosomal elements have been the subject of a number of recent reviews (WATANABE, (1963), (1971); MEYNELL, MEYNELL and DATTA (1968); ANDERSON (1968); NOVICK (1969); BOUANCHAUD (1969); MITSUHASHI (1970)); many of the reports presented at this Symposium have concerned the genetic and epidemiological aspects of R-factors.

During the past few years, there has been increasing emphasis in certain laboratories on investigations of the molecular nature and more generally, the *molecular biology* of R-factors. In part, such studies have been stimulated by the anticipation that an understanding of the biology of R-factors in molecular terms may lead to methods for control of drug resistance by selective inhibition of R-factor replication, by interference with R-factor genetic expression, by prevention of R-factor formation, or by suppression of transfer of drug resistance. Investigations carried out in our laboratory have been concerned with defining how R-factors are constituted, what their molecular relationship to other extrachromosomal elements is, how they originate, and how they regulate synthesis of the DNA, RNA, and protein required for the transfer and expression of drug resistance. The present communication reviews certain of these experiments.

Over the years there has been considerable controversy about the molecular nature of R-factors (ANDERSON, (1969); WATANABE (1969)). Transduction experiments which WATANABE and FUKASAWA (1960) carried out a decade ago led these investigators to propose that R-factors consist of a transfer unit (RTF segment), that controls transmission of the plasmid, linearly linked (as shown in Figure 1A) to drug resistance determinants, which carry genetic information specifying resistance to antimicrobial agents. Later studies by Anderson and his collaborators (ANDERSON and LEWIS (1965); ANDERSON

(1966)) showed that the transfer units of at least certain classes of R-factors can be transmitted alone (Figure 1B) as well as in combination with resistance determinants. Furthermore, Anderson and his colleagues found that ordinarily non-transmissible R-determinants can interact with transfer units (although not necessarily covalently as depicted in this figure), which are then able to accomplish transfer of resistance by con-

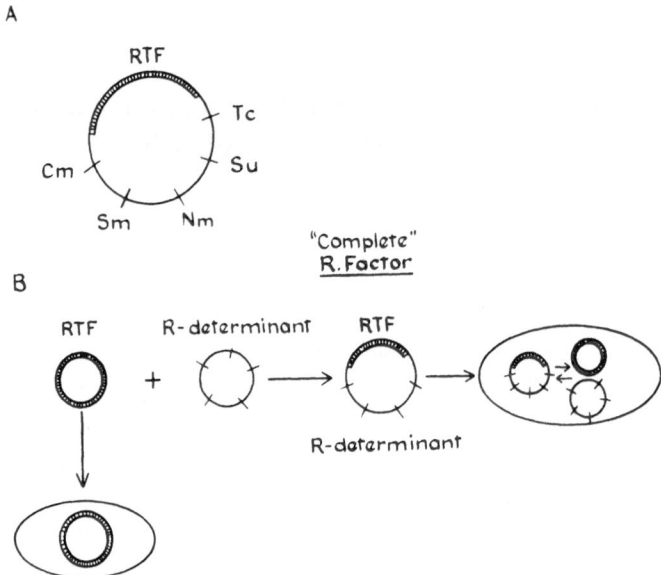

Fig. 1 Models for the molecular structure of R-factors. (A) Watanabe and Fukasawa model (1961) showing covalent linkage between transfer (RTF) unit and resistance determinant unit of R-factor. (B) Variation of Anderson and Lewis (1965) model, showing autonomously replicating transfer and R-determinant units able to interact with each other, and also showing the ability of RTF unit to be transferred separately. In Class I R-factors (see text) the interaction between the transfer and R-determinant units occurs by covalent linkage in *E. coli.*

jugation. Once within the recipient cell, the linked transfer and resistance units can replicate autonomously.

The earliest studies of the molecular nature of R-factors, which were carried out by Falkow and by Rownd and their respective collaborators (FALKOW, CITARELLA, WOHL-HIETER and WATANABE (1966); ROWND, NAKAYA and NAKAMURA (1966)), indicated that heterogeneous satellite bands of DNA are associated with the presence of R-factors in *Proteus mirabilis* and certain other bacterial species. However, because the plasmid DNA was not intact in these studies, it could not be determined whether the several component bands of R-factor satellite DNA identified by cesium chloride centrifugation reflected intramolecular heterogeneity within a single fragmented R-factor species, or whether R-factor DNA in *Proteus* consists of functionally associated but physically distinct subunits. More recently developed procedures have made it possible to obtain high molecular weight DNA from bacteria by detergent lysis and phenol extraction (DAVERN (1966); BAZARAL and HELINSKI (1968)), and to accomplish separation of DNA species having only small differences in nucleotide base composition (NANDI, WANG and DAVIDSON (1966)).

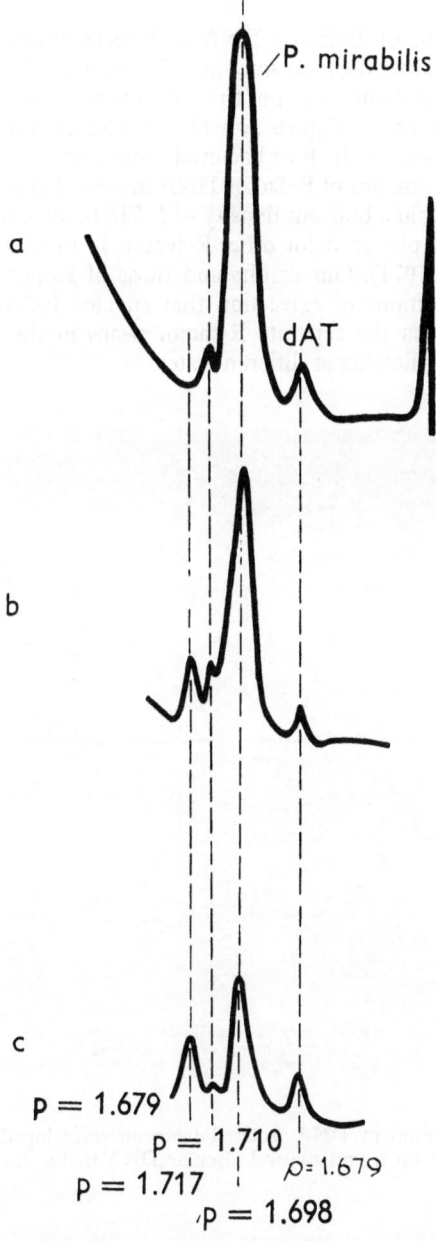

Fig. 2 Cesium chloride centrifugation of DNA isolated from *Proteus mirabilis* (PM 1) carrying the R-factor R6. The conditions for bacterial growth and isolation of DNA have been described elsewhere (Cohen and Miller, (1970a)). High molecular weight DNA was isolated by detergent lysis of (a) early logarithmic phase culture (cell density $= 3 \times 10^8$/ml), (b) late log phase-early stationary phase culture (cell density $- 1 \times 10^9$/ml), or (c) culture which had been shaking for eight hours in stationary phase. d(A$-$T) polynucleotide polymer was used as a density marker ($\rho = 1.679$ gm/cm^3).

Molecular Nature of R-Factors in Proteus mirabilis

Our initial investigations of R-factor DNA in *Proteus* (COHEN (1969); COHEN and MILLER (1970a)) indicated that the total amount of R-factor DNA and the relative amount of each of the satellite band components of this DNA varied markedly at different stages of bacterial growth, as seen in Figure 2, which shows cesium chloride equilibrium centrifugation DNA profiles. As the host bacterial growth proceeded from logarithmic to stationary phase, the total amount of R-factor DNA increased and the component peak of this satellite DNA banding at a buoyant density of 1. 718 became increasingly prominent. Similar findings have been observed for other R-factors in *Proteus* by ROWND (1970) and by KOPECKO and PUNCH (1971). Our results and those of KOPECKO and PUNCH, which were obtained using conditions of extraction that enabled isolation of high molecular weight DNA suggested that the separate R-factor peaks might represent autonomous DNA units which were replicating at different rates.

Fig. 3 Electron photomicrograph of DNA isolated from an early logarithmic phase culture of PM 1—R6. This field shows open and twisted circular DNA molecules having contour lengths of 5 μm and 28 μm.

Using the cesium sulfate-mercury gradient centrifugation technique that was developed by NANDI et al. (1965), we resolved the 1.710 peak into two separate DNA species. Additional study of the 1.718 peak indicated that it consisted of a homogenous DNA species. Electron photomicrographs of each of the separated R-factor DNA component species showed non-linear molecules appearing as both closed, tightly twisted coils and relaxed (open) circles (Figure 3). The contour lengths and buoyant densities observed for the largest of the three circular DNA species (Table 1) agreed with those values that would result from the joining of two smaller units of the observed buoyant densities and contour lengths. Most simply interpreted, these findings suggested that the large DNA circle might represent a composite of the two smaller units. Similar conclusions were reached independently by NISIOKA, MITANI, and CLOWES (1969) for other R-factors, and by SILVER and FALKOW (1970) for R1.

Table 1

SUMMARY OF R-FACTOR SPECIES ISOLATED FROM *PROTEUS MIRABILIS*

Buoyant Density in CsCl gm/cm^3	R-Factor		
	R6	R1	
	Contour Length	Contour Length	Calculated MW
$\varrho = 1.709$	26 $-31\,\mu$	28 $\pm 1\ \mu$	55 $\times 10^6$ daltons
$\varrho = 1.711$	31 $-38\,\mu$	33 $\pm 0.8\,\mu$	65 $\times 10^6$ daltons
$\varrho = 1.717-1.718$	3.8$-7\ \mu$	5 $\pm 0.5\,\mu$	9.5 $\times 10^6$ daltons

Table 1. Summary of R-factor DNA species isolated from *Proteus mirabilis*. The conditions for calculation of buoyant densities in CsCl and for determination of contour lengths have been described elsewhere (Cohen and Miller, (1970a)). Approximate molecular weights of R1 DNA species were calculated from contour lengths using a relationship of 1.96 daltons per μm (MacHattie, Berns and Thomas, (1965)). Values shown for contour lengths indicate one standard deviation. As indicated previously, substantial heterogeneity was observed for R6 but not for R1 DNA molecules.

R-Factor DNA Species Isolated from E. coli

The methods used to accomplish separation of R-factor DNA from *Proteus* could not be used in *E. coli*, since the buoyant densities of the *E. coli* chromosome and R-factor DNA are virtually identical. However, the circularity of R-factor DNA provided a means of achieving this separation (COHEN and MILLER (1969)). Vinograd and his collaborators have shown that covalently closed circular DNA has enhanced resistance to both heat and alkali denaturation, and that the interaction of closed circular DNA with ethidium bromide and certain other intercalative dyes enables its separation from linear or from nicked circular DNA. These properties of circular R-factor DNA were utilized for its identification and isolation in *E. coli* (COHEN and MILLER (1969). As seen in Figure 4, the buoyant density of a non-denaturable circular fraction of the DNA isolated from the R$^+$ host remained unchanged as a consequence of treatment at pH 12.3, while the density of the major chromosomal portion of the DNA increased following alkali treatment. No non-denaturable DNA fraction was observed in the R$^-$ host. As shown in part (e) of this figure, preparative centrifugation of tritium-labeled DNA from the R$^+$ host in the presence of ethidium bromide revealed a peak banding at a buoyant density shown by Vinograd and his collaborators (VINOGRAD, LEBOWITZ, RADLOFF, WATSON and LAIPIS (1965); RADLOFF, BAUER and VINOGRAD (1967)) to be characteristic of covalently closed circular DNA. The R$^-$ host showed only chromosomal DNA. This technique and the bulk nitrocellulose absorption procedure which we have described elsewhere (COHEN and MILLER (1969)) enabled us to physically separate circular DNA from the *E. coli* chromosome for electron microscope and ultracentrifugation studies.

In contrast to the three distinct R-factor DNA species found in *Proteus*, we observed that more than 98% of the closed circular DNA isolated from *E. coli* carrying either R1 or R6 was contained in a single class of closed and relaxed circular molecules banding at a buoyant density of 1.711 gm/cm^3, and having a molecular weight of approximately

65×10^6 daltons. The predominant molecular species isolated from *E. coli*, which is shown in Figure 5, expressed both resistance and transfer functions of the R-factor in this host, and was indistinguishable in buoyant density and molecular weight from the largest of the three R-factor species identified in *Proteus*.

These findings also were consistent with the view that at least certain R-factors are formed by reversible covalent linkage of plasmids that separately harbor either resistance or transfer functions. CAMPBELL (1969) has suggested that the apparently conflicting genetic experiments of WATANABE on one hand and of ANDERSON on the other can be

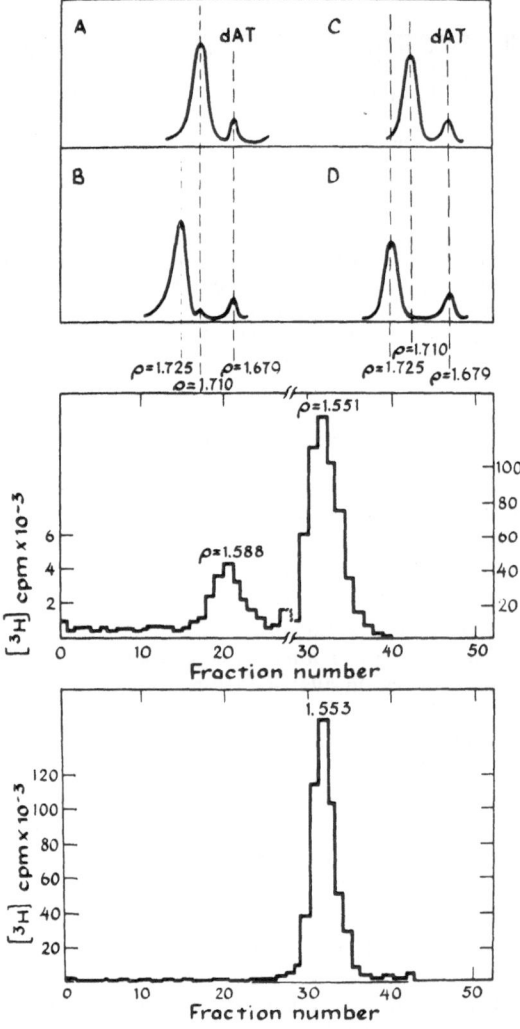

Fig. 4 Identification and isolation of closed circular R-factor DNA from *E. coli*. Analytical centrifugation of C34—R6 DNA (a) before treatment with NaOH at pH 12.3, and (b) following treatment. DNA isolated from the R⁻ parent strain and centrifuged under identical conditions is shown before alkali treatment (c), and after alkali treatment (d). (e) Preparative centrifugation of C34—R6 DNA labelled with methyl-³H-thymidine, isolated by detergent lysis, and centrifuged in cesium chloride in the presence of ethidium bromide, as previously reported (Cohen and Miller, (1970a)). Preparative centrifugation of DNA isolated from the R⁻ parent strain is shown in (f).

reconciled by a model which is formally similar to the one proposed for integrative recombination of the temperate bacteriophage λ into the *E. coli* chromosome (CAMPBELL (1962)). According to this scheme, in *Proteus* the RFT and R-determinant units can exist as independently replicating plasmids, as well as in combination with each other to form

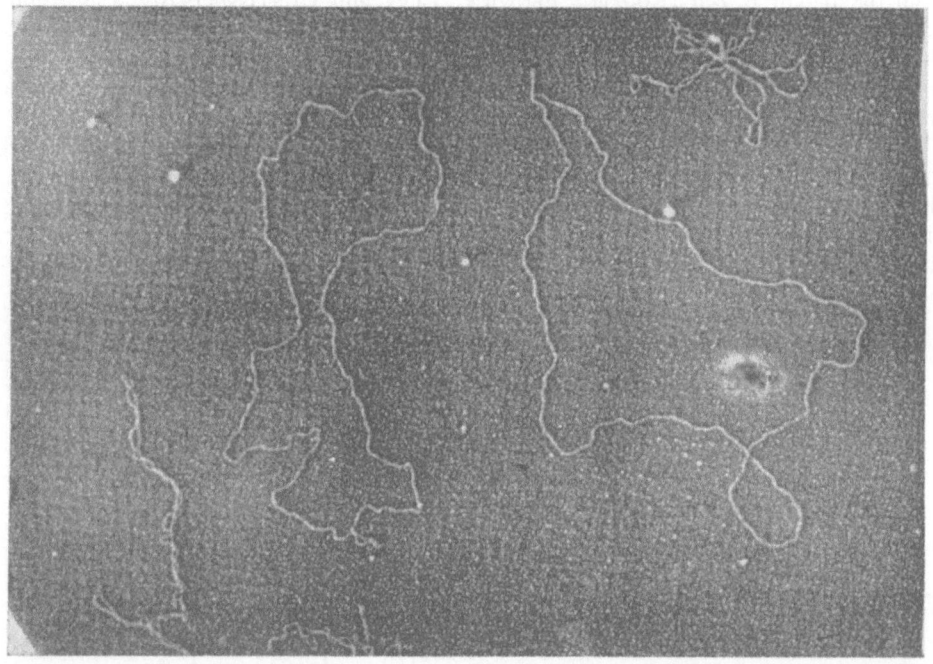

Fig. 5 Circular R-1 DNA isolated from *E. coli*.This DNA species, which was present as both covalently closed, tightly twisted coils and nicked or open circles, represented more than 98% of the total circular DNA obrained from *E. coli* carrying the R-factor R1. The average length of 20 open circular molecules measured $33 \pm 1 \mu$m, which is equivalent to a molecular weight of 65×10^6 daltons.

the "complete R-factor". In *E. coli* on the other hand, covalent association of RTF and R-determinant plasmids into the complete R-factor is more stringently controlled and little dissociation occurs.

Recent work by Anderson and Clowes (personal communication) has suggested that there are two different molecular classes of R-factors: Class I R-factors demonstrate covalent bonding between the R-determinant and transfer-factor plasmids in *E. coli*, but the two units are dissociable in certain other bacterial species. In Class II R-factors, the component plasmids remain independent of each other and occupy different cellular attachment sites, even in *E. coli*. All of the R-factors we have described here belong to Class I.

Catenated Forms of R-Factor DNA

Although the ethidium bromide-cesium chloride centrifugation and nitrocellulose absorption methods have proved useful for isolation of circular R-factor DNA from *E. coli*, these procedures necessarily select against other (non-circular) forms of R-factor

DNA that might also be present. Recently, we have utilized the "minicell" mutant of *E. coli* described by Adler and his collaborators (ADLER, FISHER, COHEN and HARDIGREE (1967)) for isolation of R-factor DNA species by biological rather than physical means (COHEN, SHARP, SILVER and McCOUBREY (1971a & b)). R-factors and other plasmids can segregate into minicells at the time when these spheres are budded off from the parent *E. coli* (ROOZEN, FENWICK, LEVY and CURTISS (1970); LEVY and NORMAN (1970); INSELBURG (1970), (1971); KASS and YARMOLINSKY (1970); ROOZEN, FENWICK and CURTISS (1971); COHEN et al (1971a & b)), and the minicells (which contain the R-factor but lack chromosomal DNA) can then be separated from normal sized *E. coli* by sequential differential and sucrose gradient centrifugation.

Study of R-factor DNA isolated from minicells led to our discovery that commonly studied R-factors such as R1 and R6 can exist in catenated form, as well as in the covalently closed circular forms that we and others had previously observed. As VINOGRAD and his collaborators have shown (HUDSON and VINOGRAD (1967); CLAYTON and VINOGRAD (1967)), catenanes consisting of closed circular DNA molecules which are topologically

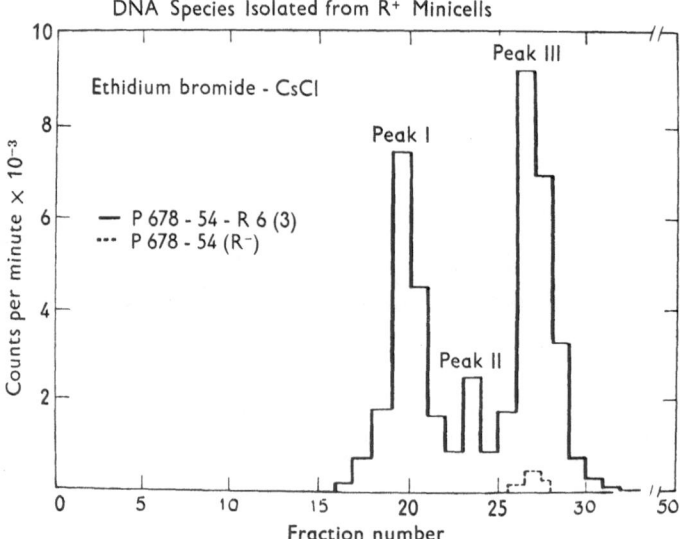

Fig. 6 Ethidium bromide-cesium chloride centrifugation profile showing an intermediate-banding peak containing catenated R-factor DNA isolated from *E. coli* minicells. Peak I contained closed circular monomeric and catenated (see Figure 8) forms of R-factor DNA. Peak II consisted primarily of catenated (interlocking) circular R-factor DNA molecules in doubly open and singly open form. Peak III contained open monomeric circles as well as some linear DNA fragments. A small amount of DNA was obtainable from R⁻ minicells (dotted line), and this consisted entirely of linear fragments banding at the same position as Peak III. Procedures used for isolation and purification of minicells, and for centrifugation, collection, and assay of ³H-labelled DNA have been described elsewhere (Cohen et al (1971b)).

linked to open or nicked circular molecules band at a buoyant density in ethidium bromide-cesium chloride gradients which is intermediate to the densities of closed circular and non-circular DNA. Figure 6 shows such a catenated R-factor DNA peak in a preparation of R6 (3) DNA isolated from *E. coli* minicells. Similar peaks of catenated R-factor DNA were obtained from minicells carrying R6, R1, and R100. Catenated DNA has previously been observed in mitochondrial DNA preparations obtained from several sources (Pikó, Blair, Tyler and Vinograd (1968)), and in *Salmonella* infected with phage P22, but the molecular mechanism of catenane formation is presently unknown. It is of interest, however, that an fi⁻ penicillinase-producing plasmid which has the unusual ability to replicate under relaxed control in *E. coli* also can exist in catenated form (Kontomichalou, Mitani and Clowes (1970)).

Figure 7 shows an electron photomicrograph of catenated R-factor DNA molecules

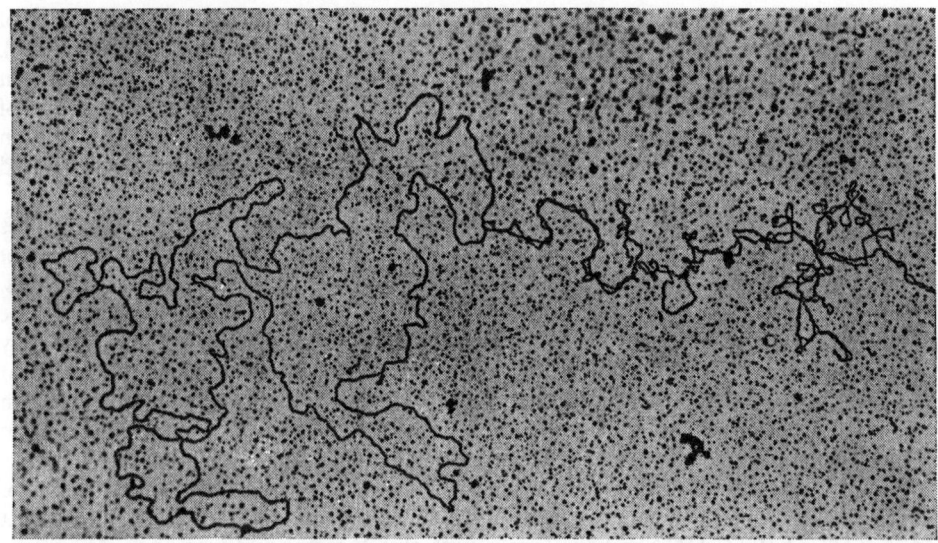

Fig. 7 Electron photomicrograph of catenated R6(3) DNA molecules isolated from *E. coli* minicells. The catenane shown consists of a closed circular supercoiled molecule interlocked with an open, nicked circular molecule. The conditions used for preparation of DNA samples for electron microscopy have been described by Davis, Simon, and Davidson (1971).

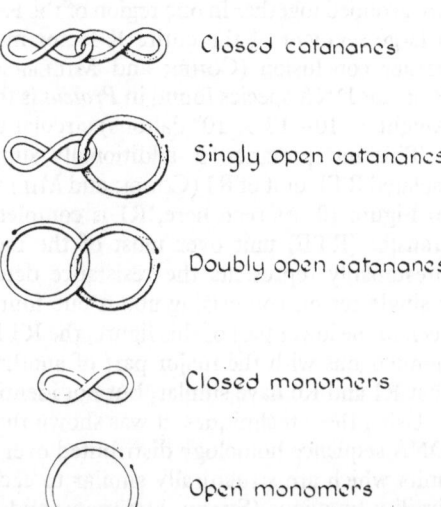

Molecular Forms of R6-(3) DNA

Closed catenanes

Singly open catenanes

Doubly open catenanes

Closed monomers

Open monomers

Fig. 8 Diagrammatic representation of the various forms of R6(3) DNA isolated from *E. coli* minicells. Monomeric and catenated forms in combinations of closed and open circles are represented here. The most prevalent forms observed were monomers (Cohen *et al* (1971)).

277

isolated from *E. coli* minicells. This catenane consists of a closed supercoiled circular molecule interlocked with an open nicked circular molecule. In addition to such catenanes consisting of interlocking nicked circular and closed circular molecules, other forms of R-factor DNA were also isolated from minicells (COHEN *et al.* (1971a & b)). These are shown diagrammatically in Figure 8.

Electron Microscope Heteroduplex Studies of R-Factor DNA Sequence Homology

Some time ago, we were able to isolate and purify the separated transfer units of R-factors R1 and R6 from antibiotic-sensitive *E. coli* (COHEN and MILLER (1970a & b)). These studies showed that each RTF unit had a size and buoyant density identical to that of the satellite DNA peak banding at 1.709 in *Proteus* and having a molecular weight of aproximately 55×10^6 daltons. It was thus concluded that the $10-12$ million dalton R-factor DNA species, which could replicate independently but could not be transferred as a separate entity represented the resistance determinant unit.

Recently, we have been using the electron microscope heteroduplex techniques described by DAVIS and DAVIDSON (1968) to study the molecular relationship of R-factor component units to each other, to different R-factors, and to other plasmids. With this technique, homologous regions of two different DNA species can be distinguished as double-stranded segments of DNA, whereas areas of non-homology appear as single DNA strands. Thus, the procedure enables localization of regions of homology and non-homology present in different plasmids and provides information which is useful in understanding the molecular relationship of various R-factors and R-factor component units to each other, and to other bacterial plasmids.

Figure 9 shows an electron photomicrograph and tracing of a DNA-DNA hybrid of R6(3) and an F-factor. It was determined from this and similar photomicrographs that $44 \pm 3.5\%$ of R6(3) DNA is homologous with this F-factor and *vice versa*. Moreover, these data indicate that homology between these two plasmids is restricted *entirely* to one-half of the R-factor DNA, and that it is interrupted occasionally by small loops of non-homology. Since it appears probable from the work of WILLETTS (1969; 1970) and OHTSUBO, NISHIMURA and HIROTA (1970) that R-factors and F-factors have the same or similar conjugation systems, our results imply that all of the genes coding for fertility are grouped together in one region of the R-factor molecule and that this region constitutes a large segment of the entire R-factor molecule. These results are consistent with our earlier conclusion (COHEN and MILLER (1970a)), that the larger of the two circular R-factor DNA species found in *Proteus* is the transfer unit, and that the smaller (molecular weight $= 10-12 \times 10^6$ daltons) circular species carries resistance determinants.

This interpretation is additionally supported by experiments carried out with the isolated RTF unit of R1 (COHEN and MILLER (1970b)), which are shown diagrammatically in Figure 10. As seen here, R1 is completely homologous with its isolated and purified transfer (RTF) unit over most of the molecule. The region of non-homology, which presumably represents the resistance determinant part of R-factor R1, is localized to a single region comprising about one-fourth the length of the "complete R-factor". As seen in the lower part of this figure, the RTF unit of R1 was also largely but not completely homologous with the major part of another R-factor, R6(4). Thus, it can be concluded that R1 and R6 have similar, but not identical, transfer units.

Using these techniques, it was shown that several different fi$^+$ R-factors have extensive DNA sequence homology distributed over their entire length and that they have transfer units which are structurally similar to each other and to the F-factor region specifying fertility functions (SHARP, DAVIDSON and COHEN (1971)). In contrast, an fi$^-$ R-factor which has been studied contains almost totally different DNA sequences. From these results, it appears likely that large regions of the DNA sequence of various fi⁺ R-factors we have studied originate from a common precursor, and that F-factors share the same precursor. Fi⁻ R-factors appear to be of a different origin.

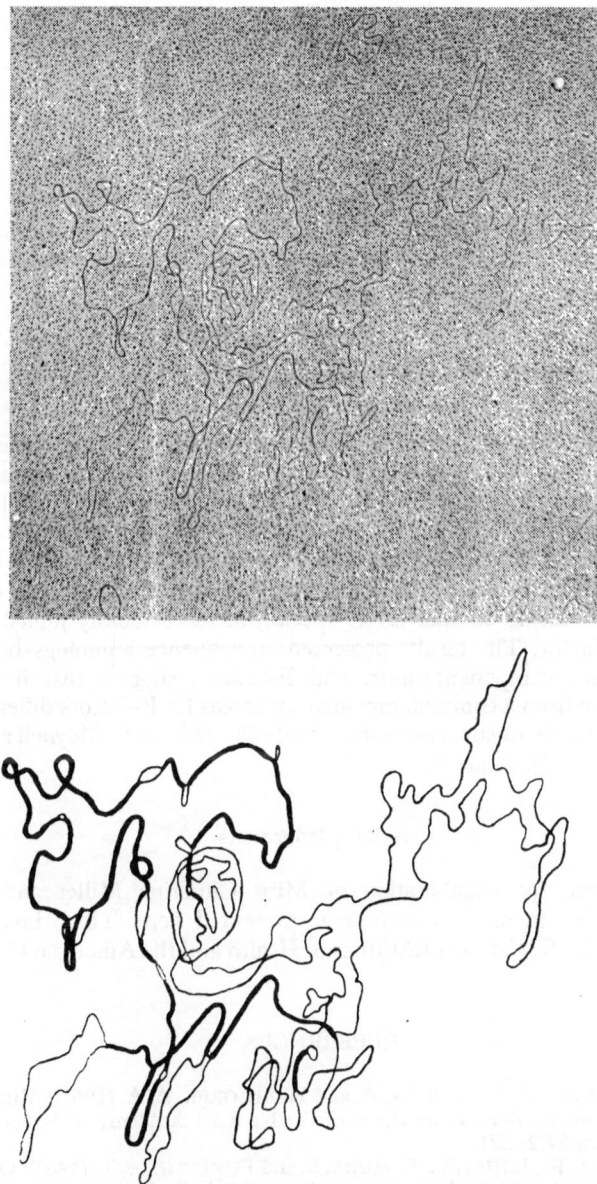

Fig. 9 Electron photomicrograph and tracing of a DNA-DNA hybrid of R6(3) and an F-factor. DNA-DNA hybridization and preparation of samples for electron microscopy were carried out as indicated by Davis and associates (1971). The tracing of the hybrid DNA molecule formed by the R- and F-factors shows double stranded regions of homology (heavy lines) and single stranded regions of non-homology (light lines). This figure is taken from Sharp, Davidson, and Cohen (in preparation).

279

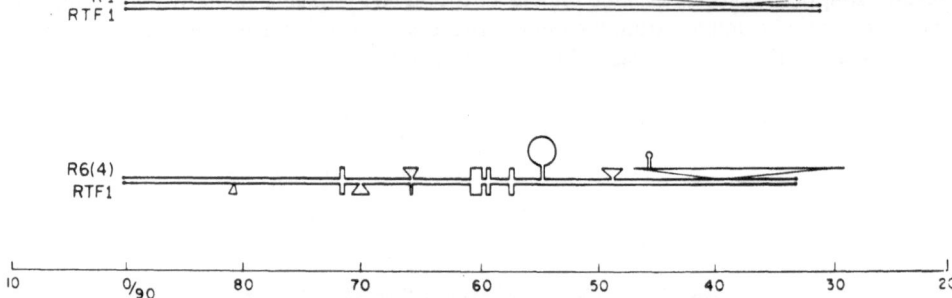

Fig. 10 Diagrammatic representation of electron microscope heteroduplex experiments showing the extent of homology of RTF 1 (the isolated transfer unit of R1 (Cohen and Miller (1970b)) with the "complete" R-factor R1, and with another R-factor (R6−4). This figure is taken from Sharp, Davidson, and Cohen (in preparation).

SUMMARY

Our findings indicate that certain fi+ R-factors (e. g., R1, R6) are formed by reversible covalent linkage of plasmids that separately harbor either resistance or transfer functions. In *E. coli*, such R-factors are represented almost entirely by a single circular DNA species containing the covalently linked transfer unit and drug resistance determinant unit. Under special circumstances, catenated (interlocking) forms of circular R-factor DNA molecules are observed. In *Proteus mirabilis*, the RTF and R-determinants units can exist as separate autonomously replicating circular DNA species, or as covalently joined components of the complete R-factor. The results presented on sequence homology between different R-factors, R-factor component units, and F-factors, suggest that fi+ R-factors and F-factors originate from a common precursor, whereas fi− R-factors differ not only in the specificity of the repressor substances they synthesize (Meynell, Meynell and Data (1968) but in their entire DNA sequence.

Acknowledgments

We acknowledge the collaboration of Miss Christine Miller and Miss Annette McCoubrey on certain of the experiments presented here. These investigations were supported by the U. S. National Institutes of Health and the American Cancer Society.

REFERENCES

ADLER, H. I., FISHER, W. D., COHEN, A. and HARDIGREE, A. A. (1967): Miniature *Escherichia coli* Cells Deficient in DNA. Proceedings of the National Academy of Sciences of the United States of America, **57/2**, 321.

AKIBA, T., KOYAMA, K., ISHIKI, Y., KIMURA, S. and FUKUSHIMA, T. (1960): On the mechanism of the development of multiple-drug-resistant clones of *Shigella*. Japanese Journal of Microbiology, **4/2**, 219.

ANDERSON, E. S. (1966): A Rapid Screening Test for Transfer Factors in Drug-sensitive Enterobacteriaceae. Nature, **208/5014**, 1016.

ANDERSON, E. S. (1968): The Ecology of Transferable Drug Resistance in the Enterobacteria. In: *Annual Review of Microbiology*, *Vol.* **22**, pp. 131−180. Editors: C. E. Clifton, S. Raffel and M. P. Starr. Annual Reviews, Inc., Palo Alto, Calif.

ANDERSON, E. S. (1969): Ecology and Epidemiology of Transferable Drug Resistance. In: *Bacterial Episomes and Plasmids, A Ciba Foundation Symposium*, pp. 102—115. Editors: G. E. W. Wolstenholme and M. O'Connor. Little, Brown & Co., Boston, Mass.

ANDERSON, E. S. and LEWIS, M. J. (1965): Characterization of a Transfer Factor Associated with Drug Resistance in *Salmonella typhimurium*. Nature, **208/5013**, 843.

BAZARAL, M. and HELINSKI, D. R. (1968): Circular DNA Forms of Colicinogenic Factors E1, E2 and E3 from *Escherichia coli*. Journal of Molecular Biology, **36/2**, 185.

BOUANCHAUD, D. H. (1969): La Résistance Extra-Chromosomique aux Antibiotiques (quelques aspects génétiques et épidémiologiques). Bulletin de l'Institut Pasteur, **67/4**, 684.

CAMPBELL, A. M. (1962): Episomes. In: *Advances in Genetics, Vol.* **11**, pp. 101—145. Editors: E. W. Caspari and J. M. Thoday. Academic Press, New York, N. Y.

CAMPBELL, A. (1969): Discussion of "Ecology and Epidemiology of Transferable Drug Resistance" by E. S. Anderson. In: *Bacterial Episomes and Plasmids, A Ciba Foundation Symposium*, pp. 117. Editors: G. E. W. Wolstenholme and M. O'Connor. Little, Brown & Co., Boston, Mass.

CLAYTON, D. A. and VINOGRAD, J. (1967): Circular Dimer and Catenate Forms of Mitochondrial DNA in Human Leukaemic Leucocytes. Nature, **216/5116**, 652.

COHEN, S. N. (1969): Isolation and Characterization of R-Factor DNA. Bacteriological Proceedings, **69/49**.

COHEN, S. N. and MILLER, C. A. (1969): Multiple Molecular Species of Circular R-factor DNA isolated from *Escherichia coli*. Nature. **224/5226**, 1273.

COHEN, S. N. and MILLER, C. A. (1970a): Non-chromosomal Antibiotic Resistance in Bacteria, II. Molecular Nature of R-factors isolated from *Proteus mirabilis* and *Escherichia coli*. Journal of Molecular Biology, **50/3**, 671.

COHEN, S. N. and MILLER, C. A.(1970b): Non-chromosomal Antibiotic Resistance in Bacteria, III. Isolation of the Discrete Transfer Unit of the R-Factor R1. Proceedings of the National Academy of Sciences of the United States of America, **67/2**, 510.

COHEN, S. N., SILVER, R. P., SHARP, P. A. and McCOUBREY, A. E. (1971a): Studies on the Molecular Nature of R Factors. In: *The Problems of Drug-Resistant Pathogenic Bacteria, Annals of the New York Academy of Sciences, Vol.* **182**, pp. 172—187. Editors: E. L. Dulaney and A. I. Laskin. New York Academy of Sciences, New York, N. Y.

COHEN, S. N., SILVER, R. P., McCOUBREY, A. E. and SHARP, P. A. (1971b): Isolation of Catenated Forms of R Factor DNA from Minicells. Nature New Biology, **231/25**, 249.

DAVERN, C. I. (1966): Isolation of the DNA of the *E. coli*. Chromosome in One Piece. Proceedings of the National Academy of Sciences of the United States of America, **55/4**, 792.

DAVIS, R. W. and DAVIDSON, N. (1968): Electron-Microscopic Visualization of Deletion Mutations. Proceedings of the National Academy of Sciences of the United States of America, **60/1**, 243.

DAVIS, R. W., SIMON, M. and DAVIDSON, N. (1971): Electron Microscope Heteroduplex Methods for Mapping Regions of Base Sequence Homology in Nucleic Acids. In: *Methods in Enzymology, Vol.* **21** — *Nucleic Acids*, pp. 413—428. Editors: L. Grossman and K. Moldave. Academic Press, New York, N. Y.

FALKOW, S., CITARELLA, R. V., WOHLHIETER, J. A. and WATANABE, T. (1966): The Molecular Nature of R-Factors. Journal of Molecular Biology, **17/1**, 102.

HUDSON, B. and VINOGRAD, J. (1967): Catenated Circular DNA Molecules in HeLa Cell Mitochondria. Nature, **216/5116**, 647.

INSELBURG, J. (1970): Segregation into and Replication of Plasmid Deoxyribonucleic Acid in Chromosomeless Segregants of *Escherichia coli*. Journal of Bacteriology, **102/3**, 642.

INSELBURG, J. (1971): R Factor Deoxyribonucleic Acid in Chromosomeless Progeny of *Escherichia coli*. Journal of Bacteriology, **105/2**, 620.

KASS, L. R. and YARMOLINSKY, M. B. (1970): Segregation of Functional Sex Factor into Minicells. Proceedings of the National Academy of Sciences of the United States of America, **66/3**, 815.

KONTOMICHALOU, P., MITANI, M. and CLOWES, R. C. (1970): Circular R-Factor Molecules Controlling Penicillinase Synthesis, Replicating in *Escherichia coli* Under Either Relaxed or Stringent Control. Journal of Bacteriology, **104/1**, 34.

KOPECKO, D. J. and PUNCH, J. D. (1971): Regulation of R-Factor Replication in *Proteus mirabilis*. In: *The Problems of Drug-Resistant Pathogenic Bacteria, Annals of the New York Academy of Sciences, Vol.* **182**, pp. 207—216. Editors: E. L. Dulaney and A. I. Laskin, New York Academy of Sciences, New York, N. Y.

LEVY, S. B. and NORMAN, P. (1970): Segregation of Transferable R Factors into *Escherichia coli* Minicells. Nature, **227/5258**, 606.

MACHATTIE, L. A., BERNS, M. I. and THOMAS, C. A., Jr. (1965): Electron Microscopy of DNA from *Hemophilus influenzae*. Journal of Molecular Biology, **11/3**, 648.

MEYNELL, E., MEYNELL, G. G. and DATTA, N. (1968): Phylogenetic Relationships of Drug-Resistance Factors and Other Transmissible Bacterial Plasmids. Bacteriological Reviews, 32/1, 55.

MITSUHASHI, S. (1971): Epidemiology and Genetics of R Factors. In: *The Problems of Drug-Resistant Pathogenic Bacteria, Annals of the New York Academy of Sciences*, Vol. 182, pp. 141–152. Editors: E. L. Dulaney and A. I. Laskin. New York Academy of Sciences, New York, N. Y.

NANDI, U. S., WANG, J. C. and DAVIDSON, N. (1965): Separation of Deoxyribonucleic Acids by Hg(II) Binding and Cs_2SO_4 Density-Gradient Centrifugation. Biochemistry, 4/9, 1687.

NOVICK, R. P. (1969): Extrachromosomal Inheritance in Bacteria. Bacteriological Reviews, 33/2, 210.

OCHIAI, K., YAMANAKA, T., KIMURA, K. and SAWADA, O. (1959): Studies of inheritance of drug resistance between *Shigella* strains and *Escherichia coli* strains (in Japanese). Nippon Iji Shimpo, 1861/page 34.

OHTSUBO, E., NISHIMURA, Y. and HIROTA, Y. (1970): Transfer-Defective Mutants of Sex Factors in *Escherichia coli*. I. Defective Mutants and Complementation Analysis. Genetics. 64/2, 173.

PIKÓ, L., BLAIR, D. G., TYLER, A. and VINOGRAD, J. (1968): Cytoplasmic DNA in the Unfertilized Sea Urchin Egg: Physical Properties of Circular Mitochondrial DNA and the Occurrence of Catenated Forms. Proceedings of the National Academy of Sciences of the Unites States of America, 59/3, 838.

RADLOFF, R., BAUER, W. and VINOGRAD, J. (1967): A Dye-Buoyant-Density Method for the Detection and Isolation of Closed Circular Duplex DNA: The Closed Circular DNA in HeLa Cells. Proceedings of the National Academy of Sciences of the United States of America, 57/5, 1514.

ROOZEN, K. J., FENWICK, R. G. Jr., LEVY, S. and CURTISS, R. III (1970): Characterization of DNA isolated from Minicells of Plasmid-Harboring Minicell-Producing Strains of *Escherichia coli K* 12. Genetics Supplement, 64/2, Part 2, S54.

ROOZEN, K. J., FENWICK, R. G. Jr., and CURTISS, R. III (1971): Synthesis of Ribonucleic Acid and Protein in Plasmid-Containing Minicells of *Escherichia coli K 12*. Journal of Bacteriology, 107/1, 21.

ROWND, R. (1970): The Molecular Nature and the Control of the Replication of R Factors. In: *Symposium on Infectious Multiple Drug Resistance: Genetics, Molecular Nature, and Clinical Implications of R Factors*. pp. 17–33. U.S. Government Printing Office, Washington, D. C.

ROWND, R., NAKAYA, R. and NAKAMURA, A. (1966): Molecular Nature of the Drug-resistance Factors of the Enterobacteriaceae. Journal of Molecular Biology, 17/2, 376.

SHARP. P. A., DAVIDSON, N. and COHEN, S. N. (1971): A Study of the DNA Sequence Homology between Plasmids of *E. coli*. Federation Proceedings, 30/3 (II), 1054Ab.

SILVER, R. P. and FALKOW, S. (1970): Specific Labeling and Physical Characterization of R-Factor Deoxyribonucleic Acid in *Escherichia coli*. Journal of Bacteriology, 104/1, 331.

VINOGRAD, J., LEBOWITS, J., RADLOFF, R., WATSON, R. and LAIPIS, P. (1965): The Twisted Circular Form of Polyoma Viral DNA. Proceedings of the National Academy of Sciences of the United States of America, 53/5, 1104.

WATANABE, T. (1963): Infective Heredity of Multiple Drug Resistance in Bacteria. Bacteriological Reviews, 27/1, 87.

WATANABE, T. (1969): Transferable Drug Resistance: The Nature of the Problem. In: *Bacterial Episomes and Plasmids, A Ciba Foundation Symposium*, pp. 81–97. Editors: G. E. W. Wolstenholme and M. O'Connor. Little, Brown & Co., Boston, Mass.

WATANABE, T. (1971): The Origin of R Factors. In: *The Problems of Drug-Resistant Pathogenic Bacteria, Annals of the New York Academy of Sciences*, Vol. 182, pp. 126–140. Editors: E. L. Dulaney and A. I. Laskin. New York Academy of Sciences, New York, N. Y.

WATANABE, T. and FUKASAWA, T. (1960): "Resistance transfer factor", an episome in Enterobacteriaceae. Biochemical and Biophysical Research Communications, 3/6, 660.

WILLETTS, N. S. (1970): The Genetics of Sexual Transfer by F and R Factors in *E. coli*. In: *Abstracts of the Tenth International Congress for Microbiology*, pp. 203. Mexico City, Mexico.

WILLETTS, N. S. (1971): Plasmid Specificity of Two Proteins required for Conjugation in *E. coli* K12. Nature New Biology, 230/14, 183.

MOLECULAR NATURE OF BACTERIAL PLASMIDS

R. CLOWES

Division of Biology, The University of Texas at Dallas, Texas, U.S.A.

Genetics of plasmid genes

It has been clearly realized for many years that R factors are representative of a group of elements, the bacterial plasmids, including sex factors and colicin factors, which are closely related in many basic properties.

The genetics and linkage of a number of plasmid-borne genes of various bacterial plasmids are shown in Tables I and II. Plasmid-borne genes are not linked to chromosomal markers, since plasmids exist extrachromosomally and are not normally integrated in the chromosome (CLOWES, 1964, NOVICK, 1969) (one major exception of course being λ). Linkage of a series of plasmid genes therefore refers to their linkage with each other, that is, whether or not they are *cointegrated* within the same extrachromosomal plasmid molecule.

Table 1

TRANSFER AND LOSS OF PLASMID GENES (COINTEGRATED PLASMIDS)

Plasmid	Conjugal Transfer		Loss		Transduction	
F-*lac*$^+$	100% μ^r-lac$^+$	(a)	100% μ^r-lac$^-$	(b)	?	
ColV	100% μ^r-Col$^+$	(a)	100% μ^r-Col$^-$	(c)	?	
FVB*trycys*	>90%(FVB*trycys*)$^+$	(d)	>90%(FVB*trycys*)$^-$	(d)	c. 90%(FVB*trycys*)$^+$	(d)
222(S-C-T)	100%(S-C-T)$^+$	(e)	100%(S-C-T)$^-$	(f)	100%(S-C-T)$^+$	(g)
Δ-T	100% Δ+T^R	(h)	?		0% Δ+T^R	(j)
PII(pen-Hg-ero)	—		c. 90%pen^{r}Hg^{r}ero^r	(k)	c. 99.9%pen^{r}Hg^{r}ero^r	(k)

(a)	Clowes and Moody (1966)	(f)	Watanabe and Fukasawa (1961a)
(b)	Clowes, Moody and Pritchard (1965)	(g)	Watanabe and Fukasawa (1961b)
(c)	Macfarren and Clowes (1967)	(h)	Anderson and Lewis (1965)
(d)	Fredericq (1969)	(j)	Anderson and Perret (1967)
(e)	Watanabe and Fukasawa (1960)	(k)	Novick and Richmond (1965)

Table 1 shows data from a group of plasmids termed *plasmid cointegrates*. The plasmid cointegrates typically show co-transfer and co-elimination of their genes. Thus, by either conjugation or transduction, all or most, of the plasmid genes are transferred simultaneously. (Cotransduction can of course only be expected between pairs of genes situated near enough on the same DNA fragment to be incorporated in the same bacteriophage particle, but when it does occur it is the only critical genetic criterion of cointegration of two plasmid genes on the same molecular structure.) The plasmid genes of this group are frequently lost 'en bloc', either by spontaneous segregation or by "curing" although partial loss can also occur.

Table 2 shows data from another group of plasmids termed *plasmid aggregates* which show contrasting characteristics. (In this group are included what would normally be

Table 2

TRANSFER AND LOSS OF PLASMID GENES (AGGREGATED PLASMIDS)

Plasmid	Conjugal transfer		Loss	
FE1	100% FE1 (2% F; 2% E1)	(a)	100% F <0.1% E1	(b)
FE2	99.0% F 1% FE2 (0.1% E2)	(a)	?	
ΔS	99% Δ 4% Δ+S (0.1% S)	(c)	?	
ΔA	96% Δ 4% Δ+S (0.4% A)	(c)	?	

(a) Clowes (1964)
(b) Clowes, Moody and Pritchard (1965)
(c) Anderson and Lewis (1965)

regarded as independent pairs of plasmids such as F and ColE1 as well as less clearly defined systems such as ΔS). In this group, conjugal co-transfer of pairs of plasmid genes is not always observed, although it can sometimes occur at high frequency and is not therefore a reliable criterion. For example, with F⁺ColE1⁺ donors, about 100% of the recipient cells acquire both characters in a normal mating. Nevertheless, interrupted mating after short periods of contact (shown in parentheses), leads to cells to which either one or other factor has been independently transferred. In all cases investigated, 'curing' leads to independent elimination of markers. For example, 100% of the F⁺ColE1⁺ cells can be cured of F without any observable loss of the E1 factor. F⁺ColE2⁺ donor cells are more typical of this group. ColE2 is not nearly as well mobilized by F as is ColE1, so that after a normal 2 hour period of contact, although 99% of the recipients acquire F, only about 1% in addition acquire ColE2. It is again necessary to resort to interrupted

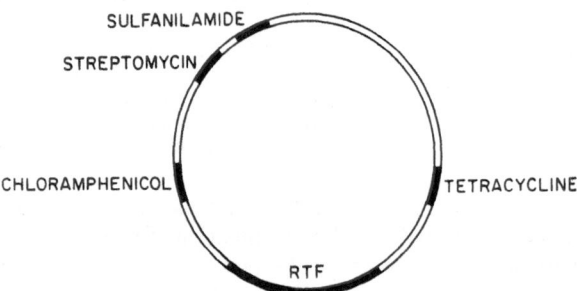

Fig. 1 Circular genetic map of the 222/R factor proposed by WATANABE (1967) on the basis of transduction data.

mating in order to identify the small number of the cells that acquire ColE2 only (0.1%).

Some of the systems analyzed by ANDERSON, for example those that involve the transfer factor Δ and the drug resistance marker S, show a clear-cut parallel with F⁺ColE2⁺ donors in conjugal transfer; most of the recipients receive only the transfer factor Δ, a small number receive in addition the drug-resistance marker S, and only with interrupted mating is transfer of S in the absence of Δ observed. ΔA is similar to ΔS with a slightly more efficient co-transfer of Δ and A.

Some of the data shown for *plasmid cointegrates* has been used to derive circular linkage summarizes tranduction data of the R factor 222 (Fig. 1) and similar maps have been made for a number of these plasmids. For example, WATANABE's circular map (1967) derived by deletion analysis for Frédéricq's composite ColVColB*trpcys*-R plasmid (1969) and the PII penicillinase plasmid from *Staphylococcus aureus* mapped by NOVICK (1969). In each case, the genetic data is consistent with the integration of a group of genes within a single genetic structure (cointegration). This has led to some controversy about the molecular nature of other plasmid systems, having the properties of *plasmid aggregates* and exemplified by the ΔAST system of E. S. ANDERSON (1969).

Molecular Models for Plasmids

An important question is therefore, "What consitutes an R factor?" Can the molecular nature of all R factors be characterized by a single circular DNA molecule shown as a 'plasmid cointegrate' in Fig. 2 in which the transfer (or sex factor) genes, are incorporated within the same molecule as drug-resistance genes; or in fact, can several extrachromo-somal genetic elements exist independently in the cell as a 'plasmid aggregate' (one at least with transfer properties and others carrying drug resistance genes and being non-

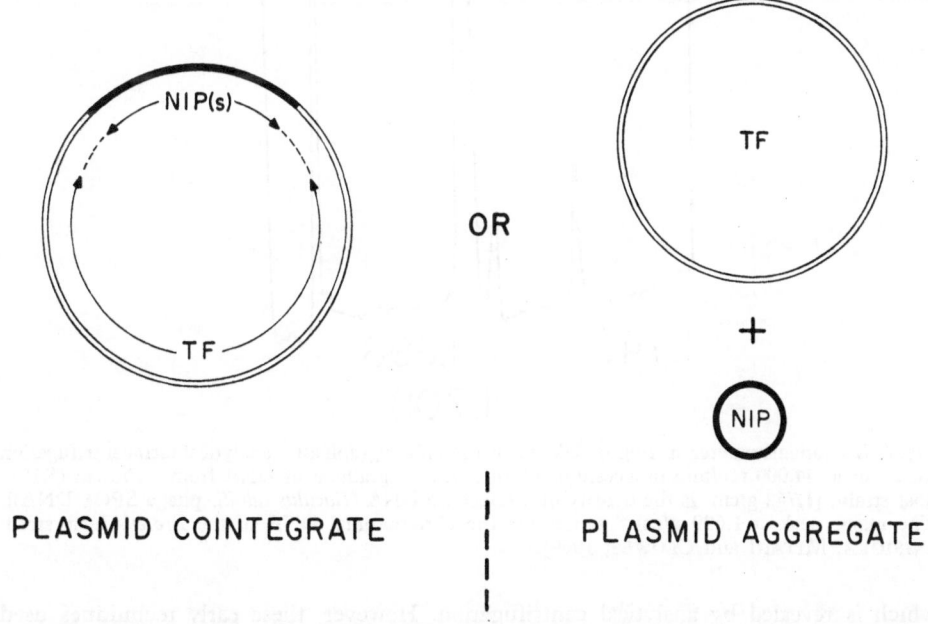

Fig. 2 Alternative molecular models for bacterial plasmids. TF represents the genetic region controlling "transfer factor" properties. NIP represents a "non-infectious plasmid", controlling genes for colicinogeny or drug resistance.

infectious) and, collectively show R factor properties? In this situation although co-transfer might occur, in general the molecules would be independently transferred and lost and, in particular, would be transduced independently. An answer to this question obviously depends upon a knowledge of the molecular nature of plasmids.

Molecular studies of plasmids

Early studies on the molecular nature of plasmids by MARMUR, ROWND, FALKOW, BARON, SCHILDKRAUT and DOTY (1961) exploited the ability of plasmids to transfer between various bacterial strains which are unrelated phylogenetically. Some of these hosts have a different guanine-cytosine (GC) composition in their DNA to that of the plasmid. Hence in this host the plasmid DNA can be separated and distinguished from the host DNA by the difference in density arising from these GC composition differences,

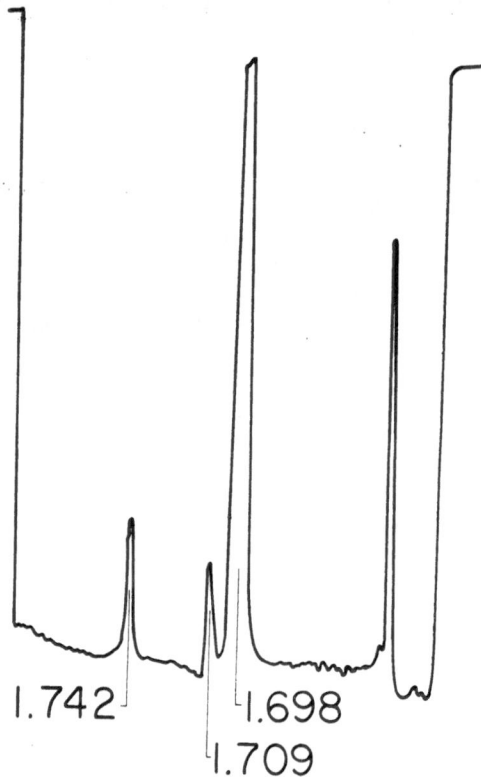

Fig. 3 Microdensitometer tracing of UV adsorption photograph after analytical ultracentrifugation for 27 hr at 44,000 rev/min in a cesium chloride density gradient of DNA from a *Proteus* (R15)+ host strain. [1.742 g/cm³ is the density of a reference DNA (*Bacillus subtilis* phage SPO1 DNA)]. The major peak at 1.699 g/cm⁻³ represents the chromosomal DNA of the *Proteus* host strain (NISIOKA, MITANI and CLOWES, 1969).

which is revealed by analytical centrifugation. However, these early techniques used methods to extract the DNA which led to its fragmentation.

More recent methods permit the isolation of intact non-fragmented plasmid DNA (HICKSON, ROTH and HELINSKI, 1967). Our first experiments (NISIOKA, MITANI and

CLOWES, 1969) used these methods to separate R factor DNA from *Proteus* host strains carrying factors 222 or R15, kindly provided by Dr. WATANABE. This separated DNA is then visualized by electron microscopy. We use the Kleinschmidt/Lang monolayer spreading technique (LANG, BUJARD, WOLFF and RUSSELL, 1967) to tease out the DNA on a surface film so that its contour length and hence its molecular weight can be determined.

In fact, when DNA from the Proteus (R15)[+] strain was sedimented by this method, it gave rise to a single-peaked satellite as shown in Fig. 3. Separation of the plasmid DNA by preparative centrifugation permitted samples from the satellite peak to be examined by electron microscopy. (A typical EM picture of R-factor DNA (Fig. 4a) shows the DNA

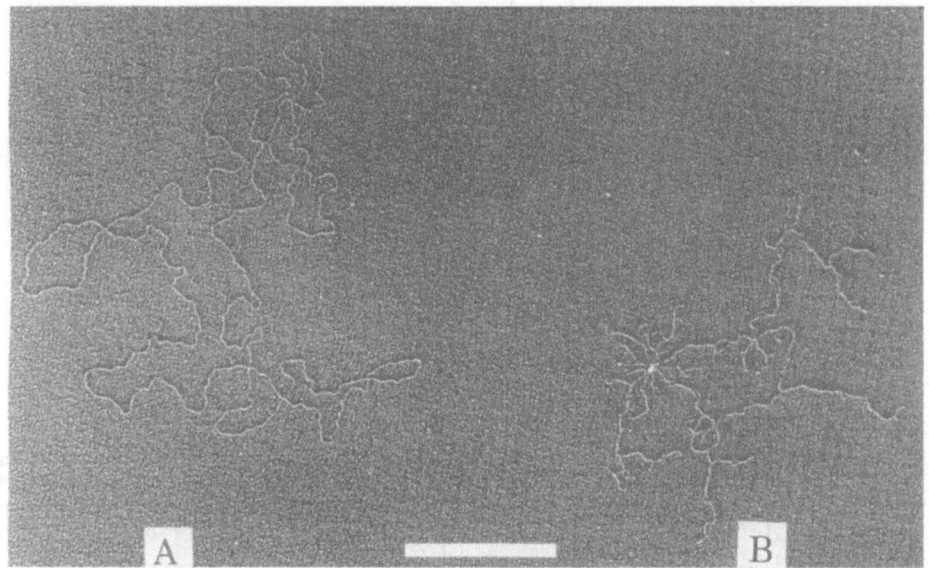

Fig. 4 Electron micrograph of R-factor DNA (222). (A) Open circular and (B) supertwisted (covalently-closed-circular) molecules. Bar represents 1μ. DNA spread by technique of Kleinschmidt and Zahn (1959) from 0.15M ammonium acetate and shadowed in two right angled directions with platinum. Photograph and preparation by courtesy of Dr. Christine Smith.

molecules to be formed of closed loops (so-called 'circular' molecules)). The contour length around a number of these loops was measured and within experimental error was found to be the same (19μ). R15 was therefore identified as an unimolecular species of DNA of about 45 million MW (assuming that 1 micron of DNA has 207×10^4 atomic mass units (LANG, 1970)) and is typical of a number of plasmids we have examined (NISIOKA et al., 1969).

In contrast, Fig. 5 shows an analytical, density-gradient profile of the 222 R-factor, an *fi*[+] factor, in which the satellite band, instead of having a single peak as with R15, and which had shown a double-peaked band in earlier experiments of FALKOW, CITARELLA, WOHLEITER and WATANABE (1966) can be seen here to have at least three peaks with densities at 1.708, 1.711 and 1.717 g/cm³. The corresponding preparative centrifugation gradient of 222 is shown in Fig. 6, samples from peaks A, B, and C being taken for electron microscopy. The contour lengths of the DNA molecules from each of these three fractions were found to differ, with a mean at about 28, 34 and 6μ respectively.

A summary of these contour length and density measurements is shown in Fig. 7 where it can be seen that the band with the heaviest density, 1.717 g/cm³, yielded 6μ molecules;

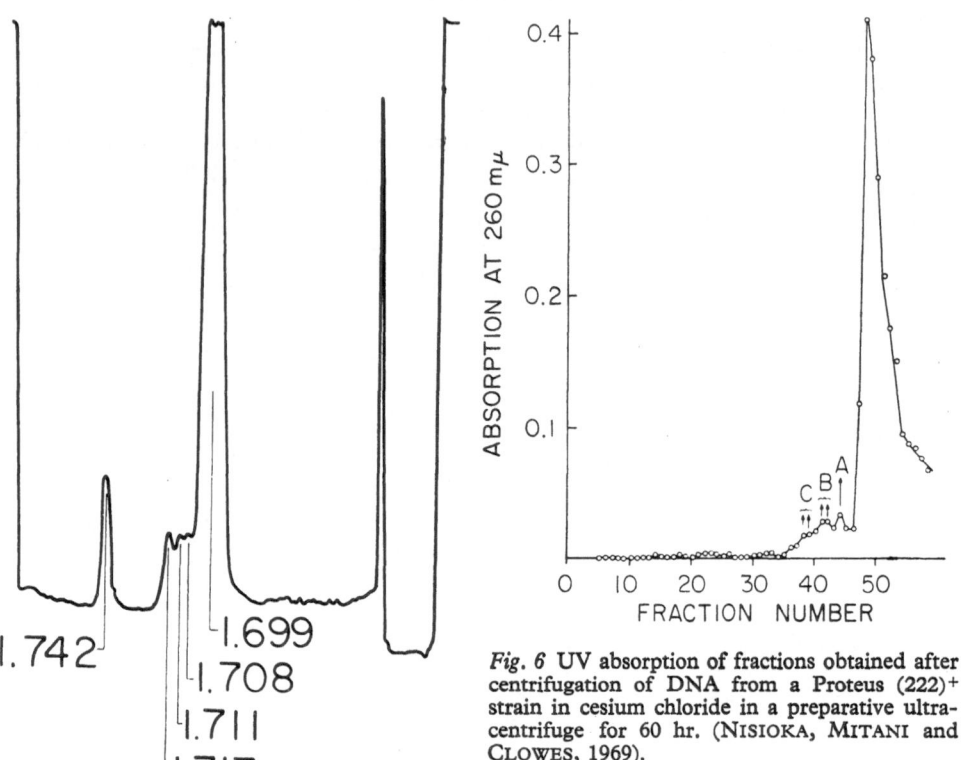

Fig. 6 UV absorption of fractions obtained after centrifugation of DNA from a Proteus (222)⁺ strain in cesium chloride in a preparative ultracentrifuge for 60 hr. (NISIOKA, MITANI and CLOWES, 1969).

Fig. 5 Microdensitometer tracing of UV adsorption photograph after analytical ultracentrifugation for 27 hr at 44,000 rev/min in a cesium chloride density gradient of DNA from a *Proteus* (222)⁺ host strain. [1.742 g/cm³ is the density of a reference DNA (*Bacillus subtilis* phage SPO1 DNA).] The major peak at 1.699 g/cm⁻³ represents the chromosomal DNA of the *Proteus* host strain (NISIOKA, MITANI and CLOWES, 1969).

the band with the medium density, 1.711 g/cm³, yielded 34μ molecules, and the band with the lowest density (1.708 g/cm³) yielded molecules of 28μ, although in this band there were also some molecules of 34μ. (Note that the peaks are about the same size and thus represent about the same amounts of DNA). Thus, within experimental error, the sum of the sizes of the two smaller molecules equals the size of the largest molecule, which is of an intermediate density to the two smaller.

From these results, it was concluded that the 222 factor is normally a composite molecule which separates in *Proteus* to two smaller molecules (Fig. 8). All three molecules were inferred to replicate independently from the fact that the amount of DNA in the 6μ peak is equivalent to that under each of the other two peaks, indicating that since the 6μ molecules are about 1/5 the size of the others, their numbers must be about five times greater than those of the large ones. These amounts cannot be explained on the basis

288

of segregation without invoking further replication of this 6μ segregant. We suggested that this segregation might indicate a reversal of a recombination event which may have occurred during the evolution of 222 (NISIOKA et al., 1969).

One drawback of using host strains such as *Proteus*, which are not the natural hosts, is that any indication of instability, such as is seen with the 222 factor, cannot necessarily be taken as characteristic of normal behavior. Ideally, it would be important to isolate

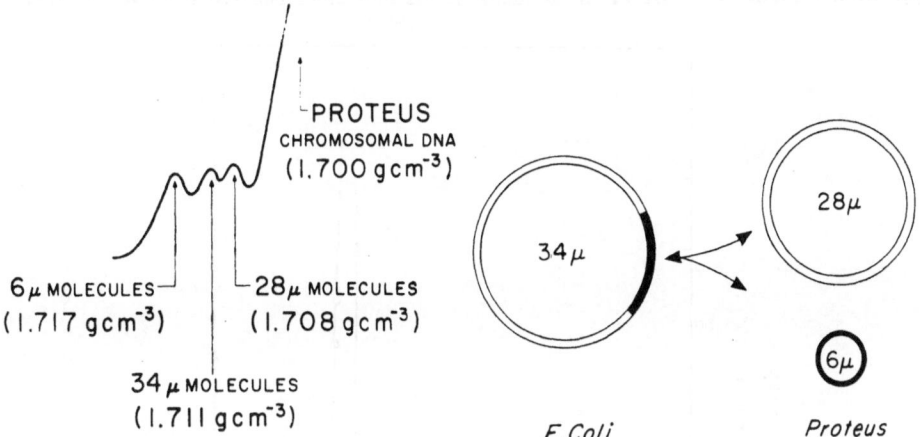

Fig. 7 Diagramatic representation of satellite peaks of 222/DNA Isolated forms Proteus host strain indicating densities and contour lengths of molecules measured (NISIOKA, MITANI and CLOWES, 1969).

Fig. 8 Possible alternate molecular forms of 222 R factor as a composite (34μ) molecule in *E. coli* which separates in *Proteus* into two component replicons of 28μ and 6μ.

bacterial plasmids and identify their molecular nature from those strains that are their normal hosts. For most plasmids we have worked with, these hosts would be enterobacterial strains such as *Escherichia coli*.

Electron microscopy of R-factor DNA had also shown many molecules in a tightly-twisted (supertwisted) form (Fig. 4b), in addition to the circular molecules whose contour lengths could be measured. The proportion of circular molecules to the supertwisted molecules increased with storage as well as by treatment with small amounts of DNAse.

Ethidium bromide (EB) was shown by RADLOFF, BAUER and VINOGRAD (1967) to intercalate between adjacent base-pairs of DNA. In so doing the helix is untwisted and the DNA duplex is extended, thus lowering its density. Uptake of ethidium bromide occurs to the same extent in the open circular form (a circular molecule in which one of the circular strands is covalently intact and the other is broken — an example is the molecule in Fig. 4A) or the linear double-stranded form, and this results in the same extension and decrease in their densities. In contrast, uptake of ethidium bromide into supertwisted DNA (in which both DNA strands are covalently-closed) is limited because of the restriction in rotation of the two chains about each other, due to the absence of a free end of rotation. Thus, extension of covalently-closed circular (CCC) molecules is less in EB than the other two forms and its density is lowered to a lesser degree. Hence, in ethidium bromide, the CCC (supertwisted) form is denser and can thus be separated from the two other double-stranded forms in the absence of any differences in base ratio.

Fig. 9 shows a density-gradient profile in ethidium bromide, cesium chloride of a mixture of DNA from two *E. coli* strains, one containing an R factor and one without, each lysed with detergent and the crude lysates mixed, centrifuged and fractionated.

Fractions from the satellite peak sq separated and examined by electron microscopy shows that the DNA isolated by this method has the same contour length as that isolated by other techniques.

In the case of 222, further analytical centrifugation of the satellite DNA gave a single peak at density 1.710 g/cm³, almost identical to that found as the intermediate density peak from Proteus. The size of the R factor DNA molecules isolated from *E. coli* was

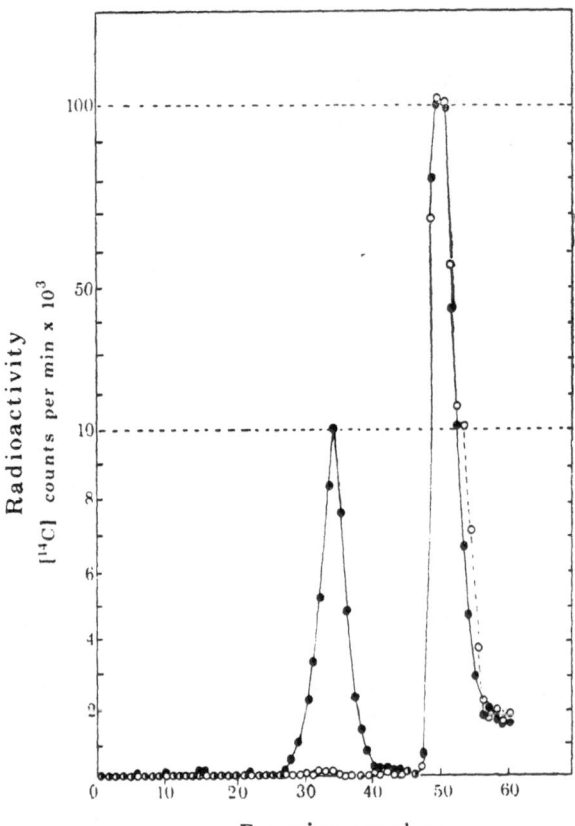

Fig. 9 Radioactivity of fractions obtained after ultracentrifugation in CsCl ethidium bromide solution of crude lysates of *E. coli* strains grown in radioactive thymidine. Open circles are from an R⁻ *E. coli* host: closed circles from the same host carrying an R factor (from NISIOKA, MITANI and CLOWES, 1970).

restricted to a single class measuring about 34μ in contour length. 222 DNA from *E. coli* is thus identified by molecular weight and by buoyant density with the largest of the three molecular species identified in *Proteus*. We would thus infer that the composite 34μ molecule is preserved intact on transfer to and replication in *E. coli*. (But after transfer to *Proteus*, it segregates into its two daughter molecules (Fig. 8) (NISIOKA, MITANI and CLOWES, 1970).)

Thus, although the 222 R factor can be concluded to be a cointegrate in *Enterobacter*, it is comprised of several plasmids which can exist as independent replicons as seen on transfer to *Proteus*. It is unlikely therefore that the drug-resistance genes of 222 have originated entirely by "gene pick-up" (since these chromosomal fragments would not be expected to be replicons) and some at least may thus be proposed to have arisen by *de novo* mutation of extrachromosomal elements.

Results by COHEN and MILLER (1970) and SILVER and FALKOW (1970) have extended our experimental data with the 222 factor to the factors R1 and R6. Both of these elements exist as single molecular species in *E. coli* at a density of about 1.710 g/cm³ and measure approximately 31 to 33μ. In *Proteus mirabilis*, both factors similarly appear to separate into two structures of similar size to those from 222, namely a large molecule of about 28μ and 1.709 g/cm³ and a small molecule of about 5μ and 1.717 g/cm³. Both these groups of workers have gone on to isolate from R1 and from R6, an *E. coli* strain carrying a DNA element similar in size and density to the largest (28μ) segregant found in *Proteus*, and which retains transfer factor properties, but no longer carries drug resistance. Both groups of workers have identified this larger molecule with the RTF element, although this does not seem to be consistent (in 222) with the isolation of segregants carrying drug resistance markers and retaining all the RTF properties and which are yet smaller in size (NISIOKA et al., 1970).

Other data showed that segregant R factor molecules which had lost some drug-resistance markers had lost a region of DNA of a specific size. Complementary segregant factors could undergo molecular recombination to regenerate molecules of the same size and drug resistance as the parental molecule. Two features therefore appear to have been demonstrated. Firstly, although many R factor plasmids are cointegrates in which the plasmid genes are carried on a single molecular structure, this structure may be separated into a number of independent molecules which are themselves replicons. Secondly, such replicons can undergo molecular recombination.

Our more recent work has turned to a series of R factor plasmids provided by E. S. ANDERSON and originating from a parental strain carrying a plasmid termed ΔAST which determines infectious resistance for ampicillin (A), streptomycin plus sulphonamide (termed collectively S), and tetracycline (T) (ANDERSON & LEWIS, 1965). From the original ΔAST strain (Fig. 10) were derived (1) a plasmid carrying infectious resistance

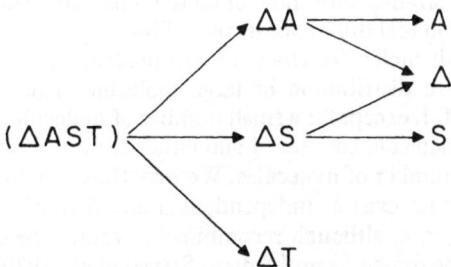

Fig. 10 Derivation of strains in ΔAST system. Δ denotes a strain with transfer factor properties and A, S and T represent non-infectious resistance to ampicillin, streptomycin (plus sulfonamide) and tetracycline respectively (ANDERSON and LEWIS, 1965).

to ampicillin and designated (ΔA); (2) another transferring infectious resistance to streptomycin plus sulphonamide (ΔS); and (3) another carrying infectious resistance to tetracycline (ΔT). From ΔA, two further factors were isolated, one carrying *non-infectious* ampicillin resistance (termed A) and the other carrying a transfer factor (Δ), shown by virtue of the fact that when grown in mixed culture with A, it can mobilize the transfer of ampicillin resistance. Similarly, ΔS segregated into two factors, S and Δ, whereas ΔT did not undergo any further segregation.

The contour length measurements of DNA from some of these plasmids are shown in Table 3. It can be seen that DNA from strains carrying Δ comprises molecules of one size only (29.8μ length, equivalent to 62 million MW). From strains carrying S, again

Table 3

CONTOUR LENGTH MEASUREMENTS OF DNA MOLECULES ISOLATED FROM
Δ^+, S$^+$, (ΔT)$^+$ AND (ΔS)$^+$ STRAINS OF *E. COLI*

Plasmid	Contour length $\pm$ SSD (μ)	MW $\times 10^6$
Δ[a]	29.8 $\pm$ 0.7	62
S[a]	2.96 $\pm$ 0.13	6
ΔS[a]	31.3 $\pm$ 1.0	65
	2.87 $\pm$ 0.14	6
ΔT[b]	32.3 $\pm$ 1.1	67

[a]SMITH, ANDERSON and CLOWES (1970)
[b]CHRISTINE SMITH (unpublished)

a unimolecular species was isolated, but of approximately 1/10 the size of Δ and of molecular weight estimated therefore as six million and thus equivalent to perhaps twenty genes. (Strains carrying A contained a small molecular species of very similar size.) In strains of ΔS, a bimodal distribution of molecules was found, corresponding in sizes to the molecules found in Δ and in S respectively. (Similarly, DNA extracted from ΔA strains formed a similar bimodal distribution of molecules) (Smith, Anderson and Clowes, 1970). In contrast, ΔT strains comprised a unimolecular species of 32.3μ length, 67 million MW (Christine Smith, unpublished observations).

From the comparison of contour length measurements of small molecules (inferred to be S) isolated from (ΔS)$^+$ strains, with those of all the molecules isolated from S$^+$ strains, we conclude that there is no real difference in size. (Similarly, when measurements of the A molecules and the small molecules from ΔA are pooled, they show one distribution group.) Moreover, the size distribution of large molecules from both ΔA or ΔS are identical with molecules of Δ, except for a small number of molecules of the size one might expect of a recombinant molecule between Δ and either A or S. However, this number is less than 5% of the total number of molecules. We may thus conclude that in ΔS strains, the majority of the molecules exist as independent Δ and S molecules and little, if any, recombination has taken place, although recombination cannot be completely excluded. A similar conclusion can be drawn from ΔA data (SMITH et al., 1970).

In contrast, in ΔT DNA, no small molecules were found, indicating that this plasmid is stable and can be represented entirely by a composite ΔT molecule. The size of ΔT is larger than Δ by a factor about the size of A or S. There is thus a nice correlation between the genetic and molecular data in this system.

ΔT therefore corresponds to 222, R1 or R6, in that it is a *plasmid cointegrate*, a single structure carrying transfer factor and drug resistance properties. In contrast, both ΔA and ΔS are clearly examples of *plasmid aggregates* in which the two DNA molecules, Δ, carrying transfer factor properties and S or A, carrying drug-resistance properties, are replicated independently in the same cell and are usually transferred, transduced or lost independently.

REGULATION OF PLASMID REPLICATION

Since we now know the size of a number of plasmids and of the *E. coli* host chromosome, if we could isolate and separate the total plasmid and chromosomal DNA from a culture of R^+ cells, we would have a clear-cut indication of the relative numbers of the plasmid per chromosome. This has been done by a number of techniques by such methods as estimating the amount of DNA either in satellite peaks in *Proteus*, or in alkaline-sucrose gradient peaks or ethidium bromide-cesium chloride satellite peaks from *E. coli*. All these estimations require the assumption that the entire plasmid DNA is isolated. They are also subject to certain, so far uncontrollable, experimental variations.

In spite of these limitations, several important features can be gained from an examination of this type of data (e. g., EB/CsCl gradients). Table 4 shows that for some

Table 4

RATIO OF SATELLITE TO CHROMOSOMAL DNA SEPARATED BY ETHIDIUM BROMIDE AND THE RELATIVE NUMBERS OF PLASMID TO CHROMOSOMAL COPIES IN *E. COLI*

Plasmid	Sat. DNA / Chrom. DNA	Copy number plasmid to chromosome	Control
R15[a]	2.5	1.4	
222[a]	5.0	1.8	
R28K[b]	4.1	2.2	Stringent
Δ[c]	2.3	0.9	
R6K[b]	15[d]	13	
	40[e]	38	Relaxed
S[c]	4.2	10	

[a] NISIOKA, MITANI and CLOWES (1970)
[b] KONTOMICHALOU, MITANI and CLOWES (1970)
[c] SMITH, ANDERSON and CLOWES (1970)
[d, e] refer to lysates from exponential and stationary cultures respectively

plasmids (e. g., R15, 222, R28K and *Δ*), the numbers of copies correspond to between one and two per chromosome. There are however a number of plasmids where this relationship clearly does not hold, where the relative numbers of copies of plasmids to chromosome are much greater and are between 10 to 40. These plasmids include the small non-infectious elements A and S and in addition the smallest plasmid so far found with sex factor activity, R6K.

Thus, although the data is crude, we can recognize two distinct classes of R factors. First, those preserving a near-unitary relationship in copy number between the factor and the chromosome and which have been termed "stringent" in the regulation of their DNA replication. Second, a group in which there are tenfold or so more copies of the R factor than chromosome and in which the replication of DNA has been termed "relaxed". A further feature of at least some relaxed-regulated plasmids is that the relative numbers of copies appears to increase some threefold if lysates are made from stationary rather than from logarithmic cultures.

Other workers have previously noted relaxed replication of the 222 R factor in *Proteus* rather than in *E. coli* (Rownd, 1969). However, Table 4 shows the cointegrated form of 222 in *E. coli* to be stringent. Further analysis of the data in *Proteus* indicates that probably the large 28μ segregant remains stringent whereas the small 6μ segregant is

293

relaxed. If this interpretation is correct, the data are consistent with those already shown, that is, smaller plasmids are relaxed in replication.

Fig. 11 summarizes the molecular weights and replication control of a number of elements investigated in our laboratory. Relaxed replication seems to be characteristic

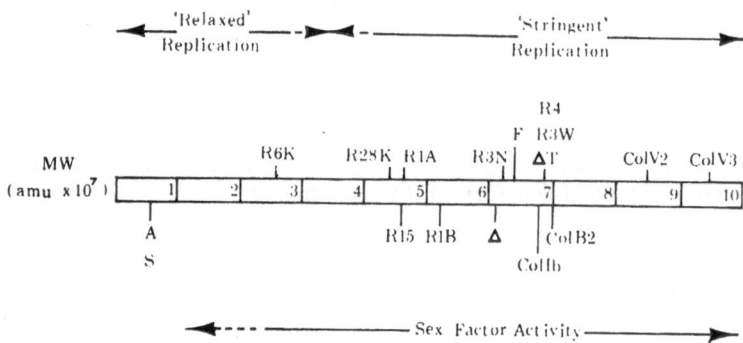

Fig. 11 Molecular weights and functional differences of bacterial plasmids isolated by ethidium bromide CsCl centrifugation and measured by contour length.

of molecules of small molecular weight, which implies that the smaller (relaxed) elements may not contain sufficient information to permit regulation in a stringent manner.

SUMMARY AND IMPLICATIONS OF MOLECULAR STRUCTURE

To summarize our conclusions on the molecular nature of plasmids; we would conclude that bacterial plasmids (and R factors in particular) represent a spectrum of entities. They range from the extreme of composite molecules in which a number of independent replicons are cointegrated in the same plasmid molecule to form a *stable plasmid cointegrate*. Examples of this are the R factors 222, R1, R6 and ΔT in *E. coli*. (ΔT would be thus more appropriately designated at Δ-T.) In the middle of the spectrum, there is what might be termed the *unstable plasmid cointegrate* in which a cointegrated plasmid tends to break down into at least two of its components, both of which are independently replicating molecules. Examples of this are 222, R1 and R6 in *Proteus*. The other extreme of plasmid structure is represented by a *plasmid aggregate* as is found in ΔA and ΔS and, as had been inferred for some time in F + ColE1 (we should thus refer to Δ + A, Δ + S). In these systems, the transfer factor properties are carried on a large molecule and the drug resistance or colicinogenic properties on a small non-infectious molecule which may frequently be transferred as a result of its being resident in the same cell as the infectious plasmid.

At the moment one can only speculate on the association between these two elements in transfer. We have previously concluded that chromosomal segments may be transferred from one bacterial strain to another by virtue of a conjugating system set up by a (ColIb) sex factor, which does not and probably cannot itself integrate in the chromosome and to which therefore is not likely to be covalently linked in transfer (CLOWES and MOODY, 1966). Similarly, it is not unlikely that non-infectious elements such as S, A, or ColE, could be transferred with Δ or ColIb or F in a similar way. Some form of homology may perhaps exist between the specific linear single-stranded fragment of the transfer factor (which is apparently transferred in a $5' \rightarrow 3'$ direction — RUPP and IHLER, 1968) and the corresponding linear strand of the non-infectious replicon.

294

The idea that R factors may arise by *de novo* mutation of molecules which were initially extrachromosomal raises interesting speculations on their evolution, and of this phenomenon as a possible general mechanism of evolution. It seems clear, at least that as an alternative evolutionary origin of R factors by a "gene pick-up" mechanism, we must consider that some drug resistance genes originate (after mutation) from elements which were extrachromosomal at the time that selective antibiotic pressure evolved the R factors in the variety and profusion that we see today. The simultaneous presence of transfer factors in the same inter-fertile population, would ensure the rapid dissemination of these small drug resistance molecules leading to systems such as $\Delta + S$ or $\Delta + A$. Later, perhaps some of these plasmid aggregates may have developed into plasmid cointegrates which are likely to be a more efficient system for the transfer of drug resistance.

Acknowledegement

This work was supported by the Public Health Service research grants GM-14394 and GM-13234 from the National Institute of General Medical Sciences.

REFERENCES

ANDERS,ON E. S. (1969): Ecology and epidemiology of transferable drug resistance. In: Bacterial Episomes and Plasmids, pp. 102–119. Editors: G. E. W. Wolstenholme and M. O'Connor. J. & A. Churchill Ltd., London.

ANDERSON, E. S. and LEWIS, M. J. (1965): Characterization of a transfer factor associated with drug resistance in Salmonella typhimurium. Nature, **208**, 843.

ANDERSON, E. S. and PERRET, D. (1967): Mobilization of transduced tetracycline resistance by the Δ transfer factor in Salmonella typhimurium and S. typhi. Nature **214**, 810.

CLOWES, R. C. (1964): Transfert génétique des facteurs colicinogènes. Annales Institut Pasteur **107/5**, 74.

CLOWES, R. C. and MOODY, E. E. M. (1966): Chromosome transfer from ,recombinationdeficient' strains of Escherichia coli K12. Genetics, **53**, 717.

CLOWES, R. C., MOODY, E. E. M. and PRITCHARD, R. H. (1965): Elimination of extrachromosomal elements in thymineless strains of Escherichia coli K12. Genetic Research (Cambridge) **6**, 147.

COHEN, S. N. and MILLER, C. A. (1970): Non-chromosomal antibiotic resistance. II. Molecular nature of R-factors isolated from Proteus mirabilis and Escherichia coli. Journal of Molecular Biology, **50**, 671. ·

FALKOW, S., CITARELLA, R. V., WOHLEITER, J. A. and WATANABE, T. (1966): The molecular nature of R factors. Journal of Molecular Biology, **17**, 102.

FREDERICQ, P. (1969): The recombination of colicinogenic factors with other episomes and plasmids. In: Bacterial Episomes and Plasmids, pp. 163–174. Editors: G. E. W. Wohlstenholme and M. O'Connor. J. & A. Churchill Ltd., London.

HICKSON, F. T., ROTH, T. R. and HELINSKI, D. R. (1967): Circular DNA forms of a bacterial sex factor. Proceedings of the National Academy of Science, United States, **58**, 1731.

KLEINSCHNMIDT, A. and ZAHN, R. K. (1959): Über Desoxyribonucleinsäure-Molekeln in Protein-Mischfilmen. Zeitschrift für Naturforschung, **14b**, 770.

KONTOTMICHALOU, P., MITANI, M. and CLOWES, R. C. (1970): Circular R-factor molecules controlling penicillinase synthesis, replicating in Escherichia coli under either relaxed or stringent control. Journal of Bacteriology, **104**, 34.

LANG, D. (1970): Molecular weights of coliphages and coliphage DNA. III. Contour length and molecular weight of DNA from bacteriophages T4, T5 and T7, and from bovine papilloma virus. Journal of Molecular Biology, **54**, 557.

LANG, D., BUJARD, H., WOLFF, B. and RUSSELL, D. (1967): Electron microscopy of size and shape of viral DNA in solutions of different ionic strengths. Journal of Molecular Biology, **23**, 163.

MACFARREN, A. C. and CLOWES, R. C. (1967): A comparative study of two F-like colicin factors, ColV2 and ColV3, in Escherichia coli K-12. Journal of Bacteriology, **94**, 365.

MARMUR, J., ROWND, R., FALKOW, S., BARON L. S., SCHILDKRAUT, C. and DOTY, P. (1961):

The nature of intergeneric episomal infection. Proceedings of the National Academy of Science, United States, **47**, 972.

NISIOKA, T., MITANI, M. and CLOWES, R. C. (1969): Composite circular forms of R-factor deoxyribonucleic acid molecules. Journal of Bacteriology, **97**, 376.

NISIOKA, T., MITANI, M. and CLOWES, R. C. (1970): Molecular recombination between R-factor deoxyribonucleic acid molecules in Escherichia coli host cells. Journal of Bacteriology, **103**, 166.

NOVICK, R. P. (1969): Extrachromosomal inheritance in bacteria. Bacteriological Reviews, **33**, 210.

NOVICK, R. P. and RICHMOND, M. H. (1965): Nature and interactions of the genetic elements governing penicillinase synthesis in Staphylococcus aureus, Journal of Bacteriology, **90**, 467.

RADLOFF, R., BAUER, W. and VINOGRAD, J. (1967): A dye-buoyant-density method for the detection of isolation of closed circular duplex DNA: the closed circular DNA in HeLa cells. Proceedings of the National Academy of Science, United States, **57**, 1514.

ROWND, R. (1969): Replication of a bacterial episome under relaxed control. Journal of Molecular Biology, **44**, 387.

RUPP, W. D. and IHLER, G. (1968): Strand selection during bacterial mating. Cold Spring Harbor Symposium on Quantiative Biology **33**, 677.

SILVER, R. P. and FALKOW, S. (1970): Specific labeling and physical characterization of R-factor deoxyribonucleic acid in Escherichia coli. Journal of Bacteriology, **104**, 331.

SMITH, C., ANDERSON, E. S. and CLOWES, R. C. (1970): Stable, composite molecular forms of an R factor. Bacteriological Proceedings, GP77.

WATANABE, T. (1967): Infectious drug resistance. Scientific American, **217**, 19.

WATANABE, T. and FUKASAWA, T. (1960): "Resistance Transfer Factor" an Episome in Enterobacteriaceae. Biochemical Biophysical Research Communications, **3**, 660.

WATANABE, T. and FUKASAWA, T. (1961a): Episome-mediated transfer of drug resistance in Enterobacteriaceae. II. Elimination of resistance factors with acridines. Journal of Bacteriology, **81**, 679.

WATANABE, T. and FUKASAWA, T. (1961b): Episome-mediated transfer of drug resistance in Enterobacteriaceae. III. Transduction of resistance factors. Journal of Bacteriology, **82**, 202.

ELIMINATION OF BACTERIAL EPISOMES BY DNA-COMPLEXING COMPOUNDS

F. E. HAHN and J. CIAK

Department of Molecular Biology Walter Reed Army Institute of Research
Washington, U. S. A.

INTRODUCTION

Our studies of the effects of DNA-complexing compounds on episomal elements of bacteria are part of a wider research program which is concerned with the biochemical, genetic and pharmacological effects of drugs and dyes which form commplexes with nucleic acids, especially with DNA.

Among these substances are chemotherapeutic drugs such as quinine, quinacrine (atebrin), chloroquine (resochin), miracil D (lucanthone) and berberine, as well as veterinary drugs such as ethidium bromide. They have the common property of acting as DNA-template poisons and inhibiting nucleic acid biosyntheses in susceptible microorganisms.

Aminoacridines as well as miracil D (HARTMAN, LEVINE, HARTMAN and BERGER, 1971) act as frameshift mutagens in bacterial viruses; on the other hand, quinacrine (JOHNSON and BACH, 1966), acridine orange, acriflavine and numerous other DNA-complexing substances (HELLER and SEVAG, 1966; BACH and JOHNSON, 1971), are "antimutagens" for bacteria, i. e. substances which reduce the frequency of spontaneous or induced chromosomal gene mutations.

Acriflavine (EPHRUSSI, HOTTINGUER and CHIMENES, 1949), berberine (MEISEL and SOKOLOVA, 1959) and ethidium bromide (SLONIMSKY, PERRODIN and CROFT, 1968) transform yeast cells quantitatively into respiratory-deficient mitochondrial "mutants" which are deficient in cytochrome oxidase (MAHLER, MEHROTRA and PERLMAN, 1971) and grow as "petite" colonies on plates (EPHRUSSI et al., 1949). Ethidium bromide evokes profound structural and compositional changes in the mitochondrial DNA of transformed yeast cells (PERLMAN and MAHLER, 1971). This shows that DNA-complexing substances can have pronounced effects on non-chromosomal genetic elements.

Such effects on episomes were first demonstrated by HIROTA and IIJIMA (1957) who found that acriflavine eliminated the F factor from F⁺ cells of *Escherichia coli* and, thereafter, by WATANABE and FUKASAWA (1961) who reported that acriflavine and acridine orange eliminated certain resistance determinants from the R-factors of multiple drug-resistant bacteria. When it was shown five years later (FALKOW, CITARELLA, WOHLHIETER and WATANABE, 1966; ROWND, NAKAYA and NAKAMURA, 1966) that R-factors are composed of DNA, the idea became apparent that the episome-eliminating action of aminoacridines represents still another instance of genetic effects of DNA-complexing compounds. Therefore, we undertook a study of the elimination of episomal elements by a series of DNA-complexing drugs and dyes. While this work was in progress,

BOUANCHAUD, SCAVIZZI and CHABBERT (1969) reported that ethidium bromide eliminated the lac$^+$ marker from F' lac in *E. coli* and certain resistance determinants from R-factors, harbored by several bacteria. An account of our work representing its state as of October 1970 has recently been published (HAHN and CIAK, 1971).

Theory of Ligand Binding to DNA]

Studies on the binding of drugs and dyes to DNA have been carried out over the past 25 years; they were placed on a firm scientific basis by the recognition of the double-helical structure of DNA (WATSON and CRICK, 1953). From a considerable amount of biophysical work, two major structural models of DNA-ligand complexes have been developed.

1. The *"stacking model"* (BRADLEY and WOLF, 1959) envisages the binding of numerous ring systems of positive charges to the periphery of the double helix by electrostatic attraction to the negatively charged phosphate groups in the phosphate-deoxyribose backbones of DNA. The prototype of such stacking ligands is acridine orange. This type of binding is characterized by a stoichiometry which exceeds one ligand molecule per 4 or 5 component nucleotides of DNA and by comparatively low apparent binding constants. Certain aliphatic polyamines such as spermine bind to DNA exclusively by peripheral electrostatic attraction (LIQUORI, COSTANTINO, CRESCENZI, ELIA, GIGLIO, PULITI, DE SANTIS SAVIONO and VITAGLIANO, 1967). These binding processes are antagonised by monovalent and, more strongly, by divalent inorganic cations. Since the neutralization of DNA phosphates by positively charged counterions will decrease or abolish the mutual charge repulsion by the negatively charged DNA phosphates, complex formation of DNA with cations increases the median thermal denaturation temperature, T_m, od DNA, i. e. it stabilizes DNA to strand separation.

2. The *"intercalation model"* envisages the insertion or "intercalation" of flat aromatic ring systems between the levels of base pairs into the DNA double helix (LERMAN, reviewed in 1964). This type of binding is characterized by a stoichiometry not exceeding one ligand molecule per two base pairs. A statistical limit of one intercalant per 4.2 DNA nucleotides (CAIRNS, 1962) has, in fact, been determined experimentally for several drugs or dyes (for example, PEACOCKE and SKERRETT, 1956) and an abstract explanation of the existence of this upper limit in which only every second base pair level can be occupied by an intercalated molecule is given by the "excluded site model" (CROTHERS, 1968) although a physical explanation of the exclusion phenomenon is still lacking. Intercalation binding occurs with significantly higher apparent association constants than outside binding.

The spaces for intercalation are created by local untwisting of the double helix by approximately 12° of rotation which causes a separation between previously adjacent base pairs of approximately 3.5 Å without a disturbance in the pattern of hydrogen bonds. This causes a lengthening of linear DNA by maximally 50 per cent (CAIRNS, 1962) when every second intercalation space is occupied and also renders DNA more rigid. Intercalation binding is relatively insensitive to antagonism by inorganic ions. To the extent to which intercalated molecules carry positive charges, these charges will help in anchoring such molecules in their intercalation sites by electrostatic attraction to DNA phosphates which, like in the case of amines attached to the outside of the double helix, stabilizes DNA to strand separation.

3. *Intercalation into supercoiled circular DNA* has come under study during the past few years (CRAWFORD and WARING, 1967; BAUER and VINOGRAD, 1968, 1970, 1971; WARING, 1970, 1971). Since the Watson-Crick helical turns and the superhelical turns in supercoiled DNA are topologically equivalent, changes in the number of Watson-Crick

turns upon multiple intercalation will change the number of superhelical turns, i. e. the "superhelix density". Systematic increases in drug concentration (in the manner of a titration of supercoiled DNA with a given drug) gradually convert supercoiled DNA into unconstrained circular DNA; upon adding further drug, this circular DNA becomes artificially supercoiled in a direction of rotation opposite to that in the original supercoiled condition (CRAWFORD and WARING, 1967). The biological role of supercoiled DNA is not well understood; for this reason, it is difficult to envisage the biological consequences of the induction of artificial supercoils in circular DNA *in vivo*. Since F' lac episomal DNA is supercoiled circular in nature (FREIFELDER and FREIFELDER, 1968a, 1968b), R-factors harbored by *E. coli* have been shown to consist of single closed circular supercoiled DNA molecules (COHEN and MILLER, 1970; SILVER and FALKOW, 1970) and mitochondrial DNA likewise is thought to be circular in structure (BILLHEIMER and AVERS, 1969), we have entertained one hypothesis (HAHN and CIAK, 1971) that the elimination of circular non-chromosomal genetic elements by intercalative substances may be a result of constraining these molecules in the form of unnatural supercoils. While our observations are in accord with this hypothesis, they do not prove it conclusively and may find a different explanation with advances in the knowledge of the molecular biology of non-chromosomal genetic elements.

Elimination by DNA-complexing of the lac$^+$ marker from F' lac episomes

In his original work on the elimination of the F-factor from *E. coli* HIROTA (1960) used a genetic recombination assay (LEDERBERG, CAVALLI-SFORZA and LEDERBERG, 1952). We worked with strain 3876 of *E. coli* K-12 which contains the F' lac episome and assayed for the percentage of lac$^-$ colonies on plates seeded with bacteria from liquid cultures

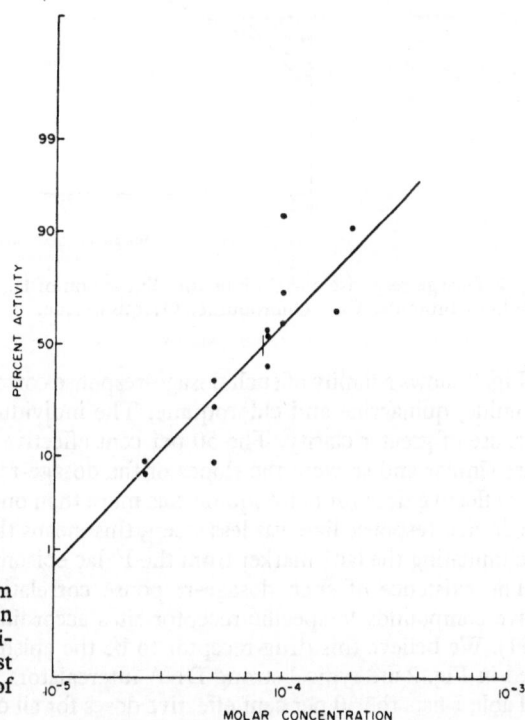

Fig. 1 Elimination of the lac$^+$ marker from F' lac containing *E. coli* 3876 grown in graded concentrations of quinacrine. Ordinate: per cents of lac$^-$ colonies on test plates. Abscissa: molar concentrations of quinacrine.

that had grown over night in the presence of graded subinhibitory concentrations of selected episome-eliminating chemicals (HAHN and CIAK, 1971). A typical set of results with quinacrine (atebrin) is shown in Fig. 1. The per cent frequency of loss of the lac$^+$ marker is expressed in per cents activity on the ordinate (which is a probability scale) as a function of the concentration of quinacrine entered on the logarithmic abscissa. This procedure amounts to a graphic probit transformation of a conventional dosage-response curve. The best straight line was fitted by the method of the least squares, according equal statistical weight to each point. From this line the 50 per cent effective dose of quinacrine was determined to be 7.2×10^{-5} M.

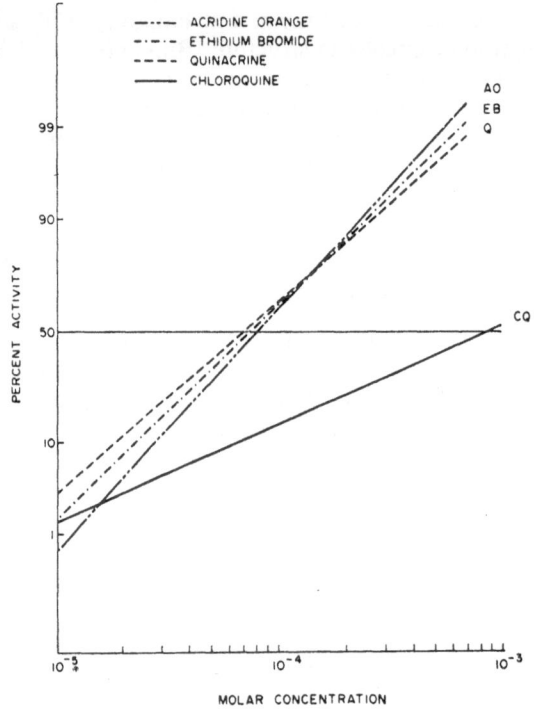

Fig. 2 Dosage response correlations for elimination of lac$^+$ as in Fig. 1. AO: acridine orange, EB: ethidium bromide, CQ: chloroquine, Q: quinacrine.

Fig. 2 shows a family of such dosage-response correlations for acridine orange, ethidium bromide, quinacrine and chloroquine. The individual points have been omitted for the purpose of greater clarity. The 50 per cent effective doses for the first three compounds were similar and so were the slopes of the dosage-response lines. In contrast, the 50 per cent effective dose for chloroquine was more than one magnitude greater and the slope of the dosage-response line was less steep; this means that chloroquine was much less active in eliminating the lac$^+$ marker from the F′ lac episome.

The existence of such dosage-response correlations is indicative of the binding of active compounds to specific receptor sites according to the law of mass action (RAND, 1971). We believe this drug receptor to be the episomal DNA since all four compounds cited in Fig. 2 are typical strong DNA intercalators.

Table 1 lists the 50 per cent effective doses for all compounds which we tested for their ability to eliminate the lac+ marker. Miracil D at the highest concentration employed did not quite produce 50 per cent elimination and the 50 per cent effective dose was estimated by extrapolation of the dosage response line. Quinine showed a trend to eliminate the lac+ marker but extrapolation to a 50 per cent effective dose could not be made with confidence. Methylene blue and p-rosaniline were completely non-active.

Table 1

FIFTY PER CENT EFFECTIVE DOSES, ED_{50}, OF COMPOUNDS ELIMINATING THE lac+ MARKER FROM *E. coli* 3876

Compound	ED_{50}
Quinacrine	7.2×10^{-5} M
Ethidium bromide	7.5×10^{-5} M
Acridine orange	8.2×10^{-5} M
Chloroquine	9.0×10^{-4} M
Miracil D*	3.3×10^{-3} M
Quinine	trend
Methylene blue	†
p-Rosaniline	†

* Extrapolated value
† No activity observed

These observations raised the question of the physical fate of the episomal DNA upon elimination of the lac+ marker. The elimination of R-factors from *Proteus mirabilis* and *E. coli* by acriflavine has been found (ROWND et al., 1966) to be accompanied by a complete physical loss of R-factor DNA from the bacteria. The transformation of yeast to "petite" mutants produces a gradation of changes in the mitochondrial DNA of these cells

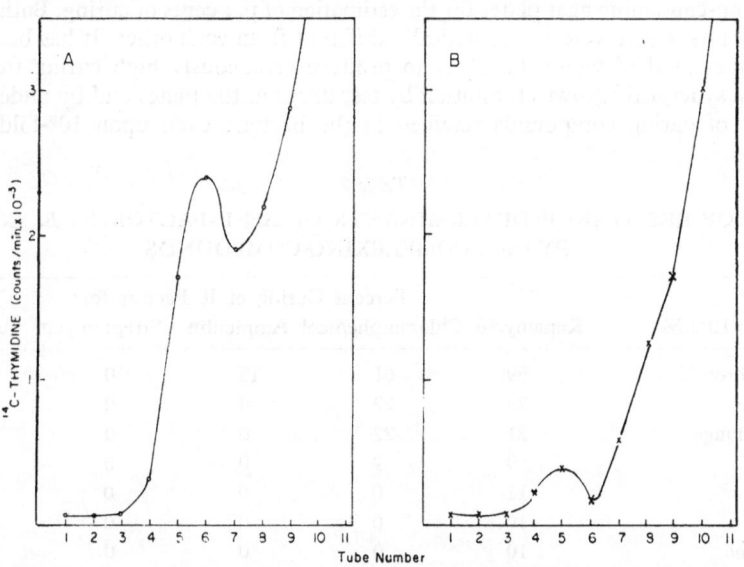

Fig. 3 Buoyant density profiles of DNA. A: from F' lac containing *E. coli* 3876; B: from the same bacterium from which lac+ has been eliminated by quinacrine.

301

(PERLMAN and MAHLER, 1971) and eventually a complete loss of mitochondrial DNA upon prolonged treatment of yeast cells with ethidium bromide (GOLDRING, GROSSMAN, KRUPNICK, CRYER and MARMUR, 1970).

When the total DNA of *E. coli* containing the F' lac episome and of the same organism from which lac+ had been eliminated with quinacrine was labelled with ^{14}C-thymidine, extracted and subjected to equilibrium centrifugation by a method (BAZARAL and HELINSKI, 1968) which has previously been used to demonstrate the circular nature of colicinogenic factors in *E. coli*, results were obtained which are shown in Fig. 3. One satellite DNA band, sedimenting like closed circular DNA, was present in the DNA mixtures from both cultures, i. e. before and after the elimination of lac+ although its radioactivities and specific gravities were different for the lac+ and lac− organisms. Certainly, the elimination of the lac+ marker by quinacrine did not result in a complete physical disappearance of episomal DNA.

Elimination of resistance determinats from an R-factor in E. coli

For this work we used strain RS-2 of *E. coli* which harbored an R-factor carrying resistance determinants for kanamycin, chloramphenicol, ampicillin, streptomycin and sulfadiazine. The organisms were grown in liquid culture in the presence of a subinhibitory concentration of 10^{-4} M of selected curing compounds, the cultures were then diluted by a factor of 10^5 and plated on agar plates either containing no drugs or containing, individually, the five drugs against which the RS-2 strain was originally resistant. The difference between the numbers of colonies on antibiotic-containing and on drug-free control plates were expressed as percentages of the numbers of total colonies on the control plates. These percentages were considered the frequencies of curing which had been attained. In a second method, the experimental cultures were plated only on antibiotic-free agar plates, these plates were incubated overnight, then flooded with broth, the bacteria of all colonies suspended and these suspensions split into aliquots and replated on drug-free and on drug-containing agar plates for the estimation of per cents of curing. Both methods yielded results which were not statistically different from each other. It has been argued that the first method would be likely to produce erroneously high curing frequencies owing to a synergistic growth inhibition by test drugs in the plates and by undetermined quantities of curing compounds retained in the bacteria even upon 10^5-fold dilution

Table 2

CURING OF RESISTANCE DETERMINANTS OF AN R-FACTOR IN *E. COLI* RS-2
BY DNA-COMPLEXING COMPOUNDS

Compound 10^{-4} M	Percent Curing of R Factors for:				
	Kanamycin	Chloramphenicol	Ampicillin	Streptomycin	Sulfadiazine
Ethidium bromide	59	61	15	0	0
Quinacrine	25	22	4	0	0
Acridine orange	21	22	0	0	0
Berberine	9	9	0	0	0
Spermine	11	0	9	0	0
Quinine	10	0	0	0	0
Chloroquine	10	0	0	0	0
p-Rosaniline	0	0	0	0	0
Methylene blue	0	0	0	0	0

prior to plating. On biochemical grounds, synergy between DNA-complexers on one hand and kanamycin, chloramphenicol or ampicillin with radically different mechanisms of action on the other, is unlikely. By carrying the mixtures of cured and uncured cells through an additional cultural passage on plates containing neither curing chemicals nor test drugs and assaying the descendants of these original cells for drug sensitivity, the argument was also methodologically invalidated.

Table 2 lists the frequencies of curing obtained by selected DNA-complexing compounds in the sequence of their relative potencies. The individual resistance determinants showed marked differences in the extents to which they were eliminated. The kanamycin determinant was most sensitive, followed by the chloramphenicol and ampicillin determinants. The determinants of streptomycin and sulfadiazine resistance were not eliminated by any of the selected compounds at the standard concentration of 10^{-4} M. ANDERSON (1968) has observed a spontaneous loss of resistance determinants to kanamycin and chloramphenicol but not to ampicillin, streptomycin and sulfonamides in a strain of *Salmonella typhimurium* harboring an R-factor.

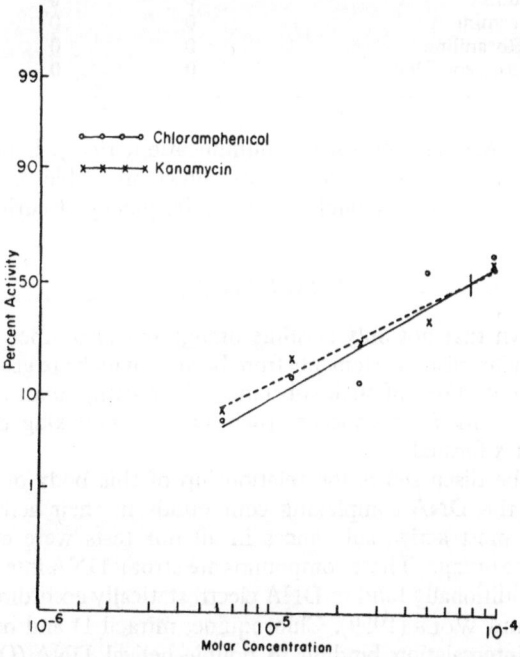

Fig. 4 Curing of resistance determinants for kanamycin and chloramphenicol in R-factor containing *E. coli* RS-2. Ordinate: frequency of curing. Abscissa: molar concentrations of ethidium bromide in whose presence the bacteria were grown.

We have developed dosage response correlations for the curing of the kanamycin and chloramphenicol resistance determinants by graded concentrations of ethidium bromide as shown in Fig. 4. The 50 per cent effective doses were identical and the slopes of the two lines were not significantly different from each other. As in the case of the elimination of the lac+ marker, the fact that a conventional dosage response correlation is observed argues in favor of the existence of discrete receptor sites for curing compounds the occupancy of which is concentration-dependent and obeys the law of mass action.

Elimination of a Gentamicin R-factor from Klebsiella pneumoniae

We obtained strain 3694 of *K. pneumoniae* from Dr. DRUBE of the Schering Corporation; this gentamicin-resistant strain was originally isolated at Georgetown University Hospital in Washington, D. C. Resistance to gentamicin of these bacteria is

Table 3

CURING OF GENTAMICIN R-FACTOR IN *KLEBSIELLA PNEUMONIAE* 3694

Compound at 10^{-4} M	Per cent curing	
	Method I	Method II
Ethidium bromide	57	47
Quinacrine	34	28
Acridine Orange	20	19
Berberine	trend	trend
Chloroquine	0	0
Quinine	0	0
Spermine	0	0
p-Rosaniline	0	0
Methylene Blue	0	0

due to an R-factor (C. MARTIN, personal communication, 1971). Experiments at curing this gentamicin resistance produced the results shown in Table 3. The two methods described above produced approximately the same frequency of curing.

DISCUSSION

Our work has shown that not only acridine orange but also other DNA-complexing compounds can eliminate episomal elements from bacteria which are grown in the presence of subinhibitory concentrations of such substances. The compounds selected have been studied by numerous workers as concerns their DNA-complexing properties and the nature of the complexes formed.

The first point to be discussed is the relationship of this body of knowledge to the relative efficiency of the DNA-complexing compounds in their action upon bacterial episomes. The three most active substances in all our tests were ethidium bromide, quinacrine and acridine orange. These compounds are strong DNA intercalators, although acridine orange can additionally bind to DNA electrostatically according to the "stacking model" of BRADLEY and WOLF (1959). Chloroquine, miracil D and berberine have also satisfied criteria for intercalation binding to double-helical DNA (O' BRIEN, ALLISON and HAHN, 1966; WEINSTEIN and HIRSCHBERG, 1971; KREY and HAHN, 1969) and quinine has been suggested to intercalate into DNA, albeit with a low stoichiometry of this binding reaction (ESTENSEN, KREY and HAHN, 1969). These four substances showed low or marginal activity against bacterial episomes. p-Rosaniline which binds to DNA but is not intercalated (NEVILLE and DAVIES, 1966) was entirely without effect. So was methylene blue which binds to both double-stranded and single-stranded DNA (HAHN and KREY, 1968). Spermine which binds to the double helix by lateral electrostatic attraction (LIQUORI et al., 1967) showed low activity in eliminating two resistance determinants from *E. coli*.

Qualitatively, the elimination of episomal elements correlates with the ability of active compounds to engage in strong intercalation binding with DNA with a high stoichiometry.

However, we have been unable to correlate, quantitatively, the antiepisomal activities of our tested compounds with any one quantitative parameter of DNA binding. Our impression is that the ability of eliminating episomal elements is a function of the extent to which DNA template poisons interfere with the replication of DNA in a given test organism.

This raises the second point to be discussed, *viz.*, the molecular mechanism underlying episome elimination. ANDERSON (1968) has proposed that the spontaneous loss of resistance determinants from R-factors is the result of a segregation during logarithmic growth, produced by an asynchrony between cell multiplication and the replication of various components of an R-factor. Although R-factors in *E. coli* have been shown to consist of single closed circular DNA molecules (COHEN and MILLER, 1970; SILVER and FALKOW, 1970) and behave as single units of genetic transmission (WATANABE, 1963), FALKOW has proposed the hypothesis that R-factors represent a recombinational assemblage of several replicons (FALKOW, TOMPKINS, SILVER, GUERRY and LE BLANC, 1971). We suggest that the segregation of resistance determinants which occured in our experiments when bacteria were grown overnight in the presence of curing compounds resembles the spontaneous segregation which ANDERSON has reported for the determinants of kanamycin and chloramphenicol resistance. The action of DNA-complexing compounds would merely enhance the natural tendency to segregation through selective inhibition of the replication of certain components of R-factors. We assume that susceptible resistance determinants whose replication is selectively inhibited by DNA template poisons are simply "left behind" in a percentage of cells during the course of cultural growth for a considerable number of generation times. These are the same resistance determinants which have shown a natural tendency to segregation by asynchrony in the absence of added selective inhibitors.

In terms of molecular pharmacology, we do not know the reasons underlying the selective toxicity of DNA-template poisons for the replication of certain resistance determinants. We have earlier (HAHN and CIAK, 1971) proposed that the circular DNA of susceptible resistance determinants may be constrained into artificial supercoils which in this conformation can not be enzymatically replicated. This proposal must remain an attractive speculation until such a time when the molecular biology of R-factors and of their replication will be understood in greater detail.

SUMMARY

1. In decreasing order of activity, quinacrine, ethidium bromide, acridine orange, chloroquine and miracil D eliminated the lac+ marker from the F' lac episome of *E. coli* when the organism was cultured in the presence of these compounds. Quinine was very slightly active and methylene blue and p-rosaniline were devoid of activity.

2. Ethidium bromide, quinacrine and acridine orange eliminated in decreasing order of frequency the resistance determinants for kanamycin, chloramphenicol and ampicillin from an R-factor in *E. coli* RS-2. Berberine, quinine, chloroquine and spermine exhibited the same low activity, while methylene blue and p-rosaniline were nonactive. Determinants of resistance to streptomycin and sulfadiazine were not cured by any of the compounds studied at the standard concentration of 10^{-4} M.

3. A gentamicin R-factor was eliminated from *K. pneumoniae* by ethidium bromide, quinacrine, acridine orange and berberine in decreasing order of activity.

4. Episome-eliminating activities of selected DNA-complexing substances could be represented in the form of probit transformations of conventional dosage response

curves suggesting that these activities were functions of the extent of occupancy of drug receptor sites, probably on episomal DNA.

5. Resistance determinants in *E. coli* which were cured at relatively high percentages (kanamycin, chloramphenicol) are known to be spontaneously lost by *Salmonella*. We propose that curing agents act by selective inhibition of the replication of susceptible episomal elements.

Acknowledgement

Figs. 1—4 have been published in Annals of the New York Academy of Sciences, *182*, 295—304 (1971).

REFERENCES

ANDERSON, E. S. (1968): The ecology of transferable drug resistance in the enterobacteria. Annual Review of Microbiology, **22**, 131.

BACH, M. K. and JOHNSON, H. G. (1971): Some studies on the antimutagenic action of polyamines. Progress in Molecular and Subcellular Biology, **2**, 329. Editor: F. E. Hahn. Springer Verlag, Berlin. Heidelberg. New York.

BAUER, W. and VINOGRAD, J. (1968): The interaction of closed circular DNA with intercalative dyes. I. The superhelix density of SV40 DNA in the presence and absence of dye. Journal of Molecular Biology, **33**, 141.

BAUER, W. and VINOGRAD, J. (1970): Interaction of closed circular DNA with intercalative dyes. II. The free energy of superhelix formation in SV40 DNA. Journal of Molecular Biology, **47**, 419.

BAUER, W. and VINOGRAD, J. (1971): The use of intercalative dyes in the study of closed circular DNA. Progress in Molecular and Subcellular Biology, **2**, 181. Editor: F. E. Hahn. Springer Verlag, Berlin. Heidelberg. New York.

BAZARAL, M. and HELINSKI, D. R. (1968): Circular forms of colicinogenic factors E1, E2 and E3 from Escherichia coli. Journal of Molecular Biology, **36**, 185.

BILLHEIMER, F. E. and AVERS, C. L. (1969): Nuclear and mitochondrial DNA from wild type and petite yeast: Circularity, length and buoyant density. Proceedings of the National Academy of Sciences of the United States of America, **64**, 739.

BOUCHANCHAUD, D., SCAVIZZI, M. R. and CHABBERT, Y. A. (1969): Elimination by ethidium bromide of antibiotic resistance in Enterobacteria and Staphylococci. Journal of General Microbiology, **54**, 417.

BRADLEY, D. F. and WOLF M. K. (1959): Aggregation of dyes bound to polyanions.Proceedings of the National Academy of Sciences of the United States of America, **45**, 944.

CAIRNS, J. (1962): The application of radioautography to the study of DNA viruses. Cold Spring Harbor Symposium of Quantitative Biology, **27**, 311.

COHEN, S. N. and MILLER, C. A. (1970): Non-chromosomal antibiotic resistance in bacteria. II. Molecular nature of R-factors isolated from Proteus mirabilis and Escherichia coli. Journal of Molecular Biology, **50**, 671.

CRAWFORD, L. V. and WARING M. J. (1967): Supercoiling of polyoma virus DNA measured by its interaction with ethidium bromide. Journal of Molecular Biology, **25/1**, 23.

CROTHERS, D. M. (1968): Calculation of binding isotherms for heterogeneous polymers. Biopolymers, **6/4**, 575.

EPHRUSSI, B., HOTTINGUER, H. and CHIMENES, A. M. (1949): Action de l'acriflavine sur les levures. 1. — La mutation „petite colonie." Annales de l'institut Pasteur, **76/4**, 351.

ESTENSEN, R. D., KREY, A. K. and HAHN, F. E. (1969): Studies on a deoxyribonucleic acid-quinine complex. Molecular Pharmacology, **5/5**, 532.

FALKOW, S., CITARELLA, R. V., WOHLHIETER, J. A. and WATANABE, T. (1966): The molecular nature of R-factors. Journal of Molecular Biology, **17**, 102.

FREIFELDER, D. (1968): Studies on Escherichia coli sex factors. III. Covalently closed F'Lac DNA molecules. Journal of Molecular Biology, **34/1**, 31.

FREIFELDER, D. R. and FREIFELDER, D. (1968) :Studies on *E. coli* sex factors. II. Some physical properties of F'Lac and F DNA. Journal of Molecular Biology, **32/1**, 25.

GOLDRING, E. S., GROSSMAN, L. I., KRUPNICK, D., CRYER, D. R. and MARMUR, J. (1970): The petite mutation in yeast. Loss of mitochondrial deoxyribonucleic acid during induction of petites with ethidium bromide. Journal of Molecular Biology, **52**, 323.

HAHN, F. E. and CIAK, J. (1971): Elimination of bacterial episomes by DNA-complexing compounds. Annals of the New York Academy of Sciences, 182, 295.

HAHN, F. E. and KREY, A. K. (1968): Deoxyribonucleic acid-induced anomalous optical rotatory dispersion of antimalarial drugs and dyes. Antimicrobial Agents and Chemotherapy — 1068, 15.

HARTMAN, P. E., LEVINE, K., HARTMAN, Z. and BERGER, H. (1971): Hycanthone: A frameshift mutagen. Science, 172, 1058.

HELLER, C. S. and SEVAG, M. G. (1966): Prevention of the emergence of drug resistance in bacteria by acridines, phenothiazines and dibenzocycloheptenes. Applied Microbiology, 14/6, 879.

HIROTA, Y. (1960): The effect of acridine dyes on mating type factors in Escherichia coli. Proceedings of the National Academy of Sciences of the United States of America, 46, 57.

HIROTA, Y. and IIJIMA, T. (1957): Acriflavine as an effective agent for eliminating F-factor in Escherichia coli. Nature, 180, 655.

JOHNSON, H. G. and BACH, M. K. (1966): The antimutagenic action of polyamines: Suppression of the mutagenic action of an E. coli mutator gene and of 2-aminopurine. Proceedings of the National Academy of Sciences of the United States of America, 55, 1453.

KREY A. K. and HAHN, F. E. (1969): Berberine: Complex with DNA. Science, 166, 757.

LEDERBERG, J., CAVALLI-SFORZA, L. L. and LEDERBERG, E. M. (1952): Sex compatibility Escherichia coli. Genetics, 37, 720.

LERMAN, L. (1964): Acridine mutagens and DNA structure. Journal of Cellular and Comparative Physiology, 64/ Supplement 1, 1.

LIQUORI, A. M., COSTANTINO, L., CRESCENZI, V., ELIA, V., GIGLIO, E., PULITI, R., De SANTIS SAVINO, M. and VITAGLIANO, V. (1967): Complexes between DNA and polyamines: A molecular model. Journal of Molecular Biology, 24, 113.

MAHLER, H. R., MEHROTRA, B. D. and PERLMAN P. S. (1971): Formation of yeast mitochondria. V. Ethidium bromide as a probe for the function of mitochondrial DNA. Progress in Molecular and Subcellular Biology, 2, 274. Editor: F. E. Hahn. Springer Verlag, Berlin. Heidelberg. New York.

MEISEL, M. N. and SOKOLOVA, T. S. (1959): Inherited cytoplasmic changes induced in yeast by acriflavine and berberine. Doklady Akademii Nauk of the Union of Socialistic Soviet Republics, 131/2, 436.

NEVILLE, D. M. and DAVIES, D. R. (1966): The interaction of acridine dyes with DNA: An x-ray diffraction and optical investigation. Journal of Molecular Biology, 17, 57.

O'BRIEN, R. L., ALLISON, J. L. and HAHN, F. E. (1966): Evidence for intercalation of chloroquine into DNA. Biochimica et Biophysica Acta, 129, 622.

PEACOCKE, A. R. and SKERRETT, J. N. H. (1956): The interaction of aminoacridines with nucleic acids. Transactions of the Faraday Society, 52, 261.

PERLMAN, P. S. and MAHLER, H. R. (1971): Molecular consequences of ethidium bromide mutagenesis. Nature New Biology, 231/18, 12.

RANG, H. P. (1971): Drug receptors and their function. Nature, 231, 91.

ROWND, R., NAKAYA, R. and NAKAMURA, A. (1966): Molecular nature of the drug-resistance factors of the Enterobacteriaceae. Journal of Molecular Biology, 17, 376.

SILVER R. P. and FALKOW, S. (1970): Specific labeling and physical characterization of R-factor deoxyribonucleic acid in Escherichia coli. Journal of Bacteriology, 104/1, 331.

SLONIMSKI, B. P., PERRODIN, G. and CROFT, J. H. (1968): Ethidium bromide induced mutation of yeast mitochondria: Complete transformation of cells into respiratory deficient non-chromosomal „petites." Biochemical and Biophysical Research Communications. 30/3, 232.

WARING, M. (1970): Variation of the supercoils in closed circular DNA by binding of antibiotics and drugs: Evidence for molecular models involving intercalation. Journal of Molecular Biology, 54, 247.

WARING, M. (1971): Binding of drugs to supercoiled circular DNA: Evidence for and against intercalation. Progress in Molecular and Subcellular Biology, 2, 216. Editor: F. E. Hahn. Springer Verlag, Berlin. Heidelberg. New York.

WATANABE, T. (1963): Infective heredity of multiple drug resistance in bacteria. Bacteriological Reviews, 27/1, 87.

WATANABE, T. and FUKASAWA, T. (1961): Episome-mediated transfer of drug resistance in Enterobacteriaceae. II. Elimination of resistance factors with acridine dyes. Journal of Bacteriology, 81/5, 679.

WATSON, J. D. and CRICK, F. H. C. (1953): The structure of DNA. Cold Spring Harbor Symposium of Quantitative Biology, 18, 123.

WEINSTEIN, I. B. and HIRSCHBERG, E. (1971): Mode of action of miracil D. Progress in Molecular and Subcellular Biology, 2, 232. Editor: F. E. Hahn. Springer Verlag, Berlin. Heidelberg. New York.

307

EFFECTS OF SUPERINFECTION IMMUNITY ON
PLASMID REPLICATION FOLLOWING CONJUGATION

D. J. LeBLANC, and S. FALKOW

Department of Microbiology, Georgetown University Schools of Medicine and Dentistry
Washington, U.S.A.

Transmissible bacterial plasmids are generally composite genetic elements composed of accessory genes carrying a variety of functions, and a transfer, or sex factor, component. Historically, most plasmids have been classified according to their auxiliary genes which, in many instances, have been responsible for their discovery. Hence, the term R factor was allocated to those plasmids which mediate transmissible multiple drug resistance among the Enterobacteriaceae, WATANABE (1963). A more specific criterion for plasmid classification, however, is provided by those genes which specify such properties as autonomous replication and conjugal transfer. For example, all naturally occurring R factors have come to be classified as fi$^+$ or fi$^-$, depending on the presence or absence of an inhibitory effect on the classical sex factor, F, WATANABE and FUKASAWA (1962) and WATANABE, NISHIDA, OGATA, ARAI and SATO (1964). Subsequently, this observation was traced to the sex factor genes controlling the biosynthesis of specific sex pili, MEYNELL and DATTA (1967). Thus, approximately 85% of all R factors have been found to synthesize sex pili which are either related to F (F-like), DATTA, LAWN and MEYNELL (1966), or related to those specified by the *Col* I sex factor (I-like), MEYNELL and LAWN (1967). Recently, Iyer has established another fi$^-$ class of R factors, termed Ike-like, as a distinct subgroup, KHATOON and IYER (1971), and, other classes of fi$^-$ R factors are likely (DATTA, personal communication).

Perhaps the most specific criterion of the relatedness between two plasmids is their inability to coexist stably in the same host cell. This phenomenon, loosely referred to as superinfection immunity, MEYNELL and DATTA (1969) and NOVICK (1969), appears to be a reflection of two distinct phenomena — plasmid incompatibility and entry exclusion. Entry exclusion is postulated to be due to a sex factor-linked gene which determines a specific cell barrier that prevents the transfer of DNA between cells carrying isogenic, or very closely related, plasmids. This cell barrier, whatever it may be, is not totally effective, however, and superinfecting DNA may enter a small proportion of the cells in a recipient population. Upon circumvention of the barrier imposed by entry exclusion, the superinfecting plasmid may still have to contend with its inherent incompatibility with the resident plasmid. The most common explanation for incompatibility is based on the replicon hypothesis, JACOB, BRENNER and CUZIN (1963), which suggests that every autonomous replicon must be attached to a structural component of the cell, a "maintenance site," which is required for replication as well as for distribution of replicas. Thus, very closely related plasmids may require the same "maintenance site" and would have to compete for this site. According to this hypothesis, then, incompatibility would be reflected in the failure of the superinfecting DNA, or the resident plasmid, to replicate normally in the recipient cell.

Data presently available on superinfection immunity has been derived, for the most part, from genetic studies. A technique for the specific labeling of sex factor DNA, initially developed by the FREIFELDERS for F, FREIFELDER (1968) and FREIFELDER and FREIFELDER (1968), and previously employed by us for following the replication of R factor DNA in *Escherichia coli*, FALKOW, TOMPKINS, SILVER, GUERRY and LE BLANC (1971) and SILVER and FALKOW (1970), seemed suitable for a molecular approach to superinfection immunity. The system consists of a male cell which is prototrophic for thymine synthesis and resistant to 5BU, and thus unable to incorporate exogenous thymine, and a female which is auxotrophic for thymine and unable to repair lesions produced by a heavy dose of ultraviolet light. The irradiated female remains competent as a conjugal partner and is able to accept extrachromosomal DNA from a donor cell. Replication of the transferred plasmid occurs in the female and, if the mating is performed in the presence of ^{3}H-thymine, the major net incorporation of label will be found in the plasmid. The successful labeling of a transmissible plasmid in this system is dependent on a high frequency of conjugal transfer. Therefore, the derepressed R factor, R1drd19 (*sul, str, cam, kan, penZ*), MEYNELL and DATTA (1967), previously obtained from DATTA, was used for our experiments.

A preliminary experiment, using this system, consisted of following the fate of DNA transferred from a donor strain to various recipients harboring isogenic, related and unrelated plasmids. Recipient cells (strain AB2500, Thy$^-$, UV^S) were prepared that carried the isogenic resistance transfer factor (RTF) from R1drd; the fi$^+$ R factor, 222; the fi$^-$ R factor, N3; and the sex factor, F. Each of these recipients, in the exponential phase of growth, were irradiated and mated, in the presence of 1 μg/ml of ^{3}H-thymine, with the same population of donor cells carrying the fi$^+$ R factor, R1drd. The results, corrected for incorporation by male and female alone, are summarized in Table I. Also included in this table, for comparison, are the results of an experiment in which the same

Table 1

^{3}H-THYMINE INCORPORATION VS. MATING FREQUENCIES DURING
RS2 × AB2500 (WITH VARIOUS PLASMIDS) MATINGS

Recipient	Pilus type produced by recipient plasmid	Relative incorporation[1] of label	Relative transfer[2] frequency of donor plasmid
AB2500	—	100	100
AB2500 N$_3$	Ike-like	73	60
AB2500 F$^+$	F-like	24	4
AB2500 (222)	F-like	18	0.24
AB2500 RTF	F-like	11	0.0009

1. Recipient cells in the exponential phase of growth were irradiated and mixed with aliquots of a single R1drd donor cell population in glucose-casamino acids medium containing 1 μg/ml of ^{3}H-thymine (18.1 C/mM) and incubated at 37 °C. The male and female controls were grown individually but were treated identically otherwise. After 60 minutes of mating, 50 μl samples were removed and assayed for trichloroacetic acid precipitable radioactivity. The net incorporation during the R$^+$ × F$^-$ mating, obtained by subtracting the incorporation by RS2 and AB2500 alone from the incorporation by the mated mixture, was 1.5 × 10^4 CPM.

2. Nalidixic acid sensitive donors (final concentration 3.5 × 10^7 cells/ml) were mixed with nalidixic acid resistant recipients (final concentration 1−2 × 10^8 cells/ml) in a minimal salts medium supplemented with casamino acids and glucose and incubated at 37°C. After 30 minutes, exconjugants were selected for resistance to nalidixic acid, chloramphenicol, ampicillin and kanamycin. The transfer frequency of the R1 plasmid to AB2500 F$^-$ was 9.1 × 10^{-2}.

recipients, unirradiated and in the presence of nonradioactive thymine, were mated with a similar population of donors and selected for inheritance of the donor resistance genes.

The net incorporation of label in the mating between the F-like donor and the unrelated Ike-like (N3) recipient was nearly as efficient as observed for the R1 X F⁻ mating. We attribute the small difference in incorporation of label, and in genetic transfer frequency, to host-controlled restriction, WATANABE, NISHIDA, OGATA, ARAI and SATO (1964) and WATANABE, TAKANO, ARAI, NISHIDA and SATO (1966). There was, however, a marked reduction in the net incorporation of label by recipients bearing F⁺, 222 and the isogenic sex factor, RTF. The correlation between the extent of genetic transfer and the net incorporation of label was excellent with respect to those recipients which were F⁻, or carried the N3 or F⁺ resident plasmid. In contrast, although the level of DNA replication was basically similar in recipients harboring F⁺, 222 and RTF resident plasmids, the eventual recovery of R1 in the 222 and RTF recipients was further reduced by some 50 to 1000-fold. We interpret these data to mean that the reduction in incorporation for a recipient bearing F⁺ purely reflects the phenomenon of entry exclusion. It would seem that the presence of F⁺ in the cell acts to either prevent the physical entry of the R1 DNA or, if the R1 DNA enters the cell it is usually not replicated. The limited amount of replication of the superinfecting DNA within the F⁺ cell, however, does generally lead to the successful establishment of R1. Thus, as has been reported many times previously, WATANABE and FUKASAWA (1962) and MEYNELL and DATTA (1967), F and an R factor are compatible even though they mutually practice entry exclusion against one another.

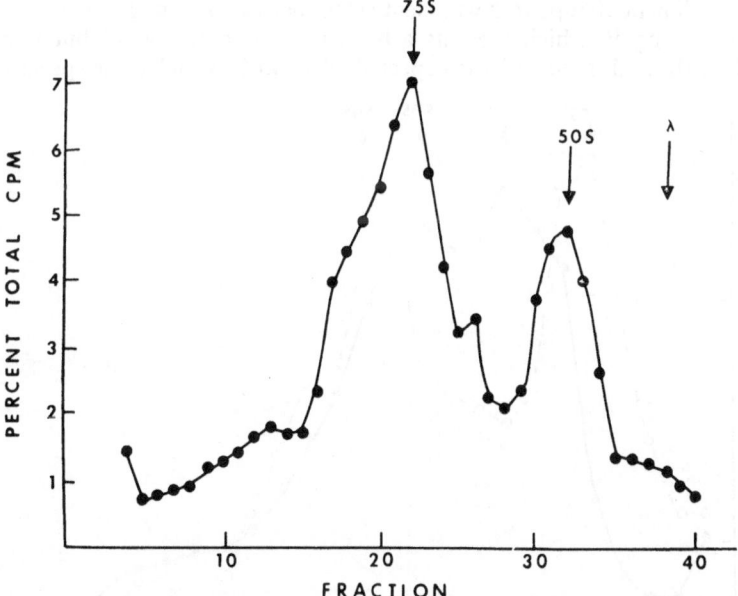

Fig. 1 Sedimentation of R factor DNA in neutral sucrose after 60 minutes of an R_1 × F⁻ mating. Cells removed from the mating mixture after 60 minutes were lysed, and 300 µl of the lysate was layered over a 5—20% sucrose gradient. Centrifugation was carried out for 2 1/2 hours at 25,000 rev/min (80,900 × g) at 20°C in the SW27 rotor (1.59 cm × 10.16 cm buckets) of a Spinco preparative ultracentrifuge. Twelve drop fractions were collected through a hole punctured in the bottom of the tube. The fractions were precipitated with trichloroacetic acid, collected on membrane filtres and counted. Linear monomers of ¹⁴C-thymine labeled λ bacteriophage DNA were added as a sedimentation reference (34S).

311

In the case of the 222 and RTF recipients, however, while very nearly the same levels of entry exclusion is evident as occurs in the F$^+$ situation, the difference between the amount of label incorporated and the eventual recovery of R1 in the recipients is a reflection of the phenomenon of incompatibility. The data, therefore, fully support the contention that entry exclusion and incompatability represent two distinct phenomena. While they may operate from the same gene cluster, it appears that they are directed against different stages of transfer replication — entry exclusion at a very early stage and incompatibility at some stage thereafter. A further distinction between the two phenomena was likewise seen when the DNA which was synthesized within compatible and incompatible recipients was isolated and characterized.

Figure 1 shows the results obtained when cells from an R1 × F$^-$ mating, after 60 minutes in the presence of ^{3}H-thymine, were lysed, deproteinized and centrifuged, together with linear monomers of ^{14}C lambda DNA, in a 5—20% linear sucrose gradient. Most of the ^{3}H-DNA sediments in two distinct peaks that are calculated, relative to the lambda DNA (34S), to have values of 50S and 75S. Earlier studies had shown that these peaks represented an open ring (50S) and a covalently closed ring (75S) of double stranded DNA with a molecular weight of approximately 64×10^6 daltons, SILVER and FALKOW (1970). It has also been previously demonstrated, FALKOW, TOMPKINS, SILVER, GUERRY, and LE BLANC (1971) that labeled material which is derived from the bacterial hosts sediments well behind the 34S lambda marker, and contributes insignificantly to the total amounts of R factor material. When DNA from an R1 × N3 mating, which exhibits neither entry exclusion nor incompatibility, was examined on neutral sucrose the sedimentation pattern was identical to that seen for the R1 × F$^-$ mating. The recipient harboring F, which presents a barrier to the entry of R1 but is genetically compatible with it, also showed the expected 50S and 75S molecular species, although

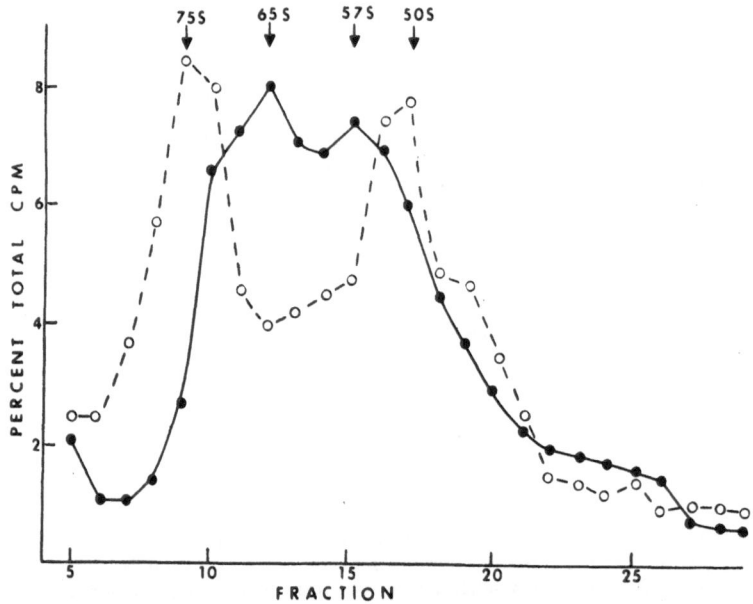

Fig. 2 Sedimentation of R factor DNA in neutral sucrose after 60 minutes of an R1 × RTF mating (homologous mating). The cells were treated as described in the legend to Figure 1 except that the λ DNA was replaced by ^{14}C DNA obtained from a 60-minute R1 × F$^-$ mating. ●———● ^{3}H-DNA; o— —o ^{14}C-DNA.

the total amount of DNA synthesized during this mating was only about 20% of that synthesized by the F⁻ recipient. As can be seen in Figure 2, the DNA synthesized by a recipient carrying the incompatible isogenic plasmid presented a totally different picture. Instead of the 50S and 75S peaks associated with replication in compatible hosts, most of the labeled DNA was represented in two peaks corresponding to sedimentation values of 65S and 57S. Since these two peaks were generally separated by only 2 or 3 fractions from the 75S and 50S regions of the gradient, the lambda marker was replaced by C^{14} DNA derived from a 60-minute compatible mating. The relationship, 65S to 57S, was calculated to be precisely what one would expect for an open ring and linear form of a *dimer* of the 64×10^6 dalton R1 plasmid. However, it was also possible that these species represented catenated molecules. At any rate, the production of these molecular species suggested that incompatibility is associated with a mechanism that either produces aberrant replicative forms, or causes the accumulation of normal replicative intermediates which ordinarily are present in very small amounts at any one time.

The Rolling Circle Model of GILBERT and DRESSLER (1968), which proposes an asymmetric mode of replication for DNA, has been applied to explain the replication of plasmid DNA, as well as chromosomes and bacteriophages. Replication begins, in this model, by breaking one strand of a parental duplex ring. The other ring strand remains intact and becomes essentially a master template rolling off many complementary copies. An interesting feature of this model, in terms of our data, was the potential to generate a concatenated long chain. Failure to cut such chains into unit length molecules could, perhaps, explain the presence of 57S and 65S material in neutral sucrose gradients of DNA from incompatible hosts. However, the possibility that these species represented dimers could be explained by a symmetrical replication scheme, which can be a variant of the Rolling Circle Model, WATSON (1970). This model, in which both strands are nicked, is characterized by elongation of both strands. If the elongation occurs in opposite directions the replicating molecule is the product of two rolling circles in opposite directions. As the growing points move the whole way around the circle, the elongated strands eventually become double length and the ends of the daughter strands are in a position to be joined into the origins of the parental strands. In short, a replicative intermediate would be a double sized duplex ring. One can then evoke specific endonucleases to form two monomeric DNA linear forms which can intrinsically circularize, followed by the covalent sealing of both strands by a ligase. The unavailability of the proposed specific endonuclease to a superinfecting incompatible plasmid could result in the accumulation of dimers, represented by the 57S and 65S peaks. On the other hand, replication of a superinfecting plasmid at a highly reduced rate in an incompatible host might also result in a predominance of the intermediate dimers after 60 minutes of mating.

If incompatibility is, at least partially, associated with a mechanism which results in a reduction in the rate of plasmid replication, other molecular species associated with normal replication should also be observed in neutral sucrose gradients of DNA from incompatible matings. In fact, significant amounts of 50S and 44S, a linear monomer of the R1 plasmid rarely seen after 60 minutes in a compatible mating, were detected in some gradients. Although a distinct 75S peak was not observed in such gradients, as much as 10% of the total label had been detected in the region of the gradient corresponding to a sedimentation value of 75S. In order to determine whether this material represented covalently closed rings, we made use of the fact that such molecules undergo a smaller change in buoyant density than that which occurs with linear or open ring structures following interactions with the intercalative dye, ethidium bromide, RADLOFF, BAUER and Vinograd (1967) and Vinograd, Lebowitz, Radloff, Watson and Laipis (1965). When material from a deproteinized lysate from a 60-minute isogenic mating was centrifuged to equilibrium in cesium chloride-ethidium bromide, a peak corresponding to approximately 8% of the total label was observed at a buoyant density which is characteristic of covalently closed duples DNA (Figure 3). Thus, this correlated well

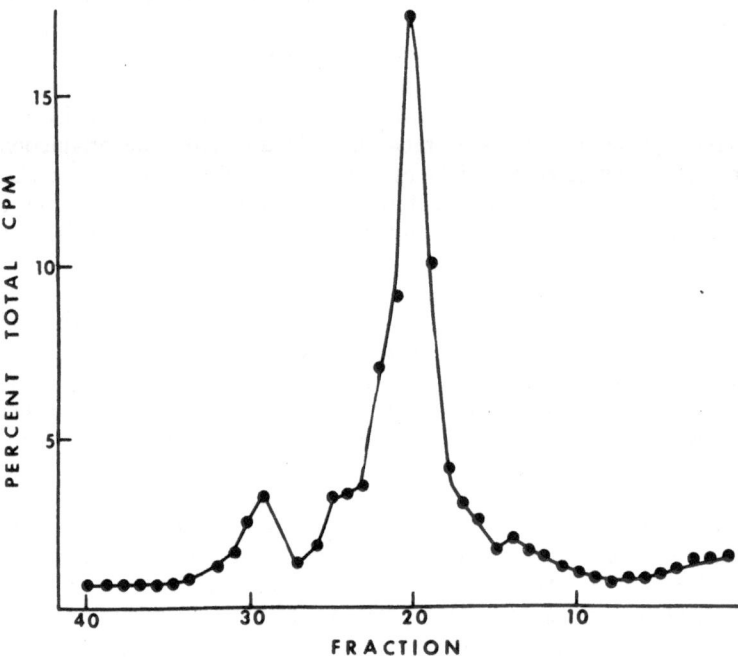

Fig. 3 Demonstration of covalently closed ring DNA after 60 minutes of an R1 × RTF mating. Cells removed from the mating mixture after 60 minutes were lysed, and 500 μl was centrifuged to equilibrium in cesium chloride-ethidium bromide. Centrifugation was carried out for 38 hours at 44,000 rev/min (125,000 × g) in the type 65 fixed-angle rotor of a Spinco preparative ultracentrifuge. Forty 10-drop fractions were collected from the top of the tube with an Auto Densi-flow apparatus (Buchler Instruments). Precipitation of fractions was as described in the legend to Figure 1.

with the observation that up to 10% of the DNA synthesized after 60 minutes of an incompatible mating sediments in the 75S region of a neutral sucrose gradient. In contrast to this, more than 30% of the label from a compatible mating was represented by covalently closed rings after the same period of time (Figure 4). These data were consistent with the idea that incompatibility might be characterized by a reduced rate of plasmid synthesis. However, the production of normal end-products during the isogenic mating could also be interpreted as a reflection of a small percentage of compatible cells in a predominantly incompatible recipient culture.

The possibility that the 57S and 65S species seen in neutral sucrose gradients of DNA from an incompatible mating represented catenated molecules was greatly diminished by the results of the ethidium bromide experiment illustrated in Figure 3. Such molecular species would be expected to have a buoyant density in ethidium bromide intermediate between covalently closed rings and linear, or open ring, molecules. Although label was present at such a density, it represented less than 6% of the total label in the gradient, accounting for much less than a third of either the 57S or 65S species.

If these two molecules species were normal replicative intermediates, and constituted the majority of the DNA present after 60 minutes of mating only because of a reduced rate of synthesis in an incompatible host, then at a later time in the mating, such species should be converted to a normal replicative end-product, that is, the 75S covalently closed ring. In addition, at an earlier time in the mating, precursors of the 57S and 65 species, e. g., the 44S linear monomer or perhaps the 50S nicked monomeric ring, might

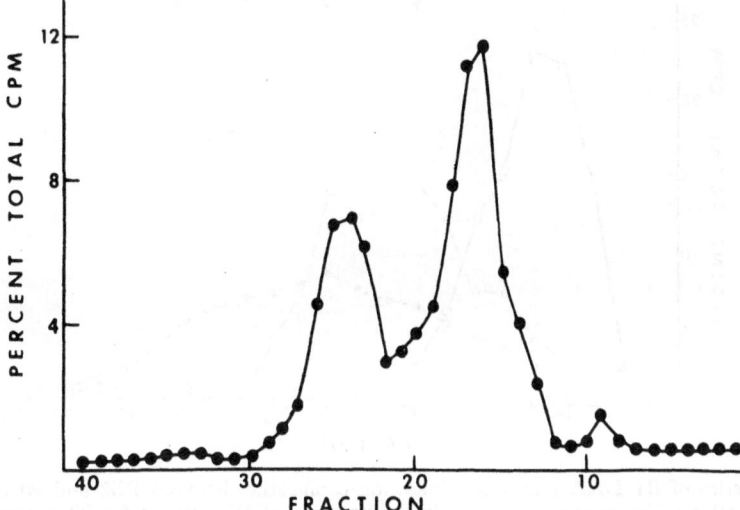

Fig. 4 Demonstration of covalently closed ring DNA after 60 minutes of an R1 × F⁻ mating. The procedure was as described in the legend to Figure 3.

be observed. Consequently, an experiment was designed to follow, over an extended period of time, the fate of radiolabel incorporated early in a mating. Cells harboring the isogenic plasmid R1 (donor) and the RTF derived from R1 (recipient) were mated in the presence of ³H-thymine for 20 minutes (pulse) after which time a 200-fold excess of nonradioactive thymine was added (chase). At various times after the chase samples were removed, lysed and examined on neutral sucrose gradients. The results of this experiment are illustrated in Figure 5.

Ten minutes after the chase, 30 minutes after mating, there was a rather broad distribution of radioactivity, with significant amounts of material ranging from the 44S linear monomer to the 65S presumptive open ring dimer. Thirty minutes later, 60 minutes after mating, the *net* effect of continuous replicative activity, obtained by subtracting the percent of label in each fraction of the 30 minute gradient from the corresponding fractions in the 60 minute gradient, was reflected in the accumulation of 57S and 65S species. However, during the interval between 60 minutes and 90 minutes of mating, well over 60% of the net change in labeled DNA was represented by a shift to 75S covalently closed monomeric rings.

These data clearly show that replication of superinfecting plasmid DNA in an incompatible host ultimately leads to the production of normal replicative end-products. If the 57S and 65S species, representing most of the ³H-DNA after 60 minutes of mating, are actually dimers, then these results are also consistent with a symmetrical replication mechanism involving a double sized duplex ring as a replicative intermediate. Preliminary physical studies suggest that the 65S species is indeed a dimer, closed by hydrogen bonding of cohesive ends.

The question still remaining was whether replication in a compatible host also proceeds by the same symmetric scheme, or is such a mechanism unique to replication following an incompatible mating? Reexamination of several neutral sucrose gradients prepared from

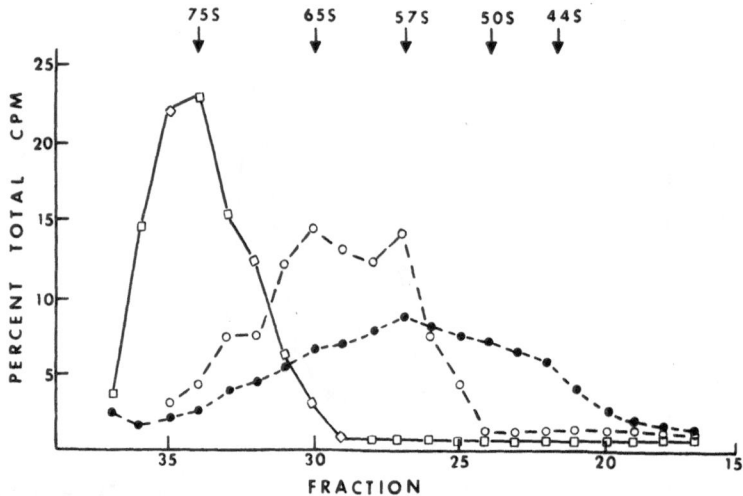

Fig. 5 Kinetics of R1 DNA replication following conjugation between RS2 and AB2500 RTF (isogenic mating). The cells were mated in the presence of ^{3}H-thymine for 20 minutes (pulse) followed by the addition of an excess of nonradioactive thymine (chase). At 10, 40 and 70 minutes after the chase (30, 60 and 90 minutes after mating) samples were removed and examined on neutral sucrose gradients as described in the legend to Figure 1. Twelve drop fractions were collected from the top od the tube as described in the legend to Figure 3.
●— — —● 30 minutes after mating
○— — —○ *net* change in radiolabeled DNA between 30 minutes and 60 minutes of mating.
□———□ *net* change in radiolabeled DNA between 60 minutes and 90 minutes of mating.

lysates of 60-minute compatible matings revealed that, occasionally, small but definitely distinct peaks corresponding to a sedimentation rate of 65S were present. Such a peak can be seen in the gradient illustrated in Figure 1. It therefore seemed possible that a pulse-chase experiment, similar to that which was performed for an isogenic mating, might reveal the presence of intermediate forms during early stages of a compatible mating. Figure 6 shows the results of such an experiment. At the time of chase, 20 minutes after mating, the predominant species observed was the 44S linear monomer, with lesser amounts of label in the regions corresponding to an open monomeric ring (50S) and a linear dimer (57S). In addition, a small peak representing the putative open dimeric ring (65S) was also present. During the next 20 minutes of mating the net result of replication was represented by a displacement of the radiolabel to the area of the gradient between 65S and 75S sedimentation rates, with the bulk of the label in the region of 65S. The difference between 40 minutes and 60 minutes after mating was reflected in a definite shift to the 75S covalently closed ring. Although the presence of a 57S intermediate species was not clearly demonstrated in this experiment, the existence of a 65S molecular species during replication in a compatible host was unmistakable. We have previously estimated that the average time for a single R factor molecule to replicate, under normal conditions, from a linear form to a covalently closed ring is between 2.5 and 3.0 minutes. Thus, we

316

would not expect more than a fleeting glance at these replicative intermediates. On the other hand, the replication time of the same plasmid in an incompatible host is calculated to be between 35 and 40 minutes, based on the sequence of events observed in the pulse-chase experiment with such an incompatible recipient.

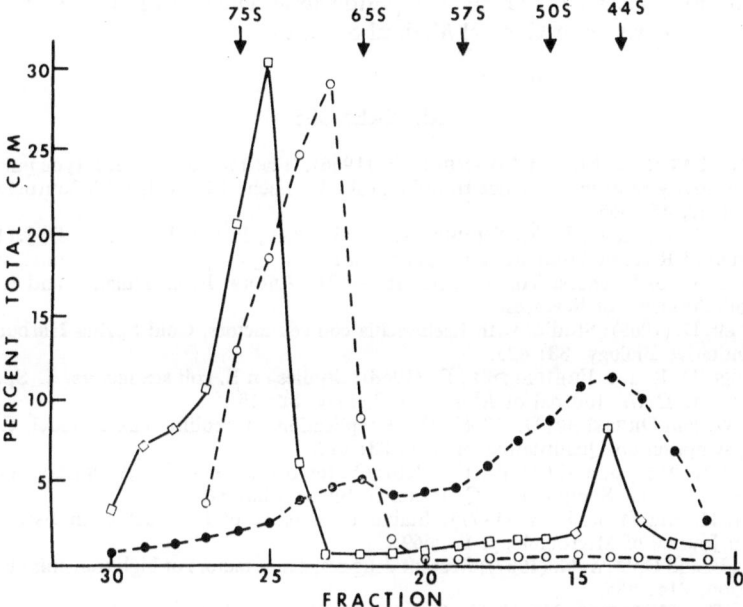

Fig. 6 Kinetics of R1 DNA replication following conjugation between RS2 and AB2500. The procedure was the same as described in the legend to Figure 5 except that samples were taken at 0, 20 and 40 minutes after the chase (20, 40 and 60 minutes after mating).
●––––● 20 minutes after mating
○––––○ *net* change in radiolabeled DNA between 20 minutes and 40 minutes of mating
□———□ *net* change between 40 minutes and 60 minutes of mating.

The data presented in this paper, with respect to the replication of plasmid DNA following conjugation, are consistent with a symmetrical replication scheme involving a double sized duplex ring as a replicative intermediate, which is subsequently converted to two covalently closed monomers. The data further suggest that the phenomenon of incompatibility is, at least partially, characterized by a 14 to 16-fold reduction in the rate of synthesis of superinfecting DNA in an incompatible host. These results are not inconsistent with the "maintenance site" hypothesis generally used to explain incompatibility, since the reduced rate of synthesis could be a reflection of the unavailability of such a site to the superinfecting DNA. Furthermore, it is unlikely that incompatibility can be entirely accounted for by such a reduced rate of replication since the estimated time for replication of the superinfecting plasmid in an incompatible host (35—40 minutes) is still less than the generation time of the host (65 minutes). However, if a structural cell component is required for distribution of replicas to daughter cells following cellular division, lack of attachment to such a structure by a superinfecting plasmid would diminish its chances of being inherited by the progeny of the host. Experiments designed to determine the role of the bacterial membrane in the replication of plasmid DNA in compatible and incompatible hosts are currently in progress in our laboratory.

Le BLANC, D. J., FALKOW, S.

Acknowledgments

This work was supported by grant GB13031 from the National Science Foundation; contract DADA 67-C7061, under sponsorship of the Commission on Enteric Infections of the Armed Forces Epidemiological Board, and by United States Public Health Service Grant GM36120-02. D. J. LeBlanc is a postdoctoral fellow of the United States Public Health Service Division of General Medical Sciences.

REFERENCES

DATTA, N., LAWN, A. M. and MEYNELL, E. (1966): The relationship of F type piliation and F phage sensitivity to drug resistance transfer in R⁺ F⁻ Escherichia coli K12. Journal of General Microbiology, **45**: 365.

FALKOW, S., TOMPKINS, L. S., SILVER, R. P., GUERRY, P. and LEBLANC, D. J. (1971): The Replication of R factor DNA in Escherichia coli following conjugation. In: Annals of the New York Academy of Sciences, Vol. 182, pp. 153—171. Editors: E. L. Dulaney and A. I. Laskin. New York Academy of Sciences.

FREIFELDER, D. (1968): Studies with Escherichia coli sex factors. Cold Spring Harbor Symposia on Quantitative Biology, **33**: 425.

FREIFELDER, D. R. and FREIFELDER, D. (1968): Studies on E. coli sex factors. I. Specific labeling of F' lac DNA. Journal of Molecular Biology, **32**: 15.

GILBERT, W. and DRESSLER, D. (1968): DNA replication: the rolling circle model. Cold Spring Harbor Symposia on Quantitative Biology, **33**: 473.

JACOB, F., BRENNER, S. and CUZIN, F. (1968): On the regulation of DNA replication in bacteria. Cold Spring Harbor Symposia on Quantitative Biology, **28**: 329.

KHATOON, H. and IYER, R. V. (1971): Stable coexistence of Rfi⁻ factors in Escherichia coli. Canadian Journal of Microbiology, **17**: 669.

MEYNELL, E. and DATTA, N. (1967): Mutant drug resistance factors of high transmissibility. Nature, London, **214**: 885.

MEYNELL, E. and DATTA, N. (1969): Sex factor activity of drug-resistance actors. In: Bacterial Episomes and Plasmids, a Ciba Foundation Symposium, pp. 120—135. Editors: G. E. W. Wolstenholme and M. O'Connor. J. & A. Churchill Ltd., London.

MEYNELL, G. G. and LAWN, A. M. (1967): Sex pili and common pili in the conjugational transfer of colicin factor Ib by Salmonella typhimurium. Genetical Research, **9**: 359.

NOVICK, R. P. (1969): Extrachromosomal inheritance in bacteria. Bacteriological Reviews, **33**: 210.

RADLOFF, R., BAUER, W. and VINOGRAD, J. (1967): A dye buoyant density method for the detection and isolation of closed circular duplex DNA: The closed circular DNA in HeLa cells. Proceedings of the National Academy of Sciences of the United States of America, **57**: 1514.

SILVER, R. P. and FALKOW, S. (1970): Specific labeling and physical characterization of R factor DNA in Escherichia coli. Journal of Bacteriology, **104**: 331.

VINOGRAD, J., LEBOWITZ, J., RADLOFF, R. WATSON, R. and LAIPIS, P. (1965): The twisted circular form of Polyoma viral DNA. Proceedings of the National Academy of Sciences of the United States of America, **53**: 1104.

WATANABE, T. (1963): Infective heredity of multiple drug resistance in bacteria. Bacteriological Reviews, **27**: 87.

WATANABE, T. and FUKASAWA, T. (1962): Episome-mediated transfer of drug resistance in Enterobacteriaceae. IV. Interactions between resistance transfer factor and F factor in Escherichia coli K12. Journal of Bacteriolgy, **83**: 727.

WATANABE, T., NISHIDA, H., OGATA, C., ARAI, T. and SATO, S. (1964): Episome-mediated transfer of drug resistance in Enterobacteriaceae. VII. Two types of naturally occurring R factors. Journal of Bacteriology, **88**: 716.

WATANABE, T., TAKANO, T., ARAI, T., NISHIDA, H. and SATO, S. (1966): Episomes-mediated transfer of drug resistance in Enterobacteriaceae. X. Restriction and modification of phages by fi⁻ R factors. Journal of Bacteriology, **92**: 477.

WATSON, J. D. (1970): The replication of DNA. In: Molecular Biology of the Gene, 2nd ed., Chapter 9, pp. 288—291. W. A. Benjamin, Inc., New York, N. Y.

318

STUDIES ON THE REGULATION OF THE CHLORAMPHENICOL ACETYL TRANSFERASE MEDIATED BY R FACTORS*

D. H. SMITH,+ J. H. HARWOOD and F. A. RUBIN

Departments of Bacteriology and Immunology and Pediatrics, Harvard Medical School, Division of Infectious Disease, Children's Hospital Medical Center, Boston, Mass., U.S.A.

INTRODUCTION

The fact that the levels of resistances mediated by R factors depends on the host cell and the individual R factor has been known since the earliest studies of these genetic elements (WATANABE, 1963). It was not possible to investigate the mechanism for these differences, however, until the biochemical basis for the resistances were defined. This situation changed with the recent delineation of an enzymatic basis for many of the R factor-mediated resistances.

Several diverse observations of the synthesis of R factor-mediated drug inactivating enzymes have recently been published. The synthesis of chloramphenicol acetyl transferase (CAT) (SHAW, 1967; SUZUKI, OKAMOTO, 1966), streptomycin adenylate transferase (SAT) (UMEZAWA, TAKASAWA, OKANISHI and UTAHARA, 1968; YAMADA, TIPPER and DAVIES, 1968; HARWOOD and SMITH, 1969), streptomycin phosphorylase (OZANNE, BENVENISTE, TIPPER and DAVIES, 1969), kanamycin acetyl transferase (UMEZAWA, OKANISHI, UTAHARA, MAEDA and KONDO, 1967), kanamycin phosphorylase (UMEZAWA, OKANISHI, KONDO, HAMANA, UTAHARA, MAEDA and MITSUHASHI, 1967), β-lactamase (DATTA and KONTOMICHALOU, 1965), and gentamicin adenylate transferase (BENVENISTE and DAVIES, 1971) is constitutive, as defined by the absence of any difference in the enzyme activity in extracts of cells grown with or without drug. The fact that the substrate does not induce a drug-inactivating enzyme provides only an operational definition, however, and does not indicate that the synthesis is truly constitutive. The synthesis of Krebs cycle and amino acid-activating enzymes have classically been assumed to be constitutive; however, it is now known that α-ketogluterate dehydrogenase, for example, is induced by acetate or glutamate (AMARSINGHAM and DAVIS, 1965) and that amino acid activating enzymes are depressed during growth under amino acid limitation (WILLIAMS and NEIDHARDT, 1969). Furthermore, the R factor-mediated resistance to tetracycline is inducible by the drug and certain analogues with little antibacterial activity (IZAKI, KIUCHI and ARIMA, 1966; FRANKLIN, 1967).

The level of SAT (SMITH, JANJIGIAN, PRESCOTT and ANDERSON, 1970; BENVENISTE, YAMADA and DAVIES, 1970), CAT (SHAW, 1967; SUZUKI and OKAMOTO, 1967), and β-lactamase (DATTA and KONTOMICHALOU, 1965; KONTOMICHALOU, 1967; SMITH,

* These studies were supported in part by Public Health Service Grant AI-08362 from the National Institute of Allergy and Infectious Diseases.
+ David H. Smith is the recipient of the Career Development Award AI-20376 from the National Institute of Allergy and Infectious Diseases.

319

1969; JACK and RICHMOND, 1970; FULLERBROOK, ELSON and SLOCOMBE, 1970) in cell-free extracts has been found to depend on the host cell and the R factor. The R factors TEM, 7268, and 1818, for example, produce 907, 125 and 29 m units/10^9 *Escherichia coli* K_{12} respectively, but the activity produced by each in *Proteus mirabilis* is only 1/20-1/100th as great (SMITH, 1969). These observations are all the more striking since there is 1 copy of the R factor per *E. coli* but multiple copies in each *P. mirabilis* cell (ROWND, NAKAYA and NAKAMURA, 1966); and the activities of β-lactamase (and CAT) correlate directly with the amount of R factor-specific DNA (FALKOW, HAAPALA and SILVER, 1969). The activity of β-lactamase in R^+ *E. coli* correlates with the growth rate of the bacteria (BURMAN, NORDSTRÖM and BOMAN, 1968), but this effect could not explain the differences between the enzyme levels observed in Proteus and *E. coli*.

Despite these obvious multiple-factor effects on R factor enzyme activities, little attempt has been made to study systematically mutants of a given R factor. Mutant R factors that produce lower levels of SAT than the parent and that transfer this phenotype conjugally have been isolated (SMITH et al., 1970) but no attempt was made to determine the genetic basis for this phenotype. No convincing evidence has been cited for the isolation of a mutant R factor that is conjugally transferable and that produces more drug-inactivating enzyme than does its parent. Thus, the findings with tetracycline resistance provide the only concrete evidence for the existence of regulatory loci on R factors. Mutants of a regulatory type can be selected, however, from β-lactamase-positive *E. coli* (ERICKSSON-GRENNBERG, BOMAN, JANSSON and THOREN, 1965) and *P. mirabilis* that produce CAT with properties nearly identical to that of R factors (JACOBSEN and SHAW, 1970).

With this background, it seemed that an investigation of the regulation of R factor-mediated enzymes might provide further insight into the control of "constitutive" enzyme synthesis, and the biology of R factors. Accordingly, studies on the regulation of CAT have been initiated; this manuscript summarizes the results of certain of these studies, some of which have been published elsewhere (HARWOOD and SMITH, 1971; RUBIN and SMITH, submitted for publication).

MATERIALS AND METHODS

E. coli K_{12} AB1932-1 (F⁻lac⁻Nal⁻B₁⁻xyl⁻lac⁻arg⁻met⁻T₆ʳ) and AB1157 (F⁻B₁⁻thr⁻leu⁻arg⁻pro⁻his⁻lac⁻gal⁻ara⁻xyl⁻mtl⁻mal⁻T₆ʳλ-Strʳ) have been described (MARSH and SMITH, 1969; WALTON and SMITH, 1969); strains 3000 (HfrH CR⁺) and LA 12G (HfrH B₁⁻CR⁻) were obtained from B. MAGASANIK; AB 257 (F⁻B₁⁻met⁻CR⁺) and PC⁻¹(F⁻B₁⁻met⁻CR⁻) from H. V. RICKENBERG; 1100 (F⁻B₁⁻) and 5336 (F⁻B₁⁻adenylcyclase deficient) from I. PASTAN; W1485 (F⁻thy⁻/P₁Cm) from S. FALKOW; *Proteus mirabilis* 997 (nic⁻) from W. V. Shaw; *P. mirabilis* 13 (nic⁻leu⁻) was isolated from the urine of a patient seen in this hospital with urinary tract infection. The origin and patterns of resistance mediated by the R factors studied are summarized in Table 1.

Microbiological Methods

Bacteria were incubated in minimal medium A (DAVIS and MINGOLI, 1950), modified by the omission of citrate and supplemented with carbohydrates or other nutrients as indicated, trypticase soy broth or MNB broth (8 gr nutrient broth per liter of medium A). These media were solidified, when indicated, with 15 grams agar per liter.

The methods used for the conjugal transfer of R factors and routine testing of patterns of drug resistance have been described (MARSH and SMITH, 1969; HARWOOD and

SMITH, 1970; RUBIN and SMITH, submitted for publication). Cells for enzyme extracts were cultured and prepared as described (HARWOOD and SMITH, 1970); incubation in test media exceeded 5—6 generations to insure that "permanent" and not "transient" repression of enzyme synthesis by glucose was studied. Resistance of individual strains

Table 1

ORIGIN AND PATTERNS OF RESISTANCE MEDIATED BY R FACTORS

R factor	Origin Specimen	Bacterial Species	Patterns of Resistance*	Reference
JJ1	Unknown	*E. coli*	Mer Sul Cml	Harwood and Smith, 1970
RK$_5$	Sputum	Klebsiella	Mer Sul Str Cml Tet Amp lac	Pitt and Smith, 1970
B$_{22}$	Blood	*E. coli*	Mer Sul Str Cml Tet Amp	Smith and Harwood, unpublished observations
B$_{30}$	Blood	*E. coli*	Mer Sul Str Cml Tet Amp	Smith and Harwood, unpublished observations
B$_{68}$	Blood	Klebsiella	Cml Amp	Smith and Harwood, unpublished observations
CI116	Stool	Klebsiella	Mer Sul Str Cml Tet Amp	Smith and Harwood, unpublished observations
CI121	Blood	Klebsiella	Mer Sul Str Cml	Smith and Harwood, unpublished observations
U143	Urine	*E. coli*	Mer Sul Str Cml Tet Amp	Smith and Harwood, unpublished observations

* The presentation of resistance patterns are for convenience and do not indicate genetic linkages.

was assayed by diluting cells in A medium, plating about 300 colonies on plates of test medium containing increasing concentrations of test drugs, incubating overnight at 37° C, and counting viable cells. The survival rate was determined by comparison to the number of viable cells on drug-free medium. Mutant bacteria were selected without or following exposure to either N-methyl-N'-nitro-N-nitrosoguanidine (ADELBERG, MANDEL and CHEN, 1965), 2-aminopurine or UV (SCHWARTZ and BECKWITH, 1969). R⁻ segregants were selected after incubation in sodium dodecyl sulfate (TOMEADA, INUZUKA, KUBO and NAKAMURA, 1968). *E. coli* were treated with Tris and EDTA (LEIVE, 1965) to render them permeable to certain compounds.

Biochemical Methods

CAT was assayed by a colorimetric method (SHAW and BRODSKY, 1968); β-galactosidase by either a velocity (HARWOOD and SMITH, 1970) or static method (PARDEE, JACOB and MONOD, 1959); and protein by the method of LOWRY, ROSEBROUGH, FARR and RANDALL, 1951.

Chemicals

Drugs and chemicals were the highest grade commercially available.

RESULTS

Effect of Carbon Source on CAT Activity

The relationship between the growth rate of an R+ E. coli and the specific activity (s. a.) of CAT in culture extracts was evaluated in initial experiments. E. coli 1932/JJ1 was cultured in minimal medium supplemented with various nutrients such that a 4-fold range of growth rates was obtained. The s. a. of CAT generally correlated to the doubling times of the cells, but that of cells grown in glucose was consistently lower than expected, if CAT was regulated only by growth rate. The contribution of the carbon source and growth rate to the s. a. of CAT was then examined in 2 pairs of cultures incubated in minimal medium with either succinate or glucose, one pair of which was supplemented

Table 2

EFFECT OF GROWTH RATE AND CARBON SOURCE ON CAT ACTIVITY

Medium			
Carbon Source 0.2%	Supplement 0.2%	Doubling time (hr.)	CAT Activity
Succinate	—	1.5	2640
Succinate	Tryptone	0.8	2320
Glucose	—	1.0	1010
Glucose	Tryptone	0.6	690

with tryptone. The results (Table 2) indicated that the effect of growth rate is insignificant compared to that produced by the presence of glucose in the medium.

An explanation for this "glucose effect" was then sought: it might have been trivial — e. g. glucose may markedly enhance the segregation of the R factor — or CAT might be regulated by catabolite repression. The former explanation was ruled out by the observation that the frequency of segregation of the R factor, JJ1, was < 3% and similar when the strain was incubated 10—12 generations in minimal medium supplemented

Table 3

RELATIONSHIP BETWEEN CAT ACTIVITY AND CARBON SOURCE

Carbon Source 0.2%	CAT Activity
Glycerol	4560
Glucose	780
Glucose-6-phosphate	980
Arabinose	1460
Mannitol	1520
Rhamnose	3120

with either glucose or succinate. The results presented in Table 3 indicate, moreover, that carbon source directly influences the s. a. of CAT, with the most potent inhibition being produced by those sugars known to produce catabolite repression.

Because catabolite repression of CAT was not predicted on the basis of the known function of the enzyme, a series of experiments were conducted on the CAT activities in R+ strains of two "catabolite repression-insensitive" mutants of E. coli K$_{12}$ (LOOMIS and MAGASANIK, 1965; HSIE and RICKENBERG, 1966). Although neither of these mutant strains is known to be defective in any function specifically essential for catabolite repression, the usual reduction in the level of several catabolic enzymes (β-galactosidase, amylomaltase, tryptophanase) in cells grown on glucose (when compared to glycerol) is less severe in the CR$^-$ mutants than in their CR$^+$ parents (HSIE and RICKENBERG, 1966; RICKENBERG, HSIE and JANECEK, 1968; LOOMIS and MAGASANIK, 1965). These mutants therefore offered an operational method for testing the prediction that CAT is catabolite repressible. The results of several experiments indicated that growth in glucose affected the activity of CAT and (the internal control) β-galactosidase of the CR$^-$ (JJ1 strains only slightly) compared to that of the CR$^+$/JJ1 strains. These findings were thus consistent with the proposal that CAT is subject to catabolite repression.

Table 4

EFFECT OF CARBON SOURCE AND cAMP ON CAT ACTIVITIES OF DIFFERENT R FACTORS

| R factor Code | Medium Supplements | | CAT Activity* |
	Carbon Source (0.2%)	cAMP (10mM)	
B$_{22}$	Glycerol	−	1549
	Glucose	−	442
	Glucose	+	2227
B$_{30}$	Glycerol	−	1738
	Glucose	−	407
	Glucose	+	1944
B$_{68}$	Glycerol	−	3121
	Glucose	−	2708
	Glucose	+	27494
CI 116	Glycerol	−	1234
	Glucose	−	546
	Glucose	+	3118
CI 121	Glycerol	−	2088
	Glucose	−	700
	Glucose	+	2096
RK$_5$	Glycerol	−	546
	Glucose	−	256
	Glucose	+	1348
U 143	Glycerol	−	1195
	Glucose	−	380
	Glucose	+	1521

* All R factors were transferred conjugally to *E. doli* 1100; the bacteria were grown overnight and diluted in A medium containing the designated cultures; cAMP was added in mid-exponential growth, and after about 3 additional generation times, the cells were harvested for the preparation of extracts and assays.

In order to rule out the possibility that this phenomenon was unique to the R factor and *E. coli* host strains studied, the effect of glucose on the s. a. of CAT produced by JJ1 in other strains and by other R factors was investigated. Similar results were obtained with JJ1 in each of 6 other *E. coli* K$_{12}$ strains. The data presented in Table 4 indicate that the s. a. of CAT varies with the R factor, but in glucose-grown cells it is lower than in glycerol-grown cells, regardless of the origin or drug-resistance patterns of the R factor.

Attention was then directed to the mechanisms for this "glucose-effect". The observation that (i) neither glucose or glucose-6-phosphate added directly to an *in vitro* CAT reaction at a final concentration of 0.2% produced a significant change in enzyme activity; and (ii) the level of CAT activity produced by mixtures of extracts of glucose and glycerol-grown cells was additive indicated that glucose affected the synthesis and not just the activity of CAT. Since CAT activity may reflect the number of copies of the R factor per cell (FALKOW et al., 1969), the observed "glucose-effect"could be at the level of R factor replication. The number of R factors per *E. coli* chromosome has been reported to be about 1 (ROWND, et al., 1966), but the cells for that study were grown in a rich broth containing glucose. This problem was therefore approached with a strain of *E. coli* infected with P_1Cm, the defective phage formed by a recombination of P_1 and an R factor (KONDO and MITSUHASHI, 1964) that contains, at least, the CAT structural locus

Table 5

EFFECT OF CARBON SOURCE AND cAMP ON CAT
PRODUCED BY P_1Cm

Medium Supplements		CAT Activity*
Carbon Source (0.2%)	cAMP (10mM)	
Glycerol	—	345
Glucose	—	87
Glucose	+	237

* Conditions of cultures were those described in Table 4, except that *E. coli* W1485/P_1Cm was used.

(KONDO, HAAPALA and FALKOW, 1970). *E. coli* grown either in glucose or glycerol contain only 1 copy of this extrachromosomal plasmid (FALKOW, personal communication). The data in Table 5 indicate that the CAT activity in such cells is lower when they are grown in glucose than in glycerol. Thus, the phenomenon under study is not produced by the enhancement of R factor replication and a gene-dosage effect.

Table 6

RELATION BETWEEN ENZYME LEVELS AND NUCLEOTIDES

Medium Supplements			Specific Activities*	
Carbon Source (0.2%)	IPTG	Nucleotide (3mM)	β-Gal	CAT
Glycerol	+	—	480	509
Glucose	—	—	8	199
Glucose	+	—	260	260
Glucose	+	cAMP (3′5′)	605	563
Glucose	+	cAMP (3′5′) (no EDTA-Tris)	551	446
Glucose	+	5′ AMP	273	172
Glucose	+	ATP	275	193
Glucose	+	cGMP (3′5′)	259	151
Glucose	+	cUMP (2′3′)	238	222
Glucose	+	cCMP (2′3′)	214	195

* *E. coli* 1100/JJ1 was used; the cells were cultured as in Table 4, but were exposed to cAMP for 2 generation times.

The Effect of Cyclic (3'5') AMP on CAT Activity

Current investigations have indicated that cyclic (3'5') AMP and certain protein factors play a critical role in the mediation of catabolite repression (PERLMAN and PASTAN, 1968; ULLMAN and MONOD, 1968; PERLMAN, DE CROMBRUGGHE and PASTAN, 1969; ZUBAY, SCHWARTZ and BECKWITH, 1970; EMMER, DE CROMBRUGGHE, PASTAN and PERLMAN, 1970). The results of experiments summarized in Table 6 indicate that in *E. coli* 1100/JJ1, treated with EDTA-Tris to enhance permeability, the s. a. of CAT (and β-galactosidase) was enhanced by cyclic (3'5') AMP but not by other cyclic or adenyl nucleotides. The Tris-EDTA treatment positively affected the cyclic AMP enhancement, but it was not needed: cyclic AMP enhanced CAT activity in untreated cells (Table 6). The data presented in Figures 1 and 2 indicate that the concentration of, and duration of exposure

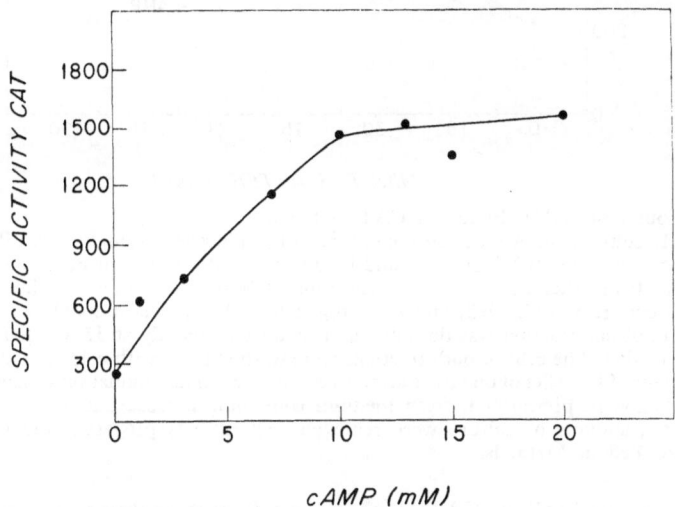

Fig. 1 Relation of cAMP Concentration to CAT Activity.
E. coli 1100/JJ1 was grown overnight in A medium containing glucose, diluted in fresh medium, and suplemented with various concentrations of cAMP in mid-exponential growth; 1 generation time later, the cells were harvested for the preparation of extracts and assays.

to, cyclic AMP were important to the cyclic AMP effect on CAT activity. The effect appeared to be maximal at 10 mM (with non-EDTA treated cells) and increased throughout a 90 minute incubation. Parallel experiments indicated that maximum enhancement of β-galactosidase activity was attained with 3 mM cyclic AMP. The results of the time course experiment reflected the impermeability of *E. coli* to cyclic AMP rather than a delay in activation of intracellular mechanisms: washing the cultures 15 minutes after exposure to cyclic AMP eliminated subsequent enhancement (Figure 2). The effect of cyclic AMP, like that of glucose, was realized with all R factors studied (Table 4). In certain cultures, the nucleotide produced a level of CAT activity that was greater than that of glycerol grown cells; the effect with B68 was indeed spectacular. This effect was associated, in each case, with growth inhibition: the doubling time of 1100 (B68, for example was 76 minutes in minimal glucose while that of a parallel culture containing 10mM cyclic AMP was 100 minutes. The final cell mass attained by the culture was also decreased by the nucleotide. This growth inhibition was specific for cyclic 3'5' AMP and certain R factors, but its basis remains undefined at present.

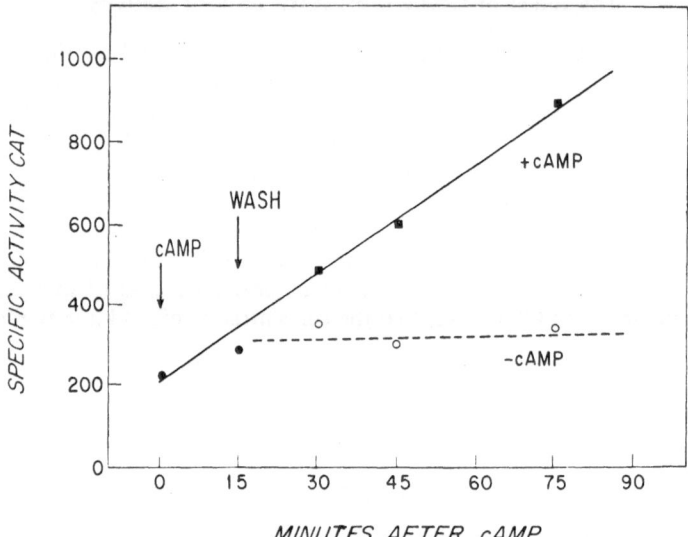

Fig. 2 Time Course of cAMP Effect on CAT Activity.
E. coli 1100/JJ1, cultured in A medium containing 0,1% glucose overnight was diluted 10 fold in fresh medium containing 0.2% glucose, and incubated until the optical density (490 mμ) was 0.115. Cyclic AMP was then added to a concentration of 10mM, and after 15 minutes of further incubation, the culture was divided, and centrifuged for 20 minutes at 20,000 × g at 4 °C; the supernatant fluid of one fraction was decanted and incubated sterilely at 37 °C, that of the other fraction was discarded. The cells of both fractions were washed twice with cold A medium containing no supplements. The pellet of one fraction was resuspended in its original supernatant fluid, that of the other fraction in prewarmed, fresh medium containing glucose but not cyclic AMP. At periodic intervals, aliquots of culture were removed, cell extracts prepared, and CAT activity assayed, as described in Methods.

The role of cyclic AMP on CAT synthesis was further explored in a mutant strain of *E. coli* K_{12} deficient in cyclic AMP because of a deficiency in adenyl cyclase (PERLMAN and PASTAN, 1969). The R factor JJ1 was transferred by conjugation to the mutant strain, 5336, at the same frequency as to the parent, 1100; furthermore, the frequency of segregation of JJ1 was low and similar in both strains. These data support the concept that cyclic AMP, like glukose, affects CAT activity at the level of translation or transcription

Table 7

EFFECT OF CYCLIC 3'5' AMP ON ENZYME ACTIVITIES

Strain	Medium Supplements		Specific Activities	
	Carbon Source (0.4%)	Nucleotide (3mM)	β-Gal	CAT
1100/JJ1 (WT parent)	Glycerol	5' AMP	4950	3000
	Glycerol	cyclic AMP	6100	4300
	Glucose	5' AMP	2550	980
	Glucose	cyclic AMP	5150	4450
5336/JJ1 (Adenyl cyclase deficient mutant)	Glucose	5' AMP	84	260
	Glucose	cyclic AMP	4750	7000

not replication. The activities of both CAT and β-galactosidase in *E. coli* 5336/JJ1 were lower by approximately 60 and 12 fold respectively than in 1100/JJ1, and they were increased back to unrepressed basal levels by cyclic AMP (Table 7).

These results provide strong evidence that the synthesis of CAT by R factors in *E. coli* K_{12} is subject to cyclic AMP-mediated catabolite repression.

Effect of Catabolite Repression on Chloramphenicol Resistance

Since CAT appears to be the primary, if not the sole basis for the R factor mediated Cml resistance, the metabolic effects that alter the intracellular concentration of CAT might be expected to affect the cell's resistance to Cml. Although differences in levels of resistance were not found under all test conditions, a definite effect on Cml resistance by glucose and cyclic AMP was reproducibly demonstrated in preliminary experiments in which the cells were grown in medium supplemented with different sugars and

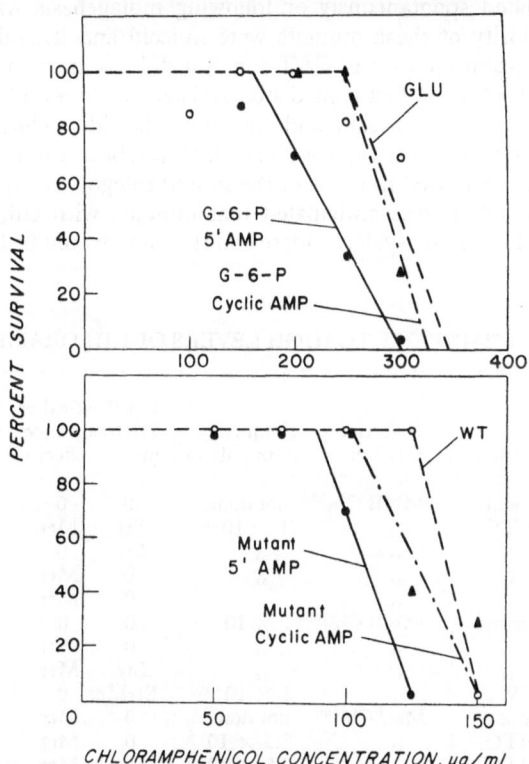

Fig. 3 Effect of Growth Conditions on Chloramphenicol Resistance.
E. coli 3000/JJ1 was grown at least 4 generations in MNB-supplemented with either glucose (GLU) or glucose-6-phosphate (G-6-P), 0.2%, with or without nucleotide, 3mM, diluted in iced A medium without carbon source and plated on MacConkey agar containing increasing concentrations of drug; viable colonies were counted after a 3 day incubation at 37°C. Lower: An experiment with the above design was performed using *E. coli* 1100/JJ1 (Wild Type) and 5336/JJ1 (adenyl cyclase deficient mutant) grown in MNB supplemented with nucleotides at 3mM.

nucleotides, and the ability of single cells to form colonies was assayed (Figure 3). These experiments were undertaken prior to the definition of the concentration of cyclic AMP needed for optimal enhancement of CAT activity; greater differences in resistance may be demonstrable if higher concentrations of cyclic AMP are employed. The effect of including test sugars in the drug agar, as well as the growth medium, is also being studied.

Selection of Mutants of R⁺ E. coli Resistant to High Levels of Cml

Since the s. a. of CAT in R⁺ E. coli is reflected in the level of Cml resistance, the isolation and characterization of mutants resistant to high levels of Cml and producing increased levels of CAT was initiated. It was anticipated that not all mutants with this phenotype would produce high levels of CAT. For example, mutations leading to an alteration in permeability to Cml would be expected to enhance the resistance mediated by CAT, and those producing increased levels of intracellular cyclic AMP, or protein(s) involved in cyclic AMP action, should produce increased resistance and CAT activity.

The first series of mutants were selected from E. coli 3000/JJ1. No highly Cml^r mutants were obtained following mutagenesis with 2-aminopurine. Nine mutants with increased resistance were isolated spontaneously or following mutagenesis with UV or nitroso-guanidine. The majority of these mutants were mucoid and irregular in morphology; none showed a significant increase in CAT s. a. nor did any transfer by conjugation the Cml phenotype with other R factor-mediated resistances. Some of these mutants had increased resistance to streptomycin and mercuric chloride, while many were more susceptible to mercuric chloride (Table 8). They have not been studied further.

In order to obviate undesired mutants of the second category mentioned above, E. coli 5336/JJ1 was employed. It was anticipated that mutants with enhanced cyclic AMP would have increased levels of β-galactosidase and therefore would be lac⁺ on MacConkey

Table 8

MUTANTS RESISTANT TO HIGH LEVELS OF CHLORAMPHENICOL[a]

Parent strain	Mutant name	Mutagen	Selective medium	Frequency in population	Levels of other JJ1 Resistances incr.	decr.	Increase in CmAT s. a.	High Chl resist. Transferable to AB1932−1 with JJ1
3000/J11	8	spont.	MNB Chl^{500}	not done	0	0	±	0
,,	H1	NTG	,,	1×10^{-5}	Str	Mer	0	0
,,	H10	,,	,,	,,	Str	0	0	0
,,	B2	,,	,,	,,	0	Mer	0	0
,,	F3	,,	,,	,,	0	Mer	0	0
,,	33	spont.	MNB Chl^{1000}	2×10^{-8}	0	0	0	0
,,	34	,,	,,	,,	0	Mer	0	0
,,	35	,,	,,	,,	Str	Mer	0	0
,,	40−2a	UV	,,	1×10^{-10}	StrMer	0	±	0
5336/JJ1	44	spont.	Mac^{b}Chl^{500}	not done	0	Mer	0	0
,,	45	NTG	,,	7.5×10^{-8}	0	Mer	+	0
,,	46	NTG	,,	2.5×10^{-8}	Str	Mer	+++^{c}	0
,,	58	UV	,,	3×10^{-9}	Str	Mer	+++	0
,,	59	UV	,,	1×10^{-8}	0	Mer	+++	0

[a] Levels of mutants' resistance were ascertained by doing Chl-, Str-, and Mer- profiles on MNB agar plates and comparing these to the drug profile of the unmutagenized parent strain.

[b] Mac = MacConkey lactose agar

[c] +++ denotes CmAT s.a. 3 times higher than in parent.

328

drug media. Five lac⁻ mutants were isolated at low frequencies on agar containing 500 μg/ml Cml; of these, none transferred by conjugation the enhanced level of Cml resistance; 3 had levels of CAT about 3 times that of the parent 5336/JJ1 but none had an increase in levels of β-galactosidase (Table 9). *E. coli* AB1932-1, infected with the

Table 9

Cml RESISTANCE AND CAT ACTIVITIES OF *E. COLI* 5336 AND DERIVATIVES

Strain	Cml Resistance	CAT Activity[b]
5336	> 5 <10[a]	0 (< 0.5)
5336−461[d]	> 5 <10	0 (< 1.4)
5336/JJ1	100[c]	325
5336−461/JJ1	200	645
5336−461/JJ1−46	300	1085

[a] μg drug/ml, MIC measured by tube dilution in trypticase soy broth.
[b] cells grown in trypticase soy broth and harvested in log phase.
[c] profile on MNB Chl agar; highest Chl concentration in μg/ml where 100% of plated cells formed colonies after 3 da. at 37°C.
[d] 5336−461 was an R⁻ segregant of 5336−461/JJ1−46.

R factor, JJ1-46, of one of these mutant cells, 5336-46, had the same pattern and level of resistance as did the same strain infected with the parent R factor. A R⁻ segregant of 5336-46 produced no CAT and was equally as susceptible to Cml as the parent *E. coli* 5336. (Table 9) Reinfection of 5336-461 with a copy of the parent R factor, JJ1, yielded a strain with a level of Cml resistance and CAT that was significantly greater than that produced by 5336/JJ1 (Table 9); the level of Str resistance, however, was identical in the mutant and parent cell. These findings suggest that the *E. coli* chromosome is able to enhance the production of a specific R factor product. Further studies of these particular strains are in progress.

Effect of Glucose and Cyclic AMP on CAT Synthesis in Proteus mirabilis

In order to determine the role of the host bacteria on CAT activity and the effects mediated by glucose and cyclic AMP, the s. a. of CAT produced by JJ1 in *E. coli* K_{12} and *Proteus mirabilis* were compared. The strains of *P. mirabilis* studied were of further interest since they are presumably R⁻ but produce CAT, and single-step mutants selected for high level Cml resistance have increased levels of CAT. The CAT of one of these strains, PM997, has been found to be nearly identical to that produced by R factors (JACOBSEN and SHAW, 1970). The effect of glucose and cyclic AMP on the *P. mirabilis* CAT was therefore studied in parallel; the catabolite repressibility of β-galactosidase produced by an F-lac factor was studied as a control.

The results summarized in Table 10 indicate that (i) the transfer by conjugation of JJ1 into *P. mirabilis* increased CAT activity; (ii) *P. mirabilis* that produced CAT gave rise to mutants that grew on 100 μg/ml Cml and produced elevated levels of CAT; (iii) the levels of CAT produced by 2 independently isolated strains of *P. mirabilis* differed markedly; (iv) the levels of CAT produced by R⁻ and R⁺ *P. mirabilis* grown in glucose were approximately 20% lower than that of cells grown in glycerol; glucose decreased by at least 250% the level of CAT produced by the same R factor in *E. coli* before, and after, its conjugal transfer into *P. mirabilis*; (v) the levels of CAT produced by the same R factor in *P. mirabilis* were approximately 0.2 (when cells were grown in glucose), and 0.4 (when

Table 10

RELATIONSHIP BETWEEN CAT LEVELS AND BACTERIAL STRAINS

Bacterial Strain	Carbon Source (.4%)	S.A.CAT[a]
Proteus mirabilis 13	Glucose	4
	Glycerol	4
Proteus mirabilis 13/JJ1[c]	Glucose	156
	Glycerol	190
Proteus mirabilis 13−1[b,c]	Glucose	1408
	Glycerol	1968
Proteus mirabilis 997	Glucose	8
	Glycerol	8
Proteus mirabilis 997/JJ1[c]	Glucose	172
	Glycerol	191
Proteus mirabilis 997−2[b,c]	Glucose	236
	Glycerol	272
E. coli K_{12} AB1932−1	Glucose	1
	Glycerol	1
E. coli K_{12} AB1932−1/JJ1[c]	Glucose	383
	Glycerol	988
E. coli K_{12} AB1932−1/JJ1−1[c,d]	Glucose	344
	Glycerol	986
E. coli K_{12} AB1932−1/JJ1−2[c,e]	Glucose	354
	Glycerol	864

a nmoles p-nitro-m-carboxythiophenol produced per min. per mg protein.
b spontaneous mutant selected on MacConkey agar containing 100 μg chloramphenicol/ml.
c grown in 5−25 μg chloramphenicol/ml broth.
d JJ1 after conjugal transfer from *Proteus mirabilis* 13/JJ1.
e JJ1 after conjugal transfer from *Proteus mirabilis* 997/JJ1.

Table 11

RELATIONSHIP BETWEEN THE S.A. OF β-GALACTOSIDASE AND BACTERIAL STRAINS

Bacterial Strain	Carbon Source (.2%) and IPTG	S.A. β-gal[a]
E. coli K_{12} AB1932−1	Glucose	3
	Glycerol	3
E. coli K_{12} AB1932−1/F lac	Glucose	81
	Glycerol	246
E. coli K_{12} AB1932−1/F lac−1[b]	Glucose	75
	Glycerol	220
P. mirabilis 997	Glucose	2
	Glycerol	1
P. mirabilis 997/F lac	Glucose	41
	Glycerol	46
P. mirabilis 997−2[c]/F lac	Glucose	33
	Glycerol	43

a nmoles o-nitrophenol produced per min. per ml at 25°C.
b F lac after conjugal transfer from *P. mirabilis* 997/F lac.
c see Table 10.

grown in glycerol) of that produced by *E. coli*. The induced level of β-galactosidase was also lower in *P. mirabilis* than in *E. coli*, and it was not markedly affected by glucose (Table 11). Attempts to impose more severe catabolite repression (as defined in *E. coli*) by growing *P. mirabilis* in glucose-6-phosphate were unsuccessful since the studied strains could not grow with this sugar as the sole carbon source. Furthermore, negative results were realized with the addition of cyclic AMP to the medium of R+ *P. mirabilis*; these findings cannot be interpreted, however, since there was no indication that the cells were permeable to the nucleotide.

DISCUSSION

These studies were initiated to define the basis for the regulation of the R factor-mediated enzyme, chloramphenicol acetyl transferase. This enzyme was selected because it can be quantitatively assayed with ease, and it is the sole basis for chloramphenicol resistance mediated by R factors (MISE and SUZUKI, 1968). The results indicate that CAT synthesis, unlike β-lactamase, is not affected markedly by the growth rate of host bacteria. CAT, however, is regulated by cyclic 3'5' AMP-mediated catabolite repression which, in turn, affects the level of bacterial resistance to Cml.

The finding that CAT is regulated by catabolite repression was somewhat unexpected in that this form of regulation is not generally reported with "constitutive" enzymes, and CAT had not been previously considered to mediate a catabolic function. If CAT is assumed to have evolved in bacteria as a detoxifying enzyme in response to growth-inhibitory concentrations of chloramphenicol in the environment, it may be useful to compare these findings with the thiogalactoside transacetylase, coded by the *lac* operon of *E. coli*. Also catabolite repressible, this enzyme's function has remained a matter for speculation since it is not essential for growth on lactose (Fox, BECKWITH, EPSTEIN and SIGNER, 1966). Galactosides are known to inhibit the growth of *E. coli* (von HOFSTEIN, 1961), and acetylated IPTG is not accumulated by *E. coli*. WILSON and KASHKEUT (1969) have recently reported that *E. coli* actively transport IPTG (or thiomethylgalacto-side), acetylate it, and lose it into the medium. Mutants lacking thiogalactoside t ans-acetylase concentrate but cannot acetylate galactosides, resulting in the marked intracellular accumulation of free galactoside. These observations have been cited as support for Zabin's (1963) proposal that the "true function" in the cell of thiogalactoside transacetylase, is to inactivate toxic glycosides.

Considerable evidence indicates that cyclic 3'5' AMP mediates catabolite repression, and that glucose depresses the synthesis of involved enzymes by decreasing the intracellular content of cyclic AMP. Evidence has also been presented that catabolite regulation of the *lac* operon requires a protein mediator (ZUBAY et al., 1970; EMMER et al.), in addition to cyclic AMP, and an intact promoter region. (PASTAN and PERLMAN, 1968; SILVER-STONE, MAGASANIK, REZIKOFF, MILLER and BECKWITH, 1969). Although the activity of β-galactosidase has been found, in these studies, to be more sensitive than that of CAT, the mechanisms involved in the catabolite repression of the 2 enzymes by *E. coli* may be similar. The finding that CAT synthesis in all Chl^r R+ *E. coli* studied, including that produced by P$_1$Cm, is so regulated indicates that the catabolite sensitive site must be so closely located to the structural locus for CAT, that its integrity has not been grossly interrupted by the genetic events that have led to its recombination into certain R factors, and from one of these, into a defective P$_1$ phage.

The lack of quantitative correspondence between CAT activity and the level of Cml resistance is perhaps not surprising. Whereas the synthesis of CAT may relate directly to available cyclic AMP, other factors undoubtedly play a role in the cell's resistance to

Cml. *E. coli* 3000, for example, is somewhat more Cml resistant when grown on glucose than on glycerol. It is therefore reasonable to expect this effect to mask (or subdue) the phenotypic expression of the "glucose effect" on CAT activity in *E. coli* 3000/JJ1. Furthermore, as indicated in Results, these findings were made during preliminary studies; future studies with more appropriate experimental design may alter the observed results.

Attempts to isolate (regulatory) mutants, of the R factor JJ1 that produce high levels of CAT have thus far been unsuccessful. This result may be evidence of some basic genetic property of this R factor, rather than poor luck or lack of persistence. SHAW and BRODSKY (1968), working with a different R factor, found on purification of CAT from R+ *E. coli* that the enzyme constitutes about 0.5% of the total bacterial protein. One class of the desired highly Cml^r mutants would be expected to include mutations in the CAT promoter region that would have an increased affinity for RNA polymerase. It is therefore worth noting that a (presumed) promoter mutation of the *i* repressor region of the lac operon (MÜLLER-HILL, CRAPO and GILBERT, 1968) increased the fraction of total *E. coli* protein that was repressor protein from approximately 0.001% to only 0.01%. It is thus possible that the mRNA for CAT is already being synthesized at a relatively high rate and that the CAT promoter of JJ1 cannot accommodate further mRNA, even with the potential number of base changes produced by the mutagens employed in these studies.

Mutants 5336-46 most probably has one or more lesions of the bacterial chromosome that allow for higher levels of CAT activity than that produced by the parent cell. This effect was relatively specific since neither the levels of β-galactosidase nor Str resistance was increased. The basis for this genotype remains undefined, but the mutant appears qualitatively analogous to the mutant *S. aureus* isolated by COHEN and SWEENEY (1968) in which the β-lactamase activity produced by a wild type plasmid was increased 100-fold.

The results obtained with JJ1 in *P. mirabilis* provide only further support that the host cell affects the level of CAT. The absence of the same quantitative "glucose effect" as seen in *E. coli* extends previous observations on catabolite repression in *P. mirabilis* (COLBY, MARTIN and HU, 1968), but unfortunately does not delineate if this species is capable of catabolite repression (perhaps with other carbon sources); likewise, the negative effect with cyclic AMP may only reflect that *P. mirabilis* is impermeable to the nucleotide. Finally, the current observations do not provide any genetic evidence regarding the possible origin in Proteus of the CAT region of R factors.

The catabolite repression of CAT raises the question of similar regulation of other R factor enzymes. The results of other experiments indicate that SAT is also catabolite repressed (HARWOOD and SMITH, 1971), but insufficient data has been obtained to determine if the SAT and CAT structural loci are part of a single operon with a single promoter. Genetic maps of certain fi+ R factors have indicated that the structural loci for chloramphenicol and streptomycin resistance (and therefore for CAT and SAT respectively) are linked (WATANABE, 1966; HASHIMOTO, IYOBE and MITSUHASHI, 1969). Considerable evidence indicate that these structural loci may exist independently of one another, and as indicated in Tables 4 and 5, the synthesis of CAT is catabolite repressible regardless of its linkage to the region for Str resistance. If there is a common promoter, therefore, it must be linked closely to the CAT structural region; study of SAT produced by R factors with a deleted CAT region should help resolve this question. Catabolite repression of R factor-mediated enzymes is not universal, however. Neither the β-lactamase produced by *E. coli* harboring the R factor R_1 (BURMAN et al., 1968) nor the gentamicin adenylate transferase (OTTO and SMITH, unpublished data) are catabolite repressible, and the levels of resistance mediated by JJ1 to mercuric chloride and sulfonamide were similar in the *E. coli* strain, deficient in adenyl cyclase, and its parent strain (HARWOOD and SMITH, unpublished observations).

Future studies should provide further insight into the control of other R factor-mediated drug-inactivating enzymes by catabolite repression, as well as a more detailed analysis of the biochemical and genetic mechanisms involved in this regulation of CAT and SAT.

REFERENCES

ADELBERG, E. A., MANDEL, M. and CHEN, G. C. C. (1965): Optimal conditions for mutagenesis by N-methyl-N'-nitro-N-nitrosoguanidine in Escherichia coli. Biochemical and Biophysical Research Communications, 18, 788.

AMARASINGHAM, C. R. and DAVIS, B. D. (1965): Regulation of α-ketoglutarate dehydrogenase formation in E. coli. Journal of Biological Chemistry, 240, 3664.

BENVENISTE, R., and DAVIES, J. (1971): R-factor mediated gentamicin resistance: A new enzyme which modifies aminoglycoside antibiotics. Federation of European Biochemical Societies Letters, 14, 586.

BENVENISTE, R., YAMADA, T. and DAVIES, J. (1970): Enzymatic adenylylation of streptomycin and spectinomycin in Escherichia coli carrying resistance factors. Infection and Immunity, 1, 109.

BURMAN, L. G., NORDSTRÖM, K. and BOMAN, H. G. (1968): Resistance of Escherichia coli to penicillins. V. Physiological comparison of two isogenic strains, one with chromosomally and one with episomally mediated ampicillin resistance. Journal of Bacteriology, 96, 438.

COHEN, S. and SWEENEY, H. M. (1968): Constitutive penicillinase formation in Staphylococcus aureus owing to a mutation unliked to the penicillinase plasmid. Journal of Bacteriology, 95, 1368.

COLBY, C. C., Jr., MARTIN, F. D. and HU, A. S. L. (1968): Catabolite repression of the synthesis of β-galactosidase in Proteus mirabilis F-lac. Biochimica et Biophysica Acta, 157, 159.

DATTA, N. and KONTOMICHALOU, P. (1965): Penicillinase synthesis controlled by infectious R factors in Enterobacteriaceae. Nature, 208/5007, 239.

DAVIS, B. D. and MINGIOLI, E. S. (1954): Mutants of Escherichia coli requiring methionine or vitamin B_{12}. Journal of Bacteriology, 60, 17.

EMMER, B., DECROMBRUGGHE, PASTAN, I. and PERLMAN, R. (1970): Cyclic AMP receptor protein of E. coli Its role in the synthesis of inducible enzymes. Proceedings of the National Academy of Sciences (U.S.A.), 66, 480.

ERIKSSON-GRENNBERG, K. G., BOMAN, H. G., TORBJÖRN JANSSON, J. A. and THOREN, S. (1965): Resistance of Escherichia coli to penicillins. I. Genetic study of some ampicillin-resistant mutants. Journal of Bacteriology, 90, 54.

FALKOW, S., HAAPALA, D. K. and SILVER, R. P. (1969): Relationships between extra chromosomal elements. In: Bacterial Episomes and Plasmids, 1st edition, pp. 136−162. Editors: G.E.W. Wolstenholme and M. O'Connor. Little, Brown and Company, Boston, Massachusetts.

FOX, C. F., BECKWITH, R., EPSTEIN, W. and SINGER, E. R. (1966): Transposition of the lac region of Escherichia coli. II. On the role of thiogalactoside transacetylase in lactose metabolism. Journal of Molecular Biology, 19, 576.

FRANKLIN, T. J. (1967): Resistance of Escherichia coli to tetracyclines. Changes in permeability to tetracyclines in Escherichia coli bearing transferable resistance factors. Biochemical Journal, 105, 371.

FULLBROOK, P. D., ELSON S. W. and SLOCOMBE, B. (1970): R-factor mediated β-lactamase in Pseudomonas aeruginosa. Nature, 226, 1054.

HARWOOD, J. H. and SMITH, D. H. (1969): Resistance factor-mediated streptomycin resistance. Journal of Bacteriology, 97, 1262.

HARWOOD, J. H. and SMITH, D. H. (1971): Catabolite repression of chloramphenicol acetyl transferase synthesis in E. coli K_{12}. Biochemical and Biophysical Research Communications, 42, 57.

HASHIMOTO, H., IYOBE, S. and MITSUHASHI, S. (1969): Unstable mutants of R factor. Japanese Journal of Microbiology, 13, 343.

VON HOFSTEIN, B. (1961): The inhibitory effect of galactosides on the growth of Escherichia coli. Biochimica et Biophysica Acta, 48, 164.

HSIE, A. W. and RICKENBERG, H. V. (1966): A mutant of Escherichia coli deficient in phosphenol-pyruvate carboxykinase activity. Biochemical and Biophysical Research Communications, 25, 676.

IZAKI, K., KIUCHI, K. and ARIMA, K. (1966): Specificity and mechanism of tetracycline resistance in a multiple drug resistant strain of Escherichia coli. Journal of Bacteriology, 91, 628.

JACK, G. W. and RICHMOND, M. H. (1970): A comparative study of eight distinct β-lactamases synthesized by gram-negative bacteria. Journal of General Microbiology, 61, 43.

JACOBSEN, H. W. Jr. and SHAW, W. V. (1970): Chloramphenicol resistance in nonepisomal Proteus mirabilis. Bacteriological Proceedings — 1970, pg. 60.

KONDO, E. and MITSUHASHI, S. (1964): Drug resistance of enteric bacteria. IV. Active transducing bacteriophage P1CM produced by the combination of R-factor with bacteriophage P1. Journal of Bacteriology, 88, 1266.

KONDO, E., HAAPALA, D. K. and FALKOW, S. (1970): The production of chloramphenicol acetyltransferase by bacteriophage P1CM. Journal of Virology, 40, 431.

KONTOMICHALOU, P. (1967): Transmissible extrachromosomal resistance to the penicillins in E. coli K12 and Falkow's Proteus host. 5th International Congress on Chemotherapy, 4, 251.

LEIVE, L. (1965): Actinomycin sensitivity in Escherichia coli produced by EDTA. Biochemical and Biophysical Research Communications, 18, 13.

LOOMIS, W. F., Jr. and MAGASANIK, B. (1964): Genetic control of catabolite repression of the lac operon in Escherichia coli. Biochemical and Biophysical Research Communications, 27, 230.

LOWRY, O. H., ROSEBROUGH, N. J., FARR, A. L. and RANDALL, R. J. (1951): Protein measurement with Folin phenol reagent. Journal of Biological Chemistry, 193, 265.

MARSH, E. B., Jr. and SMITH, D. H. (1969): R factors improving survival of Escherichia coli K12 after ultraviolet irradiation. Journal of Bacteriology, 100, 128.

MÜLLER-HILL, CRAPO, L. and GILBERT, W. (1968): Mutants that make more lac repressor. Proceedings of the National Academy of Sciences (U.S.A.), 59, 1259.

OZANNE, B., BENVENISTE, R., TIPPER, D. and DAVIES, J. (1969): Aminoglycoside antibiotics: Inactivation by phosphorylation in Escherichia coli carrying R factors. Journal of Bacteriology, 100, 1144.

PARDEE, A. B., JACOB, F. and MONODO, J. (1959): The genetic control and cytoplasmic expression of "inducibility" in the synthesis of β-galactosidase by E. coli. Journal of Molecular Biology, 1, 165.

PASTAN, I. and PERLMAN, R. G. (1968): The role of the lac promotor locus in the regulation of β-galactosidase synthesis by cyclic 3′, 5′-adenosine monophosphate. Proceedings of the National Academy of Sciences (U.S.A.), 61, 1336.

PERLMAN, R. and PASTAN, I. (1968): Cyclic 3′5′ AMP: Stimulation of β-galactosidase and tryptophanase induction in E. coli. Biochemical and Biophysical Research Communications, 30, 556.

PERLMAN, R. and PASTAN, I. (1969): Pleotropic deficiency of carbohydrate utilization in an adenyl cyclase deficient mutant of E. coli. Biochemical and Biophysical Research Communications. 37, 151.

PERLMAN, R. L., DE CROMBRUGGH, E. B. and PASTAN, I. (1969): Cyclic AMP regulates catabolite and transient repression in E. coli. Nature, 223, 810.

RICKENBERG, H. V., HSIE, A. W. and JANECEK, J. (1968): The CR mutation and catabolite repression in Escherichia coli. Biochemical and Biophysical Research Communications 31, 603.

ROWND, R., NAKAY, R. and NAKAMURA, A. (1966): Molecular nature of the drugresistance factors of the Enterobacteriaceae. Journal of Molecular Biology, 17, 376.

SHAW, W. V. (1967): The enzymatic chloramphenicol acetylation of chloramphenicol by extracts of R factor-resistant Escherichia coli. Journal of Biological Chemistry, 242, 687.

SHAW, W. V. and BRODSKY, R. F. (1968): Characterization of chloramphenicol acetyltransferase from Staphylococcus aureus. Journal of Bacteriology, 95, 28.

SILVERSTONE, A. E., MAGASANIK, B., REZNIKOFF, W. S., MILLER, J. H. and BECKWITH, J. R. (1969): Catabolite sensitive site of the lac operon. Nature, 221, 1012.

SMITH, J. T. (1969): R-factor gene expression in gram-negative bacteria. Journal of General Microbiology, 55, 109.

SMITH, D. H., JANJIGIAN, J. A., PRESCOTT, N. and ANDERSON, P. W. (1970): Resistance factor-mediated spectinomycin resistance. Infection and Immunity, 1, 120.

SUZUKI, Y. and OKAMOTO, S. (1967): The enzymatic acetylation of chloramphenicol by the multiple drug-resistant Escherichia coli carrying R factor. Journal of Biological Chemistry, 242, 4722.

TOMOEDA, M., INUZUKA, M., KUBO, N. and NAKAMURA, S. (1968): Effective elimination of drug resistant and sex factors in Escherichia coli by sodium dodecyl sulfate. Journal of Bacteriology, 95, 1078.

ULLMAN, H. and MONOD, J. (1968): Cyclic AMP as an antagonist of catabolite repression in Escherichia coli. Federation of European Biochemical Societies Letters, 2, 57.

UMEZAWA, H., OKANISHI, M., KONDO, S., HAMANA, K., UTAHARA, R., MAEDA, K. and MITSUHASHI, S. (1967): Phosphorylative inactivation of aminoglycosidic antibiotics by Escherichia coli carrying R factor. Science, 157, 1559.

UMEZAWA, H., OKANISHI, M., UTAHARA, R., MAEDA, K. and KONDO, S. (1967): Isolation and structure of kanamycin inactivated by a cell-free system of kanamycinresistant Escherichia coli. Journal of Antibiotics Ser. A., **20**, 136.

UMEZAWA, H., TAKASAWA, S., OKANISHI, M. and UTAHARA, R. (1968): Adenylylstreptomycin, a product of streptomycin inactivated by carrying R factor. Journal of Antibiotics, **21**, 81.

WALTON, J. R. and SMITH, D. H. (1969): New Hemolysin (γ) produced by Escherichia coli. Journal of Bacteriology, **98**, 304.

WATANABE, T. (1963): Infective heredity of multiple drug resistance in bacteria. Bacteriological Reviews, **27**, 87.

WILLIAMS, L. S. and NEIDHARDT, F. C. (1969): Synthesis and inactivation of aminoacyl-transfer RNA synthetases during growth of E. coli. Journal of Molecular Biology, **43**, 529.

WILSON, T. H. and KASHKET, E. R. (1969): Isolation and properties of thiologalactoside transacety-lase-negative mutants of Escherichia coli. Biochimica et Biophysica Acta, **173**, 501.

YAMADA, T., TIPPER, D. and DAVIES, J. (1968): Enzymatic inactivation of streptomycin by R factor-resistant Escherichia coli. Nature, **219**, 288.

ZABIN, I. (1963): Galactoside transport in relation to bacterial genetics and protein synthesis. Federation Proceedings, **22**, 27.

ZUBAY, G., SCHWARTZ, D. and BECKWITH, J. (1970): Mechanism of activation of catabolite-sensi-tive genes: A positive control system. Proceedings of the National Academy of Sciences, **66**, 104.

ENZYMATIC INACTIVATION OF AMINOGLYCOSIDE ANTIBIOTICS BY RESISTANT STRAINS OF BACTERIA

S. MITSUHASHI, F. KOBAYASHI,* M. YAMAGUCHI,
K. O'HARA, and M. KONO**

Department of Microbiology, School of Medicine Gunma University, Maebashi, Japan

The enzymatic inactivation of chemotherapeutic agents is considered to be one of the mechanisms of drug resistance in bacteria. The inactivation of aminoglycosides has been studied extensively by many investigators, with three mechanisms being involved in the inactivation, i. e., acetylation, adenylylation and phosphorylation.

Inactivation by phosphorylation. It was reported that kanamycin (KM), paromomycin and neomycin were inactivated by enzymes prepared from resistant strains and that the 3-hydroxyl group of the amino sugars was phosphorylated (KOBAYASHI et al., 1971a; OKAMOTO, SUZUKI, 1965; OZANNE et al. 1969; UMEZAWA et al., 1967a; UMEZAWA et al., 1967b; UMEZAWA et al., 1968b). It was also found that the hydroxyl group on C-3 of the N-methylglucosamine moiety in dihydrostreptomycin (SM) was phosphorylated by enzymes prepared from either *Escherichia coli* R+ (OZANNE et al., 1969; UMEZAWA et al., 1967b) or *Pseudomonas aeruginosa* (DOI et al. 1968a; KAWABE et al., 1971a; KAWABE, MITSUHASHI, 1971b; KOBAYASHI et al., 1971b; KOBAYASHI, 1971c). We reported (KOBAYASHI, 1971a) that a KM-phosphorylating enzyme from a resistant strain of *P. aeruginosa* inactivated paromomycin, mannosylparomomycin, aminodeoxy-kanamycin and neomycin but did not inactivate lividomycin (LV) (ODA et al., 1971), gentamicin (GM) C components (WEINSTEIN, 1964), and a new kanamycin DKB (UMEZAWA, 1968b), which were known to be devoid of a hydroxyl group at position 3 of the amino sugar. Therefore, the chemical structure where it is devoid of the 3-hydroxyl group of the amino sugar, is considered to be of biological significance.

It was found recently that the lividomycin was inactivated by enzymes prepared from resistant strains of *P. aeruginosa* (KOBAYASHI et al., 1971d) and *E. coli* R+ (YAMAGUCHI, 1971) by a mechanism involved in the formation of a monophosphorylated product of the drug, resulting in the loss of antibacterial activity. The inactivated product was converted into the original antibiotic by treatment with alkaline phosphatase. The enzymes transferred the labeled phosphate from γ^{32}P-labeled adenosine triphosphate (ATP) of lividomycin. The analytical data indicated that LV was monophosphorylated on the hydroxyl group of the drug. The phosphorylated position of LV is currently being determined and will be described elsewhere. By contrast, we have not isolated thus far bacterial strains capable of phosphorylating gentamicin C components. The sugar of GM is a 2,3,4,6-tetradeoxy-amino sugar, i. e., purpurosamine, and contains no hydroxyl groups in the rings, indicating that this fact is of biological significance. Antibacterial activity of various aminoglycosides toward *P. aeruginosa* is shown in Fig. 1.

Present adress. * Tokyo Research Laboratories, Kowa Co., Higashimurayama, Tokyo.
** Tokyo College of Pharmacy, Tokyo.

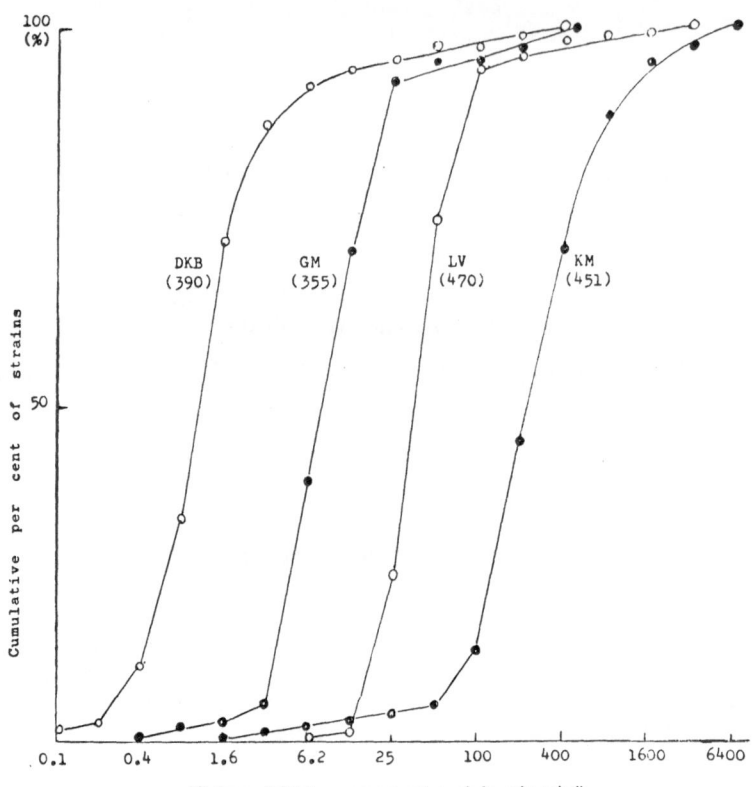

DKB
(390)

GM
(355)

LV
(470)

KM
(451)

Minimum inhibitory concetration of drug (mcg/ml)

Parenthesis indicates the number of bacterial strains examined

Fig. 1 Antibacterial activity of aminoglycosides against *Pseudomonas aeruginosa*

Table 1.

INACTIVATION OF GENTAMICIN C COMPONENTS BY CELL-FREE EXTRACTS FROM RESISTANT STRAINS

S-105 fraction[a] from	MIC[b] (mcg/ml)	Percent of inactivation		
		C_1	C_2	C_{1a}
K. pneumoniae 3020	200	100	100	95
K. pneumoniae 3694	100	98.8	99.5	80
E. coli ML1410 RM100+	25	99.3	98.5	95
K. pneumoniae 2970	1.6	0	0	0
E. coli ML1410	0.2	0	0	0

The inactivating reaction was carried out at 30 C for 1 hour and the remaining activity of the antibiotics was assayed by a paper disk method using *Bacillus subtilis*. Reaction mixture consisted of 0.3 ml of the S-105 fraction (20 mg protein per ml), 0.1 ml of 40 mM ATP, 0.1 ml of 1 mM antibiotic and 0.5 ml of TMK solution (M/10 tris buffer containing 0.06 M KCl, 0.01 M magnesium acetate and 0.006 M 2-mercaptoethanol, pH 7.8). An RM100 factor was isolated from *K. pneumoniae* 3694 and was conjugally transferred to *E. coli* ML1410.

ᵃ The bacterial cell suspension was disrupted sonically at 20 Kc. After treatment with deoxyribonuclease, the sonicated suspension was centrifuged at 105,000 × g for 60 minutes and the supernatant was dialyzed for 2 hours against cold TMK solution. The solution was designated as the S-105 fraction.

ᵇ The minimum inhibitory concentration (MIC) is defined as the least amount of antibiotic (gentamicin C complex) required to prevent growth.

Inactivation by adenylylation. It was reported that streptomycin was inactivated by enzymes prepared from *E. coli* R⁺ (UMEZAWA, et al., 1968a, YAMADA et al., 1968) and *Staphylococcus aureus* (KAWABE, MITSUHASHI, 1971b) by a mechanism involving the formation of an adenylylated product. Recent studies have disclosed that gentamicin C components are inactivated by another mechanism involving the formation of adenylyla- ted products of the drugs by enzymes prepared from GM-resistant strains of *Klebsiella pneumoniae* (KOBAYASHI et al., 1971). Drug resistance of *K. pneumoniae* 3694 was found to be transmissible by conjugation and was transferred to *E. coli* ML1410. The transmissible drug resistance factor RM100 was capable of conferring 6 drug-resistance including sulfanilamide, chloramphenicol, tetracycline, streptomycin, kanamycin and gentamicin C complex. To know the inactivation mechanism, γ-^{32}P-labeled ATP and 8-^{14}C-labeled ATP were used, demonstrating the incorporation of ^{14}C-labeled component of ATP into gentamicin C components but not of ^{32}P. These data indicated that the inactivation of gentamicin C components was caused by the formation of an adenylylated product (Table 1).

Inactivation by acetylation. It was reported that kanamycins A and B were inactivated by a mechanism involving the formation of 6-N-acetylkanamycin (UMEZAWA et al., 1967a). We reported that gentamicins C_1, C_{1a} and C_2, were inactivated by enzymes from resistant strains of *P. aeruginosa* involving the formation of acetylated products of gentamicins (MITSUHASHI et al., 1971). It was reported that an enzyme prepared from a KM-resistant strain of *E. coli* carrying either NR79 or R5, in the presence of ^{14}C-acetyl coenzyme A, transferred the labeled acetate to kanamycin A, B, neomycins B and C, gentamicins C_{1a} and C_2, but gentamicin C_1, paromomycin and gentamicin A were not acetylated(1). These data however cannot account for the resistance mechanism of clinical isolates, because *E. coli* NR79⁺ and *E. coli* R5⁺ are sensitive to gentamicins. Sisomicin(SS) was isolated from fermentation broth of *Micromonospora iyoensis* (WEINSTEIN et al. 1970) and the antibacterial spectrum appeared to be quite similar to that of gentamicins. This antibiotic was found to be inactivated by the formation of an acetylated product (O'HARA et al. 1971). The inactivating activity was lost without ATP or without both coenzyme A(CoA) and acetate, but restored completely by addition of the three agents, i. e., ATP, CoA and acetate. But these three agents could be replaced by acetyl coenzyme A. It was found that the enzyme, in the presence of ^{14}C-acetyl coenzyme A, transferred the labeled acetate to the drug (Table 2). These results indicated that SS was inactivated by a mechanism involving the formation of an acetylated product. The inactivated position of each of the gentamicin C components is still being elucidated and will be described elsewhere. The results of inactivation of aminoglycosides are summarized in Table 3.

Table 2.

INACTIVATION OF SISOMICIN BY CELL-FREE EXTRACTS FROM RESISTANT STRAINS OF *P. AERUGINOSA*

S-105 fraction from		MIC[a] (mcg/ml)	Per cent of [b] SS inactivation
P. aeruginosa	269	200	100
P. aeruginosa	314	50	100
P. aeruginosa	315	200	100
P. aeruginosa	1567	12.5	0

The reaction mixture consisted of 0.3 ml of the S-105 fraction (20 mg protein per ml), 0.2 ml of 1 mM acetyl CoA, 01. ml of 1mM antibiotic solution and 0.3 ml of TMK solution. *a* and *b*; see the footnote of Table 1.

Table 3.

INACTIVATION OF VARIOUS AMINOGLYCOSIDES BY RESISTANT
INACTIVATION OF VARIOUS AMINOGLYCOSIDES BY RESISTANT STRAINS

Drug	Microorganism	Mechanism of inactivation	Reference
Streptomycin	*E. coli* R+	Adenylylation	Umezawa et al. (1968a) Yamada et al. (1968)
		Phosphorylation	Ozanne et al. (1969)
	P. aeruginosa	Phosphorylation	Doi et al. (1968) Kobayashi et al. (1971a,b,c) Kawabe et al. (1971a)
	S. aureus	Adenylylation	Kawabe et al. (1971b)
Kanamycins	*E. coli* R+	Acetylation (A and B) Phosphorylation (A, B and C)	Umezawa et al. (1967a) Umezawa et al. (1967b)
	P. aeruginosa	Phosphorylation	Umezawa et al. (1968b) Doi et al. (1968a) Kobayashi et al. (1971a)
	S. aureus	Phosphorylation	Doi et al. (1968b)
Lividomycin	*P. aeruginosa*	Phosphorylation	Kobayashi et al. (1971a, 1971d)
	E. coli R+	Phosphorylation	Yamaguchi et al. (1971)
Gentamicin C components	*P. aeruginosa* *E. coli* NR79+	Acetylation (C_1, C_{1a} and C_2) Acetylation (C_{1a} and C_2)	Mitsuhashi et al. (1971a) Benveniste and Davis (1971)
	K. Pneumoniae	Adenylylation (C_1, C_{1a} and C_2)	Kobayashi et al. (1971e)
	E. coli R+	Adenylylation (C_1, C_{1a} and C_2)	Kobayashi et al. (1971e)
Sisomicin	*P. aeruginosa*	Acetylation	Mitsuhashi et al. (1971b) O'Hara et al. (1971)
Nebramycin factor 6	*E. coli* R+	Acetylation	Benveniste and Davis (1971)

REFERENCES

BENBENISTE, R., and J. DAVIS (1977): Biochemistry **10**: 1787—1796.

DOI, O., M. OGURA, N. TANAKA, and H. UMEZAWA (1968): Appl. Microbiol. **16**: 1276—1281.

DOI, O., M. MIYAMOTO, N. TANAKA, and H. UMEZAWA (1968b): App. Microbiol. **16**: 1282—1284.

KAWABE, H., F. KOBAYASHI, M. YAMAGUCHI, R. UTAHARA, and S. MITSUHASHI (1971a): J. Antibiotics **24** : 651—652.

KAWABE, H., and S. MITSUHASHI (1971b): Japan. J. Microbiol. **15** : 545—548.

KOBAYASHI, F., M. YAMAGUCHI, and S. MITSUHASHI. 1971a. Jap. J. Microbiol. **15**: 265—272.

KOBAYASHI, F., M. YAMAGUCHI, and S. MITSUHASHI (1971b): Jap. J. Microbiol. **15**: 381—382.

KOBAYASHI, F., M. YAMAGUCHI, J. SATO, and S. MITSUHASH I(1971c): Jap. J. Microbiol. in press.

KOBAYASHI, F., M. YAMAGUCHI, and S. MITSUHASHI (1971d): J. Bacteriol. in press.

KOBAYASHI, F., M. YAMAGUCHI, J. EDA, F. HIGASHI, and S. MITSUHASHI. 1971. J. Antibiotics in press.

MITSUHASHI, S., F. KOBAYASHI, and M. YAMAGUCHI (1971): J. Antibiotics **24**: 400—401.

ODA, T., T. MORI, Y. KYOTANI, and N. MASAHITO (1971): J. Antibiotics in press.

O'HARA, K,, M. KONO, and S. MITSUHASHI (1971): J. Antibiotics in press.

OKAMOTO, S., and Y. SUZUKI (1965): Nature **208**: 1301—1303.

OZANNE, B., R. BEVVENISTE, D. TIPPER, and J. DAVIES (1969): J. Bacteriol. **100**: 1144—1146.

UMEZAWA, H., M. OKANISHI, R. UTAHARA, K. MAEDA, and S. KONDO (1967a): J. Antibiotics 20: 136—141.

UMEZAWA, H., M. OKANISHI, S. KONDO, K. HAMANA, R. UTAHARA. K. MAEDA, and S. MITSUHASHI (1967b): Science 157: 1559—1561.

UMEZAWA, H., S. TAKASAWA, M. OKANISHI, and R. UTAHARA (1968a): J. Antibiotics 21: 81—82.

UMEZAWA, H., O. DOI, M. OGURA, S. KONDO, and N. TANAKA (1968b). J. Antibiotics 21: 154—155.

UMEZAWA, H., T. TAKEUCHI, S. UMEZAWA, and T. TSUCHIYA (1971): Presented at the VIIth International Congress of Chemotherapy, Prague.

WEINSTEIN, M. J., G. M. LUEDEMANN, E. M. ODEN, and G. H. WAGMAN (1964): In Antimicrobial Agents and Chemotherapv — 1963: 1—13.

WEINSTEIN, M. J., J. A. MARQUEZ, R. T. TESTA, G. H. WAGMAN, E. M. ODEN, and J. A. WAITZ (1970): J. Antibiotics 23: 551—554.

YAMADA, T., D. TIPPER, and J. DAVIES (1968): Nature 219: 288—291.

YAMAGUCHI, M., F. KOBAYASHI, and S. MITSUHASHI (1971): Procc. of the 44th Annual Meeting of Japan Bacteriol. Ass., p. 49, Tokyo; Antimicrobial Agents and Chemotherapy. in press.

R FACTORS-DETERMINED CHANGES IN PERMEABILITY OF E. COLI TOWARDS RIFAMPICIN AND OTHER ANTIBIOTICS

S. RIVA, A. M. FIETTA AND L. G. SILVESTRI

Laboratori di Microbiologia — Gruppo Lepetit — Milano.

and E. ROMERO

Istituto di Microbiologia — Univestita di Pavia — Pavia, Italy.

Transmissible extrachromosomal elements in the *Enterobacteriaceae* can exhibit a number of properties like: fertility (Novick, 1969), autonomous replication (Jacob, Brenner, Cuzin, 1963), restriction of certain bacteriophages (Curtiss, 1969), the synthesis of sexpili (Brinton, Gemski, Carnahan, 1964) and in addition they can carry genes determining antibiotic resistance (Watanabe, 1963).

We report here of a new property associated with some R-factors: *E. coli* cells harbouring R-factors exhibit an increased sensitivity towards rifampicin and towards some other antibiotics. We have evidence indicating that this effect is due to a surface alteration that renders the cell envelope more permeable to rifampicin and to other drugs. (Babinet, Condamine, 1968; Tocchini-Valentini, Marino, Colvill, 1968; Rebussay, Zillig, 1969).

Rifampicin has a bactericidal effect by acting on DNA-dependent RNA polymerase and it has been shown that *rif-r* mutants contain an altered RNA polymerase exhibiting an increased resistance to the drug *in vitro* (Babinet, Condamine, 1968; Tocchini-Valentini, Marino, Colvill, 1968; Rebussay, Zillig, 1969). Wild type *E. coli* is,

Table 1

EFFECT OF SOME R-FACTORS ON RIFAMPICIN-RESISTANCE OF J 53 rif-r 14

Names and markers of the R factors		Number of J 53 *rif-r* 14 R$^+$ recombinants in 0.1 ml of mating mixture plated	
		without rifampicin	with rifampicin 100 μg/ml.
R 163	*drd* (*Tc Km col I fi$^-$*)	4.1×10^5	3
R 538—*1 drd*	(*Cm Sm Su fi$^+$*)	1.3×10^5	1.2×10^5
R 538—*2 drd*	(*Tc Sm fi$^-$*)	2.2×10^5	0
R 136	*drd* (*Tc Su fi$^+$*)	4.9×10^5	3.8×10^3
R 143	(*Tc Km col I fi$^-$*)	4.1×10^4	2.4×10^2
R 64	(*Tc Sm Su fi$^-$*)	8.9×10^4	9.0×10
R 192	(*Tc Cm Sm Su fi$^+$*)	1.1×10^4	8.5×10^3

A *rif-r* mutant of the J 53 strain (metF$^-$, proA$^-$, F$^-$) was isolated on 100 μg/ml rifampicin. This *rif-r* mutant has been crossed with seven strains of J 62 (proA$^-$, his$^-$, try$^-$, lac$^-$, F$^-$) each carrying a different R factor. R$^+$ recombinants have been isolated by plating the mating mixture on minimal agar containing proline, methionine and lactose, and the R$^+$ selecting drug, with and without 100 μg/ml. rifampicin. Mating mixture: 0.05 ml. of the donor + 0.5 ml. of the recipient strains (overnight cultures) diluted to 20 ml. and incubated overnight at 37°C with shaking.

however, poorly permeable to rifampicin, the *in vivo* minimal inhibitory concentration (MIC) being 10—50 times higher than the concentration necessary to inhibit the RNA polymerase *in vitro*. This is also true for most low level *rif-r* mutants.

When an R factor is introduced into a *rif-r* strain, the resulting *rif-r* (R+) recombinants behave in general as more sensitive to rifampicin. Table I shows such an effect with one *rif-r* mutant; it can be seen that with some R factors less than 1% of the cells are able to form colonies on rifampicin-supplemented agar, while with some others there is no detectable effect.

Although most of our experiments to understand the mechanism of this effect have been done with the R163 *drd* (Km, Tc, Col I, fi−) factor, the same property is shared by other R-factors both of the fi− and of the fi+ type.

Table 2

LIST OF STRAINS USED

Strains	Genetic Markers	*rif-r* Mutants
J 53	met F− pro A− nal−r F−	*rif-r* 14, 30, 44, 53, 46
J 62	pro A− his− try− lac− F−	
JC 1569	ppc− his− leu− arg G− met B− rec− lac− F−	*rif-r* 8, 25
AB 1206	thi− pro− his− str-r tsx− del. (ilv-arg H)/F'14	*rif-r* 4, 2
AJ 4	arg G− met B− lac Z−$_{Y14}$ recA$_1^-$ rif-0/KLF10 *rif-r*	

J 62 and J 53 from R. Meynell, JC 1569 and AB 1206 from T. Yura, AJ 4 from S. Austin and J. Scaife.

A certain number of *E. coli* spontaneous *rif-r* mutants (listed in Table II) have been crossed with a donor strain containing the R163 factor. R+ recombinants have been obtained by plating on selective plates and clones grown from individual colonies. The minimum inhibitory concentrations of rifampicin of *rif-r* strains and their R+ derivatives have been determined by colony counting on nutrient agar plates containing increasing concentrations of rifampicin. The results are shown in Fig. 1. The R-factor considerably lowers the level of resistance in several *rif-r* mutants; however, in some others with very high resistance no effect is detectable probably because of the high resistance of the enzyme and of the limited solubility of rifampicin (about 2000 μg/ml).

Fig. 2 shows that, also in R+ strains, the primary target of rifampicin is the RNA synthesis as indicated by the immediate block of uracil incorporation.

Although these observations bear some resemblance with the observation according to which mutations to rifampicin resistance are recessive to wild type alleles carried by F' (AUSTIN, SCAIFE, 1970; YURA, IGARASHI, MASUKATA, 1969), we have not been able

▶

Fig. 1 Inhibition of colony forming ability by rifampicin in R− and R+ *rif-r* mutants. Overnight cultures were plated on Penassay (Difco) plates containing the indicated concentrations of rifampicin and the colonies were counted after 48 hrs of incubation at 37°C. ●, R−; ○, R+; ⊕, *rif-r* × R+ *rif-r* × R+ : 0.1 ml of the appropriate dilutions of the mating mixture were plated on agar with rifampicin and the R+ selective drug (Kanamycin 200 μg/ml).
a) *E. coli* AJ 4 *rif-o/rif-r*, b) *E. coli* JC 1569 *rif:r* 8, c) *E. coli* JC1569 *rif-r* 25, d) *E. coli* J 53 *rif-r* 44 Some of the experimental points are not represented in the graphs.

344

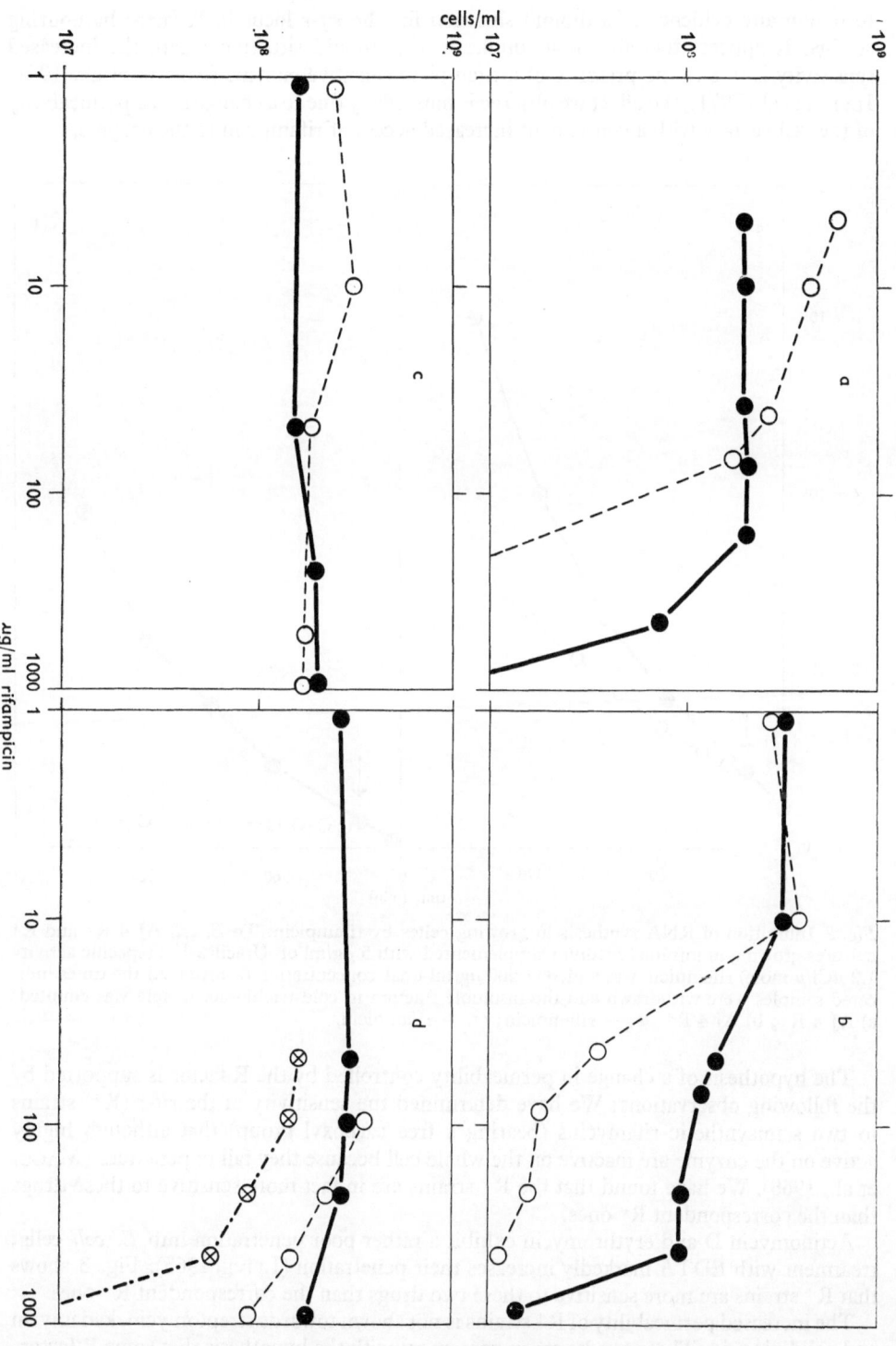

to obtain any evidence of a diploid situation for the *rif-r* locus in R-factor harbouring strains. It appears therefore that, unlike in the diploid situation where the increased sensitivity is due to the presence of a rifampicin sensitive enzyme (AUSTIN et al., 1971; ILYINA et al., 1971), the effect we observe is most likely due to a change in the permeability of the cell surface with a consequent increased access of rifampicin to the enzyme.

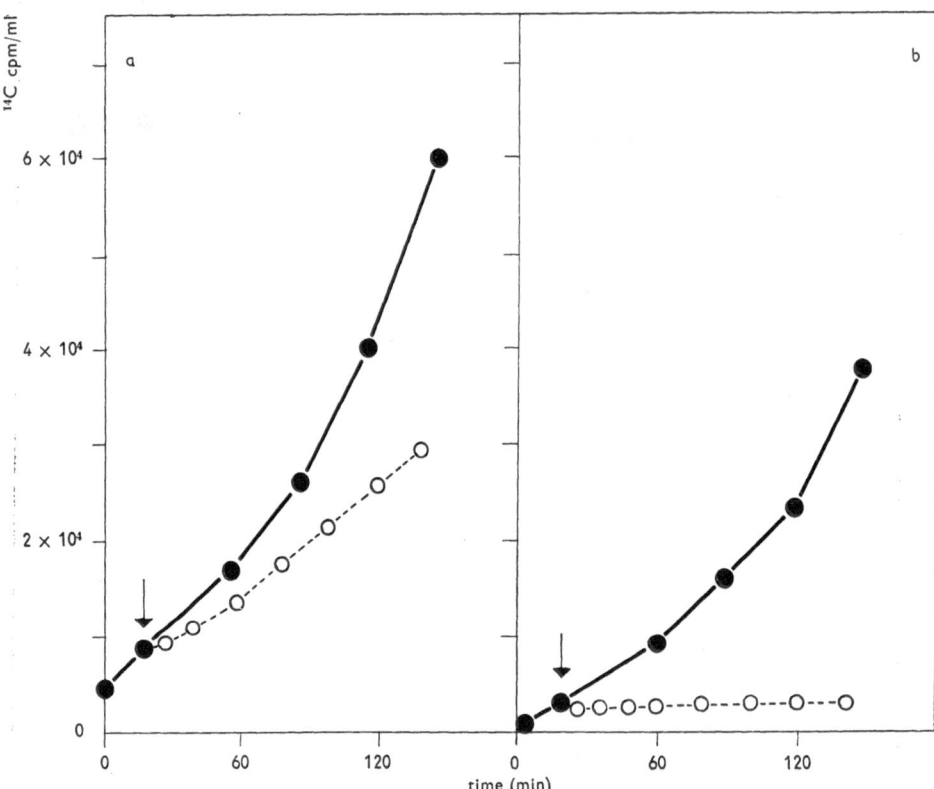

Fig. 2 Inhibition of RNA synthesis in growing celles by rifampicin. To *E. coli* AJ 4 R⁻ and R⁺ cultures growing in minimal medium supplemented with 5 μg/ml of Uracil-2-¹⁴C (specific activity 1.2 μCi/μ mole) rifampicin was added at 500 μg/ml final concentration (arrows). At the times indicated samples were withdrawn and the insoluble fraction in cold trichloracetic acid was counted: a) AJ 4 R⁻; b) AJ 4 R⁺. ●, − rifampicin; ○, + rifampicin.

The hypothesis of a change in permeability controlled by the R factor is supported by the following observations: We have determined the sensitivity of the *rif-r* (R⁺) strains to two semisynthetic rifamycins (bearing a free carboxyl group) that although highly active on the enzyme are inactive on the whole cell because they fail to penetrate (MAGGI et al., 1968). We have found that the R⁺ strains are in fact more sensitive to these drugs than the correspondent R⁻ ones.

Actinomycin D and erythromycin exhibit a rather poor penetration into *E. coli* cells; treatment with EDTA markedly increases their penetration (LEIVE, 1965). Fig. 3 shows that R⁺ strains are more sensitive to these two drugs than the correspondent R⁻ ones.

The increased permeability of R⁺ strains is not shown towards streptomycin, kanamycin and nalidixic acid. These results are in agreement with the hypothesis that some R factors

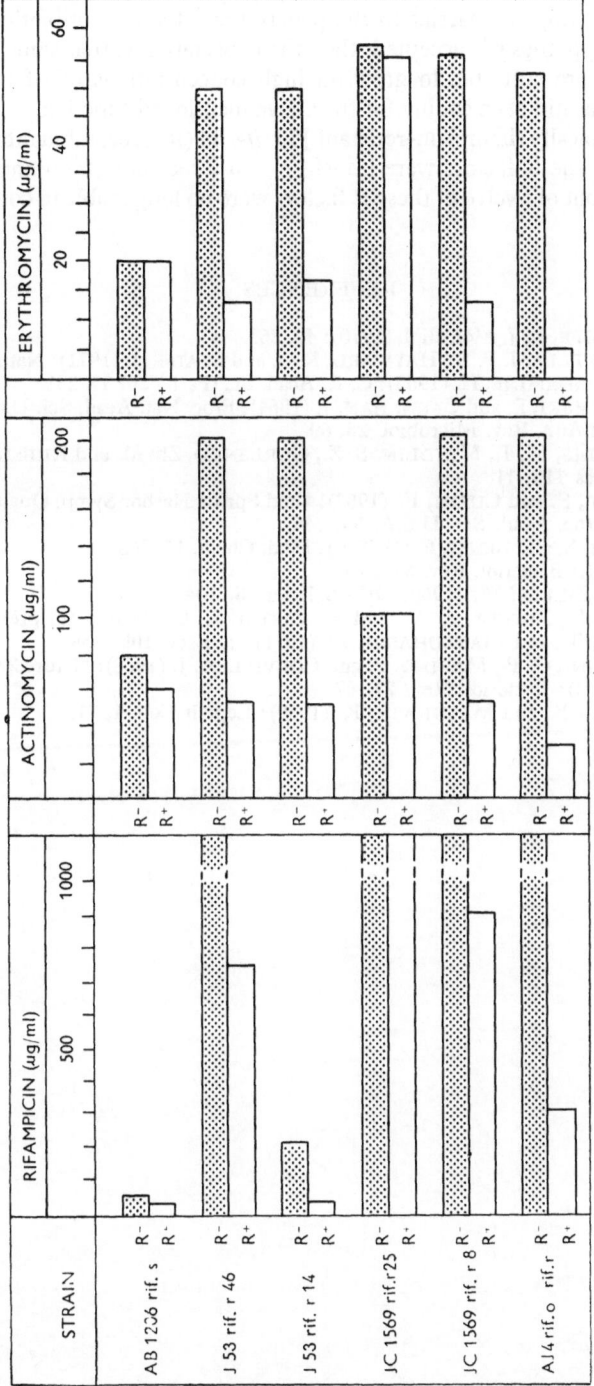

Fig. 3 Minimal inhibitory concentrations of rifampicin, actinomycin D and erythromycin in R⁻ and R⁺ *rif-r* mutants.

can code for functions that are able to alter the lipopolysaccharide backbone of the surface structure, thus lowering the barrier to the penetration of some antibiotics (TAMAKI et al., 1971). If this hypothesis is accepted, then the expectation is that some of the few R^+ recombinants that are still able to grow on high concentrations of rifampicin carry a mutation on the plasmid gene coding for the above mentioned function.

Twelve phenotypically rifampicin-resistant J53 *rif-r* 14 (R^+) recombinants were isolated. From these strains the R factors were transferred to a receptor strain and then back to J53 *rif-r* 14. Eight out of twelve of these R factors were no longer able to confer sensitivity to rifampicin.

REFERENCES

AUSTIN, S. and SCAIFE, J., J. Mol. Biol. (1970): **49**, 263.

AUSTIN, S., TITTAWELLA, I. P. B., HAYWARD, R. S. and SCAIFE, J. (1971): Nature **232**, 133.

BABINET, C. and CONDAMINE, H. (1968): C. R. Acad. Sci (Paris) **267** D, 231.

BRINTON, C. C., GEMSKI, P. and CARNAHAN, J. (1964): Proc. Nat. Acad. Sci. U.S.A. **52**, 776.

CURTISS, R. (1969): Ann. Rev. Microbiol. **23**, 69.

ILYINA, T. S., OVADIS, M. I., MINDLIN, S. Z., GORLENKO, Zh. M. and KHESIN, R. B. (1971): Mol. Gen. Genetics **110**, 118.

JACOB, F., BRENNER, S. and CUZIN, F., (1963): Cold Spring Harbor Symp. Quant. Biol. **28**, 329.

LEIVE, L. (1965): Proc. Acad. Sci. U.S.A. **53**, 745.

MAGGI, N., FÜRESZ, S. and SENSI, P. (1968): J. Med. Chem. **11**, 368.

NOVICK, R. P. (1969): Bacteriol. Rev. **33**, 210.

REBUSSAY, D. and ZILLIG, W. (1969): FEBS letters **5**, 104.

ROMERO, E., RIVA, S., FIETTA, A. M. and SILVESTRI, L. G., Nature (in press).

TAMAKI, S., SATO, T. and MATSUHASHI, M (1971): J. Bact. **105**, 868.

TOCHCINI-VALENTINI, G. P., MARINO, P. and COLVILL, A. J. (1968): Nature **220**, 275.

WATANABE, T. (1963): Bacteriol. Rev. **27**, 87.

YURA, T., IGARASHI, K. and MASUKATA, K. (1969): Lepetit Coll. **1**, 71.

GENE TRANSFER IN THE RHIZOBIUM CONJUGATION

W. HEUMANN

Institute of Microbiology — University of Erlangen, G. F. R.

The conjugation system I will discuss in this paper is not only characteristic for the genus *Rhizobium*. It applies to a taxonomically rather undefined group of bacteria which are all unified by the capacity to form starlike clusters by means of contractive fimbriae. Starforming bacteria are found in the *Rhizobiaceae* and *Pseudomonaceae* from soil and water. We tested for fertility several starforming bacteria of different origin. In almost all instances gene exchange has been found. I cannot assert that starformation is always connected with conjugation but apparently it improves the conditions for conjugation. For the fimbriae are species specific and thus elicit a very effective tool to select for compatible cells in a mixed soil population.

The strain which has been investigated in detail I have isolated 1962 from root nodules of *Lupinus luteus*, it is therefore called R. lupini. A collection of more than 700 mutants of this bacterium is available in my laboratory. Each mutant strain is characterized by one or more auxotrophic or resistant markers and by its pigmentation. The strain produces an yellow carotenoid pigment and stable pigmentation mutants are easely to produce by mutagenic treatment. These mutants make colonies of different shades of yellow, red and white. Pigment mutation is a very convenient marker for the quantitative evaluation of crossing experiments.

Early experiments which I don't want to present in detail have led to a construction of a provisional linkage map of eight auxotrophic markers. We took advantage of the pigmentation region as an easy recognizable nonselective marker. All carotenoid alleles are clustered in one chromosomal region called "car". Using parents of different color, the recombinant color class relation reveals the relative distances of the auxotrophic markers to car. The sequence of the auxotrophic markers has been defined by three- and four-point crosses. These experiments revealed the strange situation that all markers are located in one of two linkage groups with different recombination characteristics: Markers on one group are closely linked to car, they are called c (close) markers and the segment c region, markers of the other group are distantly linked to car, they are called d (distant) markers, and the segment d region. c × c crosses always exhibit recombinants with low frequency, the two parental color classes and sectored colonies, d × d crosses recombinants with high frequency (100 to 1000 times higher than c × d crosses, again the two parental color types and no sectored colonies. c × d crosses finally elicit recombinants with high frequency, with only the d parent pigmentation and no sectored colonies. Four point crosses indicate that the two regions are linked to each other to a circular structure. All new markers which had been mapped behave c or d, no intermediates are available.

The further analysis of the system was hampered by the fact that all cells are isosexual.

Differentiation into donor and recipient depends from its physiological conditions: log phase cells are donors, stationary cells are recipients. The explanation for the two regions came from one way transfer experiments. The donor fertility of cells can be eliminated. We used different procedures: SDS treatment, prolongated incubation under different conditions and so on. We don't understand the mechanism of the elimination process, but we obtained stable F⁻ clones from which we produced auxotrophic female parents by further mutagenesis.

The one way transfer experiments now possible indicated that the two chromosomal regions, defined above, are actually two chromosomal segments, whose transfer is regulated independently of each other. Accordingly four different fertility types can be defined:

Fc^+Fd^+ wild type donor
Fc^+Fd^- donor for the c region only
Fc^-Fd^+ donor for the d region only
Fc^-Fd^- recipient only

The c region transfer excludes the simultaneous d region transfer and vice versa, an unknown regulation takes care that the transfer frequency for the d region segment is 100 to 1000 times higher than for the c segment. Examples of the transfer ability of the four different fertility types are shown by the photographs of test crosses in fig. 1.

a) Demonstrates the infertility of the cross of Fc^-Fd^- strains. In b) and c) the transfer ability of Fc^+Fd^+ strains is demonstrated, whereas in d) and e) the c region only and in f) and g) the d region only are transferred. A comparison of the recombination frequency of the different crosses indicates that the yeild of recombinants is generally 100 to 1000 times higher at d region transfer than at c region transfer. The independent regulation of the transfer of those two regions, together with the different transfer frequency actually indicates the mutual transfer exclusion for the two regions. This is further proved by the observation that in crosses Fig. 1b) and c), in the lower two streaks, in which d region recombination is demonstrated by crosses, in which the donor is able to transfer both regions, only the recipient color class is found, yellow in b) and white in c). If the c region with its pigmentation alleles had been transferred simultaneously both color classes would appear.

In fig. 1 e) in the cross: $cys, car 1, Fc^+Fd^- \times ilv, car y, Fc^-Fd^-$ a small number of yellow recombinants is visible. This is unexpected since the donor transfers only its c region and ilv is a d marker, but the result is reproducible. This indicates, as I will explain later, that ilv is located proximal in the d region and that c transfer can extend into it.

What is the transfer mechanism for the two regions? One would propose to make interrupted mating experiments, according to Jacob and Wollman. But our bacteria resist to this procedure. The mating cells are very strong and irreversibly connected by fimbriae, shearing forces hardly separate the cells. The generation time of our cells is arround three hours, it is difficult to synchronize the entrance time. Finally we did not succeed to put more than two auxotrophic markers clear cut in one strain. Therefore we took advantage of our pigment factor to analyse point of origin and transfer direction of the c region.

As donor we used: pro, car 1, Fc⁺Fd⁻, which transfer its c region prototrophic into the recipient, since pro is a d marker. As recipients a collection of different car y, Fc⁻Fd⁻ mutants were used, which were known to map in the c region. The result is shown in Fig. 2.

The color class relations of each cross are represented in three columns: dark = yellow proportion, white = white proportion and striated = sectored proportion of prototrophic recombinants. We suppose that in each transfer the donor DNA molecule is interrupted by a time dependent event of increasing probability — may be by a single stranded break

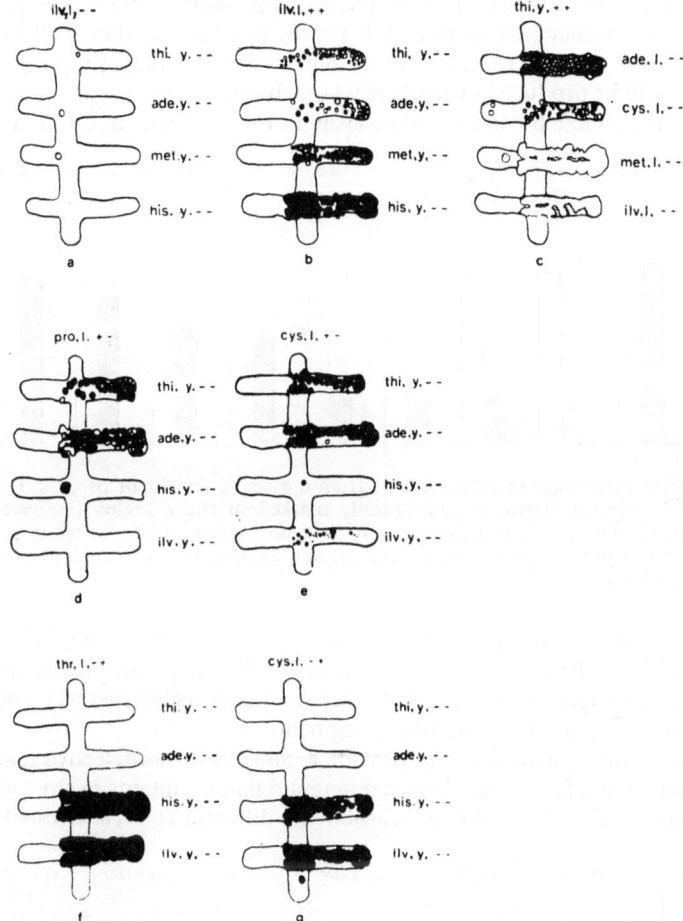

Fig. 1 Drawings of test crosses of the four different fertility types. Vertical streakes are the strains whose donor ability is tested. Always pairs of identical fertility type are used with different auxotrophic markers, one from the *c*, the other from the *d* region, e. g. *ilv* and *thi*, *pro* and *cys*, *thr* and *cys*. Horizontal streakes are standard Fc⁻Fd⁻ auxotrophic tester strains, the upper two always mapping in the *c* region, the lower two in the *d* region. Care has been taken that the two parents of each cross are differently pigmented, y = yellow and 1 = white respectively (white growth appears white, yellow growth black on the drawings). The appearance of recombinants on the right hand part of the crosses indicates *c* region transfer on the upper two streakes and *d* region transfer on the lower two streaks. Since all crosses are made with the same parental cell count the density of the recombinant growth allows a rough estimate of the transfer frequency. Abbreviations are used according to the proposal of Demerec *et al* (1966).

$$
\begin{array}{ll}
- \; - \; = \; \text{Fc}^-\text{Fd}^- & 1 = \text{car } 1 \\
+ \; + \; = \; \text{Fc}^+\text{Fd}^+ & y = \text{car } y \\
+ \; - \; = \; \text{Fc}^+\text{Fd}^- & \\
- \; + \; = \; \text{Fc}^-\text{Fd}^+ &
\end{array}
$$

during transfer replication. Each recipient strain produces recombinants with a fixed and reproducible proportion of the three color classes yellow, white and sectored. That reflects its position relative to the point of origin and to car, again under the supposition that the point of origin is fixed and the transfer is interrupted by a time depending event.

Proximal markers select for short donor pieces, distal markers for long segments. If the pigment region is somewhere located in between, proximal markers will inherit mainly the recipient color, markers close to car the donor color. The main proportion of sectored recombinants will be produced by markers whose distance to 0 is cut in halves by car. The proportion of the recipient color will raise again in recombinants of distal markers. The c

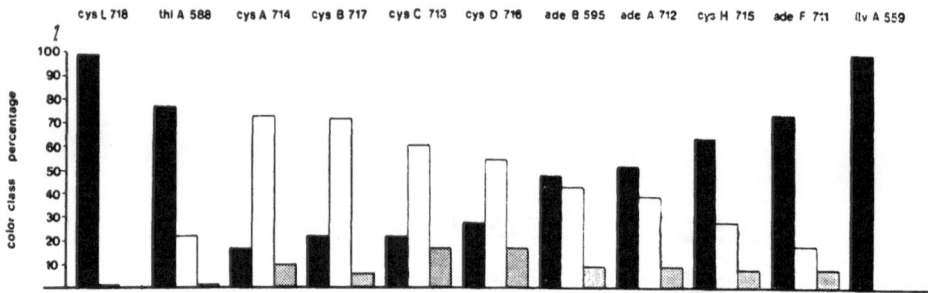

Fig. 2 Color class percentage of recombinants from crosses of the donor pro, car 1, Fc⁺Fd⁻ with yellow Fc⁻Fd⁻ recipient strains auxotrophically marked in the c region (indicated by marker and number in the figure). Dark columns = yellow proportion, white = white proportion and striated = sectored proportion of prototrophic recombinants. Abbreviations are used according to the proposal of Demerec et al. (1966).

region extends into the d region. As we will see, ilv A is a proximal d marker. It is recombined with low frequency by c region transfer. As I hope the picture shows that the color proportion analysis is a reliable procedure to map c region markers, and to indicate the transfer direction of this chromosomal segment.

Unfortunately the system does not provide a convenient nonselective marker like car for the d region. Therefore we used three different d donor mutants to cross with different recipient strains marked in the d region, again with different color, and tested the number

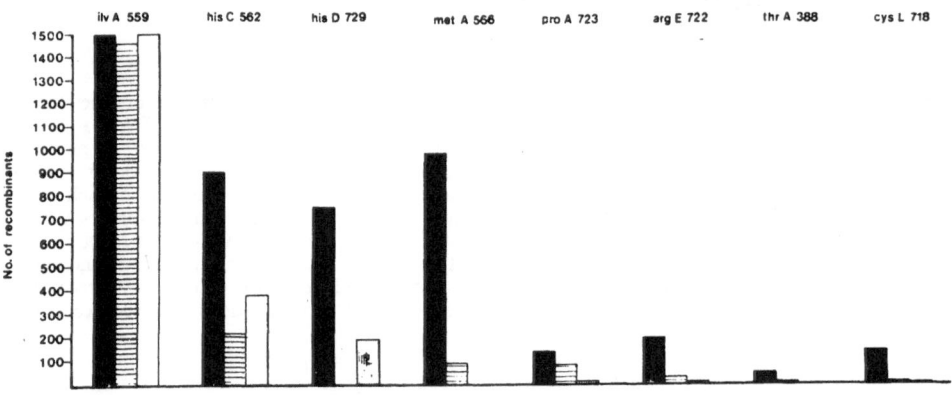

Fig. 3 Marker gradient from crosses of the donor strains
1—7, cys, car cr, Fc⁻Fd⁺ = dark columns
7—10, gab, car 1, Fc⁻Fd⁺ = horizontally hatched columns
17—1, cys, car p, Fc⁻Fd⁺ = vertically hatched columns
with Fc⁻Fd⁻ recipient strains of yellow or white pigmentation auxotrophically marked in the d region (indicated by marker and number in the figure). Abbreviations are used according to the proposal of Demerec et al. (1966.)
Strain 7—10, gab is a mutant of a R. lupini strain kindly provided by Dr. Magda Hotchkiss-Gabor.

of recombinants. If the probability for a donor segment to be transferred decreases with its length, the gradient of recombination frequency for the selected markers will reflect its distance gradient from 0.

Fig. 3 shows the result: The number of recombinants of the selected markers is represented in three differently hatched columns, one for each donor strain: dark for 1—7, cys, car, cr, Fc⁻Fd⁺, horizontal for 7—10, gab, car 1, Fc⁻Fd⁺ and vertical for 17—i, cys, car p, Fc⁻Fd⁺. The recombination gradient decreases for all combinations at the same schedule, allowing to read the marker sequence and the transfer direction. Again proximal c markers will be recombined at low frequency (1—718, cys L) indicating that d region transfer overlaps into the c region. It is worthwhile to note that different donors are differently sensitive to spontaneous break of the transferred segment. 1—7 is very effective until met, whereas 7—10 and 17—1 decrease already in his C to 1/5 th of the ilv A recombination frequency. This recombination gradient allows to define the transfer direction, but the exact marker localization can only be estimated.

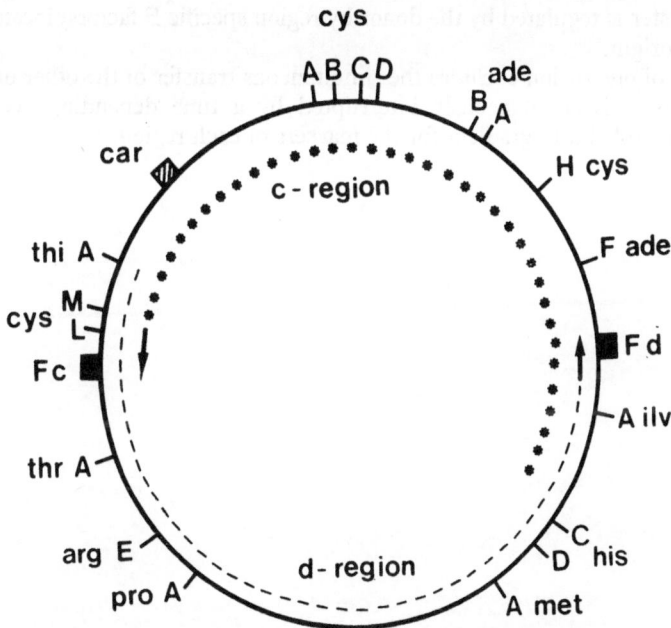

Fig. 4 Linkage map of R. lupini with the two transfer regions.

One of the main differences between enterobacteria conjugation and our system is that no fertility transfer occurs independently of the chromosome transfer. We tried therefore to map the localization of Fc and Fd by analysing its linkage to the already localized markers. To sum up the results of a long series of experiments, we found:

Fc⁺ progeny can be obtained by

        c-transfer, selection for proximal c markers
        d-transfer, selection for distal   d markers
                selection for proximal c markers

Fd+ progeny can be obtained by

> d-transfer, selection for proximal d markers
> c-transfer, selection for distal   c markers
> selection for proximal d markers.

This indicates that each F-factor is integrated on the proximal end of his own region and consequently being transferred as an early marker, probably as the first one. Fig. 4 shows the linkage map of *R. lupini* with the two transfer regions.

   Let me summarize the main characteristics of the conjugation of starforming bacteria, investigated so far:

1. Starformation is a system of species specific recognition and contact formation.
2. The conjugating cells are genetically isosexual, donor- and recipient-function during mating are determined phenotypically.
3. The chromosome is transferred in two different regions each being characterized by fixed point of origin, transfer direction and transfer frequency.
4. The transfer is regulated by the donor by region specific F factors, located close to the point of origin.
5. Transfer of one region excludes the simultaneous transfer of the other one.
6. The transfer is spontaneously interrupted by a time depending event exhibiting a transfer probability gradient for the markers of each region.

GENETIC MAPPING OF REGULATOR GENE OF PHAGE 16-3
OF RHIZOBIUM MELILOTI

L. OROSZ

Institute of Genetics, Biological Research Center, Hungarian Academy of Sciences,
Szeged, Hungary

The regulator gene (C) of 16-3 temperate phage of *Rhizobium melioti* is located on the end of chromosome (Fig. 1). The function of this regulator gene is necessary for the stability of lysogene system of Rh. meliloti and prophage 16-3 (Orosz and Sik 1970). In order to map this gene was used a three point crossing system. This system is based on that assumption that crossing a double mutant with a single one, the *wild type* recombinants were able to appeare only as a results of at least two crossingovers (Fig. 2).

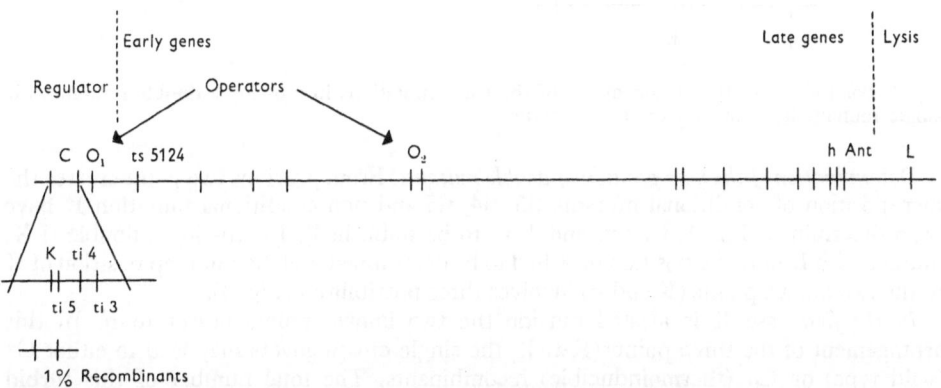

Fig. 1 Genetic map of phage 16−3 (from SIK and OROSZ, 1971., OROSZ et al. 1971). C, regulator gene., O, operator gene., ts, temperature sensitive mutation., ti, thermo inducible mutation., h, gene of tail fibers., Ant, altered antigen., L, gene of lysis.

Taking into account even the case of high negative interference the frequency of double crossingovers was much less than that of single crossingovers on the short segment of the chromosome.

The first task was to isolate double mutants and the second one to determine the map position of the two mutation of the double mutants.

Isolation of double mutants was carried out by using combination of conditional and nonconditional mutations. First temperature sensitive mutants in gene C (ti) were isolated. This so called thermoinducible (ti) mutants from turbid plaques at 28° and clear ones at 36°. The phenotype of the plaques shows that repressor is produced by ti mutants active at low temperature (lysogenisation) but not at upper temperature (no lysogenisation) (SUSSMAN, JACOB 1962, OROSZ and SIK 1970).

Into ti mutants another mutation was introduced by UV mutagenesis. This double mutants *have not repressor activity* even at 28° as it was shown by the "clear" phenotype of their plaques. (To confirm that the UV induced second mutations were located really in the gene C the complementation test was carried out between double mutants and single known mutants of gene C).

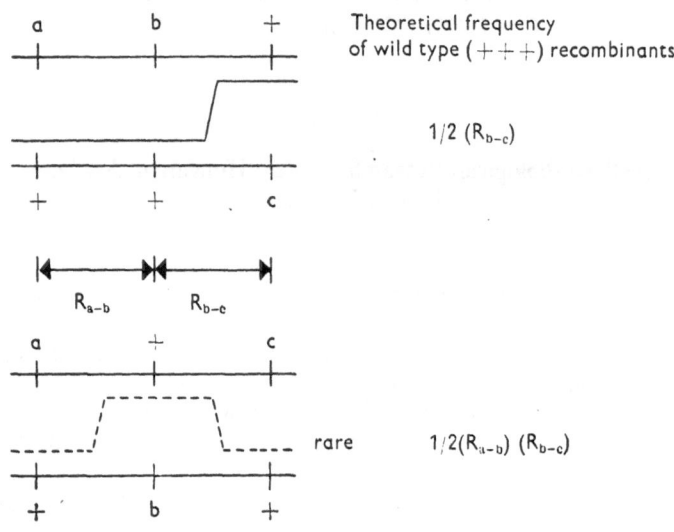

Fig. 2 Possibilities of the arrangements of the three mutations in crossing a double mutant with single mutant. R, frequency of recombination.

Determination of the map position of double mutants. From previous two point crosses the map position of conditional mutants ti3, ti4, ti5 and non conditional mutation K have been determined (Fig. 1, OROSZ and SIK, to be published). In crossing a double ti-X, mutant with K only the position of X had to be determined. Relation of map position of X to the two known points (K and ti) involves three possibilities (Fig. 3).

In the first case X is located outside the two known points nearer to *ti.* In this arrangement of the three points (K-ti-X) the single crossovers may lead to either C⁺ (wild type) or C$_{ti}$ (thermoinducible) recombinants. The total number of this turbid plaque forming recombinants at 28° corresponds to the map distance of the two non-conditional points, K and X, whereas at 36° only the C⁺ recombinants from turbid plaques and their frequency corresponds to the map distance of the two known points, K and *ti.*

In the second case X is located inside the two known points. In this arrangement (K-X-ti) the single crossovers result in C⁺ turbid plaque forming recombinants. That is why equal number of turbid plaque forming recombinants will appear both at 28° and at 36° corresponding with the map distance between K and X.

In the third case X is located outside the two known points but nearer to K. In this arrangement (X-K-ti) the double mutant "surrounds" the single mutant, therefore appearance of a C⁺ recombinant requires at least two crossovers. The frequency of C⁺ recombinants will be low, because single crossovers lead to C$_{ti}$ genotype. The frequency of C$_{ti}$ recombinants corresponds to the map distance of points K and X.

Fig. 4 shows the genetic map of gene C made by the method described above. Double mutants ti3U9, ti3U10, ti3U11, ti3U12, ti4U4, ti4U5, ti4U6, ti4U7, ti4U8, ti4Sp2, ti4Sp3, ti4Sp4, ti5U1, ti5U2, ti5U3, ti5U13, ti5U14 were crossed with single mutant K.

Fig. 5 shows the system of double mutants which can work more or less similarly to the system of deletion mutants of T4rII (BENZER 1955). (Example: let us suppose there was an *unknown single mutant* in gene C. After having crossed with the set of *known double mutants* wild type (C+) recombinants appeared in crossings with ti4U7 and ti4Sp2 but not

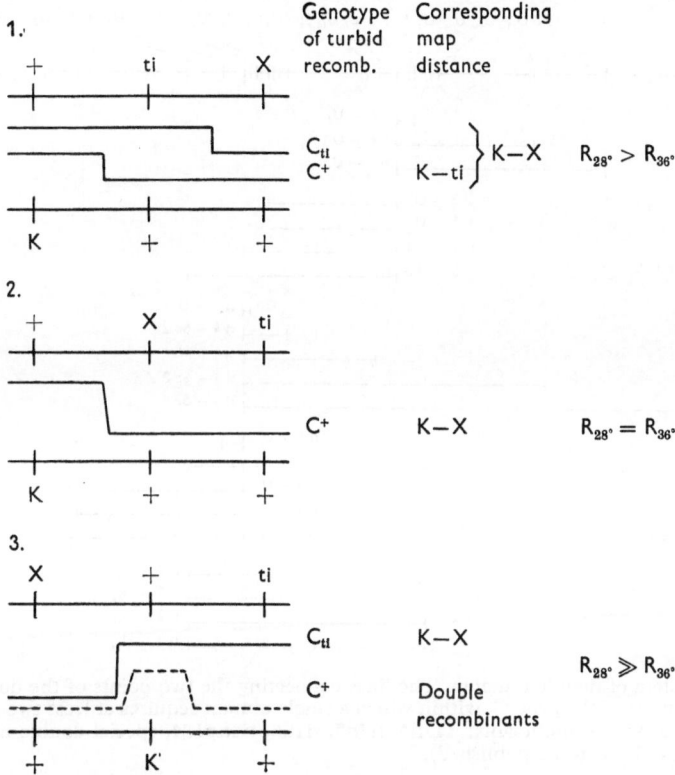

Fig. 3 The pattern of recombination in dependence of the position of the unknown point X. R, frequency of turbid recombinants. K and ti, known points.

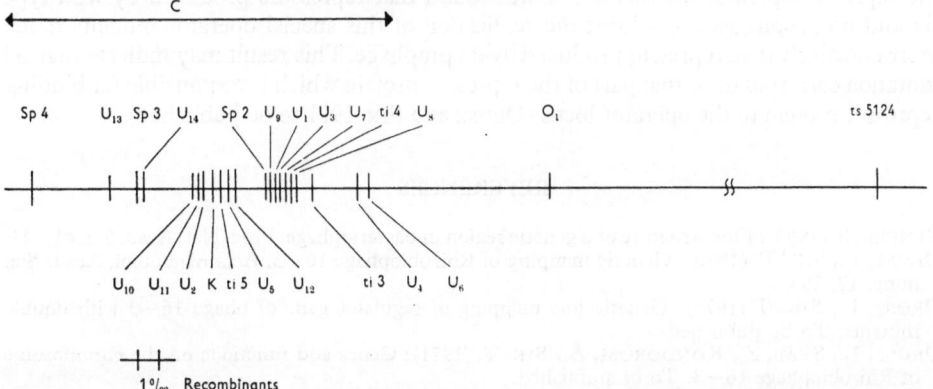

Fig. 4 The fine map of gene C. Crossing technique (OROSZ and SIK 1970). Sensitive plating of turbid recombinants (OROSZ and SIK 1971).

with ti4U5 and ti4Sp3. On the basis of this results the site of the unknown single mutation is probably between points Sp2 and U5, because single crossingovers may lead to wild type recombinants only if the unknown mutation is outside the two points of the double mutants.)

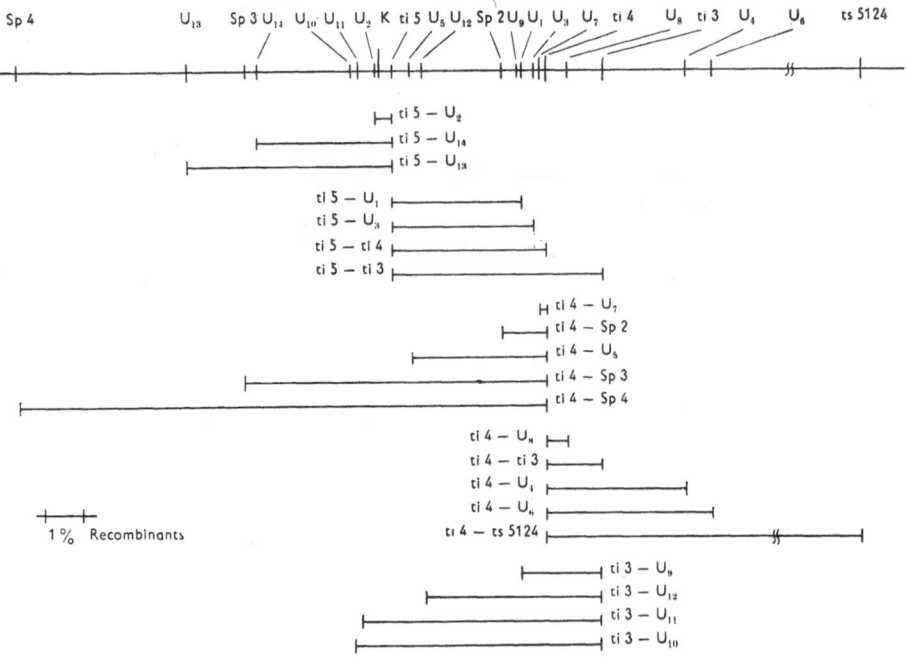

Fig. 5 The system of double mutants. The lines connecting the two points of the double mutants represent that parts of the gene C, within which a single mutant requires at least two crossingovers to produce wild type recombinants. Ti3ti4, ti3ti5, ti4ti5, ti4ts5124, special double mutants (from OROSZ and SIK, 1971, to be published).

The repressor function of wild type, ti3, ti4 and ti5 mutants was tested by superinfection of certain operator mutants in order to get indications of the effect of these mutations for the repressor-operator interaction. It was found that repressors produced by wild type ti4 and ti5 prophages can inhibit the replication of this special operator mutants much more effectively than repressor produced by ti3 prophage. This result may indicate that ti3 mutation corresponds to that part of the repressor protein which is responsible for binding repressor protein to the operator locus (OROSZ and SIK 1971 to be published).

REFERENCES

BENZER, S. (1955): Fine structure of a genetic region in bacteriophage. Proc. Nat. Acad. Sci. **41**, 344.

OROSZ, L., SIK, T. (1970): Genetic mapping of Rhizobiophage 16−3. Acta Microbiol. Acad. Sci. hung. **17**, 185.

OROSZ, L., SIK, T (1971): Genetic fine mapping of regulator gene of phage 16−3 with double mutants. To be published.

OROSZ, L., SVÁB, Z., KONDOROSI, Á., SIK, T. (1971): Genes and functions on the chromosome of Rhizobiophage 16−3. To be published.

SIK, T., OROSZ, L. (1971): Chemistry and genetics of Rhizobium phage 16−3. In press.

SUSSMAN, R., JACOB, F. (1962): Sur un systeme de repression thermosensible chez le bacteriophage d'Escherichia coli. Comptes Rendus **254**, 1516.

III.

RESISTANCE DETERMINANTS IN STAPHYLOCOCCUS AUREUS

Moderator:

SIDNEY COHEN (Chicago)

ON THE MECHANISM OF METHICILLIN RESISTANCE
IN STAPHYLOCOCCUS AUREUS

S. J. SELIGMAN

State University of New York, Downstate Medical Center, Brooklyn U.S.A.

Shortly after the introduction of methicillin, rare strains of *Staphylococcus aureus* were found resistant to this penicillinase-resistant penicillin (JEVONS, 1961). Similar strains were subsequently isolated from many parts of the world including Great Britain, Denmark, Poland, and India in situations unrelated to the use of methicillin or other antibiotics. In more recent years, methicillin-resistant staphylococci have become highly prevalent in some countries such as Denmark in which they accounted for 45% of staphylococci isolated from blood cultures (BÜLOW, 1971), but are still rarely isolated in other countries including the United States where antibiotic usage is also high. Accordingly other factors are probably also important in the dissemination of these strains.

The mechanism of methicillin resistance is not understood. Resistance does not depend upon penicillinase activity. Strains which have lost penicillinase activity may retain methicillin resistance (SELIGMAN , 1966a; DYKE, JEVONS and PARKER, 1966). Under usual test conditions, methicillin resistance is heterogeneous i. e. resistance is not uniform and a fraction of the population is highly resistant. Heterogeneity is a consequence of two different factors. The first factor is phenotypic variation in the expression of resistance and the second is mutants with large one step increases in resistance. Under certain conditions, namely with log phase cultures incubated at 33 C on hypertonic media, resistance can be increased to a uniformly high level and heterogeneity is abolished. Methicillin-resistant strains have increased resistance to all penicillins and cephalosporins (SELIGMAN and HEWITT, 1966).

A few strains of *S. aureus* have been isolated which do not have the above characteristics but are still slightly more resistant to methicillin than the typical sensitive strain. Such borderline strains do not produce highly-resistant first step mutants. They will be ignored in the subsequent discussion. *S. epidermidis* strains may have patterns of methicillin-resistance similar to coagulase-positive *S. aureus* but the resistance of Micrococci is considerably different (SELIGMAN, unpublished).

The chromosomal or extrachromosomal location of the genetic determinants oɪ restistance has been investigated. DORNBUSCH, HALLANDER and LOFQUIST (1969) found loss of methicillin resistance, of enterotoxin B and of beta hemolysin production following exposure to acridine dyes and demonstrated cotransduction of methicillin resistance and enterotoxin B production. Changes in resistance to mercury or cadmium and in production of penicillinase or beta hemolysin sometimes accompanied loss or gain of methicillin resistance. Their studies suggest that the genes for methicillin resistance and enterotoxin B production occur on a common plasmid, but the association with mercury resistance and penicillinase production is perplexing. Working with 5 methicillin-resistant isolates of phage types different from those studied by DORNBUSCH et al. (1969), I had found that, in 27 spontaneously-occurring penicillinase-negative variants selected for loss of penicillinase activity, mercury resistance was lost in all instances. Methicillin resistance remained, indicating that in the strains investigated, methicillin resistance is not on the penicillinase plasmid (SELIGMAN, 1966a). COHEN and SWEENEY (1970) were able to transduce methicillin resistance only to strains currently or previously containing a penicillinase plasmid. The kinetics of transduction following ultraviolet irradiation of phage and the failure of ethidium bromide to eliminate the marker suggested a chromosomal location. Methicillin resistance may be chromosomal in some strains but not in others and subtle interactions may involve the mercury-penicillinase plasmid and insertion of the genetic determinants of methicillin resistance.

MUTATIONS TO INCREASED RESISTANCE

A note by Knox on the production of highly resistant mutants accompanied the original description of methicillin-resistant staphylococci (KNOX, 1961; JEVONS, 1961). SUTHERLAND and ROLINSON (1965) found that strains isolated from diverse sources produced a minority population of highly resistant elements. Subsequent work confirmed that these elements were mutants (SELIGMAN, 1966b). During the course of serial sub-culture in liquid media, they may revert to the sensitivity of the parent strain. When subcultured on agar by serial passage of isolated colonies, they maintain increased resistance to methicillin. The mutant colonies are frequently smaller than the parents. Some mutants, particularly the more highly resistant ones, take several days to produce visible colonies even on antibiotic-free agar. Intracolonial sectors of more rapidly-growing organisms may appear. Sometimes they are revertants to the original sensitivity of the parent and sometimes not.

The very slow-growing mutants are what had been called G colonies or small colony variants in methicillin-sensitive staphylococci. The mutation rate to production of small colony variants is similar both in methicillin-sensitive and in resistant staphylococci. In methicillin-sensitive strains the increase in resistance is relatively small, an increase from 0.5 to 1.0 μg/ml, whereas in methicillin-resistant strains the increase is frequently from 4 μg/ml to 1000 μg/ml. A transductant to methicillin resistance, kindly supplied by Dr. SIDNEY COHEN (COHEN and SWEENEY, 1970), also produced mutants with large one step increases in methicillin resistance (SELIGMAN, unpublished).

Methicillin-resistant and sensitive staphylococci produce similar numbers of mutant colonies on exposure to various compounds including bacitracin, $BaCl_2$, crystal violet, vancomycin, cycloserine, chloramphenicol, and kanamycin. Hence the resistant strains do not possess a mutator gene which would permit them to develop rapid increase in resistance from multiple mutations.

Since both penicillin and $BaCl_2$ are known to be selective agents for the isolation of small colony variants from methicillin-sensitive staphylococci and since small colony variants may have increased resistance to methyl violet (SCHNITZER, CAMAGNI and BUCK, 1943), a number of compounds were investigated as selective agents in methicillin-resistant strains. The results indicated that mutants selected for increase in resistance to methicillin, $BaCl_2$, bacitracin, crystal violet or vancomycin may have increased resistance to other compounds (Table 1). Increases in resistance to the compounds other than methicillin were relatively small, but increases in resistance to methicillin in the methicillin-resistant strains exposed to other agents were relatively large.

These studies suggest that similar mutations result in a small increase in resistance in a methicillin-sensitive strain and a large increase in resistance in a methicillin-resistant

Table 1

SELECTION OF RESISTANT MUTANTS FROM METHICILLIN-SENSITIVE AND METHICILLIN-RESISTANT *STAPHYLOCOCCUS AUREUS*

Methicillin resistant	Selecting Agent	$\neq$ strains with increased resistance $\neq$ strains tested for resistance to given compound				
		methicillin	BaCl₂	Bacitracin	Crystal Violet	Vancomycin
13137 (penicillinase negative)	methicillin	4/4	1/1	3/4		
	BaCl₂	4/9	9/9			
	Bacitracin	9/9		8/9		
	Vancomycin	1/4				4/4
5982 (penicillinase positive)	methicillin	5/5	5/5	0/2		
	BaCl₂	3/4	7/7	0/1	1/1	
	Crystal violet	5/5		0/1	4/4	
Methicillin-sensitive 209 P	methicillin	6/6	2/2	1/6		
	BaCl₂	0/8	8/8			
	Vancomycin	0/1				1/1

strain. It is likely that several different mechanisms are involved. The mechanisms may include both changes in cell wall synthesis and in permeability. Accordingly, in experiments designed to investigate the mechanism of wild-type resistance, influence of the mutants should be scrupulously avoided (SELIGMAN, 1970).

PHENOTYPIC EXPRESSION OF RESISTANCE

CHABBERT, BAUDENS, ACAR and GERBAUD (1965) noted that differences in the phenotypic expression of resistance resulted in a heterogeneity of methicillin resistance. Some of the factors affecting phenotypic expression are growth phase of inoculum (SELIGMAN, 1970), salt concentration (BARBER, 1964), temperature (ANNEAR, 1968; SELIGMAN, 1968), magnesium (KAYSER, 1969) and other divalent cations (SELIGMAN, 1971a).

Logarithmically growing cultures are more uniformly resistant to benzylpenicillin than are stationary phase cultures (Fig. 1; SELIGMAN 1970). Log phase cultures had a gradual decline in viable count starting at .06 μg/ml. The decreased resistance of stationary phase cultures is probably related to a temperature-sensitive autolytic system (*vide infra*). Increase in phenotypic expression of resistance can be obtained by decreasing incubation temperature from 37' C to 33' C (Fig. 2; SELIGMAN, 1970). The 4 degree reduction in temperature resulted in a 32 fold increase in resistance to benzylpenicillin.

In these studies with a penicillinase-negative variant of 13137, the temperature effect on resistance to methicillin per se was modest. PARKER and HEWITT,[*] (1970), however, working with a penicillinase-producing strain, found a 16 fold increase in resistance to methicillin with decrease in temperature from 37' C to 30' C. They also found additional increase in resistance with reduction in temperature to 25' C and in further confirmation of Annear's findings (ANNEAR, 1968) they reported decrease in resistance at 43' C. At the higher temperature, resistance is very close to that for a sensitive strain.

Five % NaCl increases resistance to benzylpenicillin and to methicillin. The combination of salt and temperature results in additional phenotypic increase in resistance. Whether the salt and temperature effects have the same underlying mechanism

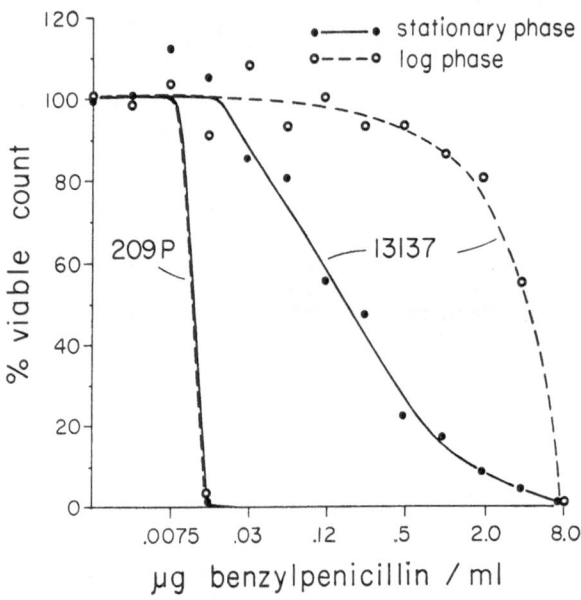

Fig. 1 Growth phase of inoculum and the percentage of colony-forming units produced on penicillin agar. The methicillin-resistant 13137 (penicillinase-negative variant) is compared with the methicillin -susceptible 209 P. Incubation was at 33° C (Antimicrobial Agents and Chemotherapy—1969, 90, 1970).

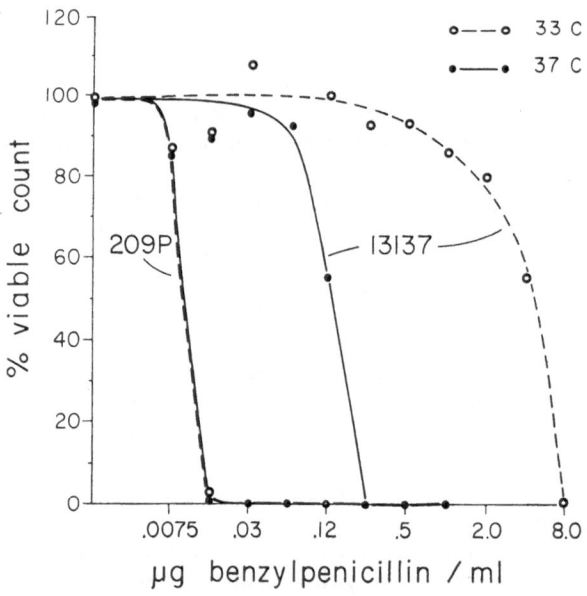

Fig. 2 Incubation temperature and growth on penicillin agar. Inocula were log phase cultures (Antimicrobial Agents and Chemotherapy—1969, 90, 1970).

is not known. BARBER (1964) suspected that salt exerted an osmotic protective effect and observed swollen coccal forms at near toxic concentrations of methicillin on hypertonic media. Methicillin-sensitive staphylococci do not have a large increase in resistance when grown on hypertonic media. Both sensitive and resistant strains, however, produce L form colonies on hypertonic media. Production of these forms should not be confused with increased resistance of cell-wall containing bacteria (SELIGMAN, 1966b).

Salt and temperature affect factors crucial to methicillin resistance. In a search for additional factors, I have been using inocula of approximately 50 colony-forming units of log phase cultures. Resistance to vancomycin and cycloserine was not affected by salt or temperature confirming that resistance to these compounds, which act on earlier stages of cell wall synthesis, is distinct from the mechanism of methicillin resistance.

Table 2

INTRINSIC RESISTANCE CONCENTRATIONS* (μg/ml) OF *STAPHYLOCOCCUS AUREUS* TO BENZYLPENICILLIN AT DIFFERENT pH AND TEMPERATURE

	Temperature	pH		
		6.0	7.0	8.0
Methicillin resistant 13137 (penicillinase-negative)	37	.06	.125	.125
	30	4	8	8
Methicillin sensitive 209 P	37	.004	.008	.015
	30	.008	.008	.015

* Highest concentration of penicillin permitting growth of 10% or more of 4 hour culture inoculated onto Trypticase Soy Agar and incubated for 1 day.

Resistance was not appreciably changed by varying pH from 6.0 to 8.0 (Table 2). SABATH and WALLACE (1971) had reported that at pH 5.2, resistance was decreased; however the methods used do not permit separation of wild-type resistance from that attributable to first step mutants.

KAYSER (1969) found that 0.1 magnesium sulphate decreased methicillin resistance. I have confirmed his results and extended them to magnesium chloride; however the

Table 3

INTRINSIC RESISTANT CONCENTRATION* OF *STAPHYLOCOCCUS AUREUS* TO METHICILLIN, MAGNESIUM, AND CALCIUM

	Methicillin Resistant		Methicillin Sensitive
	Villaluz (Donor)	451−2 (Transductant)	8325 ($\alpha\omega$) (Recipient)
Mg++ (M)	.10	.24	.24
Ca++ (M)	.60	.60	.60
Methicillin (μg/ml)	128	≥512	1
+ .08 M Mg++	0.5	≥512	0.5
+ .16 M Mg++	−	1	0.5
+ .16 M Ca++	2	2	1

* Highest concentration of methicillin or divalent cation permitting growth of 10% or more of 4 hour culture inoculated onto 5% NaCl Trypticase Soy Agar and incubated for 1 day at 30° C.

concentration of magnesium ions necessary to inhibit methicillin resistance is related to the concentration inhibitory without antibiotic (Table 3). The depicted studies involved a methicillin-resistant transductant 451-2 (kindly supplied by Dr. SIDNEY COHEN), the methicillin-resistant donor strain Villaluz, and the methicillin-sensitive recipient 8325 ($\alpha\omega$). All 3 strains are penicillinase-positive. Under the given test conditions using 5% NaCl agar and an incubation temperature of 30' C, 0.1 M Mg^{++} was the highest concentration which permitted growth of the methicillin-resistant Villaluz. A slightly lower concentration, 0.08 M was required to decrease resistance to methicillin. In contrast, the methicillin-resistant transductant was able to grow on .24 M Mg^{++}. The intrinsic resistance concentration to methicillin was not decreased by 0.08 M Mg^{++} but was markedly decreased from $\geq$ 512 μg to 1 μg by 0.16 M Mg^{++}. With calcium, both the methicillin-resistant and -sensitive strains grew on agar containing 0.6 M Ca^{++}. The other divalent cations tested, Mn^{++} and Ba^{++}, were inhibitory at much lower concentrations. However, by using near toxic concentrations, methicillin resistance could be decreased. These studies indicate that divalent cations reverse the increased methicillin resistance associated with tonicity and temperature. Whether this reversal is associated with a specific effect upon resistance or merely with increased permeability to divalent cations in methicillin-treated cells is uncertain. Preliminary studies with lysozyme and with kanamycin did not indicate increased permeability in penicillin-treated methicillin-resistant cells.

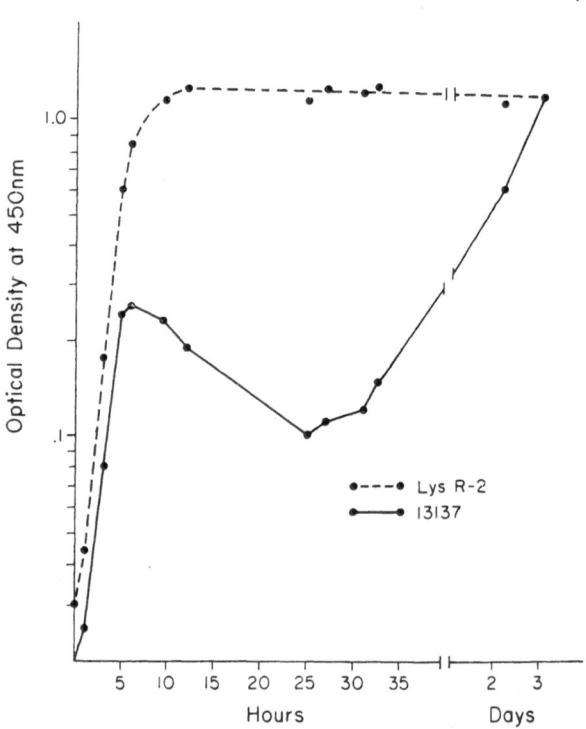

Fig. 3 Growth of 13137 and lys R-2, an autolysis-defective mutant at 33° C in a shaking water bath. (Antimicrobial Agents and Chemotherapy—1970, 218, 1971.)

AUTOLYTIC ACTIVITY AND METHICILLIN RESISTANCE

Many strains of methicillin-resistant *S. aureus* have autolytic activity manifested as decrease in optical density after overnight incubation with shaking at 33' C but not at 37' C (Fig. 3; SELIGMAN, 1971b). Some undetermined property of growth medium influences lysis since net lysis is observed with some batches of Trypticase Soy Broth (Baltimore Biological Laboratories) but not with others. The temperature-associated autolytic activity is not intimately associated with resistance. One of ten methicillin-sensitive isolates tested had similar activity. Furthermore, mutants of the methicillin-resistant strain with defect in temperature-sensitive autolytic activity are still methicillin-resistant.

SABATH, LEAF, GERSTEIN and FINLAND (1970a, b) found that strains cloned in the presence of cloxacillin which they called MR (for methicillin-resistant) had increased proportion of cells able to grow on antibiotic agar in comparison with the original MS strains. In the presence of lysostaphin, whole cells of MS lysed more rapidly than those of MR strains. They concluded that methicillin-resistant staphylococci had altered cell walls to account for the reduced rate of lysostaphin-associated lysis. In the terminology used in the present report, their MS strains correspond not only to methicillin-sensitive strains but also to wild-type methicillin-resistant strains and the MR strains correspond to the more resistant mutants. Although I have not had the opportunity to study their strains, it is possible that the MR strains in addition to being mutants with increased methicillin resistance are also autolysis deficient. The lessened rate of lysostaphin-associated lysis could be secondary to decreased autolytic activity. In a subsequent report, SABATH and WALLACE (1971) found that lysostaphin-treated cell walls (in contrast with whole cells) of MS and MR strains lysed at the same rate.

ADDITIONAL ASPECTS OF METHICILLIN RESISTANCE

Naturally-occurring methicillin-resistant *S. aureus* are found in a restricted number of phage types (PARKER and HEWITT, 1970; JESSON, ROSENDAL, BÜLOW, FABER and ERIKSEN, 1969) and are resistant to multiple unrelated antibiotics especially to streptomycin and to tetracycline. Penicillinase activity, lipase negativity (JESSON et al, 1969), temperature-sensitive autolytic activity (SELIGMAN, 1971b) and enterotoxin B production (HALLANDER and LOWELL, 1971) are other properties frequently found in methicillin-resistant strains. As demonstrated by the absence of these characteristics in some naturally-occuring strains, in methicillin-resistant transductants or in defective mutants, none are inherently connected with the mechanism of methicillin resistance but may be related to the ecological role of methicillin-resistant strains.

Binding of radioactive penicillin to methicillin-resistant staphylococci has been done in a number of laboratories but thus far few reports have been published. Preliminary results in this laboratory suggest similar degrees of binding to whole cells both in sensitive and in resistant strains at concentrations ranging from .0083 to 83 $\mu g/ml$. Binding is complete in less than 10 minutes at 0' C or at 37' C. KAYSER, BENNER, TROY and HOEPRICH (1971), however, have reported decreased binding by methicillin-resistant cells which may be significant.

DYKE (1969) and SABATH et al (1970b) found that the amino acid constituents of isolated cell walls were the same both in resistant and in sensitive strains; however the isolation of monomeric units of peptidoglycan (murein) from methicillin-resistant strains have not yet been reported.

367

SUMMARY

The mechanism of methicillin-resistance in *Staphylococcus aureus* remains an intriguing problem. The genetic determinants of resistance are transducible and presumably consist of a single gene or a cluster of closely-linked genes. Transductants possess resistance properties characteristic of the naturally-occurring strains, namely marked influence of phenotypic manipulation upon the expression of resistance and the ability to mutate in one step to considerable increases in resistance. Phenotypic expression of resistance is increased at temperatures below $37°$ C or by growth on hypertonic media. Expression is decreased by growth at higher temperatures or in the presence of near toxic concentrations of divalent cations. A variety of compounds select for mutants with increased resistance to methicillin both in methicillin-sensitive and in -resistant staphylococci. In the strains initially sensitive, the increase in resistance is relatively small (2 fold), whereas in the strains initially resistant the increase in resistance is relatively large (250 fold) suggesting that the effect of the same mutation is greatly enhanced by the previous level of resistance.

Penicillinase activity, penicillin-binding, rate of lysostaphin-induced lysis, temperature-sensitive autolysis, mutability or amino acid composition of the cell wall do not explain methicillin resistance.

Factors affecting phenotypic expression of resistance are probably the best available clues to understanding the mechanism of resistance.

Acknowledgment

These studies were supported by U. S. Public Health Service Grant Al-01074 from the National Institute of Allergy and Infectious Diseases. The technical assistance of Claire Lipp is gratefully acknowledged.

REFERENCES

ANNEAR, D. I. (1968): Effect of temperature on resistance of Staphylococcus aureus to methicillin and some other antibiotics. Medical Journal of Australia. 1, 444.

BARBER, M. (1964): Naturally occurring methicillin-resistant staphylococci. Journal of General Microbiology. 35, 183.

BÜLOW, P. (1971): Staphylococci in Danish hospitals during the last decade: Factors influencing some properties of predominant epidemic strains. Annals of the New York Academy of Sciences. 182, 21.

CHABBERT, Y. A., BAUDENS, J. G., ACAR, J. F. and GERBAUD, G. R. (1965): La resistance naturelle des staphylocoques a la methicilline et l'oxacilline. Revue d'Etudes Clinical Biologique. 10, 495.

COHEN, S. and SWEENEY, H. M. (1970): Transduction of methicillin resistance in Staphylococcus aureus dependent on an unusual specificity of the recipient strain. Journal of Bacteriology. 104, 1158.

DORNBUSCH, K., HALLANDER, H. O. and LOFQUIST, F. (1969): Extrachromosomal control of methicillin resistance and toxin production in Staphylococcus aureus. Journal of Bacteriology. 98, 351.

DYKE, K. G. H. (1969): Penicillinase production and intrinsic resistance to penicillins in methicillin-resistant cultures of Staphylococcus aureus. Journal of Medical Microbiology 2, 261.

DYKE, K. G. H., JEVONS, M. P. and PARKER, M. T. (1966): Penicillinase production and intrinsic resistance to penicillins in Staphylococcus aureus. Lancet 1, 835.

HALLANDER, H. O. and LAURELL, G. (1971): Epidemiological and clinical aspects of methicillin resistance and enteroxin production in Staphylococcus aureus. Annals of the New York Academy of Sciences 182, 98.

JESSEN, O., ROSENDAL, K., BÜLOW, P., FABER, V. and ERIKSEN, K. R. (1969): Changing staphylococci and staphylococcal infections. New England Journal of Medicine. 281, 627.

JEVONS, M. P. (1961): „Celbenin"-resistant staphylococci. British Medical Journal, 1, 124.

KAYSER, F.-H. (1969): Der Einflus des Nahrmediums auf die methicillin resistenz pathogener staphylokokken. Zeitschrift für Medizinische Mikrobiologie und Immunologie. **154**, 287.

KAYSER, F. H., BENNER, E. J., TROY, R. and HOEPRICH, P. D. (1971): Mode of resistance against β-lactam antibiotics in staphylococci. Annals of the New York Academy of Sciences **182**, 106.

KNOX, R. (1961): „Celbenin"-resistant staphylococci. British Medical Journal. **1**, 126.

PARKER, M. T. and HEWITT, J. H. (1970): Methicillin resistance in Staphylococcus aureus. Lancet. **1**, 800.

SABATH, L. D., LEAF, C. D., GERSTEIN, D. A. and FINLAND, M. (1970a): Cell walls of methicillin-resistant Staphylococcus aureus. Antimicrobial Agents and Chemotherapy—1969, 73.

SABATH, L. D., LEAF, C. D., GERSTEIN, D. A. and FINLAND, M. (1970b): Altered cell walls of Staphylococcus aureus resistant to methicillin. Nature. (London) **225**, 1074.

SABATH, L. D. and WALLACE, S. J. (1971): Factors influencing methicillin resistance in Staphylococci. Annals of the New York Academy of Sciences **182**, 258.

SCHNITZER, R. J., CAMAGNI, L. J. and BUCK, M. (1943): Resistance of small colony variants (G-forms) of a Staphylococcus towards the bacteriostatic activity of penicillin. Proceedings of the Society for Experimental Biology and Medicine. **53**, 75.

SELIGMAN, S. J. (1966a): Penicillinase-negative variants of methicillin-resistant Staphylococcus aureus. Nature (London). **209**, 994.

SELIGMAN, S. J. (1966b): Methicillin-resistant staphylococci: genetics of the minority population. Journal of General Microbiology. **42**, 315.

SELIGMAN, S. J. (1968): Phenotypic variability in penicillin resistance of hetero-resistant staphylococci. Clinical Research. **16**, 157.

SELIGMAN, S. J. (1970): Phenotypic variability in penicillin-resistance in a methicillin-resistant strain of Staphylococcus aureus. Antimicrobial Agents and Chemotherapy—1969, 90.

SELIGMAN, S. J. (1971a): Divalent cation antagonism of methicillin resistance in Staphylococcus aureus. Bacteriological Proceedings, 65.

SELIGMAN, S. J. (1971b): Autolytic activity in methicillin-resistant Staphylococcus aureus. Antimicrobial Agents and Chemotherapy—1970. 218.

SELIGMAN, S. J. and HEWITT, W. L. (1966): Resistance to penicillins and cephalosporins. Antimicrobial Agents and Chemotherapy—1965, 387.

SUTHERLAND, R. and ROLINSON, G. N. (1964): Characteristics of methicillinresistant staphylococci. Journal of Bacteriology, **87**, 887.

EXTRACHROMOSOMAL AND CHROMOSOMAL DRUG RESISTANCE IN METHICILLIN RESISTANT STAPHYLOCOCCUS AUREUS

F. H. KAYSER, M. FELIX and J. WÜST

Institute of Medical Microbiology, University of Zuerich, Switzerland

INTRODUCTION

In the last decade it has become more and more evident, that bacteria may possess besides the chromosome additional linkage groups of genes, which are referred to as extrachromosomal genetic elements. These hereditary units are structurally and functionally analogous to the chromosome, but can be characterized as extrachromosomal because of their nonessentiality and their small size (for review see NOVICK, 1969).

Extrachromosomal elements often carry determinants of resistance against chemotherapeutics. Such „resistance plasmids" mainly have been found among the *Enterobacteriaceae* and the staphylococci. Multiple drug resistance in these bacteria, which today comprise one of the main problems in clinical microbiology, is due to a great extent to extrachromosomally located genetic markers.

In *Staphylococcus* the determinants for production and regulation of the enzyme penicillinase have been found to be part of the penicillinase plasmid (NOVICK, 1963). In some strains the determinants of resistance against tetracycline (MAY, HOUGHTON and PERRET, 1964), chloramphenicol (CHABBERT, BAUDENS and GERBAUD, 1964), erythromycin (HASHIMOTO, KONO and MITSUHASHI, 1964), probably also against streptomycin (MORIMURA, WATANABE, MORI and MITSUHASHI. 1970), neomycin (CHABBERT et al., 1964), fusidic acid (EVANS and WATERWORTH, 1966), and bacitracin (BÜLOW, 1971) may be located extrachromosomally.

In this paper results about the genetics of drug resistance in methicillin resistant *S. aureus* are reported. Methicillin resistant (MR) staphylococci become more and more a problem in the hospital. 10—25 % of hospital acquired, staphylococcal infections in the Zuerich area now are caused by such strains (KAYSER and MAK, 1971). Our results indicate, that despite a variety of resistance patterns and different phage types among these bacteria, methicillin resistant staphylococci have arisen by the selection of only a few organisms, which presumably existed prior to the introduction of penicillin into therapy.

RECOGNITION OF CHROMOSOMAL AND EXTRACHROMOSOMAL RESISTANCE

The advanced state of genetic analysis in the *Enterobacteriaceae* makes it easy to determine, whether a genetic trait is part of the chromosome or located extrachromosomally. Consistent linkage to known chromosomal loci allows the conclusion, that a determinant is linked to the chromosome, whereas the absence of such linkage points to the opposite.

In addition, many species of the *Enterobacteriaceae* are able to participate in mating and to transfer plasmids, containing mostly several different markers, with high frequency from cell to cell.

Staphylococci are not well examined genetically and mating does not occurr. Therefore it is often difficult in these bacteria to establish chromosomal or extrachromosomal inheritance. NOVICK (1969) has outlined criteria for confirming plasmid or chromosomal linkage of genes. We employed some of these criteria in methicillin resistant wild strains in order to examine the genetics of drug resistance in these organisms.

Plasmid loss and „curing". In probable all bacterial strains carrying plasmids, spontaneous loss of extrachromosomal elements can occurr as a result of errors in plasmid replication or segregation. The frequency of these events can be increased by certain chemical and physical agents. (HIROTA, (1960); BAUANCHAUD, SCAVIZZI and CHABBERT (1969); WILLETS (1967); TOMOEDA, INUZUKA, KUBO and NAKAMURA (1968); JOHNSTON and RICHMOND (1970); MAY et al. (1964)). Results about spontaneous loss and curing are summarized in table 1 and 2.

Table 1

SPONTANEOUS LOSS AND ELIMINATION OF RESISTANCE MARKERS IN METHICILLIN-RESISTANT *S. AUREUS*, STRAIN E142

Treatment	Frequency of loss (%/18^h culture)					
	pen		chl		neo	
—	0.11	(A)	0.05—0.07	(A)	0.7— 2.1	(A)
acridines	0.03	(B)	0.27	(B)	5.9—98.4	(B)
ethidium bromide	10.8—55.8	(C)	0.08	(C)	1.9— 2.1	(C)
growth at 43.5°C	0.06	(D)	0.05	(D)	1.5— 2.1	(D)
storage (20 days; 20°C)	1.4—3.8	(E)	0.3—0.6	(E)	18.3—37.5	(E)

pen	A versus C: $\chi^2 = 370.1$;	$P < 0.001$
	A versus E: $\chi^2 = 40.5$;	$P < 0.001$
chl	A versus B: $\chi^2 = 4.4$;	$P = 0.05$
	A versus E: $\chi^2 = 8.5$;	$P = 0.01$
neo	A versus B: $\chi^2 = 17.1$;	$P < 0.001$
	A versus E: $\chi^2 = 79.1$;	$P < 0.001$

The determinants for penicillinase production, chloramphenicol and neomycin resistance are probable candidates for extrachromosomal location, provided, that no other genetic variations, i. e. point mutations have occurred. Such variations in general can be ruled out by the irreversibility of the event. In case of the penicillinase trait and the marker for chloramphenicol resistance, no revertants could be observed among 5×10^9 cells. However neomycin resistant cells were found at a frequency of about $10^4 / 5 \times 10^9$ bacteria. Because the rate of occurrence of these cells in a growing culture of E142neo$^-$ (4.8×10^{-7}/cell/generation) differed from the probability of loss of the neo marker in E142 (1.8×10^{-4}/cell/generation), it was concluded, that two different loci were involved.

The penicillinase trait could best be eliminated by ethidium bromide, whereas the acridine dyes as classical eliminating agents did not have any effect. Yet acridines apparently increased the occurrence of neomycin and chloramphenicol susceptible variants. A careful analysis of this effect however demonstrated that in both cases this was merely selective.

Table 2

STABILITY OF RESISTANCE MARKERS IN METHICILLIN RESISTANT *S. AUREUS*,
STRAIN E 142 AND E 420

Treatment	Frequency of loss (%/18ʰ culture)			
	meth*	ero	str	tet
—			<0.01	
acridines			<0.01	
ethidium bromide			<0.005	
rifamycin			<0.02	
sodium dodecylsulfate			<0.02	
UV irradiation			<0.02	
growth at 43.5°C			<0.005	
storage (20 days; 20°C)			<0.005	

* Additional strains examined: E208, E8. 9997P⁻. W₁P⁻. 4916.
Untreated cultures or cultures treated with the indicated chemical and physical agents were
subjected to short, controlled exposure of ultrasound, diluted and spread onto BHI agar plates.
After overnight growth, the master plates were replicated to drug containing agar. Drug susceptible
colonies were picked from the master plates and examined for drug resistance. Further details
of the methods used will be given elsewhere (Kayser (1971)).

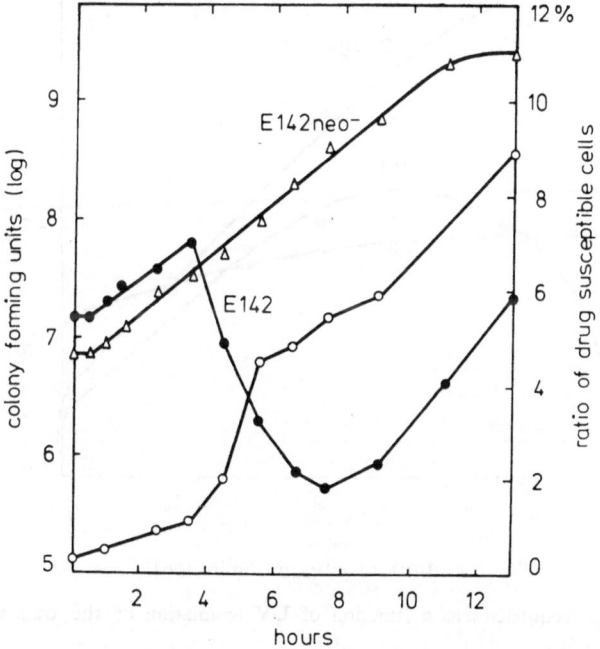

Fig. 1 Kinetics of growth and appearance of neomycin susceptible cells under the influence of
acriflavine.
Legend: △ viable counts, E142 neo⁻ (log)
● viable counts, E142 (log)
○ ratio of neomycin susceptible cells (%)
Strain E142 was inoculated into BHI broth containing 4 μg acriflavine/ml and grown in a shaking
water bath at 37°C. At appropriate time intervals, samples were withdrawn and sonicated. Viable
counts in triplicates were performed by streaking dilutions on BHI agar plates. The percentage
of neomycin susceptible cells was determined by replicating colonies from master plates on neomycin (12.5 μg/ml) containing agar.

373

The kinetics of growth and occurrence of neomycin susceptible cells in E142 under 4 μg acriflavine/ml is shown in figure 1. After an initial increase in the number of viable cells, extensive killing takes place, whereas the negative variant continues to multiply.

However not all negative variants exhibit the same degree of resistance against acriflavine as is shown in figure 1. Out of 14 neomycin susceptible clones isolated during growth in acriflavine broth, only 1 exhibited increased resistance against the dye. 9 out of 12 clones isolated without the influence of acriflavine showed resistance. The different susceptibility of the minus variants against acriflavine may explain, why the culture versus the end of growth did not turn completely into a neomycin susceptible population.

(The cells multiplying at a fast rate in the late growth phase are considered to be spontaneous acriflavine resistant mutants.)

At 1 or 2 μg acriflavine/ml, the parent is not killed but grows at a slower rate than the negative variant. On the basis of these results, a curing effect by acriflavine was not considered, although it could not be excluded. Whether a specific plasmid linked determinant of cellular susceptibility to acriflavine is involved (FALKOW, YOSHIKAWA; cited in NOVICK (1969)) — sometimes segregating from the plasmid — or a non genetic variability remains to be determined. The phenomenon demonstrates clearly, that in

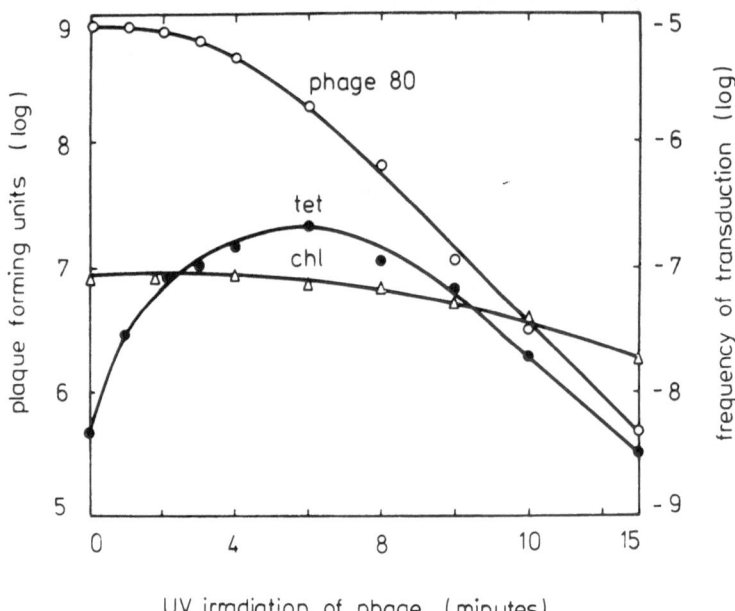

UV irradiation of phage (minutes)

Fig. 2 Transduction frequencies as a function of UV irradiation of the transducing phage 80 lysate.
Legend: ○ survival of phage 80 (log)
       ● transduction frequency of tet (log)
      △ transduction frequency of chl (log)
The frequency of transduction is expressed as number of transductants per plaque forming phage particle in the unirradiated sample.
In transductions the multiplicity of infection was 0.5 to 1. Adsorption of phage during transduction was interrupted by the addition of 0.5% sodium citrate after 30 minutes of incubation of the receptor-phage mixture, followed by centrifugation and 2 washings. No further time was allowed for phenotypic expression of resistance in the transductants. Selection was carried out by plating receptor cells in BHI soft agar on drug and 0.5 % sodium citrate containing BHI plates. (For further details see Kayser (1971)).

curing conditions much attention has to be paid to possible selective effects of the agents used.

Storage of a broth culture at room temperature proved to be the most efficient procedure to eliminate resistance markers.

Joint elimination of the determinants for penicillinase production, chloramphenicol resistance and neomycin resistance was not observed, indicating the location of these markers on separate plasmids.

Influence of ultraviolet light in transduction. It has been observed in *E. coli* (ARBER (1960) and in *Staphylococcus* (NOVICK (1963), that UV irradiation of transducing lysates increases the frequency of markers that are chromosomally integrated. This stimulation will not be seen for plasmid transduction, since it involves an enhancement of recombination. In figure 2, such a stimulation by UV is observed for the tet marker, but not for the chl marker. Table 3 summarizes the results of the stimulation experiments.

Table 3

TRANSDUCTION OF RESISTANCE DETERMINANTS FROM METHICILLIN RESISTANT S. AUREUS, STRAIN E142

Selective drug	Recipient	Transduction frequency before UV	after UV	Cotransduction	Phenotypic lag before expression of resistance
Methicillin	8325 (P524)	$<5 \times 10^{-11}$	8×10^{-10}	0/31	not observed
Erythromycin	545	4×10^{-9}	7.6×10^{-8}	0/100	observed
Streptomycin	545	$<10^{-9}$	10^{-6}	0/200	observed
Tetracycline	545	4.5×10^{-9}	1.9×10^{-7}	0/60	observed
Cadmium	N 8325 (P524)	2×10^{-7}	2.8×10^{-8}	0/100	not observed
	E142pen⁻chl⁻neo⁻	1.5×10^{-6}	—	0/50	not observed
Chloramphenicol	545	8.6×10^{-8}	7×10^{-8}	0/250	not observed
	E142pen⁻chl⁻neo⁻	2.5×10^{-7}	—	0/50	not observed

Multiplicity of infection was 0.5−1.
Frequency of transduction is expressed as number of transductants per unirradiated plaque forming phage particle. The number of colonies showing joint transduction per number examined is given under the heading "contransduction". Time allowed for phenotypic expression of resistance usually was 2 hours (BHI broth, containing 0.5 % sodium citrate). An increase in transduction frequency by a factor of 5 or more was considered as positive. For details about transduction procedure and selection see legend, figure 2.

Transduction of methicillin resistance was done according to COHEN and SWEENEY (1970). It could only be achieved with a high titre lysate of phage 80/E142 (> 10^{10} PFU/ml). Meth could not be transduced with phage 53 or 29, probably because it was not possible to get lysates with similar high titres. In transduction of markers of resistance to methicillin, tetracycline, erythromycin and streptomycin, a significant stimulation of the frequency by UV irradiation of the transducing lysate was observed, indicating their chromosomal nature. Joint transfer of the markers could not be found, suggesting their unlinkage.

Transduction of cadmium resistance/penicillinase production was not stimulated by UV light as well as transduction of the determinant for chloramphenicol resistance.

The penicillinase plasmid (P) contained the genes for regulation and production of penicillinase, extracellularity and mercury and cadmium resistance. This kind of plasmid was not only found in all methicillin resistant strains from Zuerich, but also in strains from Australia, Denmark, England, France, Germany and the United States. The chloramphenicol plasmid (Chl) did not contain other markers besides *chl* (epistatic sensitivity against acriflavine see above).

The lower susceptibility of this plasmid over the P plasmid against UV suggests its smaller size. In case of the *neo* marker, no transduction could be achieved in the system used. Presumably the plasmid is too large to be carried by phage 80. UV induced lysates from strain E142 did not transfer this marker to E142neo⁻ or other recipients.

Phenotypic lag. In transfer of recessive chromosomal markers, the selective conditions must allow the expression of the donor marker in the recipient. A good instance concerns the transduction of streptomycin resistance, which in *Staphylococcus* (KORMAN and BERMAN (1962)) happens to be recessive to susceptibility. Resistant transductants will only be found if application of the drug is withheld until segregation and the expression of resistance is complete. On the other hand, extrachromosomal resistance always has found to be dominant over susceptibility (WATANABE (1963)). Although the examination of a phenotypic lag is only a weak criterium in the demonstration of chromosomal genes, it was used here because it is easy to investigate.

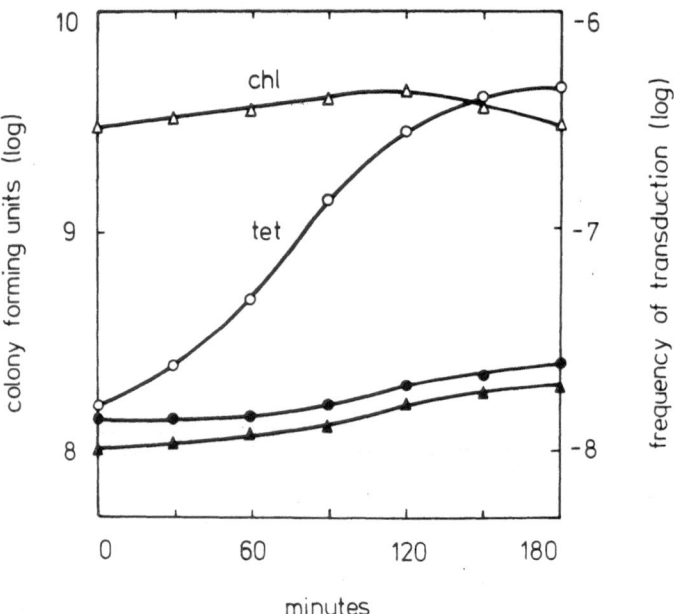

Fig. 3 Phenotypic expression of resistance determinants in transductants.
Legend: ○   transduction frequency of tet (log)
         △   transduction frequency of chl (log)
         ●▲   total viable counts during time allowed for expression of resistance (log)
In transductions, the multiplicity of infection was 0.5 to 1. The frequency of transduction is expressed as number of transductants per plaque forming phage particle. Transduction frequencies are plotted as a function of time of incubation before selection was carried out.
(For further details see footnotes, figure 2 and table 3.)

Phenotypic lag (such as in figure 3) could be observed in transduction of the *tet, ero* and str marker, and was absent in the transfer of the *chl* and *pen* marker. In case of the presumably chromosomal meth determinant, a phenotypic lag could not be observed, demonstrating the restriction of this criterium.

In summarizing it can be concluded, that the markers for methicillin, erythromycin, streptomycin and tetracycline resistance are of chromosomal nature, whereas the determinents for penicillinase production and resistance against chloramphenicol and neomycin are located extrachromosomally on separate plasmids.

ANTIBIOTYPES AND PHAGE-TYPING PATTERNS

Methicillin resistant staphylococci in the Zuerich area today are causing 20—25 % of staphylococcal infections. In 1965 when we began systematically to look for and to examine these bacteria thoroughly, the percentage was 9.8. It increased 1966 to 17.7 %, remained constant in 1967 (16.1 %), increased again 1969 to 24 % and was 20 % (98 isolates/477 staphylococcal cultures) in December 1970/January/February 1971.

MR staphylococci exclusively are isolated from the hospital environment. Among the 25 hospitals connected with the dianostic section of the institute, the university hospital is mostly afflicted by the problem. For this hospital the percentage of infections was 29.4 % in 1969 and 28 % in 1970/71. In another, smaller hospital (General Hospital, Chur), 55 % of the staphylococci isolated were found to be methicillin resistant. Phage-typing patterns of the isolates were similar, as is shown in table 4. Antibiotic resistance patterns are summarized in table 5.

Table 4

PHAGE-TYPING PATTERNS OF METHICILLIN RESISTANT *S. AUREUS*

| | Number of isolates | | | Dec. 1970 |
Phage-typing pattern	1965	1966	1967	Jan./Febr. 1971
1. Conventional group III patterns of lysis	36	99	107	70
2. Group I/group III patterns of lysis	—	—	—	1
3. 83A or 85 or 83A/85	—	2	—	1
4. 29 or 80/81	—	—	2	1
5. Conventional group III patterns of lysis (at R.T.D. = 1000)	—	1	—	19
6. Group I/group III patterns of lysis (at R.T.D. = 1000)	—	—	—	1
7. Untypable	—	1	—	2

R.T.D. = routine test dilution
Phage typing was carried out with phages of the International Typing Series as described by BLAIR and WILLIAMS (1961).

It is evident, that the majority of isolates exhibit similar patterns. Resistance against chloramphenicol and neomycin was not constantly observed, probably because spontaneous loss of these unstable determinants (see above) has occurred. Resistance against erythromycin in 86 % was of the dissociated type with cross resistance against oleandomycin after induction. In 14 % it was of the undissociated, constitutive type with cross resistance against oleandomycin, lincomycin and spiramycin.

It is assumed, that methicillin resistant staphylococci were part of the overall staphylococcal population in very low frequency before the introduction of antibiotics into medicine. These strains then became selected in the hospital environment. A first selection probably occurred by benzylpenicillin (PARKER and HEWITT (1970)). Penicillinase may be expected to protect a staphylococcus against this drug, if the population is large enough to produce sufficient enzyme. When only a few staphylococci are exposed to penicillin, the possession of an additional mechanism of intrinsic resistance might provide protection during the begin of growth. This kind of selection has worked over the years and still does so today because of the increasing use of penicillins.

Table 5

ANTIBIOTIC RESISTANCE PATTERNS OF METHICILLIN RESISTANT *S. AUREUS*

	Isolates of methicillin resistants *S. aureus*				
	1965	1966	1967	Dec. 1970 Jan./Febr. 1971	Total (%)
Su Me ETS CNP	13 (36.2)	32 (31.1)	83 (76.2)	81 (82.7)	60.4
Su Me ETS C P	18 (50.2)	57 (55.3)	16 (14.6)	3 (3.1)	27.4
Su Me ETS P	4 (11.1)	14 (13.6)	7 (6.5)	4 (4.1)	8.3
Su Me ETS NP	1 (2.5)	—	3 (2.7)	6 (6.1)	2.9
Su Me ETS CNP Nb	—	—	—	1 (1)	0.3
Su Me TS C P	—	—	—	1 (1)	0.3
Su Me TS P	—	—	—	1 (1)	0.3
Su Me S P NbRifVaFusPri	—	—	—	1 (1)	0.3
Total	36 (100)	103 (100)	109 (100)	98 (100)	

Abbreviations:
Su	=	Sulphonamides
Me	=	Methicillin
E	=	Erythromycin
T	=	Tetracycline
S	=	Streptomycin
C	=	Chloramphenicol
N	=	Neomycin
P	=	Penicillinase production
Nb	=	Novobiocin
Rif	=	Rifamycin
Va	=	Vancomycin
Fus	=	Fusidic acid
Pri	=	Pristinamycin

Antibiotypes were determined according to Bauer, Kirby, Sherris and Turck (1966). Resistance against methicillin, the sulphonamides, neomycin and the macrolides including lincomycin was determined in dilution tests on Mueller Hinton agar, supplemented in case of the sulphonamides with 5 % human blood. Resistance against the macrolides was determined in uninduced cultures and in broth cultures induced during 2 hours at 37°C with 0.1 μg erythromycin/ml. All strains were susceptible against bacitracin and gentamycin.
The figures in brackets indicate the percentage.

A second, more efficient selection occurred by the introduction of penicillinase resistant β-lactam antibiotics into therapy. Meanwhile however staphylococci in the hospital had developed resistance against other antibiotics (erythromycin, streptomycin, tetracycline, neomycin, chloramphenicol). Therefore multiply resistant, methicillin resistant staphylococci now became selected and soon formed an important part of the hospital flora in our area.

A further indication, that methicillin resistance in staphylococci stems from the selection of only a few preformed strains can be seen in the incapability to produce such strains in vitro or in experimental animal infections (Kayser, unpublished observation).

Undoubtedly further increase in the frequency of methicillin resistance will occurr. The usage of β-lactam antibiotics in the hospital is not likely to be reduced. Yet a restriction in the use of the penicillinase resistant β-lactam antibiotics for the treatment of severe staphylococcal infections is highly desirable.

SUMMARY

In methicillin resistant staphylococci, the genetics of drug resistance were examined. Spontaneous loss and „curing" by certain chemical and physical agents indicated, that the determinants for penicillinase production, chloramphenicol resistance and neomycin resistance were located on separate plasmids. The determinants for resistance against erythromycin, streptomycin, tetracycline and methicillin were found to be stable and hence probably integrated into the chromosome. The stimulation of the transduction frequency by UV irradiation of transducing lysates in case of the latter markers supported further the hypothesis of their chromosomal location. Absence of cotransduction indicated the unlinkage of these genes.

It is assumed, that MR staphylococci existed prior to the introduction of antibiotics into therapy in very low frequency. These strains were selected in the hospital, in the beginning through benzylpenicillin, later by the use of penicillinase resistant β-lactam antibiotics. This hypothesis is supported by the fact, that MR staphylococci possess similar phage typing patterns and exhibit similar antibiotypes. Most cultures are resistant against the standard chemotherapeutics. The absence of resistance against neomycin or chloramphenicol in some isolates is explained by the instability of these markers.

The restricted use of penicillinase resistant β-lactam antibiotics in staphylococcal infections that are a threat to life, is highly recommended.

REFERENCES

ARBER, W. (1960): Transduction of chromosomal genes and episomes in Escherichia coli. Virology, **11/1**, 273.

BAUANCHAUD, D. H., SCAVIZZI, M. R. and CHABBERT, A.-Y. (1969): Elimination by ethidium bromide of antibiotic resistance in enterobacteria and staphylococci. Journal of General Microbiology, **54/3**, 417.

BAUER, A. W., KIRBY, W. M. M., SHERRIS, J. C. and TURCK, T. (1966): Antibiotic susceptibility testing by a standardized single disk method. The American Journal of Clinical Pathology, **45/4**, 493.

BLAIR, J. E. and WILLIAMS, R. E. O. (1961): Phage typing of staphylococci. Bulletin of the World Health Organisation, **24/6**, 771.

BÜLOW, P. (1971): Staphylococci in danish hospitals during the last decade. Factors influencing some properties of predominant epidemic strains. Annals of the New Yorker Academy of Sciences, **182**, 21.

CHABBERT, Y. A., BAUDENS, J. G. and GERBAUD, G. R. (1964): Variations sous l'influence de l'acriflavine et transduction de la résistance à la kanamycine et au chloramphénicol chez les staphylocoques. Annales de l'Institut Pasteur, **107/5**, 678.

COHEN, S. and SWEENEY, H. M. (1970): Transduction of methicillin resistance in Staphylococcus aureus dependent on an unusual specificity of the recipient strain. Journal of Bacteriology, **104/3**, 1158.

EVANS, R. J. and WATERWORTH, P. M. (1966): Naturally occurring fusidic acid resistance in staphylococci and its linkage to other resistances. Journal of Clinical Pathology, **19/6**, 555.

HASHIMOTO, H., KONO, K. and MITSUHASHI, S. (1964): Elimination of penicillin resistance of Staphylococcus aureus by treatment with acriflavine. Journal of Bacteriology, **88/1**, 261.

HIROTA, Y. (1960): The effect of acridine dyes on mating type factors in Escherichia coli. Proceedings of the National Academy of Sciences, USA, **46/1**, 57.

JOHNSTON, J. H. and RICHMOND, M. H. (1970): The increased rate of loss of penicillinase plasmids from Staphylococcus aureus in the presence of rifampicin. Journal of General Microbiology, **60/1**, 137.

KAYSER, F. H. (1971): Elimination and transduction of resistance determinants in methicillin resistant Staphylococcus aureus. To be published.

KAYSER, F. H. and MAK, T. M. (1971): Occurrence and significance of methicillin resistant Staphylococcus aureus from 1965–1971. To be published.

KORMAN, R. Z. and BERMAN, D. T. (1962): Genetic transduction with staphylophage. Journal of Bacteriology, **84/2**, 228.

MAY, J. W., HOUGHTON, R. H. and PERRET, C. J. (1964): The effect of growth at elevated temperatures on some heritable properties of Staphylococcus aureus. Journal of General Microbiology, **37/2**, 157.

MORIMURA, M., WATANABE, K., MORI, H. and MITSUHASHI, S. (1970): Lability of streptomycin resistance in Staphylococcus aureus. Japanese Journal of Microbiology, **14/4**, 253.

NOVICK, R. P. (1963): Analysis by transduction of mutations affecting penicillinase formation in Staphylococcus aureus. Journal of General Microbiology, **33/1**, 121.

NOVICK, R. P. (1969): Extrachromosomal inheritance in bacteria. Bacteriological Reviews, **33/2**, 210.

PARKER, M. T. and HEWITT, J. H. (1970): Methicillin resistance in Staphylococcus aureus. The Lancet, I. 800.

TOMOEDA, M., INUZUKA, M. KUBO, N. and NAKAMURA, S. (1968): Effective elimination of drug resistance and sex factors in Escherichia coli by sodium dodecyl sulfate. Journal of Bacteriology, **95/3**, 1078.

WATANABE, T. (1963): Infective heredity of multiple drug resistance in bacteria. Bacteriological reviews, **27/1**, 87.

WILLETS, N. S. (1967): The elimination of Flac from E. coli. by mutagenic agents. Biochemical and Biophysical Research Communications. **27/1**, 112.

LINKAGE BETWEEN DETERMINING PENICILLINASE PRODUCTION AND BEHAVIOUR IN THE PRESENCE OF CRYSTAL VIOLET IN STAPHYLOCOCCI

J. BOROWSKI, P. JAKUBICZ

Department of Microbiology, University Medical School, Bialystok, Poland.

A variety of methods has been developed so far, for a precise differentiation of *S. aureus* strains. These include: phage typing of staphylococci, lipolytic activity assay, examination of sensitivities to antibiotics, to mercury salts and crystal violet, analysis of toxin production, evaluation of the production of penicillinase, pigment etc.

Dealing with the object stated above the crystal violet ring test (CVRT) has been devised (BOROWSKI, JAKUBICZ, 1969).

The test is based upon observation of the characteristics of growth of staphylococcus strains around the discs saturated with crystal violet. Thereby staphylococci would be divided into three groups. First, the so-called SR group is characterized by the appearance of a growth inhibition zone round the discs and of a single sharp-limited ring on the border-line of the growth. The second group designated WR, somewhat similar to this mentioned above but either with a faint violet ring or even without it. The third DR group displayed the following characteristics: a growth inhibition zone and the presence of two violet rings: one on the border-line of the growth and another a couple of millimeters outside. Between these two rings only a faintly stained growth could be seen.

The procedure was as follows. On Petri plates of 5,5 cm diameter containing 6 ml of broth-agar per dish, 1 ml amounts of an 18-hour broth culture of the strain tested were plated. The excessive volumes were removed. After drying 3 paper discs impregnated with 5, 10 and 15 mcg of crystal violet per disc were placed on the surface, on each plate. The cultures were read after a 24-hour incubation period at 37°C.

Following this method 1303 strains of *Staphylococcus aureus* were examined. This figure included 526 strains isolated from clinical specimens namely pus, feces and sputum; 514 from superficial and deep-seated wounds in out-patients; 92 Staphylococcus strains from swabs taken from farmers and 171 strains cultured from the milk.

Aside from the CVRT the following characteristics were determined in all the strains studied: their sensitivity to the antibiotics applied to routine work, penicillinase production, sensitivities to mercury chloride, crystal violet as well as their phage types.

When analysing the test the strains exhibiting the DR characteristic appeared to be the most interesting ones. They were always resistant to penicillin and to most routine antibiotics, they always produced penicillinase and generally they were resistant to mercury, an overwhelming majority was lyzed by group III phages, the remainder being not lyzed by any phage set at our disposal. The strains were lyzed neither by I nor II phage groups.

The characteristics displayed by the SR group were as follows: the strains were seldom resistant to all routine antibiotics, a majority being resistant to two or three antibiotics, only a few of them were resistant to HgCl₂, they were lyzed by all the phages employed including those of I and II groups.

The WR characteristic was seldom noticed in the strains tested. Staphylococci belonging to this group were mostly sensitive to mercury, did not produce penicillinase and generally they were sensitive to most routine antibiotics.

The DR characteristics were only exhibited by staphylococci isolated from clinical specimens. They were recorded in 31,2% of these strains. The SR staphylococci made 62,2% and those WR 6,6% only. Among all the other strains 91% were SR.

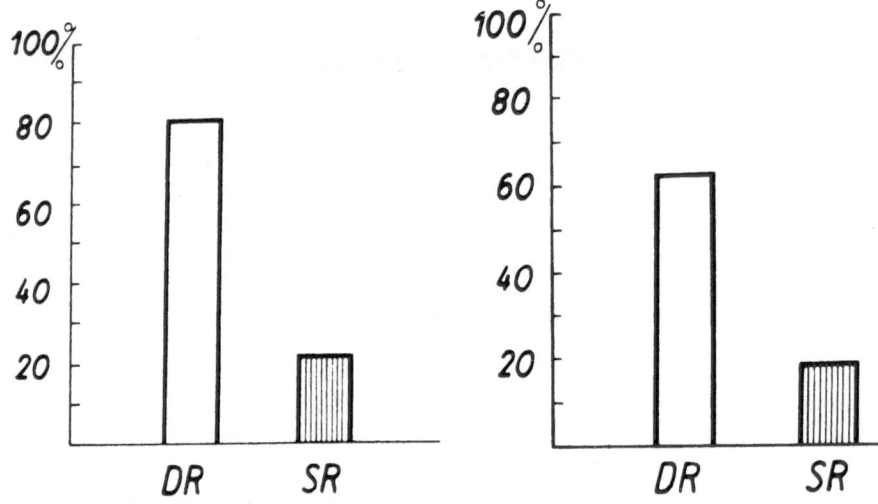

Fig. 1 Percentages of antibiotic multiresistant strains among DR and SR staphylococci.

Fig. 2 Distribution of the III AD phage group strains amog DR and SR staphylococci.

Among the PP strains isolated from clinical specimens 63% were resistant to all the routine antibiotics tested, whereas in those SR the percentages approximated 19 %.

84% of the DR strains were lyzed by III group phages while only 22,5% of those SR were.

Summarizing it may be concluded that the test we have devised can be employed as one more method for the differentiation of staphylococci.

Our attention was next focused on the genetic factors that determine the appearance of the DR characteristics. To study this, a chosen strain of *Staphylococcus* among strains belonging to the DR group, resistant to routine antibiotics, HgCl₂, crystal violet and producing penicillinase was grown at 45°C. Every day it was inoculated into a fresh broth. The appearance of penicillinase-negative mutants was estimated by the starch-penicilliniodine plate method according to BOROWSKI (1964). To employ this technique the strain tested was isolated on agar plates containing starch. After an overnight incubation semi-liquid agar with starch and penicillin G was poured on the plates followed by Lugol solution. The penicillinase-negative colonies could be easily found as they did not decolorize the medium.

The characteristics of the mutants thus obtained were as follows: abolished penicillinase production and thus sensitivity to penicillin G, they became sensitive to HgCl₂, more sensitive to crystal violet and finally the most interesting feature they displayed — they did not grow in the characteristic manner of the DR strains, that time they grew as the SR strains.

As it may be concluded the loss of the DR characteristics was associated with the loss of penicillinase production as well as with the disappearance of resistance to $HgCl_2$ what is refferred to the features determined by the penicillinase plasmid (NOVICK, 1967; NOVICK, RICHMOND, 1965; NOVICK, ROTH, 1968; RICHMOND, 1965). It is distinctive that all the mutants having lost the DR characteristics became more sensitive to crystal violet.

Table 1

CHARACTERISTICS OF THE STRAIN OF S. AUREUS 288 AND ITS PENICILLINASE-NEGATIVE MUTANTS

	Parent strain	Mutants
Penicillinase production	+	−
Resistance to mercury ions	+	−
Resistance to cristal violet	+	−
Behaviour in crystal violet ring test	DR	SR
Antibiotic resistance pattern	PSCTE	SCTE
Lipase production (Tween 80)	+	+
Enterotoxin B production	+	−
Pigment production	+	−

Two possibilities arise: firstly that the DR characteristics, resistance to mercury and penicillinase production are governed by the same gene, secondly that for the features described above are responsible different genes located in their vicinity. Further studies are needed to riddle this out.

REFERENCES

BOROWSKI, J. (1964): A simple method for detection of penicillinase negative variants among large numbers of penicillinase-producing staphylococcal colonies. Zeitschrift für Allgemeine Mikrobiologie, **4**, 134.

BOROWSKI, J. and JAKUBICZ, P. (1969): A new selective crystal violet test for detection of nosocomial Staphylococcus aureus strains (in Polish). Medycyna Doświadczalna i Mikrobiologia, **21**, 344.

NOVICK, R. P. (1967): Penicillinase plasmids of Staphylococcus aureus. Federation Proceedings, **27**, 29.

NOVICK, R. P. and RICHMOND, M. H. (1965): Nature and Interactions of the Genetic Elements Governing Penicillinase Synthesis in Staphylococcus aureus. Journal of Bacteriology, **90**, 467.

NOVICK, R. P. and ROTH, Ch. (1968): Plasmid-linked Resistance to Inorganic Salts in Staphylococcus aureus. Journal of Bacteriology, **95**, 1335.

RICHMOND, M. H. (1965): Penicillinase plasmids in Staphylococcus aureus. British Medical Bulletin, **21**, 260.

INCIDENCE OF ANTIBIOTIC RESISTANT STAPHYLOCOCCI IN HUMANS FROM DIFFERENT ENVIRONMENTS IN SLOVAKIA

M. BETINOVÁ

Research Institute of Epidemiology and Microbiology, Bratislava, Czechoslovakia

It is widely accepted that an antibiotic present in an environment acts as a selective agent which enhances spreading of microbial strains resistant to the same antibiotic. We studied the incidence and susceptibility to antibiotics of coagulase-positive strains of *Staphylococcus aureus* in humans from environments in which different conditions to contacts with antibiotics were supposed. The following groups of persons were investigated in the same winter season: healthy adults from an isolated country population in central Slovakia, blood donors from Bratislava, feeders of domestic animals (poultry and pigs) on farms in south-western Slovakia where chlorotetracycline was used as a feed additive, workers of a pharmaceutical factory working in penicillin production and in chlorotetracycline production, respectively, patients and medical staff from a surgical clinic in Bratislava, and patients and personnel from a pediatric clinic in the same town. It was supposed that the probability of contacts with antibiotics was increasing gradually from group to group.

All coagulase-positive nasal staphylococci isolated from the above mentioned groups of people were tested for their susceptibility to selected antibiotics using a quantitative plate-dilution method recommended by a Committee of the World Health Organization (1961). The strains were tested for susceptibility to 8 antibiotics, namely benzylpenicillin, streptomycin, kanamycin, chlorotetracycline, erythromycin, chloramphenicol, bacitracin, and vancomycin. Strains isolated from the pediatric clinic were further tested for their sensitivity to 6 penicillins, 4 tetracyclines, 4 macrolide antibiotics and sigmamycin. Results of our findings concerning strains from individual groups have been already published in a series of papers (BETINOVÁ, 1965, 1967, 1968; BETINOVÁ and NEMEC, 1964a, 1964b, 1965, 1966). This paper is intended to compare the published results from the point of view of different environments where the staphyloccocal strains have been isolated.

Percentual incidences of carriers of coagulase-positive staphylococci in individual groups of humans are presented on Fig. 1. Practically no differences were found between the country and town populations studied, the percentual frequencies beeing 50.3 % and 49.0 % respetively. Therefore, both of them are mentioned together as the control group. No significant difference was found between incidences of strains in the control group and the group of workers from chlorotetracycline production (40.3 %). On the other hand, significantly lower incidence was found in the group of workers from penicillin production (29.5 %, $p < 0.001$) and in the group of feeders (36.1 %, $p < 0.01$). Significantly higher frequences, in comparison to the control group, were found in patients from both the surgical and pediatric clinics, the respective percentages being

80.5 % and 78.0 % (p < 0.001). Similarly, a significantly higher percentage was found in the group of the medical staff from the surgical clinic (61.5 %, p < 0.05), while data for the staff of the pediatric clinic were on the margins of significancy (62.0 %).

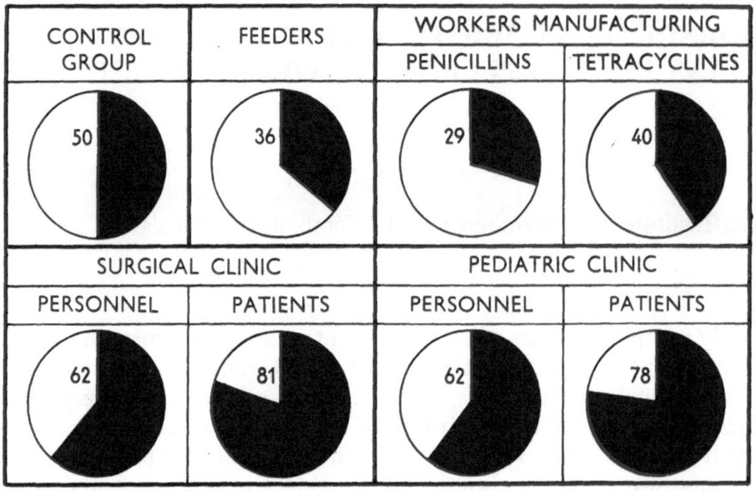

Fig. 1 Percentual frequencies of carriers of nasal staphylococci in different groups of population.

Percentual incidences of strains resistant to any of the antibiotics tested are presented on Fig. 2. Except of feeders and workers from penicillin production, significantly higher incidences of carriers of resistant strains (p < 0.001) were found in all other groups when compared with the control one. Although the percentual incidence of carriers of resistant strains in the group of feeders was similar to that in the control group, great difference was found in incidences of resistance to individual antibiotic which will be mentioned later. Low percentage of carriers of resistant strains in the group of workers in penicillin production could be in correlation with low incidence of strains at all which was shown

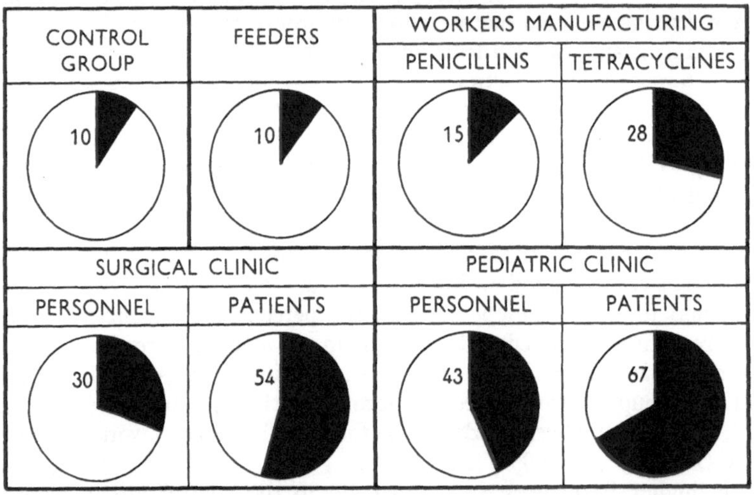

Fig. 2 Percentual frequencies of carriers of antibiotic-resistant strains of S. aureus.

on Fig. 1. The incidence of carriers of resistant staphylococci among workers in chloro-tetracycline production was similar to that among the staff of the surgical clinic. There was no significant difference in frequencies of carriers of resistant strains when the groups of the staffs of the two clinics are compared. The same can be said about the two groups of patients. On the other hand, there were significant differences between incidences of resistant strains among patients and personnel of both clinics.

A comparison of the incidences of resistance to individual antibiotics among strains, isolated from different environments, is also of interrest (Fig. 3). Of the 8 antibiotics

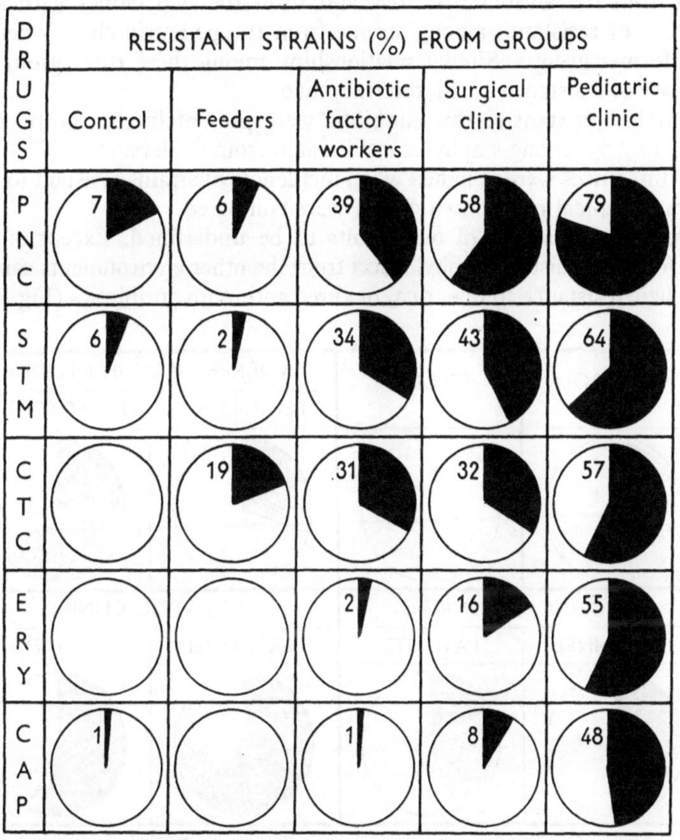

D R U G S	RESISTANT STRAINS (%) FROM GROUPS				
	Control	Feeders	Antibiotic factory workers	Surgical clinic	Pediatric clinic
P N C	7	6	39	58	79
S T M	6	2	34	43	64
C T C		19	31	32	57
E R Y			2	16	55
C A P	1		1	8	48

Fig. 3 Distribution of resistant strains from five groups according to their resistance to individual antibiotics.
Abbreviations: PNC = benzylpenicillin, STM = streptomycin, CTC = chlorotetracycline, ERY = erythromycin, CAP = chloramphenicol.

tested, resistance to 5 of them was only found. All strains were sensitive to kanamycin, vancomycin and bacitracin.

Strains resistant to benzylpenicillin, streptomycin and rarely to chloramphenicol were found in the control group. In the group of staphylococci isolated from feeders strains resistant to benzylpenicillin, streptomycin and, predominantly, to chlorotetracycline were present. Among staphylococci isolated from workers of the antibiotic factory, strains resistant to benzylpenicillin, streptomycin, chlorotetracycline, and, to a lesser extent, to erythromycin and chloramphenicol occured. There was a relatively high incidence of strains resistant to all the five antibiotics on both clinics, their percentages being in general higher on the pediatric one.

The frequency of strains resistant to benzylpenicillin, when compared with the control group, was significantly higher among staphylococci from workers of the antibiotic factory and from the two clinics ($p < 0.001$). There were also significant differences among these three groups, the incidence of resistant strains beeing highest on the pediatric clinic.

Strains resistant to streptomycin were again significantly more often found among staphylococci from the antibiotic factory and from the two clinics with significantly higher incidence of resistance among strains from the pediatric clinic when compared with the two former groups. Similar relationships among these three groups were also found in the case of resistance to chlorotetracycline.

While no strains resistant to this antibiotic were present in the control group, they were found in 19.2 % among staphylococci isolated from feeders.

Significant differences were obtained when incidences of strains resistant to erythromycin and chloramphenicol on the two clinics were compared.

There is yet another aspect of our results to be underlined. Except of the strains isolated from feeders, resistant staphylococci from the other environments can be divided according to their resistance to one, two, or three and more antibiotics (Fig. 4).

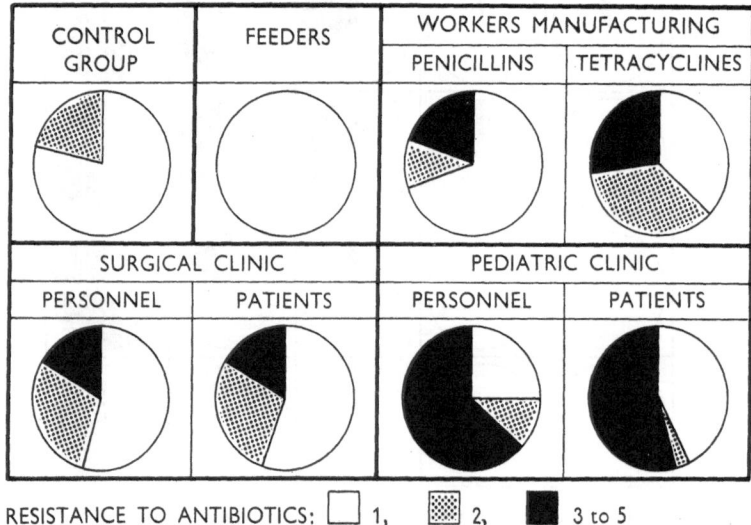

RESISTANCE TO ANTIBIOTICS: ☐ 1, ▨ 2, ■ 3 to 5

Fig. 4 Distribution of resistant staphylococci from different groups according to their resistance to one, two, and three to five antibiotics.

79.3 % of the resistant strains in the control group were resistant to one antibiotic (mostly to benzylpenicillin, fewer strains to streptomycin). The remaining 20.7 % were strain resistant to two antibiotics in two combinations: penicillin + streptomycin and streptomycin + chloramphenicol.

Among strains from feeders only strains resistant to single antibiotics were found.

A different picture was obtained with resistant staphylococci from workers of the antibiotic factory. The majority of strains (69.7 %) from penicillin production were resistant to a single antibiotic, 12.1 % to two antibiotics, and 18.2 % to three or four antibiotics. Of resistant staphylococci from chlorotetracycline production, 36.4 % were resistant to one, 27.2 % to two, and 36,4 % to three or four antibiotics.

Major differences in resistance patterns were also found on the surgical clinic. While a majority of resistant strains (58 %) isolated from patients were multiresistant (i. e. to 3 to 5 antibiotics), 22 % were resistant to two and 20 % to a single antibiotic, a majority of resistant strains (53.8 %) from the staff were resistant to a single drug, 30.8 % to two and only 15.4 % to three or four antibiotics.

In the case of resistant strains from the pediatric clinic this distribution of resistance was quite different, a majority of resistant strains from both patients and the staff showed multiresistance, the respective percentual distribution being as follows. 25.6 % and 42.8 % of strains were resistant to a single antibiotic, 9.3 % and 3.6 % were resistant to two, and 65.1 % and 53.6 % were resistant to four or five antibiotics.

It was already emphasized that resistance to antibiotics was most frequent among staphylococcal strains isolated from patients and staff of the pediatric clinic. These strains were further tested for their susceptibility to four tetracyclines, five macrolide antibiotics (sigmamycin), and, finally, to seven penicillins (BETINOVÁ, 1967, 1968).

The following results of this study should be mentioned here. A complete cross-resistance to tetracyclines of all strains originally resistant to chlorotetracycline was observed. Of the strains originally known as erythromycin-resistant, 60.7 % revealed cross-resistance to erythromycin, oleandomycin, spiramycin, and triacetyloleandomycin. Of 65 strains simultaneously resistant to tetracycline and oleandomycine only five were sensitive to sigmamycin which is a combined preparation of these two antibiotics. With penicillins, similar patterns of resistance were found in the case of benzyl- and phenoxymethyl-penicillin. Incidence of resistance to brocillin was less frequent. All strains were sensitive to meticillin and cloxacillin (orbenin).

CONCLUSION

662 coagulase-positive strains of *Staphylococcus aureus* were isolated from humans in the following environments: an isolated country population, blood donors from Bratislava, feeders from farms where chlorotetracycline was used as a feed additive, workers from an antibiotic factory, patients and staffs from surgical and a pediatric clinic. In antibiotic sensitivity patterns practically no differences were found between the country and town population. When compared with this joint control group, great differences among various environments were found in the following respects: (i) incidence of carriers of nasal staphylococci, (ii) indicence of carriers of antibiotic-resistant strains, (iii) resistance to individual antibiotics, and (iv) incidence of multiresistant strains. These findings suggest that different levels of antibiotics present in the investigated environments acted as selective agents which enhanced spreading of resistant and multiresistant strains of *S. aureus*.

REFERENCES

BETINOVÁ, M. (1965): The occurrence of pathogenic staphylococci in town and country populations of Slovakia and their sensitivity to antibiotics. (In Slovak with English summary.) Bratislavské Lekárske Listy, **45**, 147.

BETINOVÁ, M. (1967): The efficacity of biosynthetic and semisynthetic penicillins on staphylococci in vitro. (In Slovak with English summary.) Bratislavské Lekárske Listy, **47**, 21.

BETINOVÁ, M. (1968): Wirksamkeit von Tetracyclinen, Makroliden Antibiotika and Sigmamycin auf Staphylokokken in Vitro. (In Slovak with German summary.) Biológia (Bratislava), **23**, 681.

BETINOVÁ, M. and NEMEC, P. (1964a): A study of the sensitivity to antibiotics of staphylococci isolated in patients, in the nursing personnel, and in the environment of a surgical clinic. (In Slovak with English summary.) Bratislavské Lekárske Listy, **44**, 336.

BETINOVÁ, M. and NEMEC, P. (1964b): Incidence of pathogenic staphylococci in a pediatric clinic and their antibiotic sensitivity. (In Slovak with English summary.) Československá Epidemiologie, Mikrobiologie, Imunologie, **13**, 279.

BETINOVÁ, M. and NEMEC, P. (1965): Resistente Staphylokokken beim Pflegepersonal von Haustieren, denen Chlortetracyclin beigefüttert wird. (In Russian with German summary.) Biológia (Bratislava), **20**, 274.

BETINOVÁ, M. and NEMEC, P. (1966): Studium der Resistenz gegen Antibiotika bei Staphylokkenstämmen von Arbeitskräften aus der Erzeugung von Antibiotika. (In Slovak with German summary.) Biológia (Bratislava), **21**, 109.

CONCOMITANT LOSS OF MARKERS DURING ELIMINATION OF TETRACYCLINE MARKER IN STAPHYLOCOCCUS AUREUS

J. SCHINDLER

Department of Medical Microbiology and Immunology, Charles University, Prague, Czechoslovakia

Tetracycline resistant clones isolated from tetracycline sensitive populations were analyzed recently (SCHINDLER, MAREŠOVÁ, 1971). These clones carried in addition to Tet marker also erythromycin (Ery), cephaloridine (Cef), streptomycin (Stm), chloramphenicol (Clo), lincomycin (Lin) and spiramycin (Spi) markers. The influence of the elimination of Tet marker on these markers was investigated in this study.

MATERIALS AND METHODS

Tetracycline resistant strains used for isolation of Tet⁻ clones were selected from naturally occurring tetracycline sensitive strains. All 49 strains were identified as *Staphylococcus aureus*.

For selection of Tet clones, 100 ml of stationary phase culture in meat peptone broth were diluted by 400 ml of fresh meat broth. Tetracycline was added in a concentration 10 μg/ml, and cultures were then shaken in a water bath at 37°C for 18 hours. Afterwards, they were diluted to obtain isolated colonies by plating on nutrient agar plates with 10 μg/ml of tetracycline.

To obtain tetracycline sensitive mutants, Tet clones were grown in 10 ml of meat broth at 37°C and passaged three times by inoculating 0.1 ml into 10 ml of broth. Acridine orange treatment (AO) was carried out in parallel. Staphylococci were inoculated into 10 ml of broth containing 10 μg/ml of AO, and cultivated for 18 hours. Cultures were diluted and plated on nutrient agar. After 48 hours plates were replicated by means of filter paper replica discs onto nutrient agar plates containing 10 μg/ml of tetracycline and on cream agar plates. After incubation, colonies of tetracycline sensitive bacteria as well as chromogenic mutants were isolated from the master plate, purified and checked.

Sensitivity tests were performed by means of SPOFA sensitivity discs (streptomycin 30 μg, neomycin 30 μg, penicillin 10 U, chloramphenicol 30 μg, tetracycline 30 μg, erythromycin 10 μg, kanamycin 20 μg, spiramycin 20 μg, cephaloridine 10 μg, lincomycin 10 μg, novobiocin 20 μg, pristinamycin 10 μg and fusidic acid 10 μg). Strains with a zone not wider than 1 mm were read as resistant and if necessary checked on agar plate containing the respective drug. All tetracycline and erythromycin sensitivity tests were checked on agar plates containing 10 μg/ml of tetracycline and 10 μg/ml of erythromycin respectively.

Strains which were isolated from specimens as primarily tetracycline sensitive are designated TET⁻$_{(nat)}$. Selected resistant strains are designated TET⁻$_{(sel)}$, sensitive subclones obtained by treatment with AO or spontaneously are designated TET⁻$_{(el)}$. Antibiotic resistance as well as the type of chromogenesis are considered as phenotypic markers. They were designated by three-letter symbols with the first letter capitalized (DEMEREC, ADELBERG, CLARK, HARTMAN, 1966): Pen, Clo, Tet, Ery, Stm, Neo, Kan, Lin, Spi, Pri, Fus, Cef for the resistance to penicillin, chloramphenicol, tetracycline, erythromycin, streptomycin, neomycin, kanamycin, lincomycin, spiramycin, pristinamy-

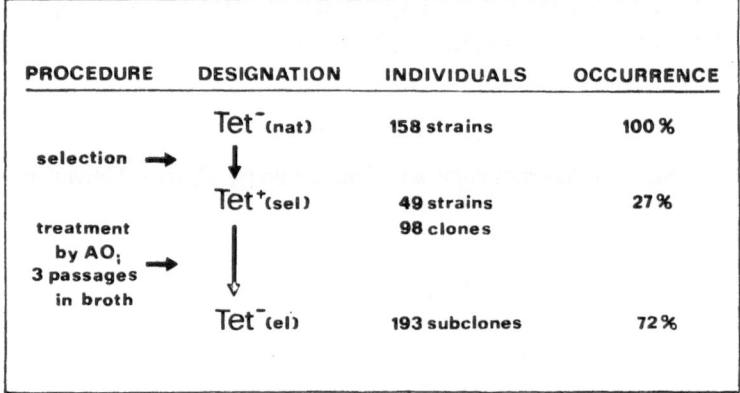

Fig. 1 Description of the experiment and the origin of bacterial clones.

cin, fusidic acid and cephaloridin respectively and Ora for orange colour of colonies on cream agar plate, Yel for yellow colour and Whi for white colour of colonies. The origin of subclones and general description of the experiment is given in Fig. 1.

RESULTS

98 tetracycline resistant clones obtained by selection of two of each of 49 naturally occurring tetracycline sensitive strains were used. In 43 strains Tet⁻ isolates were obtained. From 98 TET(sel) clones 193 Tet⁻ subclones with a different resistance pattern were obtained.

The loss of Tet was accompanied by the loss of other atb markers in 72 % of clones. More than two markers were lost in 56 % of the clones.

RMN (resistance marker number) is obtained by adding all markers present in a particular strain. The mean RMN in TET⁻(el) is 1.9. RMN in TET(sel) from which TET⁻(el) are derived is 5.1.

The distribution of RMN in TET⁻(el) subclones is demonstrated in Fig. 2. It shows two peaks — one at RMN 1 and the other at RMN 6. The former peak itself constituters 36 % of all subclones, the latter 6 %. Distribution of differential RMN (d-RMN = $RMN_{TET^-(el)} - RMN_{TET^+(sel)}$) shows that all subclones occur in the zone of negative values, with two peaks, one at number −2 and the other at −7. (Fig. 3.) This means that in almost all Tet⁻ subclones other atb markers are coeliminated. Frequencies of coelimination are given in Table 1.

It is necessary to note, that TET⁻(el) subclones change their chromogenic capacity in several instances.

72 % of Tet Yel and 7 out of 13 Tet Ora are Tet⁻Whi after elimination. In several instances, however, the chromogenic capacity is partially restored. Tet Yel → Tet⁻Ora occurs in 11 %, Tet Whi → Tet⁻Ora in 23 % of cases. No satisfactory explanation of this fact can be offered at present.

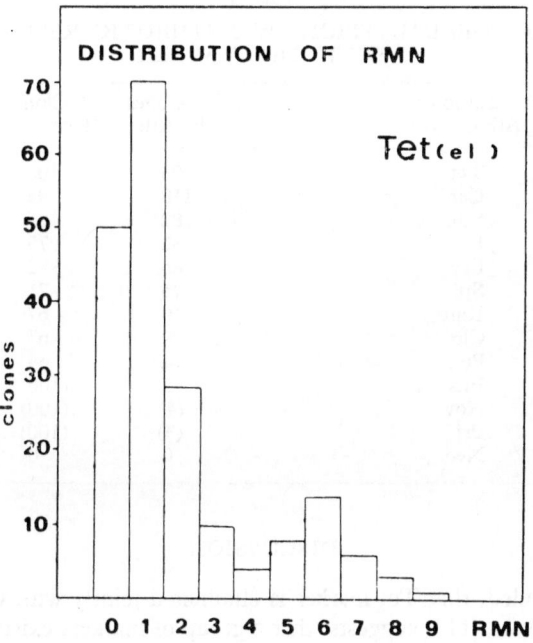

Fig. 2 Distribution RMN in Tet⁻ eliminated subclones. (RMN — resistance marker number is the sum of antibiotic resistance markers occuring in a particular clone).

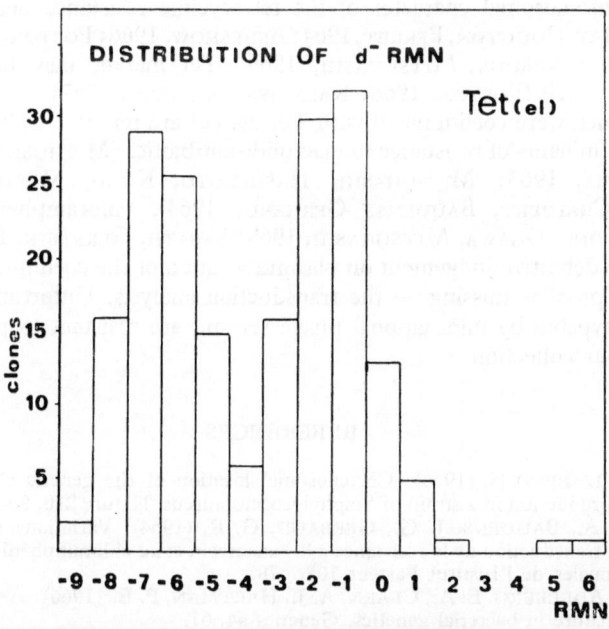

Fig. 3 Distribution od differential RMN in Tet⁻ eliminated subclones. (d⁻ RMN is obtained by sustracting of RMN Tet from RMN of Tet⁻ eliminated subclones).

393

SCHINDLER, J.

Table 1

FREQUENCIES OF COELIMINATION OF ANTIBIOTIC RESISTANCE MARKERS
WITH TET MARKER

Additional Atb marker	Tet clones Atb$^+$ Atb$^-$	Clones Tet$^-$ Atb$^-$
Tet	193	100
Cef	118	95
Stm	82	85
Lin	82	75
Ery	86	72
Spi	75	71
Kan	10	67
Clo	79	65
Pen	74	38
Fus	(3)	(100)
Nov	(4)	(100)
Pri	(3)	(100)
Neo	0	0

DISCUSSION

It may be concluded, that Tet marker is eliminated jointly with Cef, Stm, Lin, Spi, Ery, Kan, Clo markers. This suggests, that a group of markers exists, which behaves as a unit both in selection and elimination of Tet marker. The elimination occurs either spontaneously or under constraint.

It is suggested, that Tet and the above mentioned markers might be located on a plasmid.

The extrachromosomal character of the tetracycline resistance determinant is now established (MAY, HOUGTON, PERRET, 1964; ASHESHOW, 1966; POSTON, 1966; KASATIYA, BALDWIN, 1967; KASUGA, MITSUHASHI, 1968). Tet marker may be located on the chromosome as well (POSTON, 1966; KASATIYA, BALDWIN, 1967).

Markers which were coeliminated with Tet marker are reported to be extrachromosomal, e. g. determinants of resistance to macrolide antibiotics (MITHUSHASHI, MORIMURA, KONO, OSHIMA, 1963; MITSUHASHI, HASHIMOTO, KONO, MORIMURA, 1965) to kanamycin (CHABBERT, BAUDENS, GERHARD, 1964), chloramphenicol (CHABBERT et al., 1964; KONO, OGAWA, MITSUHASHI, 1968; SABATH, GERSTEIN, LODER, FINLAND, 1968). For the definitive judgement on plasmid location of the coeliminated markers one indispensable proof is missing — the transduction analysis. Unfortunately, all 98 Tet clones are untypable by international phage set and are resistant to polyvalent phages available in our collection.

REFERENCES

ASHESHOV, ELIZABETH H. (1966): Chromosomal location of the genetic elements controlling penicillinase production in a strain of Staphylococcus aureus. Nature **210**, 804.
CHABBERT, Y. A., BAUDENS, J. G., GERBAUD, G. R. (1964): Variations sous l'influence de l'acriflavin, et transduction de la resistance a la kanamycin et au chloramphénicol chez les staphylococques. Annales de l'Institut Pasteur **107**, 678.
DEMEREC, M., ADELBERG, E. A., CLARK, A. J., HARTMAN, P. E. (1966): A proposal for a uniform nomenclature in bacterial genetics. Genetics **54**, 61.
KASATIYA, S. S., BALDWIN, J. N. (1967): Nature of the determinant of tetracycline resistance in Staphylococcus aureus. Canadian Journal of Microbiology **13**, 1079.

KASUGA, T., MITSUHASHI, S. (1968): Drug resistance of staphylococci VIII. Genetic properties of resistance to tetracycline in Staphylococcus aureus E 169. Japanese Journal of Microbiology **12**, 269.

KONO, M., OGAWA, K., MITSUHASHI, S. (1968): Drug resistance of staphylococci VI. Genetic determinant for chloramphenicol resistance. Journal of Bacteriology **95**, 886.

MAY, J. W., HOUGHTON, R. H., PERRET, C. J. (1964): The effect of growth et elevated temperature on some heritable properties of Staphylococcus aureus. Journal of General Microbiology **37**, 157.

MITSUHASHI, S., HASHIMOTO, H., KONO, M., MORIMURA, M. (1968): Joint elimination and joint transduction of the determinants of penicillinase production and resistance to macrolide antibiotics. Journal of Bacteriology **89**, 988.

MITSUHASHI, S., MORIMURA, M., KONO, K., OSHIMA, H. (1963): Elimination of drug resistance of Staphylococcus aureus by treatment with acriflavine. Journal of Bacteriology **86**, 162.

NOVICK, R. P. (1969): Extrachromosomal inheritance in bacteria. Bacteriological Reviews **33**, 210.

POSTON, SUSAN M. (1966): Cellular location of the genes controlling penicillinase production and resistance to streptomycin and tetracycline in a strain of Staphylococcus aureus. Nature **210**, 802.

SABATH, L. D., GERSTEIN, D. A., LODER, B. B., FINLAND, M. (1968): Independent segregation of chloramphenicol resistance in Staphylococcus aureus. Antimicrobial agents and chemotherapy (1967), p. 264.

SCHINDLER, J., MAREŠOVÁ, A. (1971): Characteristics of tetracycline resistant clones in tetracycline sensitive populations of staphylococci. VIIth Congress of Chemotherapy, Prague, August 1971.

IV.

COLLOQUIUM
ON TETRACYCLINE RESISTANCE

Moderator:

V. KRČMÉRY (Bratislava)

ON THE MECHANISM OF TETRACYCLINE ACTION AND RESISTANCE:

Association of Tetracyclines with ribosomes and Ribosomal Subunits, studied by a Fluorometric Method

H. KERSTEN, G. FEY

Institute of Physiological Chemistry, University of Erlangen, G.F.R.

CURRENT CONCEPT OF THE MODE OF TETRACYCLINE ACTION

Since the discovery of tetracycline in 1945 by DUGGAR (Lederle laboratories) several strains of streptomyces have been found, producing antibiotics of the tetracycline group, which were chemically defined as substituted naphthacen-ring systems. Tetracyclines inhibit the growth of a wide range of microorganisms and were introduced for clinical application in 1950. Already at this time GALE and PAINE (1950) found that tetracyclines severely affect protein synthesis, results which were confirmed shortly thereafter by HAHN and WISSEMAN (1951).

Although the tetracyclines exhibit a variety of inhibitory effects in bacterial cells and also in higher organisms, the protein synthesizing system is now widely accepted to be the most sensitive target affected by the antibiotic. (For summary see FRANKLIN, 1965; LASKIN, 1967 and 1970; WEISBLUM and DAVIES, 1968). It is not possible to define precisely the molecular mechanism of action of inhibitors of protein synthesis as long as the single steps in the protein biosynthetic pathway are not known. In order to discuss the molecular mechanism of tetracycline action the current knowledge of the mechanism of protein synthesis is briefly summarized; the process of translation of mRNA into protein in bacteria can be roughly divided into three phases (LENGYEL, 1969): (1) initiation, (2) peptide chain elongation and (3) peptide chain termination.

Initiation: In the first step of initiation, the α-amino group of the chain initiator methionyl-tRNA is blocked by a formyl residue. The first intermediate in the initiation of peptide chains is a complex consisting of a 30S ribosomal-subunit; GTP, F-met-tRNA$_F$ and three initiation factors (F_1, F_2, F_3), bound to an initiation signal on mRNA abbreviated as "30S initiation complex". A 50S ribosomal subunit joins this complex to form the 70S initiation complex. The GTP molecule in this complex is cleaved into GDP and P_i. The three initiation factors F_1, F_2 and F_3 are released from the 30S subunit during or after the formation of the 70S initiation complex. The initiation phase is considered to be completed with a 70S initiation complex in which F-met-tRNA$_F$ is bound in the P site (peptidyl site) or D site (donor site) or according to KAJI (1970) site 2.

Elongation: The first step in the elongation cycle is the binding of an aminoacylated tRNA (AA-tRNA) to a specific binding site called A site (AA-tRNA binding site or acceptor site, or site 1). The AA-tRNA is first bound in a complex form consisting of AA-tRNA, a protein factor T_u and GTP. The formation of this complex involves another factor, T_s. In the next step T_u, GDP and P_i are released from the ribosome leaving the AA-tRNA at the acceptor site. In the second step of elongation a peptide bond is formed, the F-met residue is released from its linkage to $tRNA_F$ and is joined in a peptide bond with the α-amino group of AA-tRNA in the A site. The peptidyl transferase catalyzing this step is part of the 50S subunit. Recent findings from MATTHAEI (1971) suggest, that there exist three sites for incoming aminoacyl-tRNAs on the E. coli ribosome. Thus the process of peptide bond formation is even more complicated and not yet solved in detail. The third step of elongation involves a translocation of the newly formed peptidyl-tRNA from the A site to the P site. During this process the discharged tRNA is released from the ribosome and the ribosome moves the length of one codon along the mRNA. In the course of translocation a factor designated G and GTP become attached to the ribosome and the bound GTP is cleaved into GDP and P_i. G-factor, GDP and P_i are released from the ribosome. The elongation involves AA-tRNA binding, peptide bond formation and translocation. The cycles are repeated and the peptide chain grows until in the course of its movement along the mRNA a termination codon is reached by the A site of the ribosome.

Termination: Peptide chain termination signals are probably the termination codons UAA or UAG, furthermore releasing factors R_1 and R_2 and a third factor designated S or α are known to be involved in this process. The detailed mechanism of peptide chain termination is not yet known. Possible roles for R factors in termination include translation of the terminator codons, deacylation of peptidyl-tRNA and conversion of 70S ribosome into 30S and 50S subunits.

The most widely accepted concept on the interference of tetracyclines with protein synthesis is that tetracycline antibiotics inhibit bacterial protein synthesis by binding preferentially to the 30S subunit and inhibiting the binding of AA-tRNA to the specific binding site namely the A site (FRANKLIN, 1963; HIEROWSKI, 1965; SUAREZ and NATHANS, 1965; DAY, 1966; KAJI, 1966; CONNAMACHER and MANDEL, 1968; SARKAR and THACH, 1968; BODLEY and ZIEVE, 1969; MAXWELL, 1968). If tetracyclines interfere with the binding of AA-tRNA at the A site it is evident, that the antibiotic can inhibit the initiation of protein synthesis as well as the elongation of peptide chains, provided that during formation of the initiation complex F-met $tRNA_F$ is first bound to the A site. More recent experiments reveal that the A site and the P site are almost equally inhibited at low concentrations (5×10^{-5} M tetracycline) (IGARASHI and KAJI, 1970).

Tetracyclines not only interfere with the binding of F-met-$tRNA_F$ to 30S ribosomes. Interference of tetracyclines with the peptide-transfer of peptidyl tRNA to puromycin was found by ČERNÁ (1969). SCOLNICK (1968) observed an inhibition of the release of N-formylmethionine from ribosomes during the determination process. Moreover tetracyclines interfere with the effect of a certain termination factor which removes the last tRNA from the ribosome. In consequence the ribosome can not be dissociated into the subunits and ressume translation of another messenger RNA (IGARASHI et al., 1969). From the in vitro studies it seems likely that tetracyclines might affect the initiation, and/or the elongation, and/or the termination steps of protein synthesis.

Several inhibitory effects of tetracyclines were observed at concentrations of tetracyclines that correspond to greater than 100 tetracycline molecules per ribosome. An important aspect in studying the mechanism of tetracycline action is to distinguish nonspecific association of tetracycline from specific interaction with the ribosome. The widely accepted concept that tetracyclines affect protein synthesis by binding to the 30S ribosomal subunit and acting on this site of the ribosome should be revised, because binding to both 30S and 50S subunits of radioactively labeled tetracyclines has been demonstrated by DAY (1966) and MAXWELL (1968): substantial amounts of tetracyclines bind to ribosomes; a small fraction of the radioactive label is irreversibly bound; this irreversibly bound labeled material amounts to less than one molecule of drug per ribosome; the specific activity bound to the 30S subunit was found to be twice as large as the specific activity bound to the 50S subunit. Studies on the binding of radioactive tetracyclines are difficult to interpret and are not definitive especially when the radioactivity is measured in different fractions of sucrose gradients used for the separation of ribosomes. Initially bound tetracyclines might become detached from the ribosome during sucrose gradient centrifugation.

Tetracyclines are fluorescent compounds, we therefore assumed that the sensitivity of a fluorometric assay would allow to detect and to measure precisely and directly tetracycline binding to ribosomes in concentration ranges $10^{-5}-10^{-7}$ M which covers the inhibitory dosis of tetracyclines in intact cells. Independently WHITE and CANTOR (1971) measured the interaction of tetracyclines with 70S ribosomes fluorometrically.

The following investigations were carried out in order to clarify (1) whether specific binding sites exist at the 30S subunit and/or at the 50S subunit; and (2) whether tetracycline derivatives differing in biological activity differ also in their binding capacity to 70S ribosomes 50S or 30S subunits.

FLUORESCENCE CHANGES OF TETRACYCLINES IN THE PRESENCE OF RIBOSOMES AND RIBOSOMAL SUBUNITS

Specific binding of a fluorescent substrate to the active center of an enzyme is often accompanied by a significant change in fluorescens. If upon binding of tetracyclines to ribosomes changes in the fluorescens of tetracyclines occur, fluorometric measurements would allow to follow directly the interaction of tetracyclines with ribosomes. Tetracyclines

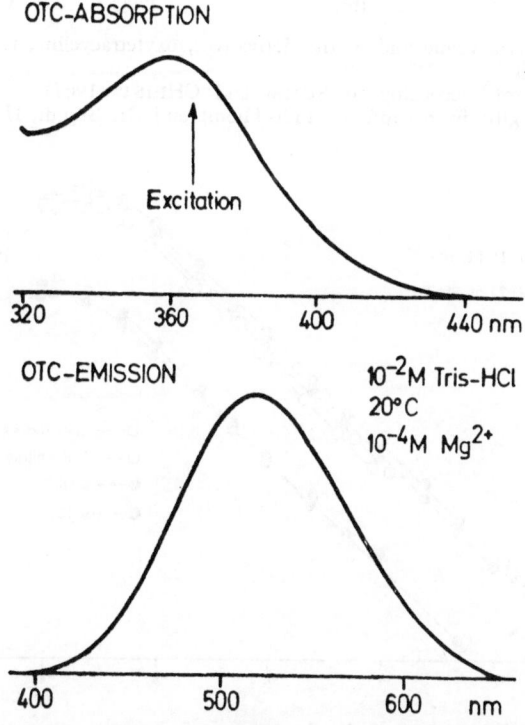

Fig. 1 Absorption- and fluorescence-spectra of oxytetracycline (OTC).

401

exhibit absorption spectra with absorption maxima near 360 nm. When tetracyclines are excitated at wave lengths close to the absorption maxima they reemitte intensively near 520 nm (fig. 1). Ribosomes and ribosomal subunits upon excitation at 366 nm show only very weak fluorescence with a maximum at 500 nm.

In the experiments to be described oxytetracycline, tetracycline-methiodide and tetracycline-nitrile were used (fig. 2). Oxytetracycline is about as active as tetracycline,

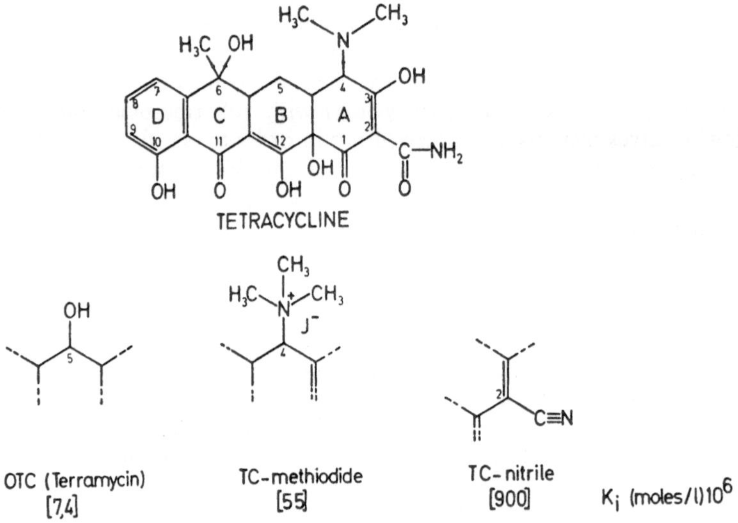

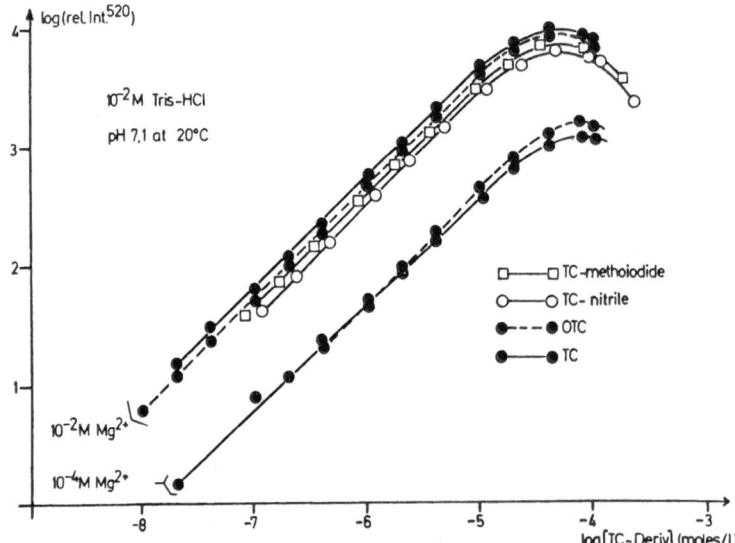

Fig. 2 Structure of tetracycline and of the derivatives, oxytetracycline, tetracycline-methiodide and tetracycline-nitrile
K_i = Inhibitor constants according to SUMM and CHRIST (1967)
The substances were gifts from Prof. Schmidt-Thome and Dr. Summ, Hoechst.

Fig. 3 Concentration dependence of the fluorescens of oxytetracycline, tetracycline-methiodide and tetracycline-nitrile measured at two different Mg^{2+} concentrations.

the methiodide is 10 times less and the nitrile 100 times less active in inhibiting microbial growth. The inhibitor constants for inhibition of poly U directed synthesis of poly phe (K_i Mol/1×10^{-6}) are 7.5 for OTC respectively 55 for the methiodide respectively 900 for the nitrile (SUMM and CHRIST, 1967). The absorption spectra and the fluorescens spectra were measured and were found to be almost identical with those of oxytetracycline.

Fluorescence intensities of oxytetracycline and the two derivatives were measured dependent on the concentration of the drug (fig. 3). Fluorescence intensity of oxytetracycline and the derivatives can be determined with accuracy down to concentrations of 5×10^{-8} M of the drug. The fluorescence studies were made at two different concentrations of Mg^{2+}, since Mg^{2+} could influence the binding of tetracyclines to ribosomes. The fluorescence of all compounds was found to be about 10 times higher increasing the Mg^{2+} concentration from 10^{-4} M to 10^{-2} M. The percentage of increase is independent of the drug concentration which is important since the measurements were made always at constant ribosome or subunit concentrations (1×10^{-6} M) and varying concentrations of the drug. The constancy in ribosome concentration avoids errors produced by light scattering.

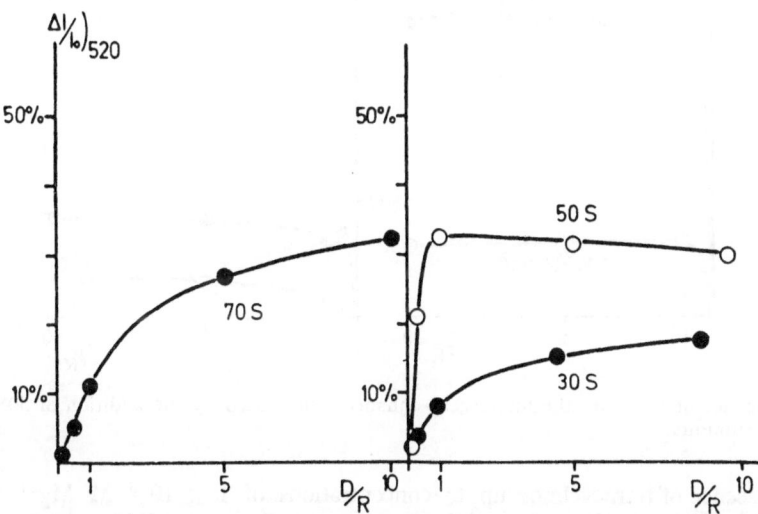

Fig. 4 Fluorescens enhancement of oxytetracycline upon addition of 70S ribosomes, 50S and 30S subunits. Measurements are made at constant ribosome concentration 1×10^{-6} M and varying concentrations of the drug. D/R molar ratios of total drug to ribosome.

70S ribosomes were purified by high speed centrifugation of the crude extract through 1 M sucrose. This removes free 30S and 50S subunits and their precursors. Ribosomal subunits were prepared from purified 70S ribosomes and separated by zonal centrifugation through sucrose gradients. The preparations used were characterized by analytical ultracentrifugation before and after fluorescens measurements; native 70S and reassociated 70S, 30S and 50S particles were tested for biological activity and were found to be active in the poly U directed synthesis of poly-phenylalanine.

The fluorescence of oxytetracycline is enhanced significantly upon addition of 70S ribosomes, 50S and 30S ribosomal subunits (fig. 4). The relative percent increase $\Delta I/I_0$

is plotted against the molar ratio of drug to ribosome respectively subunits (D/R). (ΔI = fluorescence intensity of the complex — fluorescence intensity (I_0) of the numerical sum of the components). The increase in fluorescens shows that oxytetracycline interacts with the 30S subunit, with the 50S subunit as well as with the whole 70S ribosome. In the presence of the 50S subunits enhancement is reached at a drug/ribosome ratio of 1 : 1, with the 30S subunits at a drug/ribosome ratio of about 10 : 1. The maximum fluorescence enhancement is however less with the 30S than with the 50S subunits. With respect to saturation of fluorescence increase, 70S ribosomes behave like 30S and are like the 50S subunit with respect to plateau values. Binding of tetracycline to 70S ribosomes might therefore involve binding sites at both subunits.

Decreasing the Mg^{2+} concentration in the buffer from 10^{-2} M to 5×10^{-4} M causes a four-fold increase in the enhancement of fluorescence of oxytetracycline in the presence of the 50S subunits as well as in the presence of 30S particles (fig. 5). Mg^{2+} alone increase

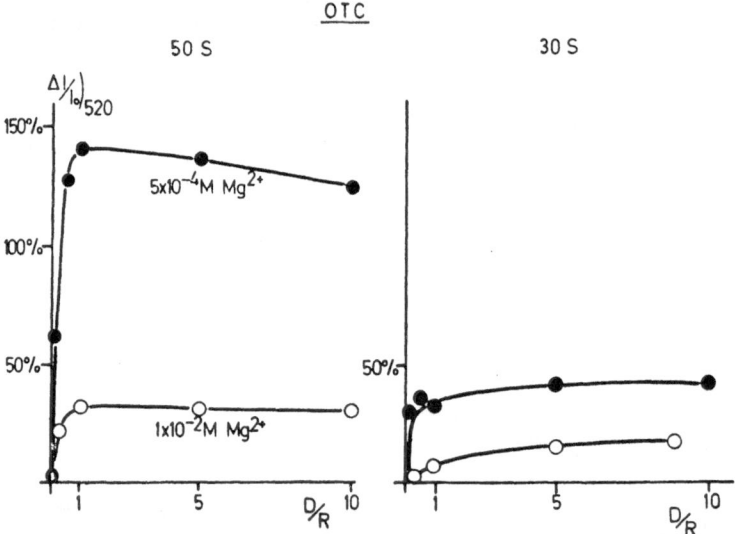

Fig. 5 Influence of Mg^{2+} on the fluorescens-enhancement caused by the addition of 50S or 30S ribosomal subunits.

the fluorescence of tetracyclines up to concentrations of 1×10^{-2} M Mg^{2+} (fig. 6), probably caused by the formation of chelate complexes between Mg^{2+} and tetracyclines. The increase in fluorescens upon removal of Mg^{2+} is however difficult to interpret since Mg^{2+} changes the conformation of tetracycline as well as that of the ribosomal subunits. WHITE and CANTOR (1971) postulated that tetracycline binding to ribosomes occurs via Mg^{2+}. If this would be the case one should expect a further fluorescence increase at raising ratios of drug/ribosome to 10^{-2} M Mg^{2+}, but this is not the case. The inhibitory biological effect of tetracyclines can be reversed by chelating metal ions especially Mg^{2+}. We assume that the Mg^{2+} complexes of tetracyclines are less effectively bound than the free compound to the ribosomes or the subunits, although Mg^{2+}, localized at specific binding sites at the ribosome might be involved in the association.

In the second type of experiments we studied whether tetracycline derivatives which are biologically less active, are also less active with respect to the interaction with 70S ribosomes or the subunits. The experiments were performed at 5×10^{-4} M Mg^{2+} and

1×10^{-2} M M^{2+}. The 30S subunit interacts with the methiodide and also with the nitrile as indicated by the fluorescence enhancement (fig. 7), although the methiodide does not enhance the fluorescence at increasing ratios of drug to ribosome to the same maximum value obtained with oxytetracycline. The nitrile shows an unusual behaviour: at low drug to ribosome ratios there is considerable increase in fluorescence which levels off to zero if the drug/ribosome ratio is raised to 10. The striking behaviour can not be

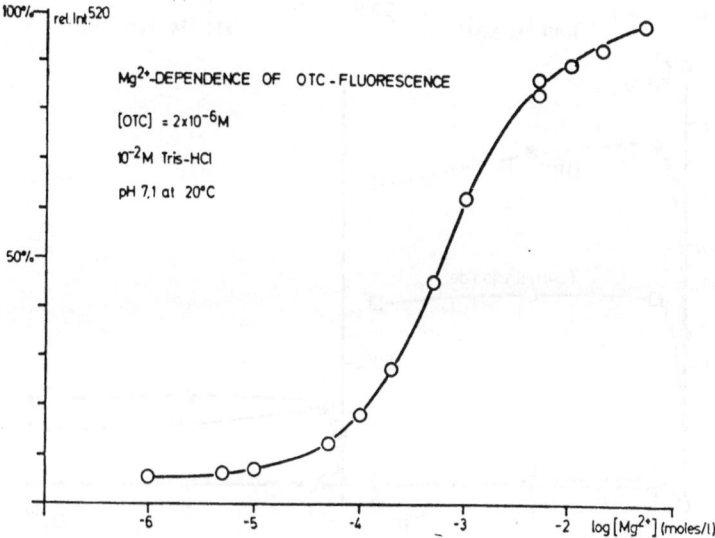

Fig. 6 Mg^{2+} dependence of oxytetracycline fluorescence.

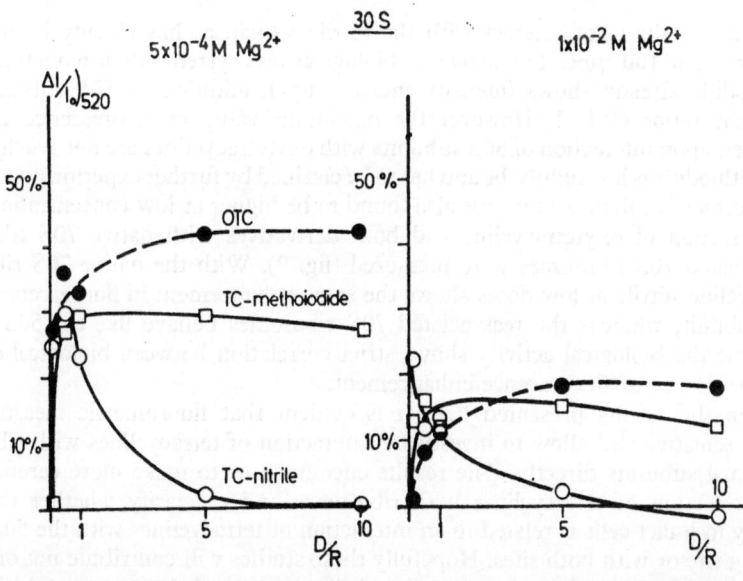

Fig. 7 Comparison of changes in the fluorescence of oxytetracycline, tetracycline-methiodide and tetracycline-nitrile upon addition of 30S subunits.

405

explained unless we assume that some unspecific binding occurs at increasing drug concentrations causing a quenching of the fluorescence. The same behaviour is observed at low and high concentrations of Mg^{2+} though fluorescence enhancement for all derivatives is considerably less.

The fluorometric data obtained upon addition of 50S subunits to oxytetracycline, the methiodide- and the nitrilederivatives (fig. 8) reflect the biological activity insofar as the

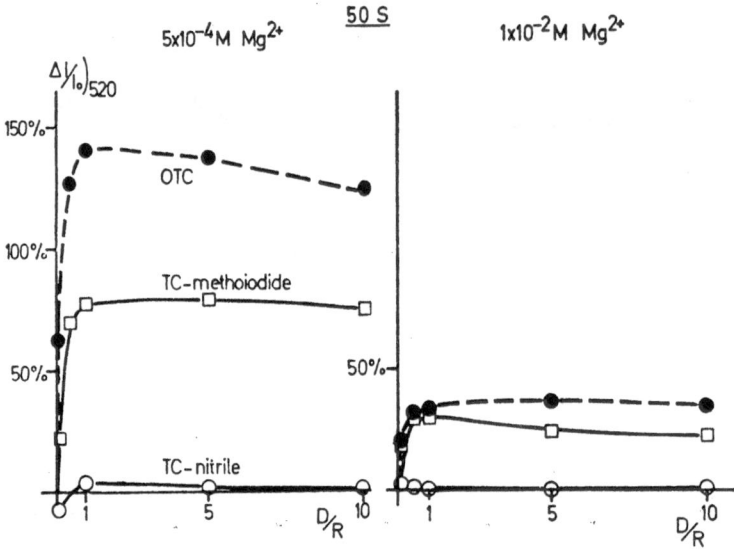

Fig. 8 Comparison of changes in the fluorescence of oxytetracycline, tetracycline-methiodide and tetracycline-nitrile upon addition of 50S subunits.

50S subunit does not interact with the nitrile which, as has already been mentioned, is more than 100 times less active in biological test systems than oxytetracycline. The methiodide already shows intensity increase upon addition of 50S subunits at drug/ribosome ratios of 1:1. However the maximum value of fluorescence enhancement obtained upon interaction of 50S subunits with oxytetracyclines are not reached. Whether the methiodide is less tightly bound has to be clarified by further experiments. The relative enhancement of fluorescence was also found to be higher at low concentrations of Mg^{2+}.

Interaction of oxytetracycline and both derivatives with native 70S ribosomes and reassociated 70S ribosomes were measured (fig. 9). With the native 70S ribosomes the tetracycline-nitrile at low doses shows the same enhancement in fluorescence as with the 30S subunit, whereas the reassociated 70S ribosomes behave like the 50S subunit. In this case the biological activity shows strict correlation between biological effectiveness and the degree of fluorescence enhancement.

From the results presented here it is evident that fluorometric measurements are highly sensitive and allow to investigate interaction of tetracyclines with ribosomes and ribosomal subunits directly. The results encourage us to make more careful studies on the interaction of tetracyclines with ribosomes and to clarify whether the biological activity in intact cells is related to an interaction of tetracyclines with the 50S or the 30S binding site or with both sites. Hopefully these studies will contribute not only to clarify the molecular mechanism of tetracycline action but also help us to get insight into the mechanisms of tetracycline resistance.

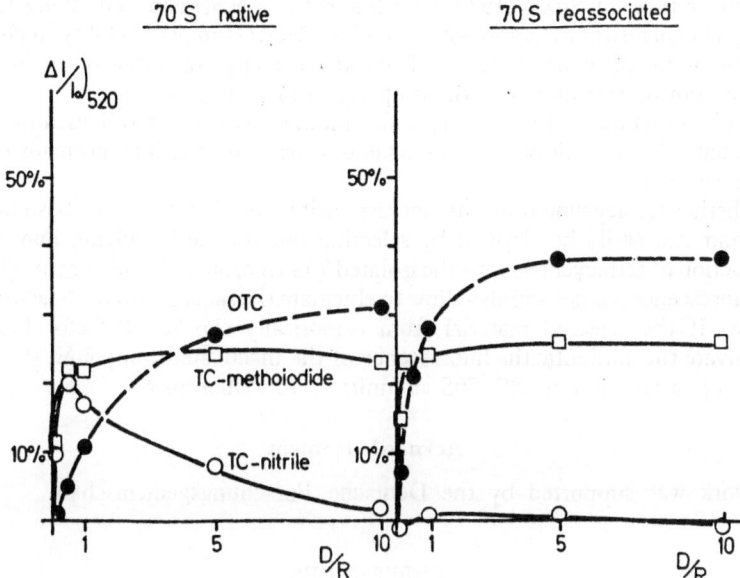

Fig. 9 Comparison of changes in the fluorescence of oxytetracycline, tetracycline-methiodide and tetracycline-nitrile upon addition of native and reassociated 70S ribosomes.

MECHANISMS OF TETRACYCLINE RESISTANCE

Three possible mechanism are discussed by which a cell can become resistant to tetracyclines. The first, and this is the most widely accepted model assumes that resistance to tetracyclines is related to a permeability defect in resistant cells such that the antibiotic is unable to reach the site of protein biosynthesis (LASKIN and CHEN, 1964; REEVE, 1968). Another type of tetracycline resistance might occur involving an alteration of ribosomal protein (s), controlled by tetracycline resistant loci at the bacterial chromosome (CRAVEN et al., 1969). This type of resistance was elucidated first for streptomycin and has been shown to involve an alteration of a certain protein in the 30S subunit, the P_{10} protein (NOMURA, 1969). Tetracyclines belong to the group of antibiotics for which extrachromosomal transferable drug resistance localized on R-factors has been shown. FRANKLIN (1971) discussed that the resistance to tetracyclines transferred by R-factors is not nessecarity due to changes in the permeability of membranes. No significant differences in the rate or extent of uptake of tetracyclines by membranes prepared from tetracycline sensitive or tetracycline resistant R-factor-bearing *E. coli* were observed.

FRANKLIN and FORSTER (1971) showed that the degree of resistance in R-bearing *E. coli* cells however could be drastically lowered by subjecting the cells to osmotic shock. It is suggested that upon osmotic shock probably an enzyme is released which in the resistant cell converts tetracycline to an inactivated form. This suggestion is based on the following findings:

Streptomycin is inactivated in R-factor containing cells by an enzyme which transfers an adenyl residue to streptomycin. It could be demonstrated that this enzyme is released upon osmotic shock from *E. coli* cells resistant to streptomycin (OZANNE et al., 1969). Enzymatically inactivated streptomycin either adenylated or phosphorylated has been shown to be unable to bind to ribosomes (YAMADA et al., 1970). These findings are

407

analoguous to those of SHAW (1970) who found the mechanism underlying R-mediated chloramphenicol resistance is also not caused by a decrease in permeability to chloramphenicol: chloramphenicol becomes acetylated and thereby converted to an inactive form which does not possess any more the property to bind to ribosomes.

It is evident that the evaluation of specific binding sites for teracyclines at the ribosomes or ribosomal subunits will be most valuable to clarify the possible mechanisms of tetracycline resistance:

(1) Whether tetracycline resistant loci responsible for alterations of ribosomal proteins might occur can easily be clarified by selecting mutants and studying fluorometrically the interaction of tetracyclines with the isolated 70S ribosome, the 50S or the 30S subunit.

(2) Fluorescence studies will also allow to elucidate the mechanism of R-factor mediated resistance. If the released material from osmotically shocked R-factor bearing cells will inactivate the antibiotic the fluorescence of the inactivated compound should not be enhanced upon addition of 30S, 50S subunits or 70S ribosomes.

Acknowledgement

The work was supported by the Deutsche Forschungsgemeinschaft.

REFERENCES

BODLEY, J. W. and F. J. ZIEVE (1969): Biochem. Biophys. Res. Commun. **36**, 463.
ČERNÁ, J., J. RYCHLÍK, P. PULKŘABEK (1969): Europ. J. Biochem. **9**, 27.
CONNAMACHER, R. H. and H. G. MANDEL (1968): Biochim. Biophys. Acta **166**, 475.
CRAVEN, C. R., R. GAVIN and T. FANNING (1969): Symposia of Quantitative Biology **34**, 134.
DAY, L. E. (1966): J. Bacteriol. **92**, 197.
FRANKLIN, T. J. (1963): Biochem. J. **87**, 449.
FRANKLIN, T. J. (1966): In Biochemical Studies of Antimicrobial Drugs Cambridge University Press, p. 192.
FRANKLIN, T. J. (1971): Biochem. J. **123**, 267.
FRANKLIN, T. J. and S. J. FORSTER (1971): Biochem. J. **121**, 287.
GALE, E. F. and T. F. PAINE (1950): Biochem. J. **47**, XXVI.
HAHN F. E. and C. L. WISSEMAN (1951): Proc. Soc. Exptl. Biol. Med. **76**, 533.
HIEROWSKI, M. (1965): Proc. Nat. Acad. Sci., Wash. **53**, 594.
IGARASHI, H., H. ISHITSUKA, Y. KURIKI and A. KAJI (1970): Progress in Antimicrobial and Anticancer Chemotherapy, **2**, 445.
KAJI, H. I., I. SUZUKI nad A. KAJI (1966): J. Biol. Chem. **241**, 1251.
LASKIN, A. J. (1967): in Antibiotics, Mechanism of Action edited by Gottlieb and Shaw, Springer Verlag Berlin, **1**, 331.
LASKIN, A. J. (1970): Progress in Antimicrobial and Anticancer Chemotherapy, **2**, 441.
LASKIN, A. J. and W. M. Chan (1964): Biochem. Biophys. Res. Comm. **14**, 137.
LENGYEL, P. (1969): Cold Spring Harbor Symposia Quant. Biol. New York **828**.
MATTHAEI, H. (1971): personell communication.
MAXWELL , I. H. (1968): Mol. Pharm. **4**, 25.
NOMURA, M., S. MIZUSHIMA, M. OZAKI, P. TRAUB and C. V. LOWRY (1969): Cold Spring Harbour Symposia on Quant. Biol. **34**, 49.
OZANNE, B., R. BENVENISTE, D. TIPPER and J. DAVIES (1969): J. Bact. **100**, 1144.
REEVE, F.C.R. (1968): Genet. Res. **11**, 303.
SHAW, W. V. (1970): Progress in Antimicrobial and Anticancer Chemotherapie **2**, 552.
SARKAR, S. and R. E. THACH (1968): Proc. Nat. Acad. Sci., Wash. **60**, 1479.
SCOLNICK, E., R. TOMPKINS, T. CASKEY and M. NIRENBERG (1968): Biochemistry **61**, 768.
SUAREZ, G. and D. NATHANS (1965): Biochem. Biophys. Res. Comm. **18**, 243.
SUMM, H. D. and O. CHRIST (1967): Arzneimittel- Forschung **17**, 1186.
WEISBLUM, B. and J. DAVIES (1968): Bacteriol. Revs. **32**, 493.
WHITE, J. P. and C. R. CANTOR (1971): J. Mol. Biol. **58**, 397.
YAMADA, T., K. KVITEK and J. DAVIES (1970): Progress in Antimicrobial and Anticancer Chemotherapy **2**, 562.

R FACTOR-DETERMINED STATES OF TETRACYCLINE RESISTANCE IN SHIGELLA FLEXNERI

SIDNEY COHEN, C. R. NATHAN and S. A. KABINS

Department of Microbiology, Michael Reese Hospital and Pritzker School of Medicine, Chicago, Ill., U.S.A.

ABSTRACT

We have reported previously that some strains of *Shigella flexneri* that bear R factor-mediated tetracycline (Te) resistance grow well on brain heart infusion agar plates containing 100 μg of Te per ml but are paradoxically susceptible to inhibition by intermediate concentrations of Te (25 to 50 μg/ml). These B$^+$ strains give a corona of growth around a Te antibiotic disk surrounded by a zone of inhibition which contains a few B$^-$ variant colonies. These variants are not paradoxically susceptible and give no zone of inhibition around Te disks.

INTRODUCTION

In current studies, we have demonstrated the paradoxical Te susceptibility of B$^+$ in dilute (10^4-10^5 cells per ml) cultures in brain heart infusion broth. Viable counts of B$^+$ cells increased more slowly in 25 μg of Te per ml than in 50 or 100 μg per ml. B$^-$ variants largely replaced B$^+$ cells cultured in 25 μg of Te per ml owing to the fact that the spontaneously occurring B$^-$ variants, once induced to maximal resistance, grew in 25 μg of Te per ml at normal rates, whereas they grew much more slowly than the B$^+$ cells at 50 μg per ml.

B$^+$ cells initiated growth in Te broth with a smaller lag than B$^-$. Thus B$^+$ cells appeared to be partially constitutive for Te resistance. This hypothesis was supported by their lesser uptake of tritiated Te.

Some strains of *Shigella flexneri* that bear R factor-mediated tetracycline (Te) resistance form colonies well on brain heart infusion agar medium containing 100 μg of Te per ml but are paradoxically inhibited by 25—50 μg of Te per ml (KABINS, COHEN, 1969). In antibiotic disk susceptibility tests these strains, designated B$^+$, give a corona of growth around the disk surrounded by a concentric zone of inhibition of 17 to 20 mm in diameter in which appear a few discrete bacterial colonies. On subculture, these variant colonies, designated B$^-$, are not paradoxically susceptible; they give no zone of inhibition in Te disk tests. Some variants give an intermediate reaction designated B$^\pm$. The B$^+$ or B$^-$ phenotype is determined by the R factor, for it is transferred with the R factor to other strains of *Shigella*. Expression of the B$^+$ phenotype is dependent on its presence in an appropriate host cell, which has been found thus far, only in some strains of *S. flexneri*. We report here additional studies on the dynamics of the growth of these organisms in the presence of Te that shed some light in this phenomenon.

MATERIALS AND METHODS

Organisms. The standard B⁺ organism, *S. flexneri* (strain 40), was a clinical isolate that had been cured of a native *fi*⁺ R factor mediating resistance to Te, streptomycin, and sulfonamides. It retained an *fi*⁻ R factor mediating resistance to sulfonamides only. It then acquired R factor R3 by conjugation from a fecal isolate of *E. coli*. (KABINS and COHEN, 1969). R3 mediated resistance to Te and streptomycin.

Antibiotic-disk susceptibility tests and R factor transfer. Procedures for these tests have been described (KABINS and COHEN, 1969).

Tetracycline-broth cultures. These were performed with brain heart infusion broth (Difco). A starter culture containing 10 ml of broth was inoculated from a stock slant and incubated with shaking at 37 C until an exponential growth curve was well established. When the culture reached an optical density of 0.3 measured in 18 mm cuvets at 540 nm in a Coleman Universal spectrophotometer, 0.3 ml was inoculated into 9.7 ml of broth containing varying concentrations of Te. At appropriate intervals samples were diluted serially in 10 fold steps in 0.01 % gelatin, 0.15 M NaCl, 0.01 M phosphate buffer pH 7.1. Colony counts were made by spotting two to four replicate 0.03 ml drops of appropriate serial 10 fold dilutions of cultures on brain heart infusion agar plates. Colonies were counted after incubation for 18 to 24 hr. From these plates individual colonies were picked at random for antibiotic disk tests to determine the Te phenotype. For experiments with Te-induced cells, the starter culture contained 5 μg of Te ml; it was incubated one hour.

Tetracycline uptake. Radioactive Te was used to determine Te uptake according to FRANKLIN (1967). Cells in late exponential phase growth in brain heart infusion broth were collected by centrifugation and washed in a pH 7.1 buffer containing per liter KH_2PO_4 5.4 gm $(NH_4)_2SO_4$ 1.2 gm, glucose 12 gm and $MgSO_4 . 7H_2O$ 0.4 gm. The cells were resuspended in buffer to give an optical density of 1.7. A 1 ml portion of a mixture of (7—³H) tetracycline (New England Nuclear or Amersham/Searle Corporation) and unlabelled antibiotic was added to 9 ml of cell suspension. After incubation for varying time at 37 C with shaking the suspension was chilled, centrifuged and Te was extracted with hot water. Aliquots were counted in a Packard scintillation spectrometer. Uptake was expressed as μg of Te per ml of a cell suspension of unit optical density (5×10^3 cells). To control for non-specific uptake, cells were incubated with labelled Te at 0.C. This was negligible in all cases.

RESULTS

Although our earlier results indicated that a B⁺ culture formed fewer colonies on brain heart infusion agar containing 25 to 50 μg of Te per ml than on agar containing 100 μg per ml, they furnished no information on relative rates of growth. We conducted comparable growth studies of B⁺ and B⁻ strains of *S. flexneri* strain 40 in brain heart infusion broth using an initial inoculum that produced barely perceptible turbidity and following the growth of the cells by changes in optical density. With relatively large inocula of this type B⁺ organisms grew well but at a progressively decrease in rate in 25, 50 and 100 μg of Te per ml without any evidence of paradoxical inhibition until growth was limited within a few hours by exhaustion of the medium.

In order to obtain a longer period of observation of the response of B⁺ and B⁻ cultures to the action of Te, we reduced the inoculum to the range of 10^4 and 10^5 organisms per ml and followed growth rates by enumeration of the number of viable organisms. An experiment of this kind is summarized in Fig. 1. An initial inoculum of 10^5 B⁺ cells from an exponential phase culture in brain heart infusion broth grew in 25 μg of Te per ml after a lag of one hr but at a progressively decreasing rate. The lag was much more prolonged in 50 μg of Te per ml but after recovery it grew more rapidly than in 25 μg. Consequently it attained the same cell density as the 25 μg culture by 10 hrs. In 100 μg

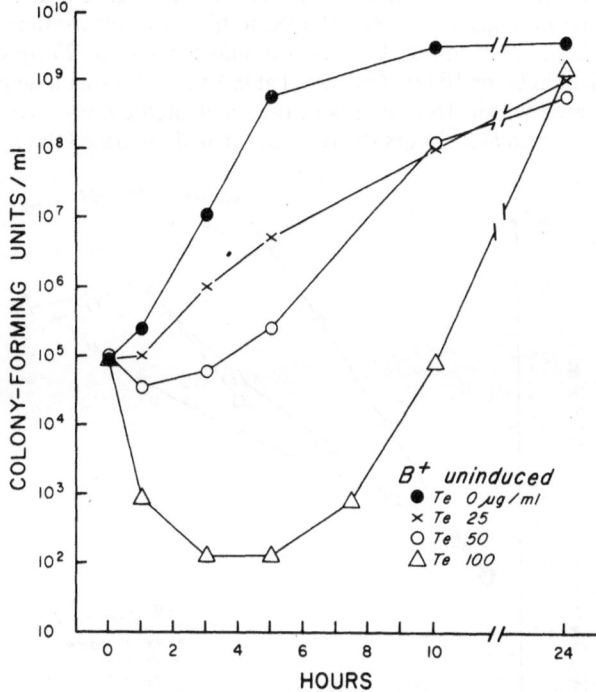

Fig. 1 Growth of uninduced B⁺ cells of *S. f.exneri* 40 in varying concentrations of Te in brain heart infusion broth.

of Te per ml the viable count first dropped about 100 fold but then growth resumed. The results of disk susceptibility tests of individual colonies taken from the viable counts at different times in experiments of this kind are listed in Table 1.

Fig. 1. indicated that there was an inducible component of Te resistance in the B⁺ organism, that is Te resistance was enhanced by prior growth of the cells in medium containing the antibiotic. This feature of Te resistance has been described for Te resistance

Table 1

EMERGENCE OF B⁻ CELLS IN B⁺ CULTURES IN Te BROTH

Time of incubation (hr)	Concentrations of Te in broth (μg/ml)					
	25		50		100	
	uninduced	induced	uninduced	induced	uninduced	induced
	proportion of B⁺ cells (%)					
10	100	40	100	100	100	100
16	90	—	100	—	100	—
24	80	6	100	100	100	100

whether associated or unassociated with R factors (3—6, 8). The degree of inducibility of the B$^+$ organism estimated from the delay in growth was slight in 25 μg per ml of Te but increased progressively in higher concentrations. Accordingly the experiment was repeated with inocula grown in brain heart infusion broth containing 5 μg of Te per ml, in which both B$^+$ and B$^-$ organisms grew at the same rate as in broth without antibiotic. When induced B$^+$ organisms were transferred to higher concentrations of Te, they grew without lag at rates much lower than control, and the rate in 25 μg of Te per ml was distinctly less than in 50 or 100 μg (Fig. 2). Table 1 indicates that a detectable proportion of B$^-$ cells appeared within 16 to 24 hrs in the unadapted culture in 25 μg of Te. In the induced culture assayed at 24 hours the B$^-$ cells virtually replaced the B$^+$ cells.

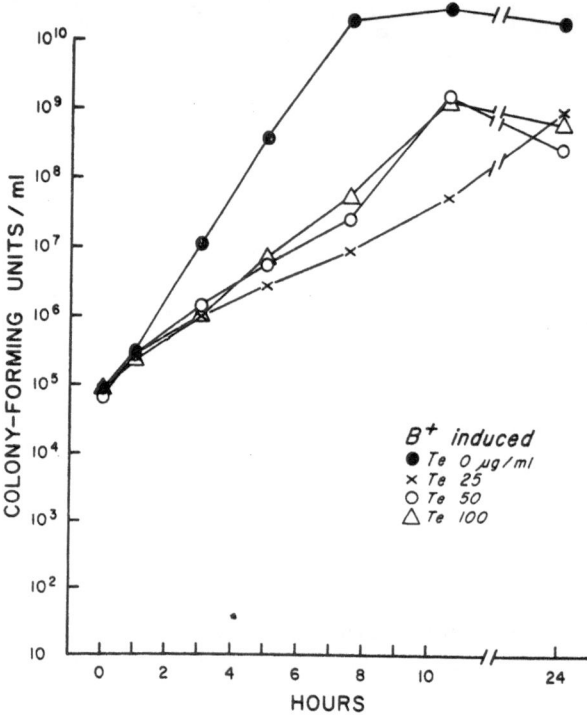

Fig. 2 Growth of induced B$^+$ cells of S. flexneri 40 in varying concentrations of Te in brain heart infusion broth.

An explanation for this change in phenotype could be deduced from the observations on the growth of B$^-$ cells in Te broth. Fig. 3 shows that uninduced B$^-$ cells were initially much more susceptible to Te than B$^+$ cells. Viable counts of uninduced B$^-$ cells dropped 1.5 logs in 25 μg of Te per ml and with 50 μg per ml the culture was almost sterilized. However, Fig. 4, shows that induced B$^-$ cells grew in 25 μg of Te per ml at a rate almost the same as the control and much more rapid than that of the B$^+$ organism. In 50 μg of Te per ml B$^-$ organisms grew more slowly, at a rate similar to that of B$^+$.

Our earlier experiments on colony formation by B$^+$ cells on Te agar indicated that the proportion of cells inoculated that formed colonies on agar containing 25 μg of Te per ml was about 10^{-4}. These colonies were for the most part B$^-$. If it is assumed that the change from B$^+$ to B$^-$ phenotype was the result of a spontaneous transition, presumably

412

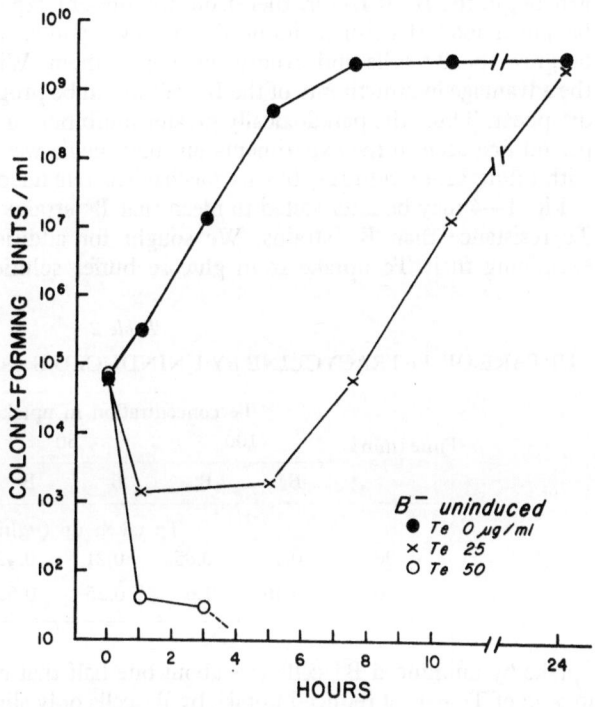

Fig. 3 Growth of uninduced B⁻ cells of *S. flexneri* 40 in varying concentrations of Te in brain heart infusion broth.

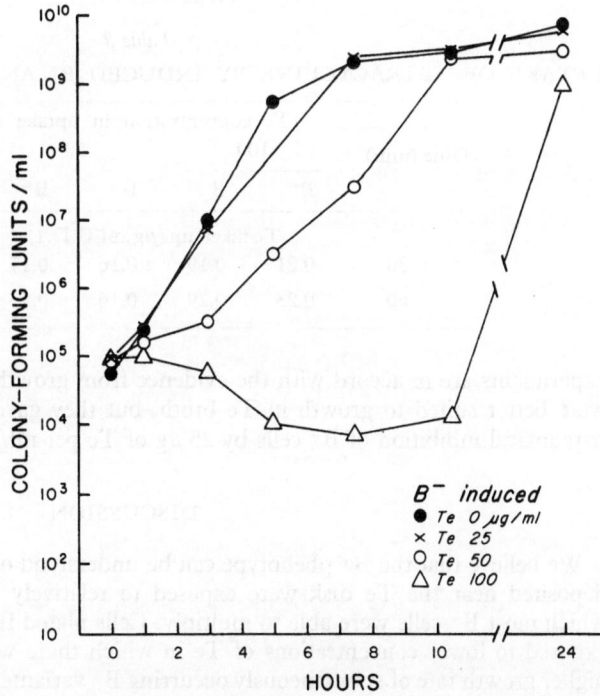

Fig. 4 Growth of induced B⁻ cells of *S. flexneri* 40 in varying concentrations of Te in brain heart infusion broth.

413

genetic, in the B⁻ R factor, then from the present experiments in broth cultures, it can be understood that, once induced, the few spontaneously occurring B⁻ cells would outgrow the B⁺ cells and eventually replace them. With higher concentrations of Te, the advantage in growth rate of the B⁻ cell would be progressively lessened and eventually disappear. Thus, the paradoxically greater inhibition of B⁺ then B⁻ cells in 25 μg of Te per ml first seen in the experiments on solid media was duplicated in these experiments with dilute broth cultures, but its mechanism remained unexplained.

Fig. 1—4 may be interpreted to mean that B⁺ strains are more nearly pre-induced for Te resistance than B⁻ strains. We sought for additional evidence on this point by examining their Te uptake from glucose buffer solutions. Table 2. indicates that Te

Table 2

UPTAKE OF TETRACYCLINE BY UNINDUCED B⁺ AND B⁻ SHIGELLA FLEXNERI

Time (min)	Te concentration in uptake buffer (μg/ml)					
	100		50		25	
	B⁺	B⁻	B⁺	B⁻	B⁺	B⁻
	Te taken up (μg/ml/O.D.1)					
30	0.42	0.85	0.21	0.42	0.10	0.18
60	0.56	1.6	0.26	0.62	0.13	0.28

uptake by uninduced B⁺ cells was about one half that of B⁻ cells. Induction by growth in 5 μg of Te per ml reduced uptake by B⁺ cells only slightly whereas uptake by induced B⁻ cells was reduced to amounts about the same as that of B⁺ cells (Table 3). These

Table 3

UPTAKE OF TETRACYCLINE BY INDUCED B⁺ AND B⁻ SHIGELLA FLEXNERI

Time (min)	Te concentration in uptake buffer (μg/ml)					
	100		50		25	
	B⁺	B⁻	B⁺	B⁻	B⁺	B⁻
	Te taken up (μg/ml/O.D.1)					
30	0.21	0.19	0.16	0.17	0.13	0.14
60	0.23	0.29	0.16	0.23	0.15	0.17

experiments are in accord with the evidence from growth experiments that the B⁺ cells were better suited to growth in Te broth, but they gave no clue to the mechanism of paradoxical inhibition of B⁺ cells by 25 μg of Te per ml.

DISCUSSION

We believe that the B⁺ phenotype can be understood on the basis of our results. Cells deposited near the Te disk were exposed to relatively high concentrations of Te, in which most B⁺ cells were able to multiply. Cells plated further away from the disk were exposed to lower concentrations of Te in which there was paradoxical inhibition. The higher growth rate of spontaneously occurring B⁻ variants in concentrations of Te around

25 μg per ml enabled them to grow as isolated colonies within the zone of inhibition of the R$^+$ organisms. The difference in uptake of Te between B$^+$ and B$^-$ cells was presumably an independent manifestation of the properties responsible for their different susceptibilities to Te, but the nature of the properties involved remained obscure.

ANNEAR (1970), ANNEAR and HUDSON (1970) observed that some strains of *Serratia* tested for susceptibility to polymyxin B or sodium colistimethate (colistin) by the disk method also exhibited a zone of growth adjacent to the disk surrounded by a zone of inhibition. Colony formation by these strains on colistin agar medium was inhibited at 2.5 to 10 μg of colistin per ml but was almost normal at higher concentrations of antibiotic. The demonstration of an optimal concentration for inhibition was not reproduced in broth medium. This observation resembles ours, but there is no way of knowing whether these similar findings with different organisms and antibiotics are mechanistically related.

Acknowledgment

This investigation was supported by Public Health Service research grant AI 07715 from the National Institute of Allergy and Infectious Diseases.

REFERENCES

ANNEAR, D. I. (1970): An optimal zone of colistin activity with Serratia marcescens. Med. J. Australia. **2**: 225−227.

ANNEAR, D. I. and J. A. HUDSON (1970): An unusual zone surrounding colistin disc in sensitivity tests of Serratia marcescens. Med. J. Australia. **1**: 840−841.

CONNAMACHER, R. H., H. G. MANDEL and F. E. HAHN (1967): Adaptation of populations of Bacillus cereus to tetracycline. Molec. Pharmocol. **3**: 586−594.

FRANKLIN, T. J. and J. M. COOK (1971): R factor with a mutation in the tetracycline resistance marker. Nature. **229**: 273−274.

FRANKLIN, T. J. (1967): Resistance of Escherichia coli to tetracyclines. Changes in permeability to tetracyclines in Escherichia coli bearing transferable resistance factors. Biochem. J. **105**: 371−378.

IZAKI, K, K. KIUCHI and K. ARIMA (1966): Specificity and mechanism of tetracycline resistance in a multiple drug resistant strain of Escherichia coli. J. Bact. **91**: 628−633.

KABINS, S. A. and S. COHEN (1969): Unusual pattern of tetracycline resistance in shigella mediated by resistance-transfer factors. Antimicrobial Agents and Chemotherapy − 1968, p. 25−29.

SOMPOLINSKY, D., T. KRAVITZ, Y. ZAIDENZAIG and N. ABRAMOVA (1970): Inducible resistance to tetracycline in Staphylococcus aureus. J. Gen. Microbiol. **62**: 341−349.

THE MOLECULAR BASIS OF TETRACYCLINE RESISTANCE IN STAPHYLOCOCCUS AUREUS

D. SOMPOLINSKY, A. WOJDANI and R. R. AVTALION

Rapaport Laboratory of Microbiology, Bar-Ilan University, Ramat Gan and
Department of Microbiology, Asaf Harofe Government Hospital, Tel-Aviv University
Medical School, Zrifin, Israel.

SUMMARY

In a lysate of a tetracycline resistant strain of *Staphylococcus aureus* an antigen has been demonstrated which was absent in a susceptible variant obtained by growth in nutrient broth with ethidium bromide. By absorption of the lysate with antiserum against the susceptible "eliminated" variant, the resistance-substance was obtained in a serologically purified state. The "resistance-antigen" was present in lysates of all but two of about twenty resistant wild strains. It was absent in lysates of eight "eliminated" clones from five resistant strains. It was likewise absent from the lysates of all but one of about twenty susceptible wild strains.

Possible explanations of these experimental results are discussed.

INTRODUCTION

Tetracyclines belong to antibiotics with least dangerous side effects, but their therapeutic usefulness is limited due to the widespread occurrence of resistant pathogenic microorganisms. New members of the tetracycline family might be expected to overcome this resistance similarly as new penicillins have proven refractory to the activity of β-lactamase. The search for such drugs would be considerably facilitated by a better understanding of the biologic substances which interact with the drug and the determinants for the affinity between the drug and these substances. In the case of many other antibiotics (penicillins, chloramphenicol, aminoglycosides), resistance depends on inactivating enzymes that can be isolated and assayed *in vitro*.

Susceptible bacteria possess at least two biologic substances with affinity to tetracyclines: 1. the uptake system that concentrates the drug intracellularly (IZAKI and ARIMA, 1965; HUTCHINGS, 1969; FRANKLIN and HIGGINSON, 1970; SOMPOLINSKY, ZAIDENZAIG, ZIEGLER-SCHLOMOWITZ and ABRAMOVA, 1970b), and 2. the ribosomal protein synthesizing machinery (LASKIN and CHAN, 1964; GOTTESMAN, 1967; SARKAR and THACH, 1968; BODLEY and ZIEVE, 1969). In resistant bacteria, two additional substances with affinity to the drug may exist: 3. the repressor of resistance (SOMPOLINSKY, KRAWITZ, ZAIDENZAIG and ABRAMOVA, 1970a), and 4. the "resistance-substance".

CRAVIN, GAVIN and FARMING (1969), pointed out that two different kinds of tetracycline (Tc)-resistant mutants can be obtained by plating susceptible cultures on Tc containing agar media. In one of them, the uptake system is altered, and the ribosomes in the other. In wild strains resistance is regularly inducible, and often borne on extrachromosomal DNA. It might therefore be expected 'that resistance is due to a macromolecular substance. We have demonstrated that lysates of the resistant *Staphylococcus aureus* 111 contain an antigen that could not be demonstrated in the susceptible strain 111-*elim* (AVTALION, ZIEGLER-SCHLOMOWITZ, WOJDANI, PERL and SOMPOLINSKY 1971). We have been able to prepare this resistance substance in an antigenically pure form and we have also obtained an antiserum specific for this substance. Furthermore, we have studied the correlation between the occurrence of this substance and resistance in a number of wild strains.

MATERIALS AND METHODS

Bacterial strains. Staphylococcus aureus 111, the relatively derepressed variant 111-der and the tetracycline susceptible eliminated variant 111-elim, have been previously described (SOMPOLINSKY et al., 1970a; SOMPOLINSKY et al., 1970b; AVTALION et al., 1971). A strain induced to high-level resistance by growth in nutrient broth with 160 μg/ml tetracycline (Tc) will be designated as 111/160. Other strains used were from pathologic human and veterinary sources. Some of the veterinary strains were dwarf colony variants (D strains), reflecting thiamine or pantothenate auxotrophy (SOMPOLINSKY, ERNST-GELLER and SEGAL, 1967; SOMPOLINSKY, GLUSKIN and ZIV, 1969).

Nutrient media. Bacto nutrient broth (NB) and nutrient agar (NA) were used throughout. For auxotrophic strains the media were enriched with one mg/liter of the appropriate vitamin.

Other methods. Methods for preparation of bacterial extracts, immunoglobulin, immunopherograms and their coloration have been described (AVTALION et al., 1971).

Fixation of proteins to insoluble matrix.

Solutions of agarose (0.4 gm per 20 ml dist. H_2O) and carboxymethylcellulose (0.2 gm per 20 ml H_2O) were adjusted to pH 3.8—3.9 with HCl/0.1 N. Dicyclohexylcarbodiimide (DCCI), 125 mg, was dissolved in one ml tetrahydrofuran. The agarose was added to carboxymethylcellulose and finally DCCI and a protein solution, containing about 0.4 gm protein, were added under stirring at 45° C. Stirring was continued at the same temperature for two hours. Thereafter, the suspension was centrifuged, and the sediment was washed several times with one liter portions of phosphate buffer (0.15 M, pH 7.2). This method has not been published earlier.

Preparation of purified resistance-antigen.

Antiserum-protein against 111-*elim* (AVTALION et al., 1971) was fixated as described above. The washed sediment was dried at 40° C, ground thoroughly and packed on a 300 mesh steel sieve. The powder that did not pass through the holes was packed into a 50 × 100 mm column. To this column 1.5 ml lysate (30 mg protein) of 111/160 was added, followed by incubation for 90 min at 37° C, and washing with phosphate buffer. The eluent was passed through a polyethylene tube from the column to a Gilson scanner of absorption at 280 nm, and from there to a fraction collector for portions of one ml. When absorption of the eluent had decreased to zero-values, washing was continued with 0.2 M glycine buffer (pH 2.4) for elution of antigen bound to antibody.

Preparation of antiserum specific for resistance antigen. Increasing amounts of lysate of the susceptible 111-*elim* strain were added to test tubes containing 0.3 ml of antiserum against 111/160. The volume was adjusted to one ml by a solution of 0.9 % NaCl. The tubes were incubated for 60 min at 45°C, and overnight at 4°C. The precipitates formed were separated by centrifugation. The supernates of each tube were examined by immunoelectrophoresis against a lysate of 111/160. With the supernates of three tubes, in the zone of maximal precipitation, only one band characteristic for the resistant 111 strain (AVTALION et al., 1971) was obtained.

RESULTS

After incubation of a lysate of 111/160 and a lysate of 111-der with anti-111-*elim* bound to carboxymethylcellulose, an essential part of the 280 nm absorbing material remained free (Fig. 1). The fractions with the highest concentration of this material were pooled and examined by immunoelectrophoresis with anti-111/160; only one clearcut precipitation band was obtained (Fig. 2). With anti-111-*elim*, no reaction was observed.

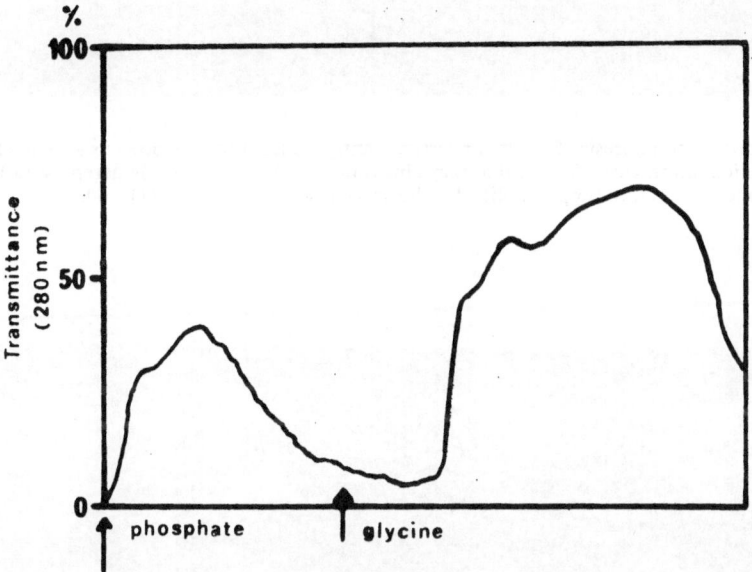

Fig. 1 Isolation of an antigen specific for tetracycline resistant strain Staphylococcus aureus 111/160. A lysate of 111/160 was added to a CMC-agarose column with activity of 111-*elim* antibody. Non-adsorbed antigen was eluted by phosphate and adsorbed by glycine.

Antiserum 111/160 after precipitation with 111-*elim* lysate, gave no clear reaction by immunoelectrophoresis with 111-*elim* lysates. With 111/160 lysate, two strong, concentric precipitation bands were obtained corresponding to slowly moving antigens (Fig. 3).

This adsorbed 111/160-serum was examined for precipitation in electropherograms of lysates of 47 staphylococcal strains isolated from human and veterinary pathological material (Table 1). Twenty-two of the strains (including 111) were resistant to Tc, i. e., the minimal inhibitory concentration (MIC) of the drug was 10 μg/ml or more. In all cases examined, the MIC could be increased significantly by subculture from NA with a subinhibitory concentration of the drug. Twenty strains gave a characteristic precipitation band with the adsorbed serum, and two were negative. The positive strains included

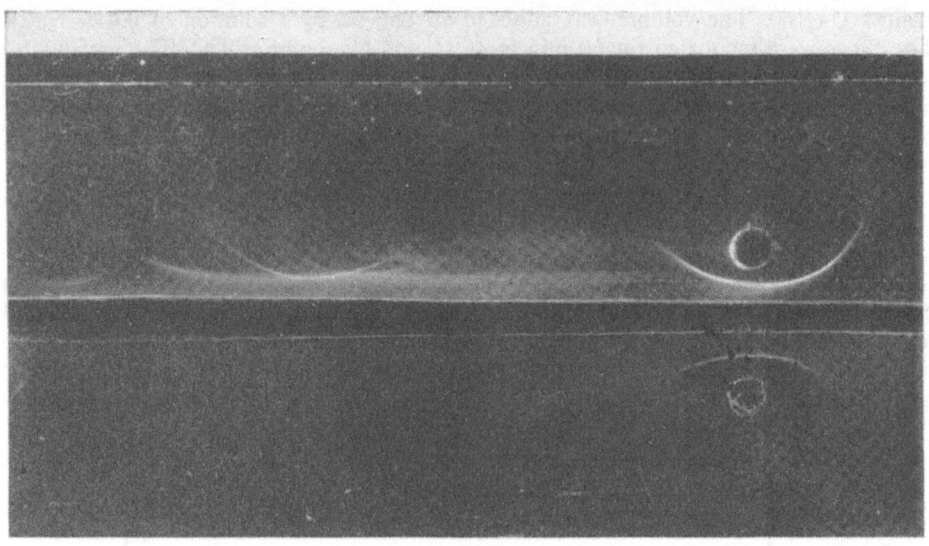

Fig. 2 Immunoelectrophoresis of isolated resistance antigens from Staphylococcus aureus 111/160, grown in nutrient broth with 160 μg/ml tetracycline (lower well) and the partly derepressed 111-der grown without tetracycline (upper well). To the groove was added anti 111/160.

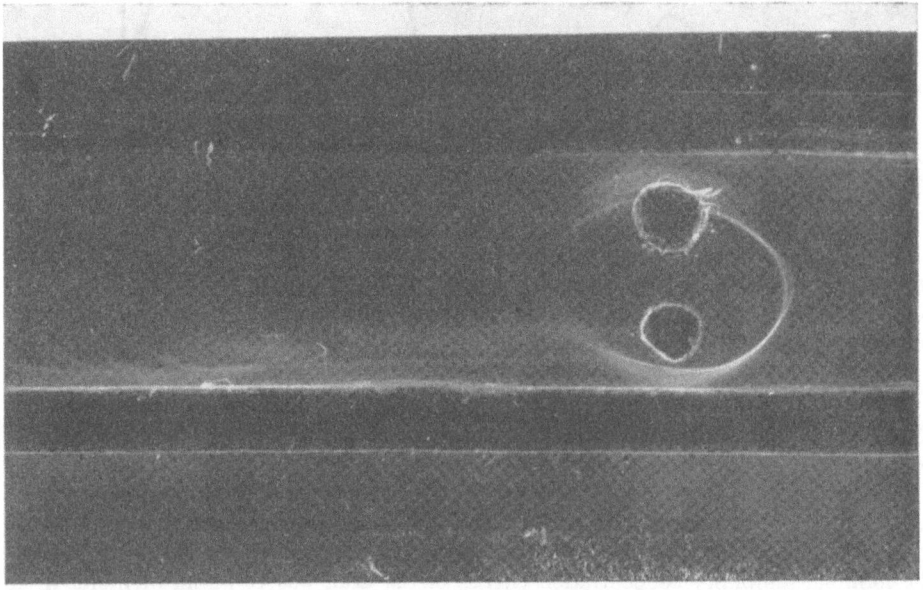

Fig. 3 Immunoelectrophoresis of lysates of Staphylococcus aureus 111/160, grown in nutrient broth with 160 μg/ml tetracycline (both wells). To the upper groove was added unadsorbed anti-111/160 and to the lower anti-111/160 adsorbed with a lysate of the susceptible strain 111-elim.

Table 1

Correspondence between resistance to tetracycline (Tc) and precipitation in electropherograms with specific anti-resistance serum (anti-111/160 adsorbed with a lysate of 111-elim). Crude extracts of the bacteria were used as antigens. The survey includes eight susceptible strains obtained from five resistant strains by elimination with ethidium bromide. Where elimination of resistance was not obtained, the number of colonies examined is added in parenthesis. The strains designated R were isolated from the upper respiratory tract of man, M from human pus, Fc and SFL from human feces, V and D from bovine mastitis milk. D-strains were auxotrophic for thiamine or pantothenate.

Strain No.	MIC*	Elimination	Reaction with anti 111/160
1 / R 45589	10	+	+
2 / R 45589 elim a	0.5		−
3 / R 45589 elim b	0.5		−
4 / Fc 13401	40	+	+
5 / Fc 13401 elim a	0.5		−
6 / Fc 13401 elim b	0.5		−
7 / V 1165	80	+	+
8 / V 1165 elim	0.5		−
9 / V 1369	80	+	+
10 / V 1369 elim	0.5		−
11 / 111	40	+	+
12 / 111 elim a	0.5		−
13 / 111 elim b	0.5		−
14 / R 45613	100	− (572 col.)	−
15 / R 45649	100	− (609 col.)	−
16 / R 46290	0.5		+
17 / R 45588	100	− (353 col.)	+
18 / R 46598	2.0		−
19 / R 46595	2.0		−
20 / R 46585	2.0		−
21 / R 46683	2.0		−
22 / R 46625	160	− (500 col.)	+
23 / M 21208	160	− (347 col.)	+
24 / M 21226	160	− (412 col.)	+
25 / M 21235	160	− (535 col.)	+
26 / M 22228	160	− (335 col.)	+
27 / R 46672	160	− (580 col.)	+
28 / M 21244	160	− (598 col.)	+
29 / M 21109	1.0		−
30 / R 46362	1.0		−
31 / R 46424	1.0		−
32 / R 46230	0.5		−
33 / M 21004	0.5		−
34 / R 46255	0.5		−
35 / R 46284	0.5		−
36 / M 20910	1.0		−
37 / SFL 13383	100	− (400 col.)	+
38 / SFL 13384	100	− (425 col.)	+
39 / M 20811	100	− (329 col.)	+
40 / M 20837	100	− (481 col.)	+
41 / M 20897	100	− (296 col.)	+
42 / V 767	160	− (210 col.)	+
43 / V 738	160	− (201 col.)	+
44 / D 3093	0.5		−
45 / D 3056	0.5		−
46 / D 2888	0.5		−
47 / D 2825	0.5		−

* Strains resistant to Tc had a minimal inhibitory concentration (MIC) of $\geq 10\ \mu g/ml$ Tc.

five in which resistance could be eliminated by growth in NB with ethidium bromide. All eight „eliminated" susceptible clones of these strains failed to show precipitation with the adsorbed serum. The positive strains included also two cultures from bovine mastitis, which showed a marked difference in relative resistance to Tc and minocycline (SOMPOLINSKY and KRAUS, in preparation). The precipitation bands of these strains merged, and the resistance material seems therefore antigenically identical. Finally, it should be noted that the two negative resistant strains, were examined repeatedly with the same result. They were not inhibited by 100 μg/ml Tc, and their behavior to different tetracyclines was similar to that of most resistant strains.

Seventeen of the wild strains were considered susceptible. The MIC of these strains was ≤ 2.0 μg/ml Tc, and in no case could resistance be increased by induction. Sixteen strains gave negative, and one of them a positive, reactions with adsorbed resistance antiserum. The precipitation band of the positive susceptible strain was clearcut, and showed identity reaction with bands of lysates of known positive strains.

DISCUSSION

When resistance to an antibacterial drug is obtained by inactivation, as is the case with penicillin, chloramphenicol and aminoglycoside antibiotics, it is expected that the resistant culture will contain a protein (enzyme) that is not present in susceptible strains. Tetracycline (Tc) resistance in staphylococci is, however probably due to a decreased ability to concentrate the drug (SOMPOLINSKY et al., 1970b) and resistance might therefore simply be due to a mutated, functionally deficient uptake system. Still, since resistance is often extrachromosomal, it might seem more attractive, though far from obligatory, to assume that it is associated with a new gene product rather than with an altered uptake system.

We have previously demonstrated that *Staphylococcus aureus* 111 contains an antigen that is not demonstrable after elimination of the resistance (AVTALION et al., 1971). We could also show that the same antigen was present in a wild, resistant strain in which resistance could not be eliminated by growth in NB with ethidium bromide or at 44°C. This antigen has now been isolated in a serologically pure state. Since it adsorbs ultraviolet light as protein and is precipitated by 90% saturated $(NH_4)_2$ SO_4, it may be essentially a protein, though preliminary analysis showed also trace amounts of sugar. An antiserum specific for this antigen has been produced. Only two out of twenty-two resistant wild strains lacked this antigen; in these two strains resistance could be due to another mechanism, or else, they might contain a functionally identical, but antigenically dissimilar, protein. Staphylococcal penicillinases exist in several antigenically distinct forms (NOVICK and RICHMOND, 1965).

It is more difficult to explain the presence of this antigen in one of the notoriously susceptible strains. One must, therefore, consider the possibility that the antigen has a function which is usually, but not always, associated with Tc-resistance. This hypothetical function must then be borne on the same plasmid as Tc-resistance, and even on the same operon, so that derepression for Tc-resistance brings about an increased synthesis of the described antigen as reported earlier (AVTALION et al., 1971). Alternatively, our strain No. 16 might have a mutated, functionally impotent, resistance gene that codes for a serologically cross-reacting material. It is also possible that the resistance system is composite and the antigen demonstrated by us is only one of its components.

At the present state of our investigations, we are unable to distinguish between these possibilities.

Acknowledgements

The authors are indebted to Prof. KURT STERN for critical reading of the manuscript. This investigation was supported by a Research grant from Bar-Ilan University and from The Medical Research Funds of the Israel Ministry of Health.

REFERENCES

AVTALION, R. R., ZIEGLER-SCHLOMOWITZ, R., WOJDANI, A., PERL, M. and SOMPOLINSKY, D. (1971): Derepressed resistance to tetracycline in Staphylococcus aureus. Microbios, 3/10−11, 165.

BODLEY, J. W. and ZIEWE, I. J. (1969): On the specificity of the two ribosomal binding sites: Studies with tetracycline. Biochemical and Biophysical Research Communications, 36/3, 463.

CRAVEN, G. R., GAVIN, R. M. and FARMING, T. (1969): The transfer RNA binding site of the 30S ribosome and the site of tetracycline inhibition. Cold Spring Harbor Symposia on Quantitative Biology, 34. 129.

FRANKLIN, T. J. and HIGGINSON, B (1970): Active accumulation of tetracycline by Escherichia coli. Biochemical Journal, 116/2, 287.

GOTTESMAN, M. E. (1967): Reaction of ribosome-bound peptidyl transfer ribonucleic acid with aminoacyl transfer ribonucleic acid or puromycin. The Journal of Biological Chemistry, 242/23, 5564.

HUTCHINGS, B. L. (1969): Tetracycline transport in Staphylococcus aureus H. Biochimica et Biophysica Acta, 174/2, 734.

IZAKI, K. and ARIMA, K. (1965): Effect of various conditions on accumulation of oxytetracycline in Escherichia coli. Journal of Bacteriology, 89/5, 1335.

LASKIN, A. I. and CHAN, W. M. (1964): Inhibition by tetracyclines of polyuridilic acid directed phenylalanine incorporation in Escherichia coli cell-free systems. Biochemical and Biophysical Research Communications, 14/2, 137.

NOVICK, R. P. and RICHMOND, M. H. (1965): Nature and interactions of the genetic elements governing penicillinase synthesis in Staphylococcus aureus. Journal of Bacteriology, 90/2, 467.

SARKAR, S. and THACH, R. E. (1968): Inhibition of formylmethioninetransfer RNA binding to ribosomes by tetracycline. Proceedings of the National Academy of Sciences of the United States of America, 60/4, 1479.

SOMPOLINSKY, D., ERNST-GELLER, Z. and SEGAL, S. J. (1967): Metabolic disorders in thiamine-less dwarf strains of Staphylococcus aureus. The Journal of General Microbiology, 48/2, 205.

SOMPOLINSKY, D., GLUSKIN, I. and ZIV, G. (1969): Pantothenate requiring dwarf colony variants of Staphylococcus aureus as the etiological agent in bovine mastitis. The Journal of Hygiene, Cambridge, 67/3, 511.

SOMPOLINSKY, D., KRAWITZ, T., ZAIDENZAIG, Y. and ABRAMOVA, N. (1970a): Inducible resistance to tetracycline in Staphylococcus aureus. The Journal of General Microbiology, 62/3, 341.

SOMPOLINSKY, D., ZAIDENZAIG, Y., ZIEGLER-SCHLOMOWITZ, R. and ABRAMOVA, N. (1970b): Mechanism of tetracycline resistance in Staphylococcus aureus. The Journal of General Microbiology, 62/3, 351.

NONGENETIC ADAPTATION OF BACILLUS CEREUS 569H TO TETRACYCLINE

R. CONNAMACHER

Department of Pharmacology University of Pittsburgh, School of Medicine, Pittsburgh, Pa. U.S.A.

Resistance of bacteria to antibiotics has been a topic of urgency since the onset of penicillin resistance. With the discovery of each new antibiotic, there has followed an emergence of resistant strains. Some of these strains depended on the presence of the antibiotic for the development of resistance. Others did not. Some drugs such as streptomycin were very prone towards development of resistance. Other drugs such as chloramphenicol were much less prone. But in each case, what had appeared to be the answer to problems in antibiotic therapy has, at least in part, been short circuited by the emergence of resistant strains.

To date, there have been two systems of adaptation that have been studied in great detail. One of these is the production of β-lactamase by penicillin-resistant bacteria (review: ASHESHOV, 1969).

GROWTH CURVES OF B CEREUS INHIBITED BY TETRACYCLINE

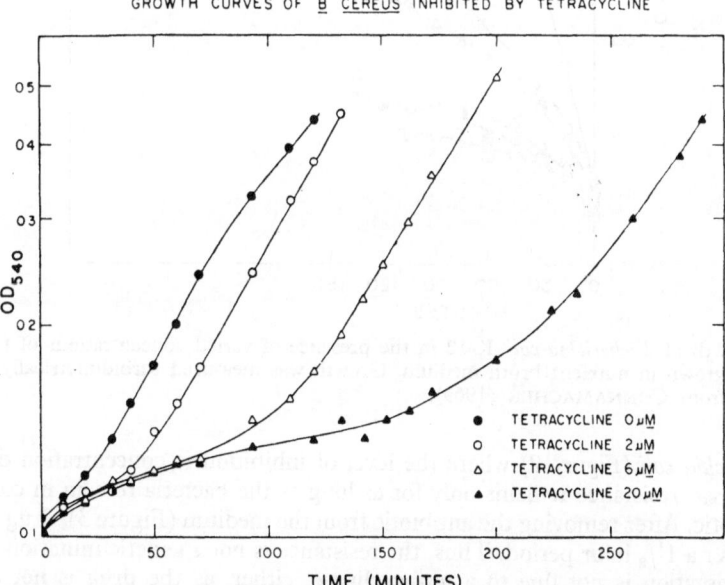

Fig. 1 Growth of *Bacillus cereus* 569H in the presence of varied concentrations of tetracycline. Cells were grown in the medium of MATTHEWS and SMITH (1952). Growth was measured turbidimetrically at 540mu. Reprinted from CONNAMACHER, MANDEL and HAHN (1967).

425

The other is the discovery and investigation of the R factor of Watanabe (rf. *The Problems of Drug-resistant Pathogenic Bacteria*) 1971. The former is an antibiotic destroyer, induced by the presence of penicillin from genes which are an inherent part of the chromosome. The latter is an episome, often present in a large percentage of a gram negative cell culture, containing the resistance factors.

The major difficulty in studying the biochemical events causing a genetic mutation resistance has been the spontaneity of that resistance. Cells became resistant, often in a single step. One can simply look for differences between two cell cultures (LAST, IZAKI and SNELL, 1969).

It is in the study of the biochemical events involved in the acquisition of resistance that the *Bacillus cereus* system has the most to offer. *B. cereus* adapts to tetracycline on coming into contact with the drug (Figure 1). This inhibition is not immediate but becomes manifest at up to 3 hours after the addition of the drug. In fact, the adaptation time varies proportionally with the drug concentration. This adaptation has been seen in all four *B. cereus* strains tested. These events are in sharp contrast to the effect of tetracycline

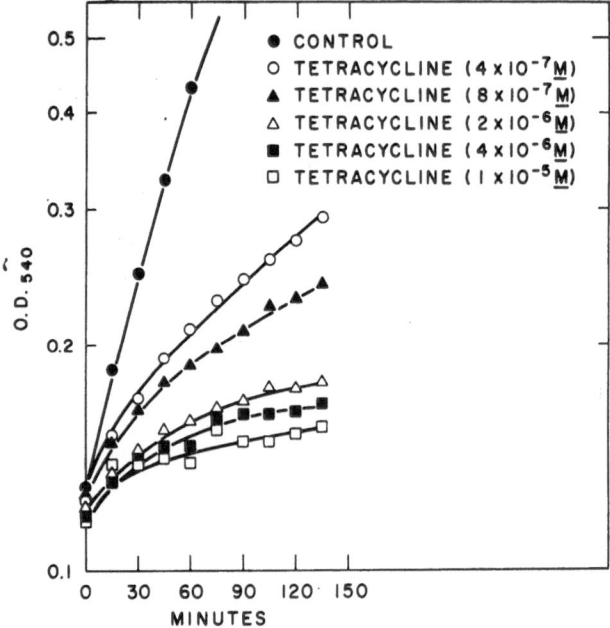

Fig. 2 Growth of *Escherichia coli* K-12 in the presence of varied concentrations of tetracycline. Cells were grown in nutrient broth medium. Growth was measured turbidimetrically at 540mu. Reprinted from CONNAMACHER (1969).

on *Escherichia coli* (Figure 2) where the level of inhibition is concentration dependent. The *B. cereus* resistance remains only for as long as the bacteria remain in contact with the antibiotic. After removing the antibiotic from the medium (Figure 3), drug sensitivity returns over a $1^1/_2$ hour period. Thus, the resistance is not a genetic mutation.

The adaptation is not due to a tetracyclinase, either, as the drug is not destroyed. Medium from cells adapted to tetracycline can inhibit fresh, untreated bacteria. Also, after cells are incubated in the presence of tritiated tetracycline for more than an hour, medium from these cultures show only a single radioactive substance as determined by paper chromatography using 70% isopropanol, pH 3.5, the system of KELLY and BUYSKE (1960), and the system of URX, VONDRACKOVA, KOVARIK, HORSKY and HEROLD (1963).

Although the time required for adaptation to take place is proportional to the concentration of tetracycline in the medium, the level of resistance is not. Inducing

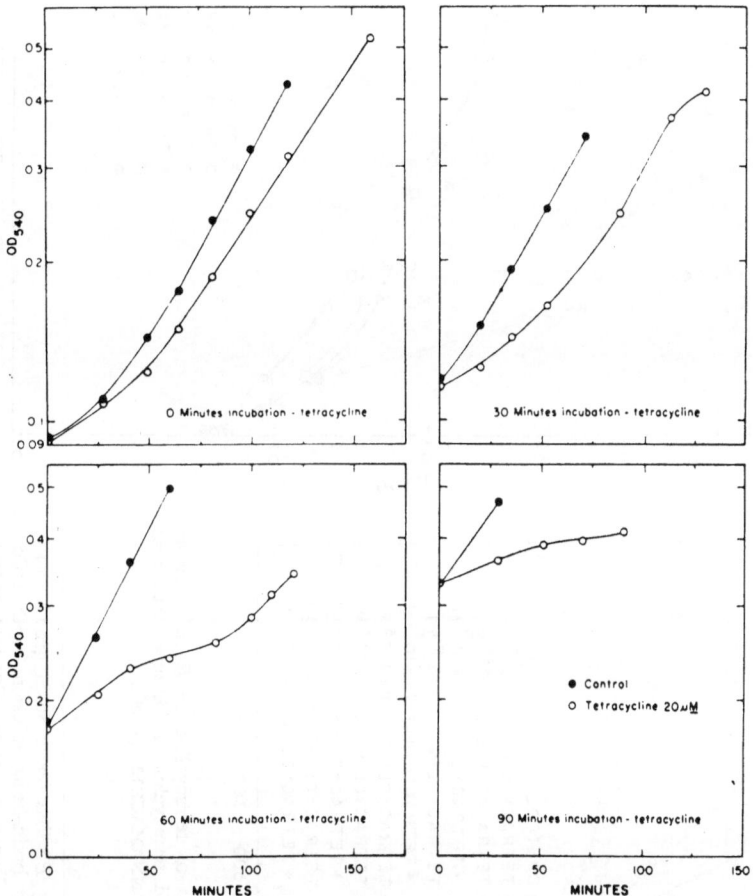

Fig. 3 Return of tetracycline sensitivity to phenotypically drug-resistant *Bacillus cereus*. Cells made resistant to 6×10^{-6}M tetracycline were resuspended in drug-free medium. At 0, 30, 60 and 90 minutes after resuspension, culture samples were removed and grown in the presence (0) or absence (•) of 2×10^{-5}M tetracycline. Reprinted from CONNAMACHER, MANDEL and HAHN (1967).

concentrations, ranging from minimum inhibitory concentration ($2 \times 10^{-6} M$) to maximum adaptable concentration ($2 \times 10^{-5} M$) all produce resistance of the same magnitude (Fig. 4). The cells remain completely resistant to concetrations greater than $2 \times 10^{-5} M$, partially resistant to $5 \times 10^{-5} M$, and sensitive to concentrations greater than $40^{-4} M$. Although such drug resistance is less than that seen in cells containing R factor, it is still sufficient to affect a normal therapeutic dose.

As might be expected from the chelative action of tetracycline, antibiotic activity on *B. cereus* is sensitive to divalent cation concentration. Cell grown in brain-heart infusion

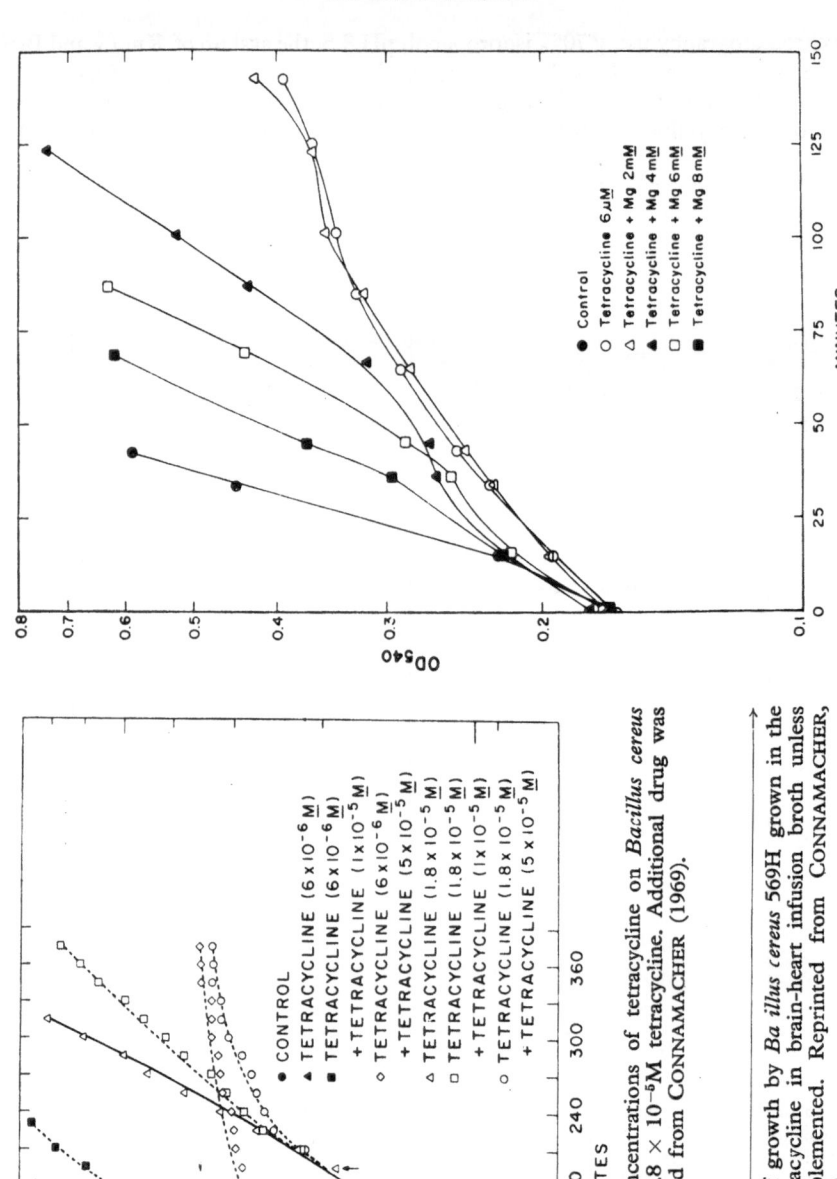

Fig. 4 Action of higher concentrations of tetracycline on *Bacillus cereus* adapted to 6×10^{-6}M or 1.8×10^{-5}M tetracycline. Additional drug was added at the arrow. Reprinted from CONNAMACHER (1969).

Fig. 5 Failure of recovery of growth by *Ba illus cereus* 569H grown in the presence of 6×10^{-6}M tetracycline in brain-heart infusion broth unless additional Mg^{++} was supplemented. Reprinted from CONNAMACHER, MANDEL and HAHN (1967).

broth, low in divalent cations, do not recover from 6×10^{-6} M tetracycline unless additional cations are added (Fig. 5). The most active cations are Mg^{++} and Ca^{++}, but this appears to be the result of their high water solubilities. The cations may work in either of two ways: They may bind the tetracycline and prevent its uptake. Most likely, they combine with the monoanionic form of the drug (JONES and MORRISON, 1962) causing a decrease in the amount of the nonionic, penetrable form. Changing the pH causes similar effects, the lower the pH, the longer the drug action. This increase in drug action also parallels an increased percentage of the drug in a nonionized form.

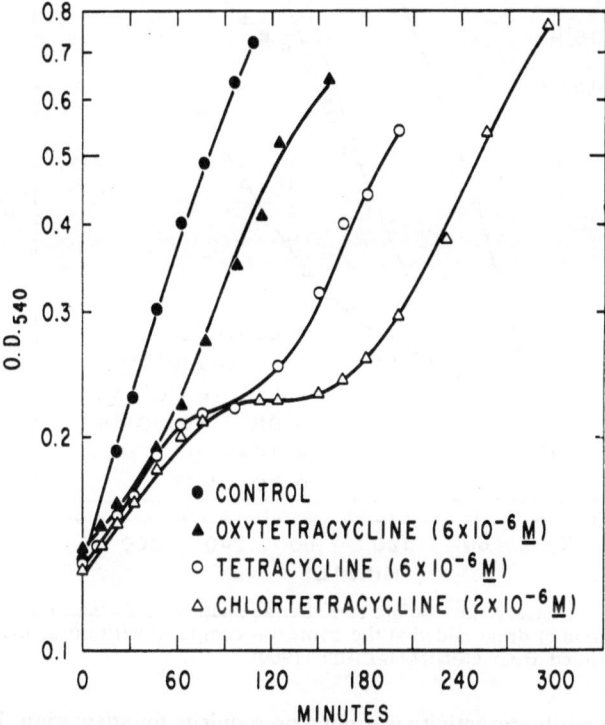

Fig. 6 Adaptation of *Bacillus cereus* 569H to different tetracyclines. Reprinted from CONNAMA-CHER (1969).

As with other tetracycline resistances, there is crossresistance among all drugs in the family. *B. cereus* adapts to tetracycline, chlortetracycline, oxytetracycline, and demethylchlortetracycline. Of these, adaptation occurs most rapidly with oxytetracycline, followed in order by tetracycline and demethylchlortetracycline. Chlortetracycline is too active against *B. cereus* to produce resistance to 6×10^{-6} M drug, but concentrations below 2×10^{-6} M show the characteristic recovery. (Figure 6.) Adaptation of *B. cereus* to 6×10^{-6} M tetracycline will protect the cells against the effects of any of the other three compounds (Figure 7).

As we just reported in Prague, the presence of tetracycline in very small concentrations is sufficient to cause adaptation. These concentrations are far below those required for inhibition of growth. This phenomenon was discovered by an indirect route. In an attempt to produce an adaptation without concomitant inhibition, we first inactivated tetracycline by incubating it at room temperature for 24—48 hours in 0.1 N sodium hydroxide. This drug was almost devoid of antibiotic activity. Pretreatment of a culture of *Bacillus cereus* with the inactivated drug prevented the action of tetracycline itself added at a later time. The identical effect could be seen if pure 4-epitetracycline, kindly supplied to us by Dr. R. G. KELLY of Lederle Laboratories, was used in place of the inactivated drug. It was

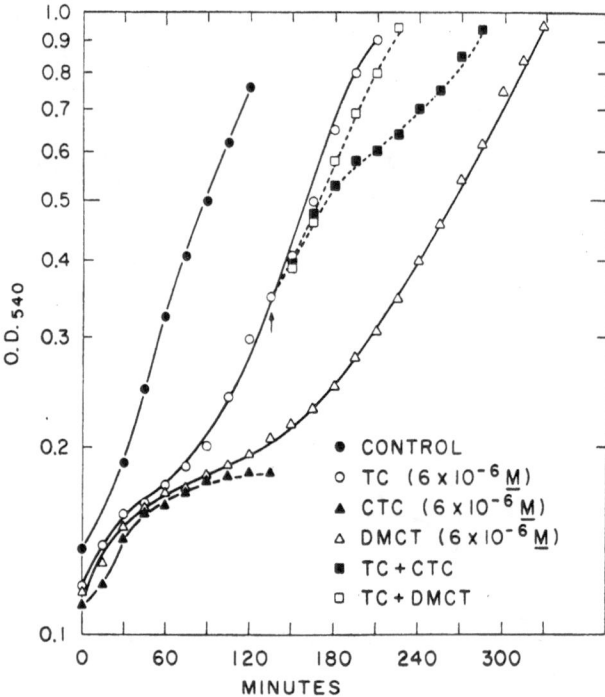

Fig. 7 Effect of several tetracyclines before and after adaptation of *Bacillus cereus* to 6 × 10⁻⁶M tetracycline. The action of drugs added at the arrow was compared with the action of drugs added at 0 minutes. Reprinted from CONNAMACHER (1969).

then apparent that antibiotic activity was not a prerequisite for adaptation. Using tritiated inactive tetracycline, it was seen that no radioactivity was accumulated by the cells, nor was it bound to ribosomes. However, the inactive and 4-epi analogs did show some activity in the amino acid incorporation system of NIRENBERG and MATTHAEI (1961). It was important to be certain that the adaptation was not due to the minute amounts of active tetracycline present in both the inactive and 4-epi analogs. It became increasingly clear, as we lowered the drug concentration, that the adaptation with the inactive or 4-epi tetracyclines could be attributed solely to trace contaminants of the active drug. The minimum concentration showing protection against 6 × 10⁻⁶ *M* tetracycline appears to be 10⁻⁹ *M* drug.

If cultures are treated with 7-³H-tetracycline and the cells assayed for radioactivity, a peculiar pattern emerges (Figure 8). Tetracycline enters the cells quickly, reaching a maximum level in 20—30 minutes. At times, the inward flux occurs so rapidly that maximum levels are seen before the first few samples are taken. Binding studies show that the drug is preferentially attached to the bacterial ribosomes (CONNAMACHER and MANDEL, 1968). Following this maximum level, there is a linear efflux of the drug from cells, at least until the bacterial recover and often for an hour thereafter. The pattern then breaks up with a variability that may be due to a trapping of the radioactivity by the cells and a self-absorption of tritium by the bacteria. Experiments were done to determine whether the effluxed material may have been metabolized and excreted. Cells were grown in the presence of 7-³H-tetracycline for 20—30 minutes. They were then centrifuged and

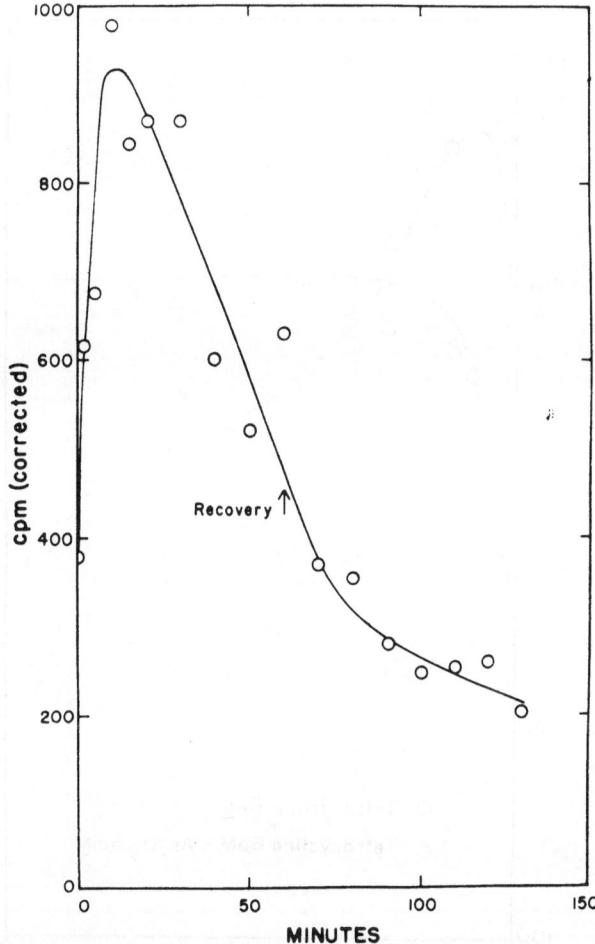

Fig. 8 Flux of 7-³H-tetracycline in and out of *Bacillus cereus* 569H. Cells were grown in casein-hydrolysate-salts medium with 6 × 10⁻⁶M 7-³H-tetracycline. At various intervals, 2ml aliquots were added to iced 0.14M. sodium chloride and filtered onto membrane filters. The counts were assayed in a windowless Nuclear-Chicago automatic planchette counter.

resuspended in drug-free medium. The cells continued to be inhibited and they continued to express their tetracycline, although recovery did appear more rapidly than in control cultures. The medium from the recovered cells was concentrated and subject to paper chromatography in the same systems mentioned earlier. Again, no metabolites of tetracycline could be found. It was concluded that the material that effluxed from the bacteria was tetracycline itself.

It was possible to experimentally vary the influx of tetraycline alone or the influx and efflux in combination but not the efflux alone. The influx was able to be changed by anything that would change the level of unbound, nonionized drug. For instance, lowering the Mg^{++} concentration of the medium, or lowering the pH of the medium increased the level of drug within the cell. The efflux pattern or slope was not affected.

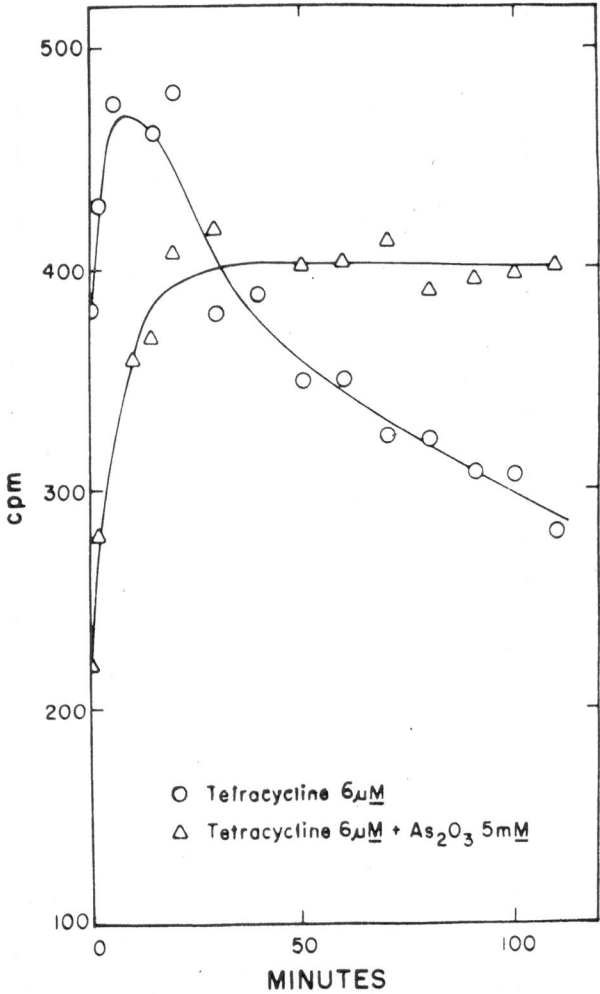

Fig. 9 Inhibition of 7-^{3}H-tetracycline influx and efflux by 10^{-3}M arsenite. Reprinted from CONNAMACHER, MANDEL and HAHN (1967).

Conversely, raising the divalent cation concentration of the medium reduced the level of radioactive drug within the cell. Recovery occurred in both cases when the intracellular drug concentration reached the same levels. On the other hand, anything that blocked the efflux of tetracycline from the cell, which included in effect anything that inhibited the energy metabolism of the cell, also reduced the level of drug acheived in the input phase. A complete block of the energy system, as with arsenite (Figure 9) changed the

432

normal influx-efflux pattern into one of diffusion controlled kinetics. The effect of lowering temperature can be seen in Figure 10. The influx at 2° is lower than at 37°. The efflux at 2° is almost completely inhibited. Once the culture was returned to the 37° bath, efflux resumed and the cells recovered.

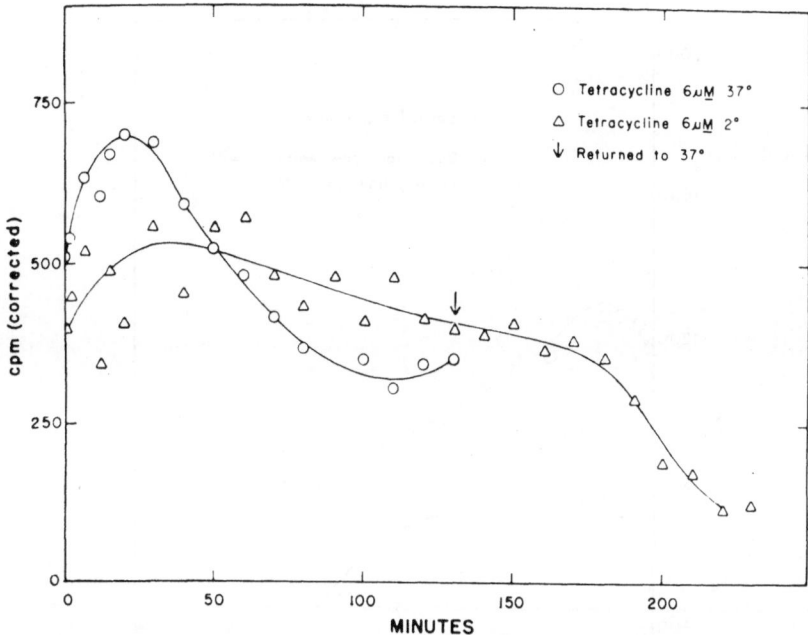

Fig. 10 Inhibition of 7-³H-tetracycline influx and efflux by reduced temperature. Reprinted from CONNAMACHER, MANDEL and HAHN (1967).

Cells which were made resistant to 6×10^{-6} M 7-³H-tetracycline had drug levels below the minimum inhibitory level. An additional 6×10^{-6} M radioactive drug did not significantly increase the intracellular antibiotic concentration (Figure 11). Thus, the resistance produced by tetracycline was correlated with an inability of the drug to enter the cell.

Preliminary data shows that tetracycline is accumulated by the cells to a level at least ten fold that of the medium. To accumulate, the drug must be bound by the tissues, actively transplanted, or both. If the drug is bound, the efflux phase must mean that the material to which it is bound is unstable and not required for cell survival or growth, its disintegration must be energy dependent, leading to the observed efflux. More likely, the efflux is a membrane transport phenomenon. If sensitive or resistant cells are broken by alumina grinding or sonication, the resultant extracts bound equivalent amounts of tetracycline (Figure 12).

In conclusion, we have described a system that adapts to a protein synthesis inhibiting antibiotic. It does not destroy the active drug. The system appears to be similar in many respects to that seen with the tetracycline R factors. But it occurs in the entire culture over a period of hours.

The influx of drug which occurs when it is added to the culture is immediate and to a level well above that of the surrounding medium. Part of that influx is diffusion dependent, but part is due to an energy-requiring system. After a period of time, that influx is cut off, and little additional drug can enter. The efflux system now becomes evident. The energy-requiring efflux will reduce the intracellular drug concentration to a level lower than the inward diffusion movement would indicate, suggesting that after

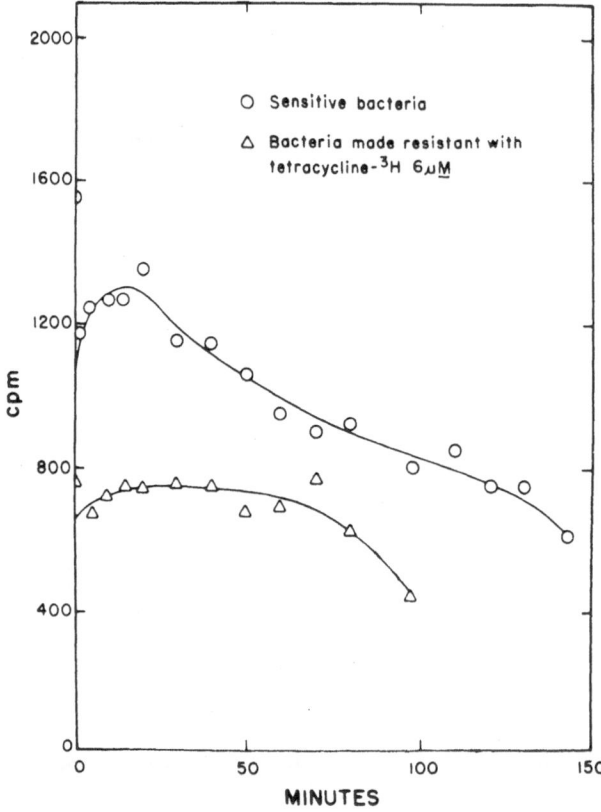

Fig. 1I Uptake of radioactivity into normal cells and into cells made resistant to the radioactive drug by incubation in casein hydrolysate medium containing 6 × 10⁻⁶M 7-³H-tetracycline. Recovery of growth of the inhibited culture occurred at 70 minutes. Reprinted from CONNAMACHER, MANDEL and HAHN (1967).

20 minutes there is indeed a block of tetracycline uptake. When the level of the drug falls below a minimal inhibitory level, recovery of growth occurs. Once the cell stops taking in drug, it has adapted, and it remains resistant to the drug for as long as the drug remains in contact with it. Removal of the drug initiates the return to drug sensitivity. The adaptation appears to be due to a change in the bacterial membrane. It appears to be induced and to require protein synthesis, because where no protein synthesis occurs, recovery also does not occur. It is not yet known whether the recovery itself or the resumption of cell protein synthesis is the primary control of recovery. In any case, there is, in *Bacillus cereus*, an opportunity to study the biochemical phenomena that lead to a depressed intake of and sensitivity to a major antibiotic agent.

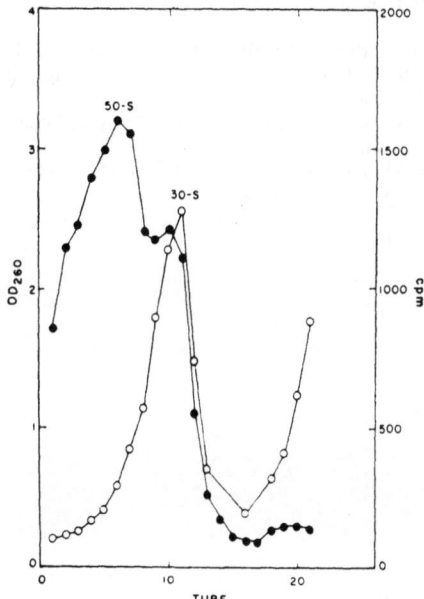 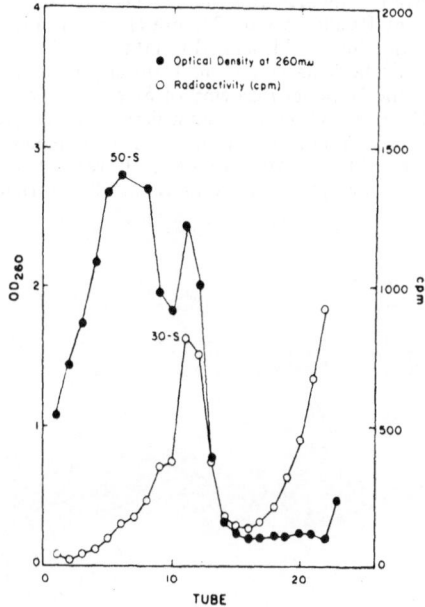

Fig. 12 Elution patterns of sucrose gradients of ribosomes from tetracycline resistant (left) and tetracycline-sensitive (right) *Bacillus cereus*. Ribosomes were dialyzed for 20 hours in the presence of 7-³H-tetracycline and then centrifuged in 10^{-4}M Mg^{++}5-20% 5ml. sucrose gradients for 150 minutes. The O.D.260 and the counts were assayed on each 0.2 ml sample. Reprinted from CONNAMACHER, MANDEL and HAHN (1967).

The author wishes to acknowledge the assistance of the following people associated with the work described above.

Dr. H. GEORGE MANDEL
Dr. FRED E. HAHN
Dr. DONG H. SHIN
Mrs. MARLEASE L. CONLEY

REFERENCES

ASHESHOV, E. (1969): The Genetics of Penicillinase Production in Staphylococcus aureus Strain P.S. 80. Journal of General Microbiology, **59**, 289.

CONNAMACHER, R. H. (1969): Specificity of Phenotypic Adaptation of Bacillus cereus to Tetracycline. Journal of General Microbiology, **55**, 275.

CONNAMACHER, R. H. (1969): Separation of the Ability of Bacillus cereus 569H to Adapt to Tetracycline and the Drug's Antimicrobial Action. Pharmacologist. **11**, 235.

CONNAMACHER, R. H. and MANDEL, H. G. (1968): Studies on the Intracellular Localization of Tetracycline in Bacteria. Biochimica et Biophysica Acta **166**, 475.

CONNAMACHER, R. H., MANDEL, H. G. and HAHN, F. E. (1967): Adaptation of Populations of Bacillus cereus to Tetracycline, Molecular Pharmacology **3/6**, 586.

JONES, J. G. and MORRISON, G. A. (1962): The Bacteriostatic Actions of Tetracycline and Oxytetracycline. Journal of Pharmacy and Pharmacology **14**, 808.

KELLY, R. G. and BUYSKE, D. A. (1960): Paper Chromatography of the Tetracyclines, Antibiotics and Chemotherapy **10**, 604.

LAST, J. A., IZAKI, K., and SNELL, J. F. (1969): The Resistance of Escherichia coli to Oxytetracycline. Canadian Journal of Microbiology, **15/9**, 1077.

MATTHEWS, R. E. F. and SMITH, J. D. (1952: Distribution of 8-azaguanine in the Nucleic Acids of Bacillus cereus. Nature (London) **177**, 271.

NIRENBERG, M. and MATTHAEI, J. H. (1961): The Dependence of Cellfree Protein Synthesis in Escherichia coli upon Naturally Occurring or Synthetic Polyribonucleotides. Proceedings of the National Academy of Sciences (Washington), **47**, 1588.

Problems of Drug-resistant Pathogenic Bacteria (1971) Annals of the New York Academy of Sciences, Volume 182. Editors: E. L. Dulaney and A. I. Laskin.

URX, M., VONDRACKOVA, J., KOVARIK, L., HORSKY, O., and HEROLD, M. (1963): Papierchromatographie der Tetracyclinstoff. Journal of Chromatography **11**, 62.

AUTHOR INDEX*

Aamarasingham C. R., 319
Aarai T., 23, 106, 132, 135, 137, 138, 309, 311
Abramova N., 405, 417, 418, 422
Acar J. F., 21
Achtman M. A., 173, 174
Adachi Y., **63**, 69, 72
Adams M. H., 192
Adelberg E. A., 321, 392
Aden D. P., 98
Adler B., 219
Adler H. I., 276
Adler S. P., 184
Aguirregoita E., **225**
Akiba T., 269
Aldag V., 145
Alexander D. C., 93
Alexander M., 145
Alicino J. F., 233
Allison J. L., 304
Allison M. J., 44
Amati P., 203
Ambler R. P., 34
Anagnostis D., 54
Anderson E. S., 14, 21, 33, 37, 41, 43, 54, 105, 132, 179, 209, 217, 246, 263, 269, 284, 285, 291, 292, 293, 295, 305
Anderson P. W., 319, 320
Annear D. I., 363, 405
Aoki T., **131**, 132, 134, 138, 139
Apirion D., 161
Arai T., 179, 183
Arber W., 182, 183, 184, 185, 186, 375
Arima K., 319, 409, 417
Armour S. E., 27
Aronowitch J., 180
Asheshov E., 394, 425
August J. T., 33
Austin S., 344, 346
Avers C. L., 299
Avtalion R. R., **417**, 418, 422
Ayliffe G. A. J., 23, 27, 263

Bach M. K., 297

Baldi M. I., m 159
Baldroin J. N., 394
Bankier J. C., 98
Bannister D., 138, 179, 180, 182, 185, 187
Baláž M., 14, 151
Baráth Z., 165, 167
Baráthová H., 165, 168
Barber M., 363, 365
Baron O., 37, 41
Bartoš J., 13
Baudens J. G., 19, 21, 364, 371, 394
Bauer A. W., 298, 378
Bauer F., 105, 111
Bauer Š., 165
Bauer W., 29, 273, 289, 313
Bazaral M., 270, 302
Beckwith J. R., 325, 331
Benner E. J., 367
Bennett J. V., 44, 115
Benveniste R., 19, 21, 28, 319, 337, 340, 407
Benzer S., 357
Berger H., 297
Berman D. T., 376
Berns M. I., 273
Berquist K. R., 117
Bertani G., 182
Best L. C., 115, 116
Betina V., **157**, 165, 167, 168
Betinová M., 167, **385**, 389
Betz-Bareau M., 204
Bialy H., 180
Biggs D. R., 166
Billheimer F. E., 299
Black W. A., 23, 27
Blair D. G., 277
Blair J. E., 377
Bobrowski M., **43**, **263**, 264
Bodley J., 162
Bodley J. W., 408
Böhme H., **217**, 219, 222
Bohuš J., 14, **151**
Boman H. G., 320, 332
Boman N. G., 245
Bond W., **115**, 119, 120
Bonner J. T., 167
Boronskij J., 40, 45

Borowski J., **43, 263, 381,** 382
Bouanchaud D. H., 19, 298, 372
Boussongant Y., 19
Boyer H. W., 183, 185, 186
Bradley D. F., 298, 304
Bradley M. O., 167
Brinton C. C. Jr., 112
Brachman P. S., 115
Braun C. B., **225**
Brenner S., 309, 343
Brian P. W., 167
Brigham K. L., 119
Broda R. F., 321, 322
Brown J. F., 115
Brzezinska M., 28
Buck M., 362
Bujard H., 278
Bulger R. J., 59
Bullock G. L., 133
Bülow P., 361, 367, 371
Bure A., 19
Burman L. G., 245, 320, 332
Burrows T. W., 41
Buyske D. A., 427

Cairns J., 298
Calendar R., 180
Camagni L. J., 262
Cantor C. R., 409, 412
Campbell A. M., 219, 274, 275
Caskey T., 408
Casal E., 54
Carnahan J., 343
Carson L. A., **115,** 120
Cavalli-Sforra L. L., 299
Celma M. L., 162
Cerami A., 159
Chabbert Y. A., **19**, 20, 21, 298, 364, 371, 372, 394
Chamberlin M., 159
Chan W. M., 407, 417
Chandra P., 159
Chen G. C. C., 321
Cherubin C., 44
Chimenes A. M., 297
Christ O., 402, 403
Christol D., 19, 29
Chou J., 233

439

440

441

SUBJECT INDEX

MEMBRANE
- its role in DNA replication 317

METHICILLIN RESISTANCE
- in S. aureus 361—369, 371—380
- extrachromosomal location of 361, 371
- is not on a plasmid 362
- increasing by mutation — 362
- selected by penicillin, BaCl₂ etc. 362
- etnerotoxin production with 361, 367, 371—380
- problems in hospitals 361, 371
- elimination of 373
- transduction of 375

MILK
- occure nce of R⁺ strains of E. coli in 15

MINICELLS
- transfer of R factors into 276—278

MOBILISATION OF
- chromosomal determinants by Col factors 203—209
- chromosomal determinants by R factors 219
- R determinants by Col factors 13—17, 147—150, 203—209

MOLECULAR NATURE OF R FACTORS
- covalently closed circles in Ps. aeruginosa 29
- of beta lactase, 247—260
- Anderson's and Watanabe's 269
- cointegrated and aggregated types 283—292
- model of 294—295

MULTIPLE DRUG RESISTANCE
- dynamics in Japan 69—73
- development from single resistance by addition 72

NEOMYCIN
- elimination of in staphylococci 372
- inactivation by acetylation 337—340
- transduction of neo plasmid in S. aureus 376

NOSOCOMIAL INFECTIONS
- changing patterns of 115
- gramnegative bacteria in 115
- air and surface sampling 115—121
- with methicillin resistant staphylococci 361, 371, 377—379

ORIGIN OF R FACTORS
- model of mutations on sex factors 294—295
- pick up of chromosomal genes 9—13

PENICILLINASE PLASMIDS
- in staphylococci from patients 60
- in penicillin- and erythromycin-resistant staphylococci 60
- not responsible for methicillin resistance 361

- in staphylococci 417, see also STAPHY-LOCOCCAL PLASMIDS

PERMEABILITY
- R factors code functions altering permeability 348
- R factors enhance p. to Flavomycin 105
- R factors enhance p. to Rifampicin 343
- to tetracyclines 417, 399
- to tetracyclines and elimination (efflux from resistant cells) 422, 425—435

PHYSICAL INTEGRITY OF PLASMIDS
- dissociates in Proteus 249, 270
- in aggregated and cointegrated plasmids 287—293

PLASMIDS IN STAPHYLOCOCCI
- of resistance to tetracyclines 391
- loss of car with tet marker 393
- loss of pen with tet 13
- to methicillin 361, 371
- for penicillinase 375
- penicillinase and crystal violet 381

PROTEIN SYNTHESIS IN BACTERIA
- effects of antibiotics on 160—163, 399—410
- effect of tetracyclines on 160, 400—401

PROTEUS
R factors in Switzerland 47
- various types of resistance spectra in 50
- dynamics of multi-resistance in two Moscow hospitals 59
- multi-resistance in West Germany 125—126
- R factors in 256—260, 272
- beta lactamase activity depending on growth phase 256
- dissociation of R factors in 260, 276 to 279
- low activity of beta-lactamase in 263
- sex factors and R determinants in 278 to 279
- R factor 222 (cointegrated), satellite peaks in 289
- CAT, constitutive synthesis in 329

PROVIDENCIA
- Gentamycin resistance factors in 20

PSEUDOMONAS AERUGINOSA
- Transfer of R factors to 9, 11, 23, 27
- Gentamycin resistance factors in 20, 337—340
- occurence of R factors in 23, 27
- new phylogenetic group of R factors 25, 28
- transfer of R factors to Rhizobium, Chromobacter, etc. 25
- R factors in strains from burns 27
- different molecular species of R factors in 28—29
- high-level beta-lactamase for carbenicillin in 28

449

452